DATE DUE

FEB 20 2012		
FEB 04 2015		
MAR 2 5 2015		
MAY 1 9 2015		
FEB 06 2018		

Occupational Therapy with Elders

STRATEGIES FOR THE COTA

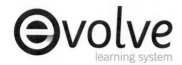 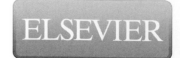
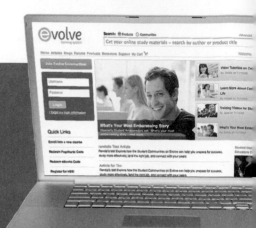

Occupational Therapy with Elders THIRD EDITION

STRATEGIES FOR THE COTA

René L. Padilla, PhD, OTR/L, FAOTA
Associate Dean for Academic and Student Affairs
School of Pharmacy and Health Professions
Creighton University
Omaha, Nebraska

Sue Byers-Connon, MS, COTA/L, ROH
Adjunct Instructor
School of Occupational Therapy
Pacific University
Hillsboro, Oregon
Adjunct Instructor
Occupational Therapy Assistant Program
Linn Benton Community College
Gresham, Oregon
OTA and GED Instructor (Retired)
Mt. Hood Community College
Gresham, Oregon

Helene L. Lohman, OTD, OTR/L
Professor
Department of Occupational Therapy
School of Pharmacy and Health Professions
Creighton University
Omaha, Nebraska

ELSEVIER
MOSBY

3251 Riverport Lane
Maryland Heights, MO 63043

OCCUPATIONAL THERAPY WITH ELDERS: STRATEGIES
FOR THE COTA

ISBN: 9780323065054

Copyright © 2012, 2004, 1998 by Mosby, Inc., an affiliate of Elsevier Inc.

"OTR" is a certification mark of the National Board for Certification in Occupational Therapy, Inc., which is registered in the United States of America. "COTA" is a certification mark of the National Board for Certification in Occupational Therapy, Inc., which is registered in the United States of America. "NBCOT" is a service and trademark of the National Board for Certification in Occupational Therapy, Inc., which is registered in the United States of America.

NBCOT did not participate in the development of this publication and has not reviewed the content for accuracy. NBCOT does not endorse or otherwise sponsor this publication, and makes no warranty, guarantee, or representation, expressed or implied, as to its accuracy or content. NBCOT does not have any financial interest in this publication, and has not contributed any financial resources.

Notice

Library of Congress Cataloging-in-Publication Data

Occupational therapy with elders : strategies for the COTA / [edited by]
Ren? L. Padilla, Sue Byers-Connon, Helene L. Lohman. — 3rd ed.
       p. ; cm.
   Includes bibliographical references and index.
   ISBN 978-0-323-06505-4 (hardback : alk. paper)
   1. Occupational therapy for older people.   2. Occupational therapy assistants.   I. Padilla, Ren? L.
II. Byers-Connon, Sue.   III. Lohman, Helene
   [DNLM: 1. Occupational Therapy.   2. Aged.   3. Rehabilitation. WB 555]
   RC953.8.O22O246 2012
   615.8′5150846—dc22

2011002407

Executive Editor: Kathy Falk
Developmental Editor: Megan Fennell
Publishing Services Manager: Peggy Fagen
Project Manager: Priya Dauntess
Book Designer: Karen Pauls

Working together to grow
libraries in developing countries

www.elsevier.com | www.bookaid.org | www.sabre.org

ELSEVIER   BOOK AID International   Sabre Foundation

Printed in the United States of America
Last digit is the print number: 9   8   7   6   5   4   3   2   1

To all our COTA colleagues who have been a vital part of our profession for many years, and to all OTA students who share in the promise of the future of occupational therapy.

René

To the Occupational Therapy Practitioners who have assisted me in my professional growth:

- *Chris Hencinski-Heideman (in memoriam), a mentor, distinguished teacher, and friend. Her generous spirit, positive attitude, and infectious smile touched so many lives.*
- *Lilian Crawford, who grounded me in the profession, teaching me the importance of the philosophical roots and historical perspective of Occupational Therapy.*
- *Robin Jones, whose professional involvement set the standard for many COTAs to become significant contributors to both state and national committees.*
- *Steve Park, whose understanding of the OTR/COTA partnership helped shaped my clinical practice.*
- *Helene Lohman and René Padilla, for believing in me and inviting me to become a part of this project.*

Sue

To my parents Mira Lee and Henry, who instilled in me the value of education; to all their friends and relatives who gave me an appreciation of their generation; and to my Aunt Jeanne, Caroline, and Ben, who live successful aging.

Helene

Shadows and Sunlight

I remember being young and wild,
Although my body forgets and betrays me.
I peer out of this aging body
With a mind that still knows
Who, when, where and how.
When did fifty
Or even sixty seem like young?
Birthdays only serve as a yardstick for the outside.
How can you measure what I feel on the inside?

My heart tears seeing friends disappear
Into places I only fear.
My memories of yesteryear seem crystal clear.
I close my eyes and feel myself running in the breeze.
The crowds along the college track applauding my triumph,
When the sound of my therapist
Cheering my toddling in a walker wakes me.
I laugh out loud
And people shake their heads as if I am half crazed.
So many losses totaling into this single moment.

The respect I had as a working man
Still fills my chest with pride.
My dearest Rosalie leaving me on Earth so quickly.
Our dreams of travel and leisurely walks are gone.
Saying goodbye to my neighborhood of 43 years,
To move into a room with a stranger.
Overhearing the hushed voices of my son and daughter
As they discuss the exorbitant costs of my care outside my door.
Then the frustrated voices in deciding who will take Dad home.

How did the tables get turned so fast?
Ironically my children become my caretakers now.
How can I express to those I love,
Do not grieve for my losses so deeply.
As I still intend to live
As best I can,
As much as you will allow me.
Keep open the windows of possibilities.
Do not shut the door of life just yet.

Yolanda Griffiths

Contributors

Marlene J. Aitken, PhD, OTR/L
Associate Professor (Retired)
Department of Occupational Therapy
School of Pharmacy and Health Professions
Creighton University
Omaha, Nebraska

Danielle Lancaster Barber
Student, MSOT
Occupational Therapy Department
College of Nursing and Health Sciences
Florida International University
Miami, Florida

Tonya Bartholomew, BSOT
Occupational Therapist
Creighton University Medical Center
Omaha, Nebraska

Rebecca Bothwell, OTR
Research Coordinator
Occupational Therapy Education
University of Kansas Medical Center
Kansas City, Kansas

Lea C. Brandt, OTD, MA, OTR/L
Program Director
The Missouri Health Professions Consortium
Clinical Assistant Professor
School of Health Professions
University of Missouri
Columbia, Missouri

Kris R. Brown, BS, OTR/L
Private Practice
Sioux City, Iowa

Leslie Brunsteter-Williams, BSOT
Formerly Staff Occupational Therapist
Acute Care, In-Patient, and Out-Patient Services
Rehabilitation Services Department
Trinity Lutheran Hospital
Kansas City, Missouri

Ann Burkhardt, OTD, OTR/L, FAOTA
Adjunct Faculty
New England Institute of Technology
Greenwich, Rhode Island
Occupational Therapist
Therapy Resource Management
Warren, Rhode Island

Kelli Coover, Pharm.D., CGP, FASCP
Assistant Professor of Pharmacy Practice
School of Pharmacy and Health Professions
Creighton University
Omaha, Nebraska

Brenda M. Coppard, PhD, OTR/L
Associate Professor and Chair
Department of Occupational Therapy
School of Pharmacy and Health Professions
Creighton University
Omaha, Nebraska

Jana K. Cragg, MA, OTR
Associate Professor
Occupational Therapy Assistant Program
St. Philip's College
San Antonio, Texas

Terryn Davis, COTA
Certified Occupational Therapy Assistant
Occupational Therapy Department
San Jose State University
San Jose, California

Michele Faulkner, Pharm.D.
Associate Professor of Pharmacy Practice
School of Pharmacy and Health Professions
Creighton University
Omaha, Nebraska

Coralie H. Glantz, OT/L, BCG, FAOTA
Co-Owner, Glantz/Richman Rehabilitation Associates
Riverwoods, Illinois

Cynthia Goodman, MS, OTR/L
Day Center Supervisor
Providence Elder
Place Gresham, Oregon

Yolanda Griffiths, OTD, OTR/L, FAOTA
Associate Professor
Department of Occupational Therapy
School of Pharmacy and Health Professions
Creighton University
Omaha, Nebraska

LTC Karoline D. Harvey, OTR
Assistant Chief and Intern Coordinator
Department of Occupational Therapy
Walter Reed Army Hospital
Washington, DC

Jessica Hatch
Student, OTD
Department of Occupational Therapy
School of Pharmacy and Health Professions
Creighton University
Omaha, Nebraska

Jean T. Hays, COTA
Instructor/Academic Fieldwork Coordinator
Occupational Therapy Assistant Program–Allied Health
St. Philip's College
San Antonio, Texas

Carly R. Hellen, BS, OTR/L
Dementia Care Consultant and Educator
Durham, New Hampshire

Tyrome Higgins, MS, COTA, ROH
Certified Occupational Therapy Assistant
Alamo Heights Rehabilitation Center
San Antonio, Texas

Ada Boone Hoerl, BS, COTA
Adjunct Professor
Division of Science and Allied Health
Sacramento City College
Sacramento, California

Yan-hua Huang, PhD, OTR/L
Assistant Professor
Occupational Therapy Department
California State University, Dominguez Hills
Carson, California

Lou Jensen, OTD, OT/L
Assistant Professor
Department of Occupational Therapy
School of Pharmacy and Health Professions
Creighton University
Omaha, Nebraska

Evelyn Z. Katz, OTR/L
Occupational Therapist
Weigel Williamson Center for Visual Rehabilitation
University of Nebraska Medical Center
Omaha, Nebraska

Mary Ellen Keith, COTA, CDRS
Adaptive Mobility Services
Orlando, Florida

Penni Jean Lavoot, COTA, CDRS, CRC
Rehabilitation Specialist
Project Threshold
Rancho Rehabilitation Engineering Center
Downey, California

Ivelisse Lazzarini, OTD, OTR/L
Former Director, Allied Health Complexity Center
Edward and Margaret Doisy School of Allied Health Professions
Saint Louis University
Saint Louis, Missouri

Michele Luther-Krug, COTA/L, SCADCM, CDRS
Driving Educator
Shepherd Center Driving Program
Atlanta, Georgia

Amy Matthews, OTD, OTR/L
Assistant Professor and Vice Chair
School of Pharmacy and Health Professions
Creighton University
Omaha, Nebraska

Tracy Milius, BSOT, OTR/L
Director of Operations
RehabVisions
Omaha, Nebraska

Deborah L. Morawski, BS, OTR/L
Owner, Achieving Independence
Abbey Physical Medicine and Rehabilitation
Grass Valley, California

Candice Mullendore, MS, OTR/L
Former Assistant Professor and Academic Fieldwork
Coordinator
Department of Occupational Therapy
School of Pharmacy and Health Professions
Creighton University
Omaha, Nebraska

Sandra Hattori Okada, MSG, OTR/L, CDRS
Gerontologist, Occupational Therapist, Certified Driver
Rehabilitation Specialist
Occupational Therapy Driving Program
Rancho Los Amigos National Rehabilitation
Downey, California

Steve Park, MS, OTR/L
Doctoral Candidate
University of Sydney
Sydney, Australia

Claire Peel, PhD, PT
Associate Dean for Academic Affairs
School of Health Related Professions
University of Alabama at Birmingham
Birmingham, Alabama

Emily Penington
OTD Student
Department of Occupational Therapy
School of Pharmacy and Health Professions
Creighton University
Omaha, Nebraska

Angela M. Peralta, COTA
Certified Occupational Therapy Assistant
Occupational Therapy
Toddler and Infant Program for Special Education
Staten Island, New York
Formerly Adjunct Instructor
Occupational Therapy Assistant Program
Touro College
New York, New York

Claudia Gaye Peyton, PhD, OTR/L, FAOTA
Associate Professor, Department of Occupational
Therapy
California State University, Dominguez Hills
Carson, California

David Plutschack
Student, OTD
Department of Occupational Therapy
School of Pharmacy and Health Professions

Creighton University
Omaha, Nebraska

Sherrell Powell, MA, OTR
Professor, Natural and Applied Science
LaGuardia Community College
City University of New York
Long Island City, New York

Nancy Richman, BS, OTR, FAOTA
Co-Owner, Glantz/Richman Rehabilitation Associates
Riverwoods, Illinois

Barbara Jo Rodrigues, MS, OTR/L
Occupational Therapy Program Director
Behavior Health Unit
Dominican Hospital
Santa Cruz, California

Michelle Rudolf
Student, OTD
Department of Occupational Therapy
School of Pharmacy and Health Professions
Creighton University
Omaha, Nebraska

Ellen Spergel, MEd, OTR
Professor, Coordinator of Occupational Therapy
Occupational Therapy Assistant Program
Rockland Community College
Suffern, New York

Sharon Stoffel, MA, OTR/L, FAOTA
Associate Professor
Occupational Science and Occupational Therapy
The College of St. Catherine
St. Paul, Minnesota

Andrea Thinnes, OTD, OTR/L
Assistant Professor
Department of Occupational Therapy
School of Pharmacy and Health Professions
Creighton University
Omaha, Nebraska

Mirtha Montejo Whaley, PhD, MPH, OTRL
Assistant Professor
Occupational Therapy Department
College of Nursing and Health Sciences
Florida International University
Miami, Florida

Preface

Certified Occupational Therapy Assistants (COTAs) continue to be a significant part of the occupational therapy workforce treating elders. The most recent American Occupational Therapy Association (AOTA) workforce and compensation survey report[1] states that skilled nursing facilities, which primarily service elders, continue to be the number one employer of COTAs. The U.S. Department of Labor's Bureau of Labor Statistics (BLS)[2] projected employment of both occupational therapists and occupational therapy assistants to increase by 30% or more between 2008 and 2018, much faster than the average for all professions. This trend has much to do with the growth of the elder population. The need for COTAs to possess a strong knowledge base that will allow them to provide the best care possible and to confidently represent the profession remains as high a priority as when we prepared the first and second editions of this text. Therefore, we have sought to include the most up-to-date information possible in order to support COTAs as they work in this important practice area.

Based on reader feedback, we retained the conceptual organization of the previous editions. The first section, Concepts of Aging, presents foundational concepts related to the experience of elders. A general discussion of aging trends, concepts, and theories is followed by a discussion of occupational therapy (OT) professional beliefs, including an introduction to the second edition of the *Occupational Therapy Practice Framework*.[3] The second section, Occupational Therapy Intervention with Elders, includes updated OT strategies that take into account the principles presented in Section One. We begin Section Two with issues related to all elders with such topics as cultural diversity, OT theories applied to elders, ethical aspects, and working with caregivers. We conclude Section Two with chapters dedicated to strategies applicable to the work with elders who have specific medical conditions.

As we prepared this third edition we remained committed to the goals that guided us in the previous editions:

- We wanted the project to acknowledge the reality of life experience of elders and be respectful of them as occupational beings. We recommitted to the use of the term "elder" as a way to prevent reducing these people to the stereotypical role of dependent patients and to dispel myths about aging.
- We continued to emphasize the importance of collaboration between the Occupational Therapist, Registered (OTR) and COTA. Our own collaboration as an editorial team continued to be

vivid example to us of the richness of such collaboration. We chose to use the titles "COTA" and "OTR" throughout the text to reflect the importance of national certification. Although recertification is not mandated by our profession, we believe strongly that it significantly contributes to maintaining standards of competent practice to provide consumers a high quality services.

- We wanted to produce a comprehensive text for both OTA students as well as practicing COTAs who wish to refresh their knowledge and for OTRs who are committed to the development of the COTA/OTR partnership.
- We wanted to highlight the important contribution COTAs make to the life of elders.
- We integrated available research evidence for effectiveness of interventions in order to enhance justification for services and advocacy for meeting elders' needs.
- We emphasized the illustration of principles and strategies through case studies and narratives using the language of the second edition of the Occupational Therapy Practice Framework[3] so that readers can easily relate their learning to real-life situations.
- We continued to ground the suggested strategies in traditional OT philosophy and practice and emphasized the kind of reasoning that should be part of all OT intervention regardless of professional level.

It remains our hope that this text will contribute to readers' knowledge so they can contribute to the improvement of life satisfaction of elders wherever they come into contact with them.

René Padilla, PhD, OTR/L, FAOTA
Sue Byers-Connon, MS, COTA/L, ROH
Helene L. Lohman, OTD, OTR/L

REFERENCES

1. The American Occupational Therapy Association (2010). 2010 AOTA workforce and compensation survey: Final report. Bethesda, MD: AOTA.
2. U.S. Department of Labor Bureau of Labor Statistics (2010). Occupational Outlook Handbook, 2010-11 edition. Last accessed November 26, 2010 at http://www.bls.gov/oco/
3. The American Occupational Therapy Association (2008). Occupational therapy practice framework: Domain and process (2nd ed.). The American Journal of Occupational Therapy (62), 625-683.

Acknowledgments

As was true in the previous edition, writing a book is not a simple process that one person can undertake alone. We wish to acknowledge many people for their contributions to this project:

- The contributing authors, for their hard work
- The individuals who reviewed the second edition and provided feedback
- Yolanda Griffiths for the moving poem that appears for the third time at the beginning of the book. We have found no better way to capture the experience of elders.
- The elders who graciously appeared in the photographs
- Kevin Callahan, COTA/L, for his photographic skill
- Megan Fennell and Kathy Falk for their patience and direction
- Judy Bergjoid at the Creighton Health Science Library for all her help with research
- The administrators and faculty of the Department of Occupational Therapy, School of Pharmacy and Health Professions at Creighton University, for their continued encouragement.

Contents

SECTION ONE   CONCEPTS OF AGING   **1**

1   AGING TRENDS AND CONCEPTS   **3**
Helene L. Lohman
Ellen Spergel
Emily Penington

**2   BIOLOGICAL AND SOCIAL THEORIES
OF AGING**   **21**
Marlene J. Aitken
Michelle Rudolf

3   THE AGING PROCESS   **31**
Mirtha Montejo Whaley
Danielle Lancaster Barber

4   PSYCHOLOGICAL ASPECTS OF AGING   **43**
Yolanda Griffiths
Andrea Thinnes

**5   AGING WELL: HEALTH PROMOTION
AND DISEASE PREVENTION**   **53**
Claudia Gaye Peyton
Yan-hua Huang

**6   THE REGULATION OF PUBLIC POLICY
FOR ELDERS**   **69**
Helene L. Lohman
Coralie H. Glantz
Nancy Richman

**SECTION TWO   OCCUPATIONAL THERAPY
INTERVENTION WITH ELDERS**   **83**

**7   OCCUPATIONAL THERAPY PRACTICE
MODELS**   **85**
René Padilla

**8   OPPORTUNITIES FOR BEST PRACTICE
IN VARIOUS SETTINGS**   **103**
Steve Park
Sue Byers-Connon

**9   CULTURAL DIVERSITY OF
THE AGING POPULATION**   **121**
René Padilla

**10   ETHICAL ASPECTS IN THE WORK
WITH ELDERS**   **135**
Lea C. Brandt

**11   WORKING WITH FAMILIES AND
CAREGIVERS OF ELDERS**   **145**
Ada Boone Hoerl
Barbara Jo Rodrigues
René Padilla
Sue Byers-Connon

**12   ADDRESSING SEXUAL ACTIVITY
OF ELDERS**   **155**
Helene L. Lohman
David Plutschack

13   USE OF MEDICATIONS BY ELDERS   **169**
Brenda M. Coppard
Kelli Coover
Michele Faulkner

14   CONSIDERATIONS OF MOBILITY   **183**
PART 1   RESTRAINT REDUCTION   **183**
Tracy Milius
Candice Mullendore
Ivelisse Lazzarini

**PART 2   WHEELCHAIR SEATING AND
POSITIONING: CONSIDERATIONS
FOR ELDERS**   **191**
Cynthia Goodman

PART 3   FALL PREVENTION   **194**
Lou Jensen
Sandra Hattori Okada

PART 4   COMMUNITY MOBILITY   **202**
Penni Jean Lavoot
Michele Luther-Krug
Mary Ellen Keith

**15   WORKING WITH ELDERS WHO HAVE
VISION IMPAIRMENTS**   **213**
Evelyn Z. Katz
Rebecca Bothwell

**16   WORKING WITH ELDERS WHO HAVE
HEARING IMPAIRMENTS**   **229**
Sharon Stoffel
Jessica Hatch

17 STRATEGIES TO MAINTAIN
   CONTINENCE IN ELDERS   241
   Kris R. Brown
   Jessica Hatch

18 DYSPHAGIA AND OTHER EATING
   AND NUTRITIONAL CONCERNS
   WITH ELDERS   251
   Deborah L. Morawski
   Terryn Davis
   René Padilla

19 WORKING WITH ELDERS WHO HAVE
   HAD CEREBROVASCULAR ACCIDENTS   263
   Deborah L. Morawski
   René Padilla

20 WORKING WITH ELDERS WHO HAVE
   DEMENTIA AND ALZHEIMER'S DISEASE   275
   Carly R. Hellen
   René Padilla

21 WORKING WITH ELDERS WHO HAVE
   PSYCHIATRIC CONDITIONS   291
   Ann Burkhardt

22 WORKING WITH ELDERS WHO HAVE
   ORTHOPEDIC CONDITIONS   299
   Brenda M. Coppard
   Tyrome Higgins
   Karoline D. Harvey
   René Padilla

23 WORKING WITH ELDERS WHO HAVE
   CARDIOVASCULAR CONDITIONS   313
   Tonya Bartholomew
   Jana K. Cragg
   Jean T. Hays
   Amy Matthews
   Claire Peel
   René Padilla

24 WORKING WITH ELDERS WHO HAVE
   PULMONARY CONDITIONS   323
   Angela M. Peralta
   Sherrell Powell
   David Plutschack

25 WORKING WITH ELDERS WHO HAVE
   ONCOLOGICAL CONDITIONS   329
   Leslie Brunsteter-Williams

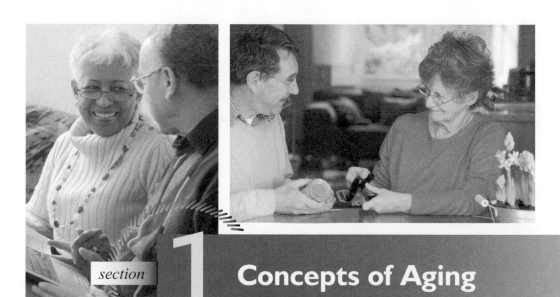

Concepts of Aging

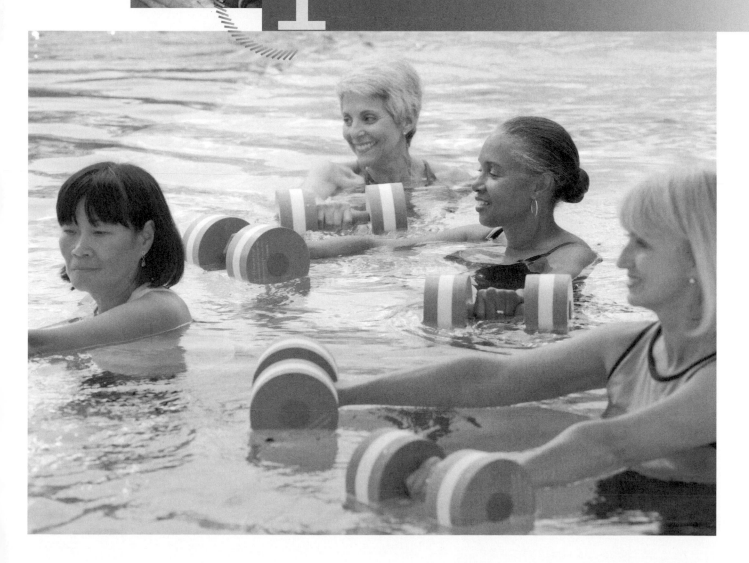

chapter 1

Aging Trends and Concepts

HELENE L. LOHMAN, ELLEN SPERGEL, AND EMILY PENINGTON

KEY TERMS

gerontology, geriatrics, cohort, health, illness, chronic illness, young old, mid old, old old, demography, trends, aging in place, intergenerational, generational cohorts (Traditionalists, Baby Boomers, Generation X, Generation Y), ageism

CHAPTER OBJECTIVES

1. Define relevant terminology regarding elders.
2. Describe the relation between aging and illness.
3. Discuss components of health and chronic illness.
4. Discuss a client-centered approach.
5. Describe the three stages of aging, and define their differences.
6. Describe the effects of growth of the elder population on society.
7. Discuss the effects of an increasingly large number of elder women on society.
8. Describe the problems and needs of the oldest old populations—that is, those elders 85 years and older, including the centenarians.
9. Describe living arrangements of elders and living trends, such as aging in place.
10. Discuss the significance of economic trends on the elderly.
11. Relate implications of demographical data for occupational therapy practice.
12. Discuss current trends impacting elders in America and implications for occupational therapy practice.
13. Describe the importance of intergenerational contact for occupational therapy intervention.
14. Explain the importance of understanding generational cohorts for intervention.
15. Describe the concept of "ageism" in today's society and the effect of the views of the American youth culture on aging.

Eric is a 25-year-old certified occupational therapy assistant (COTA) practicing in a skilled nursing home facility. He provides daily occupational therapy (OT) intervention for 5 days a week. Most of the elders are in some stage of recovery from an acute illness and are participating in OT to regain functional abilities. Many of the elders are quite frail and some have cognitive impairments. As a student, Eric observed Mark, a COTA working in an independent living facility. Mark was part of a team providing wellness programming for elders. Most of Mark's clients were quite active at the facility and in the community. Eric especially enjoyed watching Mark lead Tai Chi groups with the residents. On weekends, Eric visits his grandparents, both of whom are 75 years of age and are also independent, active members of the community. One spring break Eric had the opportunity to accompany his grandfather to an AARP advocacy meeting. He was proud to watch his grandfather and others asking questions that reflected critical thinking about policy issues. Eric often thinks about his grandparents, the elders at the AARP meeting and the independent living facility, as well as the nursing home residents. He contemplates about who are the typical elders.

Lea is a 20-year-old occupational therapy assistant student in an OTA program. As one of her course require-ments, class members participate in intergenerational book discussion groups at an independent living facility. The specific readings focus the book discussions on inter-generational values and beliefs. Lea is surprised to identify generational differences and similarities. The elder generations discuss the influences that World War II (WWII) and post-war America had on their lives. Her instructors also participate in the groups. They discuss growing up in the 1960s and 1970s and the influence of the media, the Civil Rights Movement, the Women's Movement, the assassination of President John F. Kennedy, and the Vietnam War on their generation. Lea and some of her classmates often comment on the strong influence that technology has had on their generation. All of the genera-tions commonly share the impact of the terrorist attacks on September 11, 2001, and the economic downturn of 2008. Lea notes that within each generation there are a variety of perspectives based on individual life experi-ences. These lively discussions have increased each par-ticipant's awareness of intergenerational commonalities and differences, as well as the individual uniqueness of each group member. The discussions have created a strong bond among the group members. Lea feels that as a result of participating in the intergenerational book discussion group, she will be more comfortable working with elders in a clinical practice.

Lea has a strong desire to go into practice with elders. She remembers helping her grandmother recover from a stroke. When she studied the content about elders in her course work, Lea was surprised to learn of the diversity among the elder population. She realized that just as her OTA class represents diversity among age groups and cultural groups, so does the elder population. She also recognized misconceptions she had about the elder generation. Some were based on clinical observations at a nursing home and informal observations from visits to her grandmother. One misconception was that all elders are sick and frail. Another misconception was that most elders have cognitive impairments. Through her participation in course experiences with well elders in community settings, Lea learned that many elders are healthy and active, especially the younger generation of elders (those 65 to 75 years of age). Lea also learned that cognitive impairment affects a small portion of the elder population, primarily the oldest of the old (those 85 years and older).[1]

COTAs may easily acquire a skewed image of the elder population, especially in a nursing home setting, which is the second largest area of practice for COTAs.[2] Elders in nursing homes tend to be representative of a sicker, older, and frailer elder population. Elders in nursing homes often have circulatory, cognitive, and mental disorders, and most residents require assistance with activities of daily living (ADL).[3] In reality, only 4.4% of all elders at any one time reside in nursing homes.[4] OT practice continues to change with a movement toward community-based practice, where the majority of elders reside. Therefore, COTAs must have a broader perspective about elders to work effectively with a diverse, continuously changing elder population. This chapter provides relevant background information as it relates to OT practice and to the overall elder population.

The term *gerontology* comes from the Greek terms *geron* and *lojas*, which mean "study of old men." Gerontology is often thought of as the study of the aged and can include the aging process in humans and animals. The field of gerontology is broad and includes the historical, philosophical, religious, political, psychological, anthropological, and sociological issues of the elder population. The term *geriatrics* is often used to describe medical interventions with the elderly. In OT practice, geriatrics sometimes refers to an area of clinical specialty. The term *cohort* refers to "a collection or sampling of individuals who share a common characteristic, such as members of the same age or the same sex."[5] In gerontological literature, the elder generation may also be referred to as the *elder* (or *aged*) *cohort* compared with younger cohorts. Different terms used in this book refer to the geriatric population as the *aged*, *older*, or the *elder* population.

HEALTH, ILLNESS, AND WELL-BEING

Although *health*, *illness*, and *well-being* are familiar terms, they require expanded definitions for OT practice in geriatrics. One part of a definition for *health* is "the absence of disease or other abnormal condition."[5] Few elders would be considered healthy with this general definition. However, a theory of well-being can be developed if health is considered the optimal level of functioning for a person's age and condition. Many individuals have chronic illnesses to which they have adjusted and are able to live optimally. These people should be considered as being in a state of well-being. For example, to live optimally, individuals with lifelong disabilities, such as multiple sclerosis, need health care system services such as OT home evaluations for environmental adaptations even though they are not ill. These individuals do not think of themselves as ill and may resent being labeled as "patients" and placed in this role by health care professionals.

The biological systems of elders may change. Some changes that result in disease or dysfunction may be treated through medication or surgery. Other biological changes, such as decreased balance, can be handled with environmental adaptations such as installing brighter lights in stairwells and removing loose rugs and electrical cords from traffic areas in the home. Some sensory changes can be partially resolved with glasses and hearing aids. These biological and sensory changes should not be thought of as illnesses. They are changes that elders adjust to and incorporate into their daily lives.

Chronic Illness

Many medical conditions of elders are chronic—that is, they cannot be cured, but they can be managed. The physician may not cure heart disease, but the pain and debilitating consequences can be managed for years with medications, diet, exercise, surgery, and technology. COTAs can provide ideas to help elders manage their chronic conditions to maintain involvement in occupations (see Chapter 5). In these cases it could be said that, although the disease has not been cured, the elder's life has been extended in a qualitatively meaningful way.

Most elders have a minimum of one or more chronic conditions. Recent data indicate the most prevalent conditions for elders are hypertension (53%), arthritis (49%), hearing impairments (42%), heart disease (32%), cancer (22%), diabetes (18%), visual impairments (17%), and asthma (11%).[6] The incidence of chronic illness may be greater in minority elder groups than in white elders. Blacks and Hispanics over age 65 report higher levels of diabetes than whites. Hypertension is also more prevalent among blacks than whites.[6]

The following examples illustrate the way one elder learns to adapt to a chronic illness. Henry has osteoarthritis and needs assistance with some ADL functions. He continues to maintain his apartment and values his independence. He takes frequent breaks to rest while doing housekeeping tasks. Because of his decreased endurance, he uses a lightweight upright vacuum, which also helps reduce upper extremity strain. Henry has an active social life outside of his home. He maintains mobility in the community by taking a bus to activities. Henry has osteoarthritis, a disease that cannot be cured. However, most COTAs would say that Henry is not sick.

Miriam is 89 years old. She lives with her 97-year-old husband in the same house that they moved into after they got married. She has a chronic blood condition called *thrombocytopenia*, along with osteoporosis and hearing loss. She has been admitted several times to the hospital for complications related to the thrombocytopenia. After she returns home and when she gets her energy back, she assumes her normal routine of managing cooking, housework, and walking every morning for 3 miles around the neighborhood. Through her walks she has met many of her younger neighbors and established friendships. Miriam desires to stay in her home, and she enjoys being in an intergenerational community. Again with this example most COTAs would say that Miriam is not sick.

Some health care practitioners may dismiss an elder's complaints with comments such as "It's your age; it's your problem; what do you expect from me? I can't cure you." They are likely to overlook important ways to treat and to reduce symptoms that may increase the length and quality of that elder's life. Generally, health professionals are educated to cure illness, and some may be less knowledgeable about illness management. Thus, some health care practitioners feel uncomfortable treating elders who cannot be cured, and thus in response the health care practitioners develop a dismissive approach.

The alternative to a dismissive approach is a collaborative approach, or what has been referred to in OT literature as *client-centered therapy*.[7] In this approach, emphasized in the second edition of the Occupational Therapy Practice Framework: Domain and Process,[8] registered occupational therapists (OTRs) and COTAs partner with their clients to help determine therapy goals and intervention activities. They spend time getting to know clients by hearing their stories through assessments such as the Canadian Occupational Performance Measure (COPM)[9] and making an occupational profile. An occupational profile helps gain a better understanding of the elder's personal history and viewpoints.[8] Elders are central to the management of their own health and well-being. By using a client-centered approach, elders identify meaningful intervention activities and thus are more invested in intervention.[10]

A partnership involves the OTR, COTA, and the elder working together to help determine meaningful intervention goals that enhance the elder's quality of life. The following example illustrates this partnership.

Sadie is an 86-year-old widow with arthritis and living in a senior citizen housing. Her daily life is a balance of self-maintenance, simple meal preparations, visits with neighbors in the community recreation room, telephone calls to family members, and watching television. Sadie has reported decreasing vision, weakness, and joint pain to her primary care physician. General anxiety and depression also appear to be features of her condition. She comments to her physician, "I think that I belong in a nursing home. I'm old, and I'm having difficulty taking care of myself."

Placing Sadie in a nursing home may manage some of her medical conditions, as well as provide care and social opportunities. However, the medical team also can evaluate additional supports to maintain independent living in the community if that is what Sadie really desires. The physician can adjust drug dosages for the management of Sadie's arthritis and order an OT evaluation and intervention. The OTR and COTA decide to first screen Sadie using the COPM to obtain a clearer picture of Sadie's concerns. With the COPM Sadie mentions that she would really like to remain home and identifies her main concerns as having difficulties with meal preparation and reading the newspaper. Both concerns are related to her low vision. In addition, she has difficulty getting dressed because of arthritis. On the basis of this information, the OTR, COTA, and Sadie collaborate to develop the following intervention recommendations:

1. A kitchen evaluation for suggestions for low vision
2. A lighted magnifier to improve visual function with reading
3. Arthritis education that includes joint protection and mobilization, energy conservation, work simplification, and adaptive devices to improve dressing

A client-centered approach can address the elder's chronic conditions, interests, and desires. Elders with multiple chronic diagnoses that often accompany acute conditions or changes in functional status are not unusual. When managed properly, all interventions work smoothly to improve the elder's independent status and occupational well-being. The elder may need to adjust to a different status of functioning with different occupational roles. The OT interventions suggested in the example may result in improved functional abilities in many areas of life and decreased anxiety about independent living. The accumulation of medical conditions does not necessarily lead to decreased function and increased disability. Despite the "graying of America,"[11] elder citizens are experiencing less disability and are living longer and better.[12]

THE STAGES OF AGING

What age constitutes "old age"? The federally mandated age to collect Social Security varies between 65 and 67 years based on year of birth. The age that most retirement communities set as the minimum for their residents is 55 years. At age 50 years, one can join the AARP, and by age 40 years, Americans are protected by the Age

Discrimination in Employment Act. The third stage of aging, called *senescence*, which social gerontologists define as a stage of biological decline, begins at age 30 years.

One definition of old age classifies 65 to 75 years of age as young old, 75 to 85 as mid old, and 85 and greater as old old.* This may help COTAs think of old age in terms of occupational role performance and expectations. However, COTAs should use this classification as a guideline because every person ages differently and every elder does not fit neatly into one of these three categories. Socioeconomic factors, societal changes, cultural factors, and personality considerations can largely influence the way each elder approaches aging. As the Baby Boomers enter the aging population, these categories may change and, ultimately, this generational cohort may change how aging is defined as they desire to stay youthful. Along with maintaining youthful attitudes, their life expectancy has increased.[12] Yet as the following discussion indicates, Baby Boomers will also inevitably experience changes with an aging body.

Young Old (65 to 75 years of age)

Elders who are young old may be recently retired and enjoying the results of their years of employment, their essential role as grandparents, and their continuing role as parents in the growth of their adult children. They have increased leisure time to pursue interests and to develop new ones. They may choose to do volunteer work with a community service, return to school, or travel. Some elders, however, because of economic issues or other personal reasons, will choose to remain in the workforce.[15] Others, because of family circumstances, may reassume the role of raising children with their grandchildren. The young old must often cope with chronic conditions such as osteoarthritis, hypertension, and cardiovascular disease. However, these chronic conditions are often managed medically and usually do not represent a major barrier to functioning or satisfactory occupational role performance.

Mid Old (75 to 85 years of age)

In the mid old period of life, more changes may be evident. These elders may make modifications in their occupational role performance. They may reduce or simplify their lives in various ways, including resting during the day, volunteering less, traveling less, and limiting distance of trips. They may rely more on social systems such as Meals on Wheels, public transportation, and family for some assistance with ADL (Figure 1-1). COTAs may provide interventions when necessary. The frequent loss of significant others brings affective stressors and

---

*These classifications are an adaptation of ones developed by Lazer.[13] In his work he defined four classifications of elders as "older" (55 to 64 years), "elderly" (65 to 74 years), "aged" (75 to 84 years), and "very old" (85 years and older). Earlier, Neugarten divided elders into the "young old" (55 to 74 years) and "old old" (older than 75 years).[14]

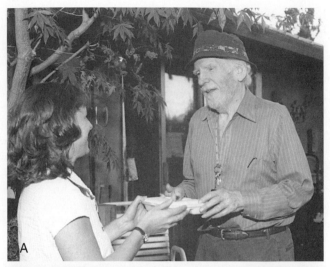

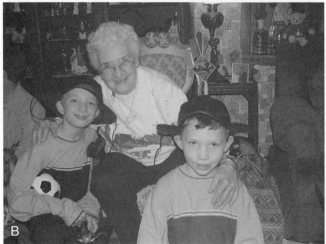

FIGURE 1-1   Lifestyle adaptations for elders. A, Some elders may use Meals on Wheels to maintain nutrition and remain in their own homes. B, Some elders may rely on family to help them remain active.

additional role changes (see Chapter 2 for a discussion of specific theories explaining the stages of aging).

Old Old (85 years of age and older)

During the old old period of life, elders may reflect on the meaning of their lives, the quality of their relationships, and their contributions to society. They may think about the losses they are experiencing and about their own deaths. This may be a time of peace and generosity; elders in the old old period of life may find it meaningful to give valued objects to loved ones who will treasure them. Conversely, it can be a period of fear and anger resulting from unresolved conflicts. Resolution of these conflicts can make this the most spiritual and fulfilling period for elders. Personal growth and reflection continue throughout life.

This time in an elder's life is usually a period of further systemic change affecting the sensory, motor, cardiac, and pulmonary systems. Chronic conditions impair self-maintenance capacities, and elders in the old old stage may need personal assistance with bathing, mobility, dressing, and money management that COTAs can provide. If these elders live independently, they may need some family member support.

An alternative health care delivery option to help frail elders primarily in the old old age group is a national demonstration project called Program for All-Inclusive Care of the Elderly (PACE). PACE addresses elders' preventive, acute, and long-term health care needs, providing medical and support services to help keep elders in their homes after they have been certified to need nursing home care.[16] PACE is financially supported by monthly capitation payments from Medicare and Medicaid or by private pay. In general, the goal of the project is to demonstrate that elders remain independent longer when their health care delivery system is sensitive and responsive to their medical, rehabilitative, social, and emotional needs. This project provides alternative models of long-term care such as adult day care, primary health care, rehabilitation, home care, transportation, housing, social services, and hospitalization. An interdisciplinary team handles case management. OTRs and COTAs are important team members with their strong skills of prevention, adaptation, and restoration of function.

As of 2008, there were 61 PACE programs operating in 29 states.[16] PACE has been demonstrated to reduce costs "by delaying nursing home care and shortening hospital stays" (p. 1).[17] It may be one answer to the ethical and economic dilemmas regarding ways to meet the increasing needs of elders as they live longer in a health care climate of declining resources and advancing technology.

DEMOGRAPHICAL DATA AND THE GROWTH OF THE AGED POPULATION

Demography is "the study of human populations, particularly the size, distribution, and characteristics of members of population groups."[5] Demographical data clearly suggest that the aged population is growing. This growth is often referred to in the literature as "the graying of America."[11] The portion of the elder population that consists of those 65 years or older comprises 12.6% of the total U.S. population. This population is expected to continue growing; it "will burgeon between the years 2010 and 2030 when the 'baby boom' generation reaches age 65" (p. 3).[4] The elder generation is projected to be 19.3% of the total population by the year 2030.[4] Minority elder populations also are growing rapidly and are projected to represent 28% of the elder population by the year 2030 compared with 18% of the elder population in 2003.[18] Future generations of elders will be more ethnically and racially variant than the current elder population. By 2050, the elder white population is projected to decline from 81% to 61% of the total elder population. The growth of

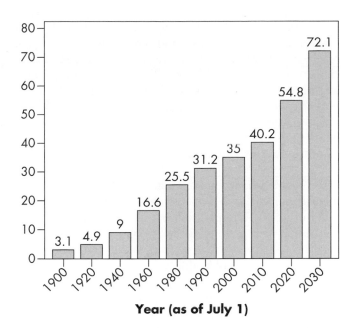

FIGURE 1-2 Number of persons age 65 years and older: 1900 to 2030. *(From Administration on Aging: Profile of older Americans, 2009, Department of Health and Human Services.)*

the minority populations will be greatest among Hispanics, who are projected to account for 18% of the elder population in 2050.[6] Many factors contribute to this significant population growth, including a declining mortality rate, advances in medicine and sanitation, improved diet, improved health expectancy with fewer chronic illnesses among Baby Boomers,[12] and improved technology. Figure 1-2 illustrates the growth of the elder population.

Accompanying the "graying of America" is a growth of the female aged population. For every 100 men older than 65 years, there are 143 women. This ratio increases with age. There are 114 women for every 100 men in the 65- to 69-year age group and 210 women for every 100 men in the 85 years and older age group.[4] Women, though, are much more likely to live with a disability, which is often defined as "having difficulty with" ADL[19] and indicates a need for OT intervention.

About 42% of women older than 65 years are widows, and there are over four times as many widows as widowers[4]; these statistics have broad sociocultural implications. A major consequence for some elder women with the loss of a spouse is an increased risk for poverty. In 2003, older single women, mostly widows, were more than twice as likely as older married women and more than three times as likely as older men to be poor or near poor.[18]

The Aging of the Aged Population

The fastest growing segment of the elder population is the 85 years and older cohort. As of 2006, elders older than 85 years numbered 5.3 million, and their size is projected to increase to 21 million by 2050.[6] The 85 years and older cohorts have their own unique needs because they may have more difficulty with physical and social functioning.[20] The 85 years and older cohorts are at risk for health problems such as cardiovascular disease and vision and hearing problems.[20] The risk for serious injuries from falling increases as aging progresses because the number of risk factors increases.[21] Risk factors for falls can include issues like having a chronic condition or poor lighting in the home.[21] In addition, the risk for severe cognitive impairment is much greater in the 85 years and older age group. Approximately 32% of those 85 years and older experience moderate to severe memory impairment compared with 5.1% of elders between 65 and 69 years of age.[22] The prevalence of Alzheimer's disease is increasing with a trend toward more elders having the condition.[23] Not surprisingly, the 85 years and older group uses a large amount of health, financial, and social services provided by public policies such as Medicare.[6] The current elder population, one of many groups of Americans who can qualify for Medicaid, spends the highest amount of Medicaid funds.[24] This large usage of federal money, along with concerns about increasing costs, may have future implications for continual modifications of public policies.

The 85 years and older age cohort is more likely to be institutionalized compared with their younger age cohorts. Although only 4.4% of the 65 years and older population are in nursing homes, 15.1% of those 85 years and older reside in institutional settings.[4] The need for long-term care is anticipated to increase as this age group grows,[25] especially for those with no living children or those living alone without other supports.

Although there are more elders among the 85 years and older population than in any age cohort who live in nursing homes and other long-term care facilities, the majority still reside in the community (Figure 1-3). Living in the community presents challenges because the need for assistance with ADL functions dramatically increases with age.[4] "ADLs include bathing, dressing, eating, and getting around the house. Instrumental activities of daily living (IADL) include preparing meals, shopping, managing money, using a telephone, doing housework, and taking medication."[4]

Many elders require a support system to have assistance with ADL. Currently, half (49%) of women 75 years and older live by themselves in households, and only 30.1% of women 75 years and older live with a spouse.[4] Many members of this age cohort also live with family members such as adult children who provide assistance with ADL functions. The majority of care in the community is provided informally by family members, usually adult daughters.[25] A future trend that may influence the type of caregiving needed for some members of the Baby Boom generation when they become the elder generation is a larger percentage of couples that are childless. These Baby Boomers should plan ahead and learn about community resources before they need them.[26]

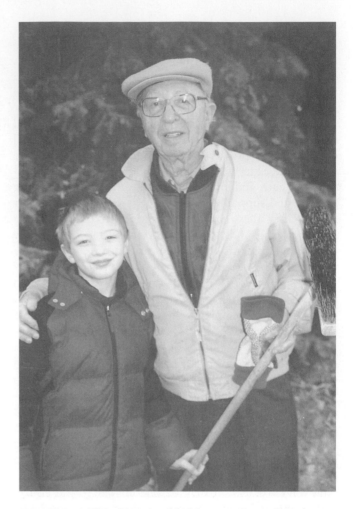

FIGURE 1-3   This 90-year-old elder remains well and active in the community.

Another important factor to consider is that some elders, particularly the old old age group, have relatively minimal formal education. However, the education level of all elders is increasing.[6] The number of elders completing a high school education increased from 24% in 1965 to 76% in 2007. Approximately 19% of elders have a baccalaureate degree or higher.[6] Knowing the educational level of their clients will help COTAs adjust or determine the instruction or training.

The Oldest of the Old: The Centenarians

An even older and more quickly growing group of elders are the centenarians, or those elders living beyond 100 years.[27,28] Researchers are fascinated about factors contributing to this longevity. Lifestyle, genes, environment, and attitude are researched contributors to longevity.[29-32] Of these factors, lifestyle appears to strongly impact longevity,[27] although further research is warranted.[30,31] Centenarians mainly experience a rapid decline in health status in their final years of life.[30] Some centenarians, though, have been in good health throughout their lives.[30,31]

Compared to younger cohorts, centenarians tend to escape or delay chronic illnesses during their lifetimes.[33]

Living Arrangements

COTAs working in geriatric practice need to consider the elder's home environment because housing problems can negatively affect the elder's physical and psychological well-being.[6] The majority of noninstitutionalized elders live in family households,[34] and 30.2% live alone.[4] Age influences living arrangements. Over half of people over age 65 live with spouses. A majority of elders living alone are women who outlive their husbands.[34]

There are a variety of living options available for elders. For elders with few economic resources, low-income housing is available. However, the number of units is limited, and there may be long waiting lists or lottery systems for applicants. Continuing Care Residential Communities and Life-Care Community Housing are other alternatives for elders with low incomes. In some cases, residents are required to contribute all of their assets. Residents have contracts for housing, supportive services, and often a continuum of services that include health and nursing homes.

Assisted living facilities are the fastest growing living option for seniors and have been available in the United States since the mid-1980s.[35] Assisted living facilities focus on frail elders or adults with disabilities. With assisted living, elders receive care management and supportive services to enable maximal independence in a homelike setting. Assisted living residents need some help to remain independent but do not require the same level of 24-hour care provided in nursing home facilities.[36] Typical residents are ambulatory 86-year-old women who require help with approximately two ADL.[37] Most residents use private funds to finance assisted living.[38] In some states, elders with less income can finance assisted living with Medicaid.[39] The growth of assisted living is attributed to the increase in the aged population, the desire of elders to have their own home and not go into nursing homes, and state policies that limit access to nursing home facilities.[38] There is much variability in the types of facilities. This variability in facilities and the expensive costs for residents are areas of discussion.[38] Additionally, because there are no federal regulations for assisted living facilities and variability in the way that states regulate them,[40] it would be beneficial for COTAs who practice in them to determine their state regulations.

Board and care homes, personal care, adult day care, adult foster care, family care, and adult congregate living facilities are other alternative care options in the community. Board and care homes service elders, many of whom have been deinstitutionalized. Adult day care is a community-based group program designed to meet the needs of functionally impaired elders. This structured, comprehensive program provides a variety of health, social, and related support services in a protective setting during any part of the day but provides less than 24-hour care. Adult foster homes are family homes or other facilities that provide residential care for elderly or physically disabled residents not related to the provider by blood or marriage. Adult congregate living facilities provide seniors with high-rise living accommodations with innovative service delivery options such as team laundry, cleaning, shopping, congregate meals, and home-delivered meals. Home health services are also available but are usually restricted to more acute episodic needs and require some level of homebound restrictions for reimbursement by Medicare.[41]

For those elders with assets, retirement communities include a variety of services such as leisure activities, congregate meals, laundry, transportation, and possibly health care. Some retirement communities may require entrance fees that could range from $20,000 to $400,000. Monthly payments may be as low as $200 or as high as $2,500.[42] In these communities, COTAs can act as activity directors, using their skills to select, analyze, and adapt activities to the abilities and interests of the residents (see Chapter 8).[43]

Aging in place or staying in one's current household with adequate support[44] is a trend expected to influence present and future elder generations.[12] Aging in place can be perceived as involving more than just an elder's home, including also the broader community[45] or an elder's context and environment.[8] Goals of aging in place is to allow elders a good quality of life by enabling them to stay in their homes and participate in their communities and to modify their homes to permit aging in place.[46] Along with aging in place is the phenomenon of Naturally Occurring Retirement Communities (NORC), which are apartments or communities comprising more than 50% of elder populations.[45] Elders living in NORCs can work together to provide enough resources to help the residents maintain a quality of life.[47] Some health care professionals are choosing to become Certified Aging in Place Specialists (CAPS). With this certification developed by the National Association of Home Builders Remodelers Council (NAHB) along with AARP, health care practitioners are trained in understanding the specific needs of elders for home modification.[48]

Aging in place is also sometimes perceived as a market-driven concept where elders in a facility receive various levels of care. Thus, an elder might start out on an independent living unit and, when his or her functional status changes, move to an assisted living unit and eventually to a nursing home unit or even an Alzheimer's disease unit, all in the same facility.[49] COTAs working in these facilities can provide continuity of care as the resident's functional status changes.

For those elders who desire to remain in their homes and communities, support services such as adult day care, meal programs, senior centers, and transportation services can help them age in place.[50] Aging in place is a trend that OT practitioners should pay close attention to for as

Yamkovenko states, "A part of the 2017 Centennial Vision of the American Occupational Therapy Association (AOTA) is to meet society's occupational needs. Occupational therapy practitioners can meet the needs of an aging population by helping them age in place, stay healthy, and lead full lives."[46]

Most of these discussed living options require having adequate financial assets and good retirement planning because long-term care is costly. In 2009, the average cost for living in an assisted living apartment was $2,825 per month or approximately $34,000 a year.[51] Nursing home yearly costs vary across the country with an average cost of $183 daily or almost $67,000 yearly for a semi-private room.[51] Medicare does not generally cover long-term care.[50] Some elders have shifted their finances to qualify for Medicaid, a program that provides some long-term care coverage for the indigent. However, the Deficit Reduction Act of 2005 now imposes a period of ineligibility for elders who give away assets or resources in order to qualify for Medicaid.[52] At the time of this writing a positive addition with health care reform is an optional benefit for long-term care support called the Community Living Assistance Services and Supports Program (CLASS). This program helps pay for nonmedical services to support community residency such as "housing modification, assistive technologies, personal assistance services and transportation" for a person with functional limitations.[53]

Most federal funds for elders go toward institutional care rather than home and community services. Funding for community services for elders comes from a variety of programs such as Medicaid and the Older Americans Act.[50,54] Long-term care insurance is an option to help people plan for their future long-term care needs. Plans differ but usually cover a variety of long-term care options such as assisted living, nursing home, Meals on Wheels, and home health. Coverage is usually based on the criteria of having difficulty with a set number of ADL. Generally, it is more financially advantageous to purchase a plan when one is younger, which results in lower premiums. Unfortunately, it is estimated that 85% of Americans over age 45 do not have any form of long-term care insurance.[55] Federal and state governments do provide tax incentives for private long-term care insurance, but primarily affluent elders actually benefit from these incentives because of the set up of tax deductions.[56]

Finally, recent data on community-resident Medicare beneficiaries suggest that over 27% had difficulty with performing ADL, and an additional 12.5% had difficulty with one or more IADL.[4] These data point to one strong reason for OT intervention in any of the discussed settings.

Economic Demographics

Most elders are not impoverished. Data from 2006 suggest that medium- and high-income elders account for more than two-thirds of the total elders.[6] The economic status of the elder population has been variable over the past 40 years. The poverty rate in 1959 for elders was 35.2%.[57] By 2003 the rate was reduced to 10.2%.[57] It is easy to see that the elder poverty rate has "declined substantially" (p. 946).[58] The current poverty rate for the elder population is 9.7%,[4] which is close to the working age population's (ages 18 to 64 years) level of poverty.[6] General indicators of becoming impoverished after retirement are work history, occupational type, residence in rural areas,[59] and preretirement income.[60] Working in professional occupations with higher earnings and cognitive requirements may result in better retirement planning.[59]

Elder women have a greater poverty rate than elder men. Approximately 12% of elder women are poor compared with 6.6% of elder men.[4] The economic statuses of elder men and women differ as a result of many factors. When they were younger, elder women of the current oldest generational cohort, the *Traditionalists*, were generally housewives or worked occasionally at paid employment. This resulted in fewer Social Security benefits and smaller or no pensions. When women become widowed, their chances of becoming impoverished increase, especially if they lose their spouse's pension funds.[58] Minority widows are especially at risk because they may have accrued fewer assets during their working years.[61]

Although there are differences across ethnic groups in rates of poverty, a wide economic disparity exists between white elders and elders of minority groups. Approximately 7.4% of white elders are poor, compared with 23.2% of black elders and 17.1% of Hispanic elders. Elder Hispanic and black women living alone have the highest poverty rates at 39.5% and 39%, respectively.[4]

Public policy influences the elder population's economic status. Social Security, which provides retirement income for elders, and Supplemental Security Income, which provides some financial support for lower income elders,[62] help elders. Ninety percent of people over age 65 live in families with income from Social Security.[6] Overall, these public policies have proven to be antipoverty measures for elders.[63]

Changes are projected to occur because of concerns related to the economic solvency of Social Security. Amendments to the Social Security Act in 1983 increased the age in which upcoming generations of elders can start receiving social security.[64] The current retirement age of 65 years will eventually increase to 67 years.[65] This change, which will be gradually phased in, is applicable to workers who are 62 years of age in the year 2000 (McBride, 1996, personal communication). The economic solvency of Social Security is related to an increasing aging population with less tax dollars in the federal budget to pay for benefits. Discussed reforms are higher taxes, less benefits, or the privatization of retirement funds. Social Security reform will be an important discussion throughout this century.[57]

Changes in the Medicare and Medicaid policy also will continue to affect the economic status of the elder population, especially if elders are required to pay more money for health care. Adding new benefits such as prescription medication may result in cutbacks in other areas of Medicare or increased costs. At the time of this writing, with health care reform some positive benefits for Medicare beneficiaries are improved coverage for prescription medication and coverage for preventive services, such as annual physicals. Yet cost cuts are planned with other areas of Medicare, such as payment adjustments for home health care agencies.[66] Other factors such as the increasing costs of health care and the general state of the American economy also influence the economic status of elders. For example, after the events of September 11, 2001, and in 2008, the stock market took a downswing, which decreased many retirement funds (see Chapter 6 for a discussion about public policy).

Additional Trends and the Influence of Aging Trends on Occupational Therapy Practice

COTAs working with elders need to be aware of aging trends. This section discusses three additional trends that impact elders and their possible influence on COTA practice. One growing trend is elders raising grandchildren. Grandparents in a parenting role can range in age from thirties to seventies.[67] Approximately 5.1 million children were living with a grandparent in 2006.[68] Grandparents raising grandchildren occurs in all socioeconomic and ethnic groups.[68] However, grandparent-headed households are more likely to be living in poverty than other family units.[67] Reasons for this phenomenon vary and can result from substance abuse, teen pregnancy, divorce, incarceration, death or disability, and the increasing number of single-parent families.[67]

Grandparents raising children can experience major challenges. For example, some elders may be dealing with their own health or financial issues along with the stresses of caregiving. It can be difficult to learn to set limits as they did with their children.[67] However, some grandparents in a parenting role may find it rewarding to provide a sense of stability and predictability for their grandchildren.[67] COTAs working with elders in this situation need to be sensitive to the demands and enjoyment of this parenting role.

A second trend will be an increase in elders remaining in the workforce. Data from 2006 indicate that 29% of workers ages 65 to 69 years old and 11% of workers age 70 years and older remain in the workforce.[6] A 2009 survey indicated that 27% of people ages 55 to 64 plan to postpone retirement,[15] and 27% of people ages 45 to 54 are seeking new jobs because of economic uncertainty. Another study by AARP found that 80% of Baby Boomers intend to continue working either for an economic reason or for self-gratification.[69] The percentages of elders remaining employed have varied over the past 40 years

with the greatest percentage occurring in the 1960s. A gradual decrease in workforce participation took place before the early 1980s.[6] Since the late 1990s, the percentage of elders remaining in the workforce has gradually increased,[6] and projections are for a continual growth of elders in the workforce, especially from the Baby Boomer generation[70] and because of economic times.[15] Many older workers choose to stay in the workplace "to feel useful and productive" and "live independently" (p. 2).[71] In addition, public policy such as changes in the Social Security Act from the 1983 amendments will influence the next generation of elders to remain in the workforce. These amendments allow increases in payment if retirement is delayed between ages 65 and 69. As discussed earlier, full Social Security benefits will be extended until a person is 67 years old.[65] The Age Discrimination in Employment Act of 1967 and its amendments along with the removal of required retirement laws also help elder workers remain in the workforce.

Though it has not been the case in the recent past, currently, most employed elders work full-time.[72] Older workers tend to have less education and make less money than younger workers, but both of these trends are changing.[72] The influence of an aging labor force on OT practice remains to be seen. However, innovative therapists may identify new areas of practice to ensure continual success of elders in the workforce.

A third trend influencing elders is the increased usage of computer technology. Approximately 41% of those age 65 and older have a computer at home, and 33% have Internet access at home.[73] The usage of computers by elders has many advantages, such as decreasing isolation and providing telemedical support.[74] Computers can assist elders with making purchases, which is a helpful benefit for those who are homebound (Figure 1-4). Adaptive computer programs aid elders with disabilities. For

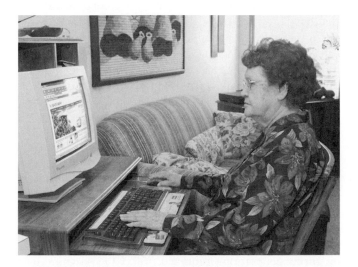

FIGURE 1-4 Elders may use computers to access the Internet to make online purchases.

example, voice programs help elders who have arthritis and have difficulty with keyboarding. Elders with low vision can benefit from many computer programs geared for their visual needs. Elders who desire more intergenerational contact can achieve this contact through e-mail and instant messaging.[74] Li and Perkins[75] found that a majority of elders have a positive view of technology and are willing to learn necessary skills, but few have taken steps to do so. COTAs can suggest computer resources in the community, such as state sites supported by the Assistive Technology Act, which provides computer training, or libraries. They can suggest appropriate software to assist elders with functional concerns and can make adaptations to allow computer usage.

In summary, these three highlighted trends are examples from many trends influencing elders. As the elder generation continues to grow and as society continues to change, it will be paramount that COTAs remain aware of aging trends and consider them in terms of society and OT practice.

Implications for Occupational Therapy Practice

Because of continued growth of the elder population, the need will increase for OTRs and COTAs working with them. The effects of all of the demographics, issues, and trends discussed in this chapter on OT practice remain to be seen. However, it can be assumed that in the future, dilemmas related to limited resources will affect the practice arena. In the coming decades, as the Baby Boom cohorts reach 85 years of age, Ericson, Toohey, and Wiener[25] expect that "burdens on families and institutions will increase substantially" (p. v). At this time, no one can predict whether there will be adequate funding and social services to meet the needs of a growing elder population and whether there will be enough health care resources to address this population's health care needs. The increasing cost of health care,[76] the ever changing economy, and the tenuous state of Social Security are current concerns that have future implications for the aged population. OT personnel will continue to be challenged to provide quality intervention in a cost-constrained environment. New models of OT geriatric care will evolve in the future, especially in community settings where the majority of elders remain. All OT personnel should be at the front end of this evolution.

INTERGENERATIONAL CONCEPTS AND GENERATIONAL COHORTS

In today's society, same-age cohorts socialize, for the most part, among themselves and have minimal intergenerational contact. When they work in a nursing home, COTAs may have little daily interaction with well elders in the community. COTAs treat elders who are often two or three generations removed. Yet COTAs must have meaningful contact, either informally or formally, with both well and frail elderly to work effectively with the elder population. Many benefits are mentioned in the literature about formal intergenerational programs. Some of these benefits include a better understanding of the elder generation from a historical perspective and their values and beliefs,[77] increased positive views of elders,[78,79] improved social skills and academic performance for youth, and increased socialization and emotional support for elders.[80]

In recent literature there has been much discussion about generational cohorts or a "group of people whose birthdates fall between specified dates and who move through life together" (p. 103).[81] Other classical defining factors of generational cohorts are being from the same area and experiencing similar historical and social events.[82] Thus, generational cohorts experience comparable social and historical occurrences that predispose them to related life perspectives.[83] From an OT standpoint context and environmental factors[8] are some considerations with a population of generational cohorts. Current generations are divided into the several groups, each with its own characteristics (Table 1-1). In reviewing this table, consider generational traits and historical/social factors that influenced the generational cohort that you are from as well as from the generations that you will work with in intervention. Table 1-1 also emphasizes concepts about approaching intervention with the current elder generations—the Traditionalist and the entering elder generation of Baby Boomers. Some consideration for intervention is how each generation approaches work, reward, communication, learning, and authority. Contemplate how you can capitalize on the generational characteristics to maximize interventions. Also, when reading this discussion, keep in mind that there is individual variation in any generational cohort based on each individual's life experiences. Individuals born closer to the end or beginning of a generational cohort may take on traits from their own or the previous or next generational cohort. So ideas presented in this discussion should be viewed as general guidelines.

Think about the influence that the Great Depression, WWII, and the Korean War had on the current oldest elder generation. That generation, the Traditionalists, which came of age during WWII, was used to the military being of their lives and therefore embrace a hierarchal approach, are formal in their interaction approach, respectful of authority, value conformity, and believe in working for the greater good.[84-86] Based on these traits, Traditionalists in an intervention situation may be very respectful and adherent to the suggestions of "the authorities" on the health care team. It will be important to ask these elders how they want to be addressed because many Traditionalists embrace a formal communication style and prefer titles, such as Mr. Jones, instead of being addressed by a first name.[87] Because the Traditionalists value formality and conformity, COTAs should be particularly cognizant of their dress and language. Additionally, Traditionalists

TABLE 1-1

Intergenerational Factors to Consider with Therapy with the Current Elder Generational Cohorts				
Generational cohort	Birth years	Historical and contextual influences	Sample characteristics	Elder generation as clients in therapy
Traditionalist (Veterans and Silent Generation)	1922-1945	Great Depression WWII Korean War Postwar building of America (GI Bill) Cold War	Appreciate hierarchal organizational structure "Chain of Command" Loyal Disciplined Value tradition and are conformers Formal in approach Articulate with writing and speaking	Respect of health care team Hard worker Adherence to intervention program Value formal communication with intervention and education Value compassionate approach Value in person communication (not technological-based)
Baby Boomer	1946-1964	Assassination of John F. Kennedy and Martin Luther King Jr. Cuban Missile Crisis Civil Rights Movement Disability Rights Movement Sexual Revolution Vietnam War Television First walk on the moon Watergate	Interactive and team players Strong work ethic and work identification Driven and ambitious High expectations of self and others Desire personal satisfaction and self-realization Value learning Value personal communication Idealistic	Work as a team in intervention (client-centered approach) Value in person communication Works hard Wants to be valued Wants to learn
Generation X	1965-1980	Fall of Berlin Wall Gulf War Challenger Space Shuttle disaster Latchkey children MTV Video games Seeding of Internet	Balance of work, family, and leisure Self-reliant Flexible and at ease with change Informal Focus on quality outcomes Desire support and encouragement Technologically strong part of their lives Value diversity Skeptical of institutions	
Generation Y (Millennial)	1981-2000	September 11 terrorist attacks Oklahoma City bombing Columbine school shooting Internet, cell phones "Baby on Board" generation	Balance of work, family, and leisure Technology large part of their lives Multitasking Success oriented Value recognition Optimistic Altruistic Politically active Social and participative Desire quick reward and feedback Educated generation Diverse generation that tolerates diversity	

Data from Fogg, P. (2008). When generations collide. *The Chronicle of Higher Education*, 54, B18-B20; Hammill, G. (2005). Mixing and managing four generations of employees. *FDU Magazine* online. Retrieved from http://www.fdu.edu/newspubs/magazine/05ws/generations.htm; Johnson, S. A., & Romanello, M. L. (2005). Generational diversity: Teaching and learning approaches. *Nurse Educator*, 30(5), 21-216; Mueller, K. (2010). *Communication from the Inside Out: Strategies for the Engaged Professional*. FA Davis; Philadelphia: Zemke, R., Raines, C., & Filipczak, B. (1999).Training Generational gaps in the classroom, 36(11), 48-54.

grew up at a time when physicians were more personal with house calls and may desire a compassionate approach.[87] Having experienced the Great Depression, Traditionalists may be frugal about spending their money, such as for adaptive equipment.

Now think about the Baby Boomer generation that came of age during a time in American history when there was much optimism, prosperity, and yet societal angst and turbulence. Growing up in a secure time of post-WWII, Baby Boomers experienced the benefits of an expanding American society with many advances in science and technology. They also experienced the assassination of President Kennedy, the Vietnam War, and related unrest. The defining events of President Kennedy's assassination and the Cuban Missile Crisis may have contributed to the Baby Boomers' focus on living for the moment and personal gratification.[12] Additionally, many societal changes were happening, such as the reformation of Congress to be more liberal, the Civil Rights Movement, and the Disability Rights Movement, along with the deinstitutionalization of people with mental illness and people with developmental disabilities. Growing up in such a prosperous time, many members of the Baby Boomer generation were more educated than those of previous generations.[12] Generational slogans developed during the youthful period of the Baby Boomers reflected their beliefs. The slogan "Make Love Not War" suggested the unrest of the time about the Vietnam War and the sexual revolution. "Don't Trust Anyone Over Thirty" reflected the distrust that the Baby Boomer generation had of people in authority. Current Baby Boomers still do not like to think of themselves as aging and desire to stay young.[12]

According to generational cohort literature, the Baby Boomer generation currently entering the aged population is very different from the present oldest of the aged population, the Traditionalists, based on their life experiences. Baby Boomers value a team approach rather than the authoritative leadership approach that the Traditionalist generation desires.[88,89] However, similar to the Traditionalists, Baby Boomers value hard work.[88] Baby Boomers are very driven in what they do, often being thought of as achievers.[86] Baby Boomers desire personal gratification with life's occupations,[89] like to learn for learning's sake,[88,90] and want to be valued.[86] Johnson and Bungum[90] found in their research that the Baby Boomer subjects wanted to learn new activities because of multiple reasons, such as providing more social options and relationships, improving health and length of life, and obtaining educational goals. Research indicates that Baby Boomers want to age in place in their homes and remain in their own communities or move to a community that is designed for their aging needs.[91]

COTAs contemplating intervention approaches with Baby Boomers, based on generational cohort theory, would recognize that elders from this generation may need to be approached differently than elders from the current generational cohort, the Traditionalists. With Baby Boomers, COTAs might strongly integrate a client-centered approach or a team partnership with intervention based on this generational cohort values about work and leadership. In addition, COTAs might recognize that Baby Boomers would want in-depth education about their condition because of valuing learning and that they may have already researched their condition before therapy. The OTR/COTA therapy team will have a strong role helping elders from the Baby Boomer generation who desire to age in place or perhaps helping design homes in communities for elders.

COTAs should familiarize themselves with the characteristics of all generations, including their own, because they may have a positive influence on intergenerational interactions. The exercise in Figure 1-5 demonstrates that each generation has certain values and attitudes that are influenced by similar generational experiences and historical events.[92] Yet each person has his or her own story to tell. This exercise can be completed as a group or individually. The exercise in Box 1-1 will help pull together concepts about working with the entering aged population of Baby Boomers.

AGEISM, MYTHS, AND STEREOTYPES ABOUT THE AGED

"If you are a man and you are prejudiced against women, you will never know how a woman feels. If you are white and you are prejudiced against blacks, you will never know how a black person feels. But if you are young and you are prejudiced against the old, you are indeed prejudiced against yourself, because you, too, will have the honor of being old someday" (Lewis).[93]

"Ageism is an attitude that discriminates, separates, stigmatizes, or otherwise disadvantages older adults on the basis of chronological age."[5] Ageism is a form of prejudice because it promotes general assumptions, or stereotypes, about a group of people. These assumptions are not true for all members of the elder population and may change to some different expressions of ageism with the Baby Boomer population. Following are some stereotypes expressed with ageism:

- Elders are useless because they can't see, hear, or remember.

BOX 1-1

Active Learning Exercise

You have been asked to be on a marketing committee to redesign an assisted living facility to meet the needs of the Baby Boomer generation. What will be your suggestions? Consider concepts of context and environment from the Occupational Therapy Practice Framework II with this exercise.[8]

Fill in the following lifelines with significant historical and personal events about yourself, someone from the generation 10 years older than you, one of your parents, and one of your grandparents. After filling in the lifeline, answer the questions below.
Refer to the following example:

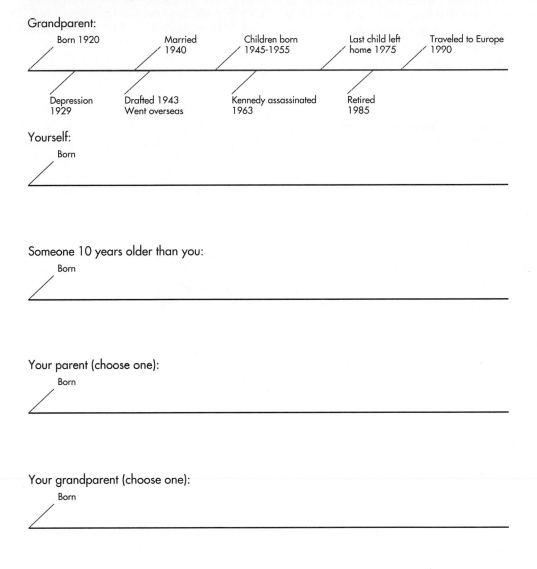

Answer the following questions:
What significant intergenerational differences did you notice between your generation, your parents' generation, your grandparents' generation, and even the generation 10 years older than you? What are some of the significant values of each generation and how were they influenced by historical events?
How might these similarities and differences between generations affect clinical treatment?

FIGURE 1-5   Lifeline exercise. *(Adapted from Davis, L. J., & Kirkland, M. (1987). ROTE: The role of occupational therapy with the elderly: Faculty guide. Rockville, MD: American Occupational Therapy Association, with permission.)*

- Elders are slow when they move about.
- Elders are in ill health.
- Elders cannot learn new things.
- Elders drain the economy rather than contribute to it; they are unproductive.
- Elders are too old to remain part of the workforce.

- Elders cannot perform or enjoy sexual activity.
- Elders prefer being with and talking with other elders.
- Elders are depressed and complain about all that is new.
- Elders are rich; or elders are poor.

Many of these statements have been challenged by research. With any stereotype, there may be a small amount of truth for some members of the group. For example, it is true that elders frequently need glasses as aging progresses; however, the need for glasses does not render an elder useless. An unfortunate result of these myths is that some elders may believe them. For example, whereas young persons may joke about becoming forgetful, elders may seriously question their cognitive abilities as a result of the stereotype that elders have trouble remembering.

These stereotypes may develop as a result of fear of the unknown, or from a lack of contact with the aged. American culture often focuses on youth. Youth is seen as beautiful, as something to aspire to and maintain at any cost. Young is sexy, and old is not.

The medical system in the United States also has been focused on youth. The goal of this system has traditionally been to find a cure for all illnesses. This goal has prompted significant contributions to the world's health care; however, the belief in a cure for all ills may conflict with the care elder citizens need. With the United States' current technological knowledge, some chronic illnesses of old age can be managed only, not cured.

In the health care system, references to ageism often occur as a response to a medical diagnosis. OT documentation that begins, "This 91-year-old female was admitted with the diagnosis of total hip replacement," may trigger preconceived ideas based on age bias, such as the opinion that the client is too old for intervention. Readers of this type of documentation may question the benefits versus risks of surgery or OT intervention for this elder.

In day-to-day interactions, language can encourage ageism. People working in the health care field may unintentionally be condescending when they refer to elders as "dear" or "sweetie." This type of "elderspeak" can contribute to more negative images of aging and lead to worse functional health over time.[94] Simply referring to a person as "the older stroke patient in Room 570" dehumanizes the person. Stating that a person is incapable of doing a task because of being old or having some deficits without a true understanding of the person's functional abilities also promotes ageism. The following story illustrates this concept. At an assisted living facility there were several elders who had mild to moderate cognitive deficits. The COTA knew each elder as a human being and had an understanding of each person's identified meaningful occupations. For elders who valued cooking, the COTA organized a cooking group followed by a party. She adapted the activity so that all of the elders would be successful. Before the cooking activity, the team leader expressed negative feelings because she felt that the elders would be incapable of cooking. The team leader was surprised to observe that the cooking activity turned out to be beneficial and successful for the elders. The leader later honestly remarked that oftentimes her feelings of being

BOX 1-2

Reflection Questions about Ageism

- How did I respond to the elders I saw today?
- Am I aware of any actions or language that I used that might promote ageism?
- Am I aware of any actions or language that others used that might promote ageism?

"protective" of the residents got in her way. Feeling protective of elders promotes ageism. A protective attitude can encourage assumptions, such as elders are incapable or elders are like children. Sometimes staff working with elders who have cognitive deficits and have regressed in their function can inadvertently talk to them in a childish manner. Unprofessional actions also can reflect ageism. One COTA who had a very full day skipped an appointment with an elder assuming that the elder had a cognitive deficit and would not remember. Later that day the elder called the COTA to inquire about what happened. The COTA learned a hard lesson from that experience about her own ageism. As these stories illustrate, reflection often helps people realize their own stereotypical beliefs and attitudes. A way to be more aware of ageism and general attitudes is to record in a journal one's feeling about contact with elders. Box 1-2 provides reflection questions about ageism that COTAs should ask themselves.

Perspectives are changing as reflected in initiatives such as the International Classification of Functioning, Disability and Health, or ICF,[95] and Healthy People 2020.[96] The ICF is an "international standard to describe and measure health and disability."[95] The ICF focuses on the impact of disability rather than cause and considers not just the disease but also the environmental context in which people live.[95]

The Occupational Therapy Practice Framework: Domain and Process, second edition, reflects perspectives from the ICF. The Practice Framework considers the intervention process within the broad "domain" of OT.[8] Similar to the ICF, the Practice Framework takes into account the influence of context and environment on occupation. Context and environment includes "cultural, personal, temporal, virtual, physical, and social" (p. 645) dimensions.[8] As Youngstrom[97] stated, "Occupational therapists [need] to understand their role within a larger societal and health context in order to position themselves in changing traditional areas and to take advantage of opportunities in emerging areas" (p. 607). In the second edition several changes were made, including considering clients as persons, organizations, or populations. (See Chapter 7 for more information about the Occupational Therapy Practice Framework.)

Healthy People 2020 envisions "a society in which all people live long, healthy lives."[96] It is based on the following four goals: (1) Attain high quality, longer lives free of preventable disease, disability, injury, and premature death; (2) achieve health equity, eliminate disparities, and improve the health of all groups; (3) create social and physical environments that promote good health for all; and (4) promote quality of life, healthy development, and healthy behaviors across all life stages.[96] All goals impact the elder population.

Many aspects of American society, including housing, employment, and recreational resources, are geared toward youth. However, that focus is slowly changing with the emergence of the senior citizen as a powerful political and economic force and with the growth of the aged population. Who knows what changes the next generation of entering elders of Baby Boomers will bring to society!

CHAPTER REVIEW QUESTIONS

1 Define the terms gerontology, geriatrics, and cohort.
2 What is the relation between aging and illness?
3 What is a client-centered approach? How might it affect client care?
4 What considerations should be taken for managing clients with chronic illnesses?
5 What factors are related to the significant population growth of the elder generation?
6 What is a result of more widows than widowers among the elder population?
7 What are some of the needs of the 85 years and older generation?
8 What does the COTA need to know about the educational level of any elder for intervention?
9 What age group has the highest poverty rate and why?
10 How has public policy influenced the economic status of elders?
11 What are some implications of the demographical data for future OT practice?
12 How do you think the three discussed trends (grandparents raising children, aging workforce, and increased computer usage) can impact OT practice?
13 How do you keep abreast of aging trends?
14 What is ageism? Provide examples of it in today's culture. How do you think expressions of ageism might differ or stay the same with an aging population of Baby Boomers?
15 What were misconceptions you had about growth of the aged population, minority elders, the old old (85 years and older), economic demographics, and living arrangements before reading this chapter?
16 What are some of your ideas about what will happen when the Baby Boomers become the elder generation?

REFERENCES

1. Burnstein, A.B., Remsburg, R.E., 2007. Estimated prevalence of people with cognitive impairment: Results from nationally representative community and institutional surveys. The Gerontologist 47, 350-354.
2. American Occupational Therapy Association. 2010 occupational therapy compensation and workforce study. AOTA Press, Bethesda, MD.
3. Jones, A.L., Dwyer, L.L., Bercovitz, A.R., Strahan, G.W., 2009. The National Nursing Home Survey: 2004 overview. National Center for Health Statistics. Vital Health Stat 13 (167).
4. U. S. Department of Health and Human Services (DHHS), 2008. A profile of older Americans http://www.hhs.gov/.
5. Mosby's Dictionary of Medicine, Nursing, and Health Professions, seventh ed. 2006. Mosby, St. Louis, MO.
6. Federal Interagency Forum on Aging-Related Statistics, 2008. Older Americans 2008: Key indicators of well-being. Federal Interagency Forum on Aging-Related Statistics.
7. Law, M., Mills, J., 1998. Client-centered occupational therapy. In: Law, M. (Ed.), Client-Centered Occupational Therapy. SLACK Inc, Thorofare, NJ, pp. 1-18.
8. American Occupational Therapy Association, 2008. Occupational therapy practice framework: Domain and process, second ed. American Journal of Occupational Therapy 62(6), 625-683.
9. Law, M., Baptiste, S., Carswell, A., McCall, M.A., Polatajko, H., Pollock, N., 1998. Canadian Occupational Performance Measure, third ed. CAOT Publications ACE, Ottawa, Ontario, Canada.
10. Law, M., 2000. Identifying occupational performance issues. In: Fearing, V.G., Clark, J. (Eds.), Individuals in Context: A Practical Guide to Client-Centered Practice. SLACK Inc, Thorofare, NJ, pp. 31-45.
11. McLean, C., 1988. The graying of America. Oregon Starter 11, 11-17.
12. Greenblatt, A., 2007. Aging Baby Boomers: The issues. CQ Researcher 17 (37), 857-887. Retrieved from http://www.agingsociety.org/agingsociety/publications/public_policy/cqboomers.pdf.
13. Lazer, W., 1985. Inside the mature market. American Demographics 7 (3), 48.
14. Neugarten, B.L., 1974. Age groups in American society and the rise of the young-old. Annals of the American Academy of Political and Social Sciences 415, 187-188.
15. Walker, B.S., 2009. Uncertain economy changes outlook on job status. AARP Bulletin Today, Retrieved from http://bulletin.aarp.org/yourmoney/work/articles/uncertain_economy_changes_outlook_on_job_status.html.
16. National PACE Association, 2009. What is PACE? Retrieved from http://www.npaonline.org/website/article.asp?id=12.
17. Petigara, T., Anderson, G., 2009, April. Program of all-inclusive care for the elderly. Health Policy Monitor. Retrieved from http://www.npaonline.org/website/download.asp?id=3034.
18. U.S. Census Bureau, 2005. 65+ in the United States: 2005. Retrieved from http://www.census.gov/prod/2006pubs/p23-209.pdf.
19. Bould, S., 2007. Oldest old. In The Encyclopedia of Health and Aging. Retrieved from http://www.sage-ereference.com.cuhsl.creighton.edu/aging/Article_n206.html.
20. Schoenborn, C.A., Heyman, K.M., 2009, July 8. Health characteristics of adults aged 55 years and over: United States, 2004-2007. National Health Report Statistics 16. Retrieved from http://www.cdc.gov/nchs/data/nhsr/nhsr016.pdf.
21. Stevens, J.A., 2006. Injury. In: Schultz, R. (Ed.), The Encyclopedia of Aging: A Comprehensive Resource in Gerontology and Geriatrics, vol. 1. fourth ed. Springer, New York, pp. 591-593.

22. Federal Interagency Forum on Aging-Related Statistics, 2006. Older Americans 2006: Key indicators of well-being. Federal Interagency Forum on Aging-Related Statistics.

23. Fernandez, A., 2009. Alzheimer's disease: Is our healthcare system ready? Retrieved from http://www.sharpbrains.com/blog/2009/09/21/alzheimers-disease-is-our-healthcare-system-ready/.

24. Sommers, A., Cohen, M., 2006. Kaiser Commission on Medicaid and the Uninsured. Medicaid's high cost enrollees: How much do they drive program spending? 1-18. Retrieved from http://www.kff.org/medicaid/upload/7490.pdf.

25. Ericson, R.W., Toohey, D., Wiener, J.M., 2007. Meeting the long-term care needs of the Baby Boomers: How changing families will affect paid helpers and institutions. The Retirement Project. The Urban Institute, Washington, DC. Retrieved from http://www.urban.org/UploadedPDF/311451_Meeting_Care.pdf.

26. Snyderman, N., 2007, May 2. Aging without children—who provides care? NBC News. Retrieved from http://www.msnbc.msn.com/id/18444782/ns/nightly_news_with_brian_williams-trading_places.

27. MacKnight, C., 2006. Centenarians. In: Schultz, R. (Ed.), The Encyclopedia of Aging: A Comprehensive Resource in Gerontology and Geriatrics, vol. 1. fourth ed. Springer, New York, pp. 196-198.

28. Poon, L.W., Jang, Y., 2007. Centenarians. In The Encyclopedia of Health & Aging. Retrieved from http://www.sage-ereference.com.cuhsl.creighton.edu/aging/Article_n55.html.

29. Adams, E.R., Nolan, V.G., Andersen, S.L., Perls, T.T., Terry, D.F., 2008. Centenarian offspring: Start healthier and stay healthier. Journal of the American Geriatrics Society 56 (11), 2089-2092.

30. Willcox, D.C., Willcox, B.J., Wang, N., He, Q., Rosenbaum, M., Suzuki, M., 2008. Life at the extreme limit: Phenotypic characteristics of supercentenarians in Okinawa. Journal of Gerontology Series A: Biological Sciences & Medical Sciences 63A (11), 1201-1208.

31. Power, C., Koch, T., Kralik, D., 2006. Exploring longevity with Australian centenarians. Geriaction 24 (4), 5-14.

32. Perls, T.T., 2006. The different paths to 100. American Journal of Clinical Nutrition 83 (Suppl. 5), 484S-487S.

33. Poon, L.W., 2005. The Georgia Centenarian Study: A study of longevity and survival of the oldest old. The University of Georgia Gerontology Center. Retrieved from http://www.geron.uga.edu/pdfs/CentStudyBooklet.pdf.

34. Angel, J.L., Lewis, E., 2007. Living arrangements. In The Encyclopedia of Health & Aging. Retrieved from http://www.sage-ereference.com.cuhsl.creighton.edu/aging/Article_n157.html.

35. Assisted Living Federation of America, 2009. Assisted living today—a brief overview of senior living care. Retrieved from http://www.alfa.org/alfa/About_ALFA.asp?SnID=1357427202.

36. Mitty, E.L., 2006. Nursing homes. In: Schultz, R. (Ed.), The Encyclopedia of Aging: A Comprehensive Resource in Gerontology and Geriatrics, vol. 2. fourth ed. Springer, New York, pp. 842-853.

37. National Center for Assisted Living, 2009. Resident profile. Retrieved from http://www.ahcancal.org/ncal/resources/Pages/ResidentProfile.aspx.

38. Hawes, C., Phillips, C.D., Hutchison, L.L., 2006. Assisted living. In: Schultz, R. (Ed.), The Encyclopedia of Aging: A Comprehensive Resource in Gerontology and Geriatrics, vol. 1. fourth ed. Springer, New York, pp. 87-91.

39. American Association of Homes and Services for the Aging, 2009. About assisted living. Retrieved from http://www.aahsa.org/article.aspx?id=3836.

40. Kreiser, J., 2006. Assisted living, erratic regulation. Retrieved from http://www.cbsnews.com/stories/2006/11/13/cbsnews_investigates/main2177892.shtml.

41. Medicare.gov, April 1, 2007. Home health compare: Medicare coverage of home health care. Retrieved from http://www.medicare.gov/HHCompare/Home.asp?dest=NAV|Home|About|MedicareCoverage#TabTop.

42. American Association of Retired Persons (AARP), 2009. Continuing care retirement communities. Retrieved from http://www.aarp.org/families/housing_choices/other_options/a2004-02-26-retirementcommunity.html.

43. Ryan, S.E., Sladyk, K., 2005. The occupational therapy assistant as activity director. In: Ryan, S.E., Sladyk, K. (Eds.), Ryan's Occupational Therapy Assistant: Principles, Practice Issues, and Techniques, fourth ed. SLACK Inc, Thorofare, NJ, pp. 517-528.

44. Mitty, E., Flores, S., 2008. Aging in place and negotiated risk agreements. Geriatric Nursing 29 (2), 94-101.

45. Black, K., 2008. Health and aging in place: Implications for community practice. Journal of Community Practice 15 (1), 79-95.

46. Yamkovenko, S., n.d. Occupational therapy: Helping America age in place. Retrieved from http://www.aota.org/News/Centennial/40313/Aging/Aging-in-Place.aspx.

47. Seniorresource.com, n.d. Aging in place. Retrieved from http://www.seniorresource.com/ageinpl.htm.

48. Ageinplace.com, n.d. Introduction to Certified Aging in Place Specialists (CAPS). http://ageinplace.com/certified-aging-in-place-specialists-caps/.

49. Seniorresource.com, 2009. Aging in place. Retrieved from http://www.seniorresource.com/ageinpl.htm#ageinpltop.

50. Agency for Healthcare Research and Quality, 2009. Your guide to choosing quality healthcare: Long-term care. Retrieved from http://www.ahrq.gov/consumer/qnt/qntltc.htm.

51. Genworth Financial, Inc, 2009. Genworth 2009 cost of care survey. Retrieved from http://www.genworth.com/content/etc/medialib/genworth_v2/pdf/ltc_cost_of_care.Par.8024.File.dat/cost_of_care.pdf.

52. Gosselin, J., 2009, September/October. Medicaid planning. Aging Well 2 (4), 26. Retrieved from http://www.agingwellmag.com/archive/083109p26.shtml.

53. Kaiser Family Foundation, 2009. Focus on health reform: The Community Living Assistance Services and Supports (CLASS) Act. Retrieved from http://www.kff.org/healthreform/upload/7996.pdf.

54. Administration on Aging, 2009. Home and community-based long-term care. Retrieved from http://www.aoa.gov/AoARoot/AoA_Programs/HCLTC/index.aspx.

55. Meiners, M.R., 2007. Long-term care insurance. In The Encyclopedia of Health & Aging. Retrieved from http://www.sage-ereference.com.cuhsl.creighton.edu/aging/Article_n163.html.

56. Baer, D., O'Brien, E., 2009. Federal and state income tax incentives for private long-term care insurance. AARP Public Policy Institute. Retrieved from http://www.aarp.org/research/ppi/ltc/ltc-ins/articles/2009-19-tax-incentives.html.

57. Clark, R.L., 2006. Economics. In: Schultz, R. (Ed.), The Encyclopedia of Aging: A Comprehensive Resource in Gerontology and Geriatrics, vol. 1. fourth ed. Springer, New York, pp. 348-351.

58. Bensing, K.M., 2006. Poverty. In: Schultz, R. (Ed.), The Encyclopedia of Aging: A Comprehensive Resource in Gerontology and Geriatrics, vol. 2. fourth ed. Springer, New York, pp. 946-949.

59. McLaughlin, D.K., Jensen, L., 2001. Work history and U.S. elders' transition into poverty. The Gerontologist 40 (4), 469-480.

60. Holden, K.C.A., Kim, M., 2001. Poverty. In: Atchley, R.C. (Ed.), The Encyclopedia of Aging: A Comprehensive Resource in Gerontology and Geriatrics, vol. 2. third ed. Springer, New York.

61. Angel, J.L., Jimenez, M.A., Angel, R.J., 2007. The economic consequences of widowhood for older minority women. The Gerontologist 47(2), 224-234.

62. Social Security Online—The official website of the U.S. Social Security Administration, 2009. Supplemental security income (SSI). Retrieved from http://www.ssa.gov/ssi/.

63. American Association of Retired Persons (AARP), 2005. How social security keeps older persons out of poverty across developed countries. AARP Public Policy Institute. Retrieved from http://assets.aarp.org/rgcenter/econ/dd118_ss_poverty.pdf.

64. Social Security Online—The official website of the U.S. Social Security Administration, n.d. Historical background and development of social security. Retrieved from http://www.ssa.gov/history/briefhistory3.html/.

65. Rix, S.E., 2006. Employment. In: Schultz, R. (Ed.), The Encyclopedia of Aging: A Comprehensive Resource in Gerontology and Geriatrics, vol. 1. fourth ed. Springer, New York, pp. 362-368.

66. Intermill, M. (n.d.). Provisions of H.R. 3590 that reduce Medicare spending. AARP Nebraska.

67. American Academy of Child & Adolescent Psychiatry, 2008. Grandparents raising grandchildren. Retrieved from http://www.aacap.org/cs/root/facts_for_families/grandparents_raising_grandchildren.

68. U.S. Census Bureau, 2008, July 7. Grandparents day 2008: Sept. 7. U.S. Census Bureau News. Retrieved from http://www.census.gov/Press-Release/www/releases/pdf/cb08ff-14_grandparents.pdf.

69. Novelli, W.E., 2002. The end of retirement. Retrieved from http://www.aarp.org/aarp/articles/novelliretirement_1.html.

70. Toossi, M., 2007, November. Labor force projections to 2016: More workers in their golden years. Monthly Labor Review. Bureau of Labor Statistics. Retrieved from http://www.bls.gov/opub/mlr/2007/11/art3full.pdf.

71. Pew Research Center, 2009, September 3. America's changing workforce: Recession turns a graying office grayer. Retrieved from http://pewsocialtrends.org/assets/pdf/americas-changing-workforce.pdf.

72. U.S. Bureau of Labor Statistics, 2008. Older workers: Spotlight on statistics. Retrieved from http://www.bls.gov/spotlight/2008/older_workers/.

73. Kaiser Family Foundation, 2005. e-Health and the elderly: How seniors use the Internet for health information. Retrieved from http://www.kff.org/entmedia/upload/e-Health-and-the-Elderly-How-Seniors-Use-the-Internet-for-Health-Information-Key-Findings-From-a-National-Survey-of-Older-Americans-Survey-Report.pdf.

74. Mundorf, N., Mundorf, J., Brownell, W., 2006. Communication technologies and older adults. In: Schultz, R. (Ed.), The Encyclopedia of Aging: A Comprehensive Resource in Gerontology and Geriatrics, vol. 1. fourth ed. Springer, New York, pp. 242-247.

75. Li, Y., Perkins, A., 2007. The impact of technological developments on the daily life of the elderly. Technology in Society 29(3), 361-368.

76. Congressional Budget Office, 2007. The long-term outlook for health care spending. Congress of the United States. Retrieved from http://www.cbo.gov/ftpdocs/87xx/doc8758/11-13-LT-Health.pdf.

77. Lohman, H., Griffiths, Y., Coppard, B., Cota, L., 2003. The power of book discussion groups in intergenerational learning. Educational Gerontology 29 (2), 103-116.

78. Chung, J.C.C., 2009. An intergenerational reminiscence programme for older adults with early dementia and youth volunteers: Values and challenges. Scandinavian Journal of Caring Science 23, 259-264. doi: 10.1111/j.1471-6712.2008.00615.x.

79. Dunham, C.C., Casadonte, D., 2009. Children's attitudes and classroom interaction in an intergenerational education program. Educational Gerontology 35 (5), 453-464.

80. Aging Initiative, 2009. Benefits of intergenerational programs. U.S. Environmental Protection Agency. Retrieved from http://www.epa.gov/aging/ia/benefits.htm.

81. Thompson, J., 2009. Generational rights and duties. In Intergenerational Justice: Rights and Responsibilities in an Intergenerational Policy. Routledge, New York, pp. 103.

82. Ryder, N.B., 1965. The cohort as a concept in the study of social change. American Sociological Review 30 (6), 843-861.

83. Sessa, V.L., Kabacoff, R.I., Deal, J., Brown. H., 2007. Generational differences in leadership values and leadership behaviors. The Psychologist-Manager Journal 10, 1-28.

84. Fogg, P., 2008. When generations collide. The Chronicle of Higher Education 54, B18-B20.

85. Johnson, S.A., Romanello, M.L., 2005. Generational diversity: Teaching and learning approaches. Nurse Educator 30 (5), 21-216.

86. Zemke, R., Raines, C., Filipczak, B., 1999. Generational gaps in the classroom. 36 (11), 48-54.

87. Mueller, K., 2010. Communication from the Inside Out: Strategies for the Engaged Professional. FA Davis, Philadelphia.

88. Coates, J., 2007. Generational learning styles. LERN Books, River Falls, Wis.

89. Hahn, J., 2009. Effectively manage a multigenerational staff. Nursing Management 40 (9), 8-10.

90. Johnson, M.L., Bungum, T., 2008. Aging adults learning new avocations: Potential increases in activity among educated Baby-Boomers. Educational Gerontology 34 (11), 970-996.

91. Metlife, 2009. New housing trends report: Most Baby Boomers prefer to age in place, but growing numbers head to age-restricted communities, say NAHB and Metlife Mature Market Institute. Retrieved from http://www.metlife.com/about/press-room/us-press-releases/2009/index.html?SCOPE=Metlife&MSHiC=65001&L=10&W=Aging%20Housing%20Place%20Whats%20in%20new%20&Pre=%3CFONT%20STYLE%3D%22background%3A%23ffff00%22%3E&Post=%3C/FONT%3E&compID=12912.

92. Davis, L.J., Kirkland, M. (Eds.), 1987. ROTE: The role of occupational therapy with the elderly: Faculty guide. Module I: Teaching Resources Gerontology in Theory and Practice. American Occupational Therapy Association, Rockville, MD, pp. 71-79.

93. Lewis, C., 1989. How the myths of aging impact rehabilitative care for the older person. Occupational Therapy Forum 10, 10, 11, 14, 15.

94. Leland, J., 2008, October 6. In "sweetie" and "dear," a hurt for the elderly. The New York Times. Retrieved from http://www.nytimes.com/2008/10/07/us/07aging.html.

95. World Health Organization, 2010. International Classification of Functioning, Disability, and Health (ICF). Retrieved from http://www.who.int/classifications/icf/en/.

96. U.S. Department of Health and Human Services (DHHS), 2009. Healthy people 2020 framework. Retrieved from http://www.healthypeople.gov/HP2020/Objectives/framework.aspx.

97. Youngstrom, M.J., 2002. The occupational therapy practice framework: The evolution of our professional language. The American Journal of Occupational Therapy 56 (6), 607-608.

chapter 2

Biological and Social Theories of Aging

MARLENE J. AITKEN AND MICHELLE RUDOLF

KEY TERMS

genetic aging, nongenetic aging, successful aging, developmental stages

CHAPTER OBJECTIVES

1. Identify the purpose and use of current theories of aging.
2. Discuss the biological theories of aging, including genetic and nongenetic theories.
3. Discuss the psychosocial theories of aging.
4. Understand the ways to apply the theories of aging to the care of elders.

Megan is a certified occupational therapy assistant (COTA) employed in an assisted living center that offers several levels of care. Her daily work involves treating elders who have a variety of diagnosed conditions and the planning of occupation-based activities. Megan has observed that although many of the elders require rehabilitation, each reacts differently to illness and the aging process. At least once a week, Megan meets with Kelly, a registered occupational therapist (OTR), for a supervision session in which they thoroughly discuss each person participating in occupational therapy (OT).

After reviewing the caseload during one particular session, Megan and Kelly began a lively discussion about the complexities of aging. Megan noted that some of the elders whom she treats as part of her caseload seem active and vigorous, whereas others seem withdrawn and lack energy to participate in therapeutic tasks. She also commented that some of the elders seem older than their chronological ages, whereas others seem to be their age or younger. Kelly encouraged Megan to review theories about aging to form a context in which to think about the elders. The next week Megan and Kelly discussed the application of the theories to their work with elders who are part of their caseloads.

Questions like Megan's regarding reasons for aging and the differences in aging can be answered in multiple ways because aging research consists of many different studies and perspectives. COTAs need to understand various theories because the theoretical concepts attempt to go beyond the data to the fundamental biological, social, or psychological processes. Furthermore, theories explain what is observed or experienced and why and how it is important.[1] A growing trend over the last 10 years has been interdisciplinary collaboration to merge profession-specific concepts into a unified theory to explain the aging phenomena.

This chapter uses the format of current biological, social, and psychological theories to provide insight on social aspects of aging. (The physical and psychological changes that occur with the aging process are described in Chapters 3 and 4.)

BIOLOGICAL THEORIES OF AGING

As many as 300 or more aging theories have been presented in the literature over the past several decades; however, not all have stood up to scrutiny and in-depth scholarly investigation.[2] The major biological theories that attempt to explain the individual differences in aging fit into one of two categories: **genetic aging**, which presumes that aging is predetermined or programmed, and **nongenetic aging**, which presumes that aging events occur randomly and accumulate with time.[3,4] Four genetic aging theories are programmed aging, somatic mutation, free radical, and neuroendocrine theories. A nongenetic theory is the wear and tear theory. One or multiple theories may explain the aging process and characteristics as a wide range of factors that may affect aging such as genetics, random events, environment, lifestyle, and/or habits.

Genetic Theories

Programmed aging

The premise of the programmed aging theories is that the human body has an inherited internal "genetic clock" that determines the beginning of the aging process. This genetic clock may manifest as a predetermined or limited number of cell divisions, called the *Hayflick limit* (also known as *replicative senescence* or *cellular senescence*).[5-8] The Hayflick limit does not affect all cells in the body as germ cells (sperm or egg), and cells in some tumors (cancer) seem to divide infinitely.[7,9] The theory of cellular aging explains why many older adults have one or multiple conditions related to decreased or impaired client factors (sensory, neuromusculoskeletal, cardiovascular, respiratory, digestive, metabolic, and reproductive) and why it is rare to find any of these impairments in a young adult.[10] The perception that cellular senescence is not programmed aging of the whole person explains why such conditions are not universal among older adults.[7]

Somatic mutation theory

According to the somatic mutation theory, stochastic (random) chromosomal changes occur as a result of miscoding, translation errors, chemical reactions, irradiation, and replication of errors; these mutations result in changes in the ribonucleic acid (RNA) deoxyribonucleic acid (DNA) code sequences.[7,9,11] Mutations of the genetic material within a cell can accumulate if the alterations are not repaired when the code is being transcribed (reading process to make the building blocks of proteins).[8] The accumulation of mutations can alter the genetic sequence of a cell in such a way that the "safe guard" to control the proliferation of cellular growth is deactivated, resulting in unrestrained cell division, sometimes leading to tumorigenesis and/or cancer.[9,12] Mutations can occur in the expression of the genetic code or the way that the code is read without directly changing the RNA or DNA sequence; the expression of the genetic code is the epigenome, and the mutations are epimutations.[7,13]

Free radical theory

The free radical theory of aging stemmed from the study of unstable atoms in living cells and the damage they caused as they tried to stabilize.[14,15] Free radicals are highly reactive because of the unpaired electron(s) that seek to be paired but, in turn, damage cells, proteins, lipids, and DNA (by altering their structures).[16] Free radicals happen naturally in the body whenever metallic ions, enzymes, or cellular materials combine with oxygen and are also introduced into the body through toxins, pollutants, and tobacco smoke. Low-level, free radical damage is theorized to accumulate over time, especially mutations in mitochondrial DNA (mtDNA), resulting in aging characteristics.[16,17] Most organisms have defense mechanisms to limit the effects of free radicals and to repair the damage left behind, but because not all of the repairs can be fixed, the damage accumulates.[11,15] The accumulated mutations of the mtDNA result from a decrease in or loss of function of the natural antioxidant defense layer in the body and cells. However, Harman[17] highlights some studies that show a decrease in the loss of mtDNA through the consumption of coenzyme Q_{10} and other antioxidants such as Ginkgo biloba. Ames[18] discusses the importance of nutrient balance, specifically of iron, copper, zinc, vitamin B_6, biotin, and pantothenate. Too much of these nutrients tend to increase oxidative stress and mtDNA damage. However, these nutrients are important for mtDNA repair

and cellular function, so too little of these nutrients decreases function and the repair of oxidative damage. The direct effect of the free radical theory on aging and dysfunction continues to be questioned and studied, but it is clear that the presence of oxidative damage from free radicals increases through the life span.[15,16]

Neuroendocrine theory

The neuroendocrine theory suggests that the central nervous system is the aging pacemaker of the body.[19,20] Modification of metabolism or reproductive function affects the life span, and the hypothalamus is predicted to be one possible starting point for neuroendocrine-related changes because it influences the regulation of the metabolic and reproductive systems.[20]

Nongenetic Theory

Wear and tear theory

The wear and tear theory proposes that cumulative damage within the body leads to the death of cells, tissues, organs, and, finally, the organism.[21] Wear and tear are natural from living things to inanimate objects, and organisms are able to repair wear and tear.[21] The wear and tear theory is studied with identical twins. Identical twins are nature's natural clones in that they have identical genotypes (genetic information); however, upon closer inspection there are phenotypic (physical) differences.[22] It was found that epigenetic differences were greater between older monozygotic twins than younger pairs, even if external variables were almost identical.[22] Cases in which the time of death varies between twins indicate that environmental factors may be as important as genetic factors in determining life span.[23] Therefore, it can be concluded that internal and external factors play roles in aging and, like other biological aging theories, wear and tear within the body accumulate through the years.[21,22]

SOCIAL THEORIES OF AGING

Longer life spans and an increased number of elders in U.S. society have resulted in greater attention to the aging process. Quality of life and successful aging are becoming important areas of study. The disengagement, activity, and continuity social theories each present a different process of aging and focus on different aspects of successful aging. The next three social theories, which consist of Erikson's and Peck's stages of psychological development and the life course, place more emphasis on the developmental stages of aging. The last social theory of aging, the theory of exchange, examines perceptions regarding the value of interactions and the ways that these perceptions affect elders' relationships.

Researchers on the major social theories of aging—activity theory, disengagement theory, and continuity theory—have not consistently demonstrated accuracy in identifying behaviors at various stages. The disengagement theory, activity theory, and continuity theory seem to manifest from each other as elaborations or "glass half full" versus "glass half empty" arguments,[24] as the following discussion illustrates.

Disengagement Theory

Disengagement occurs when people withdraw from roles or activities and reduce their activity levels or involvement.[25] While completing an interest checklist with the COTA, an elder might indicate former activities and roles with various social clubs or organizations that they found meaningful.[10] When asked for the reason for withdrawal from these activities, the elder might state that it was because of age. On the basis of their research in Kansas City, Missouri, in the 1950s, Cumming and Henry[26] theorized that the turning inward typical of aging people produces a natural and normal withdrawal from social roles and activities, an increasing preoccupation with self, and decreasing involvement with others. They perceived individual disengagement as primarily a psychological process involving withdrawal of interest and commitment. Social withdrawal was a consequence of individual disengagement, coupled with society's push for the withdrawal of the elderly manifested in such things as retirement plans and pensions.[25]

The disengagement theory resulted in increased research. The proposition of withdrawal being normal challenged the conventional wisdom that keeping active was the best way to deal with aging. Streib and Schneider[27] suggested that differential disengagement was more likely to occur than total disengagement. For example, people may withdraw from some activities but increase or maintain their involvement in others. Troll[28] found that elders often disengage into the family—that is, elders often cope with lost roles by increasing involvement with their families. Atchley and Barusch[29] present that disengagement can also be due to increased frailty or disability such as decreased visual acuity, so elders choose not to attend sports events but rather stay home to hear the news cast of the events. People are seldom completely engaged or disengaged. Rather, they strike a balance between the two states that reflects their individual preferences, often mediated by social encouragement or discouragement from others.

The frequency of disengagement is very much the product of the opportunity for continued engagement. For example, elders may wish to continue many activities, but, because they believe that other people may think they are "too old," they withdraw. For elders in facilities who think they are too old or unable to continue activities, the COTA could discuss with them doing activities that would be similar to former interests. For example, if elders are interested in gardening, they could assist with the plants in and out of their residence. If elders are interested in communicating with friends, perhaps an introduction to e-mail would be a meaningful activity.

Activity Theory

The activity theory was proposed as an alternative view of the disengagement theory to explain the psychosocial process of aging.[24] Havighurst, Neugarten, and Tobin[30] articulated an activity theory of aging, which held that unless constrained by poor health or disability, elders have the same psychological and social needs as people of middle age. Hochschild[31] presented that the changing of activities was the result of changed meaning in the activities as seen through the life span. An example is parents regularly attending PTA meetings for their child's school. As the child grows and moves away, the parents begin to read more because there is no longer meaning in the PTA meetings. Thus, the adults embrace the activity of reading for pleasure without the need to monitor children.[10] Menec[32] purported "different types of activities may have different benefits. Whereas social and productive activities may afford physical benefits, as reflected in better function and greater longevity, more solitary activities, such as reading, may have more psychological benefits by providing a sense of engagement with life" (p. 74).

The activity theory has received a great deal of criticism in that it excludes elders' physical well-being, past lifestyle, and personality attributes. It also does not account for the value or the personal meaning that the elder may find in activities. Instead, it most often quantifies the number of roles and the amount of involvement in these roles.[25,33,34] In addition, the belief that it is better to be active than inactive is a bias derived from the Western culture.[25,34] Much of OT is based on the assumption that our value of human beings comes from what we know and do, rather than on who we are and have been.[10,35]

A further component of the activity theory considers the preferences of elders and the extent to which they wish to be active. Setting aside time for quiet reflection may be equally as important as more active pursuits for some elders. COTAs should remember this when attempting to get everyone involved in an activity. Some elders may welcome participation in physical activities such as bowling and walking (Figure 2-1, A), and others may be content with listening to quiet music and reading (Figure 2-1, B).

Continuity Theory

The premise of the continuity theory is that elders adapt to changes by using strategies to maintain continuity in their lives, both internal and external. Internal continuity refers to the strategy of forming personal links between new experiences and memories of previous ones.[29,36,37] External continuity refers to interacting with familiar people and living in familiar environments.[29,37,38] According to this theory, elders should continue to live in their own homes as long as possible. If this is not possible, the family should attempt to locate housing for the elder in the same general area to maintain friendships and familiar environments. Many elders continue to be independent as long as they are in familiar surroundings. Some families have noted that once they moved their elder family member from a familiar area, the elder was confused and disoriented.

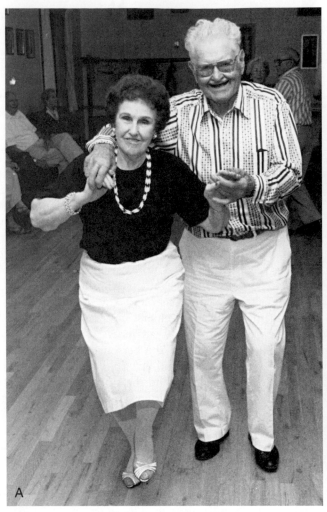
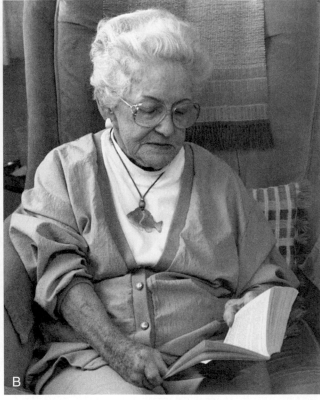

FIGURE 2-1   A, Through ongoing social interactions, elders can maintain a positive self-concept. B, This elder enjoys a sedentary activity.

Continuity of activities and environments helps the individual concentrate energies in familiar areas of activity. Practice of activities can often prevent, offset, or minimize the effects of aging. Atchley and Barusch[29] state that by maintaining the same lifestyle and residence, an older person is able to meet instrumental activities of daily living needs. Continuity of roles and activities is effective in maintaining the capacity to meet social and emotional needs for interaction and social support. Maintaining independence is important for continued good self-esteem. Continuity does not mean that nothing changes; it means that new life experiences occur, and the elder must adapt to them with familiar and persistent processes and attributes. New information is likely to produce less stress when an elder has memories of similar experiences. This may be one reason new information does not have the same weight for both younger and older generations and may help explain the reason that some elders seem more conservative than others. For example, an elder may reject learning to use a computer to order home supplies

and to be in contact with others despite being isolated in a rural location because the activity involves a new way of performing a task.

Practice should not be based on one theory but a combination of theories as they apply and are appropriate to our clients. For instance, it may be dangerous to allow an elder to withdraw by considering it a normal function of aging or to push meaningless activity with a disinterested elder. COTAs may want to discuss with elders what activities have meaning to them and allow elders to reminisce about past activities, or perform client-centered assessments such as an interest checklist or the Canadian Occupational Performance Measure.[39] The information gleaned from the individual could give COTAs more insight into a selection of activities that are most appropriate.

The activity and continuity theories are compatible with OT in that they assume that performance of meaningful activities promotes competence, independence, and well-being. Kielhofner[40] states that human beings are occupational in nature; therefore, occupation is vital for our well-being. The Model of Human Occupation incorporates this assumption and is a valuable theory of OT for aging.[40] What a person does depends on individual factors such as level of interest, values, personal causation, health, socioeconomic status, and prior occupations.

Life Span/Life Course Theory

The life span, or life course, perspective is a recent approach to human development by theorists interested in the social and behavioral processes of aging (Box 2-1). Life course is defined by Elder, Johnson, and Crosnoe[41] as "an age-graded sequence of socially defined roles and events that are enacted over historical time and place" (p. 15). This theory was influenced by the age stratification model, which emphasizes the significant variations in elders, depending on the characteristics of their birth cohort. Some researchers believe that this is not actually a theory, but rather a conceptual framework for conducting research and interpreting data.

Most elders who experienced the Great Depression seem to have a different perception of the meaning of "poor." Many elders reject offers of help because they compare what little they had in the past with what they currently have, which seems sufficient. In addition, some elders who are eligible for Social Security insurance may not accept it. This viewpoint may vary with subsequent generations of elders.

Elder, Johnson, and Crosnoe[41] reported considerable consensus on age-related progression and sequence of roles and group memberships that individuals are expected to follow as they mature and move through life. The stages of the adult life course as defined by this group are middle age, later maturity, and old age. Unlike Erikson's and Peck's stages, life course stages are related to specific chronological ages. Age norms generally define what people within a given life stage are "allowed" to do and be at certain ages. Many norms are established by long traditions. Others are often the result of compromise and negotiation. In addition, a series of assumptions related to the capabilities of the people in a given life stage underlies age norms. Thus, opportunities may be limited for some elders because others assume they are not strong enough

or lack education or experience.[29,38] Elders who achieve greatness beyond expectations for their life stages are perceived as unique or different. Their accomplishments elicit comments about their endeavors being met by a person of "their age." Many older elders, such as the current group of centenarians, are considered pioneers because few prescribed behaviors or age norms exist for them. Franklin and Tate[24] stated, "A large body of research and theoretical literature confirms that physical, cognitive, and social functioning, broadly speaking, are key factors of successful aging and that multiple lifestyle choices, behaviors, and psychosocial factors influence them" (p. 8).

Erikson's Theory of Human Development

Erik Erikson's theory of human development over the life span is one of the most influential descriptions of psychological change.[21,42] Erikson's stages of ego development are familiar to most students of psychology (Table 2-1).

Erikson's framework addresses the developmental tasks at each stage of the life cycle. The stage most commonly identified with aging is that of integrity versus despair. In this stage, the elder comes to terms with the gradual deterioration of the body but at the same time may reflect on the acquisition of wisdom associated with life experiences. Ego integrity involves the elders' ability to see life as meaningful and to accept both positive and negative personality traits without feeling threatened. Integrity provides a basis for elders approaching the end of life with a feeling of having done their best under the circumstances. Despair is the elder's rejection of self and life experiences, and it includes the realization that there is insufficient time to alter this assessment. The despairing elder is prone to depression and is afraid to die. COTAs can play a vital role in assisting elders to master this developmental stage. Helping elders develop self-empathy, the

BOX 2-1

Key Elements of the Life Span Framework

- Aging occurs from birth to death.
- Aging involves biological, social, and psychological processes.
- Experiences in aging are shaped by historical factors.

From Passuth, P., & Bengtson, V. (1988). Sociological theories of aging: Current perspectives and future directions. In J. Birren & V. Bengtson (Eds.). Emergent Theories of Aging. New York: Springer.

TABLE 2-1

Erik Erikson's Stage of Ego Development

Time period	Stage
Early infancy	Trust versus distrust
Later infancy	Autonomy versus shame and doubt
Early childhood	Initiative versus guilt
Childhood middle years	Industry versus inferiority
Adolescence	Ego identity versus role confusion
Early adulthood	Intimacy versus isolation
Middle adulthood	Generativity versus stagnation
Late adulthood	Ego integrity versus ego despair

From Erikson, E. (1985). Childhood and Society. New York: WW Norton.

ability to bounce back from change, and a focus on the completeness of their lives supports elders' efforts to deal with this life stage.

Erikson originally proposed eight stages of psychosocial development. As Erikson himself reached later life, he noted that the predominant image of old age was quite different from when he had first formulated his theory. To fit with the increasingly older population, Joan M. Erikson[43] published a ninth stage of development. This ninth stage, applicable to elders in their eighties and nineties, enhanced her husband's well-known eight-stage theory of development.[43,44] It is felt that in the ninth stage elders may also revisit unresolved crisis issues from earlier stages in a different manner. For example, elders in the ninth stage may perceive the first stage of trust versus mistrust as trust in their own physical and mental abilities with functional activities.[43] Erikson also discusses the concept of *gerotranscendence* in which elders deal with their aging selves and consider life satisfaction as they move beyond materialistic concerns to spiritual or as Lars Tornstam stated, "cosmic and transcendent" thoughts.[45]

Brown and Lewis[44] purported that the results of surveying individuals near or in the ninth stage showed a sense of peace and acceptance, decreased fear of death, closeness to those who have gone before, acceptance of the age-related changes, and increased understanding of the meaning of life. Reminiscence groups and other life review activities conducted as part of an intervention program by COTAs can be effective in helping elders work through developmental stages.

As increasing numbers of people reach very old age, tasks and other aspects of psychosocial development that were not systematically described in Erikson's original formulations are emerging. Positive resolution of crisis is the elder's confidence in the continuity of a personal contribution beyond death. For example, an elder who handcrafts rocking chairs may pass on those skills to children, who may pass them on to their children. Tasks of this stage include coping with the inevitable physical changes that accompany aging. The elder may be increasingly obliged to turn attention from the more interesting aspects of life to the demands of the body. In addition, the very old may have to shape new patterns for adapting to late life because few norms for behavior and few responsibilities are established for elders who reach a very old age. Numerous articles on persons older than 100 years show a fascination with the many activities of this fastest growing age group. Most of these elders attribute their longevity to keeping their minds, not their bodies, stimulated.[46,47]

Peck's Stages of Psychological Development

Robert Peck[48] believed that Erikson's eighth stage, integrity versus despair, was intended to "represent in a global, nonspecific way all of the psychological crises and crisis-solutions of the last forty or fifty years of life" (p. 88). He suggested that it might be more accurate and useful to

TABLE 2-2

Robert Peck's Psychological Stages in the Second Half of Life		
Time period		**Stage**
Middle age	First stage	Wisdom versus physical powers
	Second stage	Socializing versus sexualizing
	Third stage	Cathectic flexibility versus cathectic impoverishment
	Fourth stage	Mental flexibility versus mental rigidity
Old age	First stage	Ego differentiation versus work-role preoccupation
	Second stage	Body transcendence versus body preoccupation
	Third stage	Ego transcendence versus ego preoccupation

From Peck, R. (1968). Psychological developments in the second half of life. In B. Neugarten (Ed.). Middle Age and Aging. Chicago: University of Chicago Press.

take a closer look at the second half of life and divide it into several different psychological stages and adjustments (Table 2-2).

Peck[48] proposed four stages that occur in middle age and three stages in old age. He avoided establishing a chronological period for these stages, suggesting instead that they might occur in different time sequences for different individuals.

The first stage of old age is ego differentiation versus work-role preoccupation. The effect of retirement, particularly for men in their late sixties, is the issue at this stage. In U.S. culture, identity tends to be tied to the individual's work role. Retiring individuals must reappraise and redefine their worth in a broader range of role activities (Figure 2-2, A). Retirement also affects women, regardless of whether their careers were inside or outside of the home. As more working women from the Baby Boomer generation retire, it will be interesting to see how they redefine their roles. The housewife's work role changes drastically when the husband retires and is suddenly always in "her" domain (Figure 2-2, B). With economic downturns and policy changes associated with the Social Security Act, this stage may move to later years as more elders remain or return to the workforce (see the discussion on elders in the workforce in Chapter 1).

Peck[48] states that a critical requisite for successful adaptation to this stage may be the establishment of varied sets of valued activities and self-attributes. These activities and attributes allow the individual to have satisfying and worthwhile alternatives to pursue. Participation in voluntary organizations, such as the AARP, formally the American Association of Retired Persons, can provide meaningful

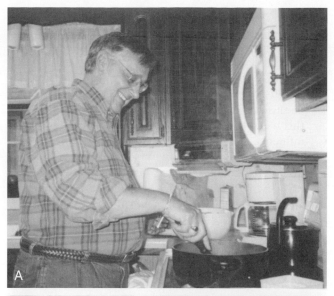

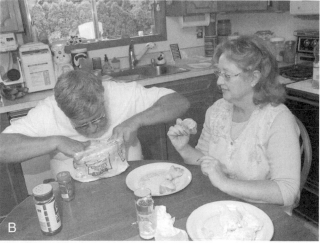

FIGURE 2-2 Changing roles. A, This retired man enjoys his new role as he prepares the family meal. B, The housewife's work role can change when the husband retires and is suddenly in "her domain." *(A Courtesy of Sue Byers-Connon, Mt. Hood Community College, Gresham, OR.)*

activities. Involvement in the AARP can be initiated as early as 50 years of age and continues after the formal work role has ended. This organization provides opportunities for driver refresher courses through AARP Driver Safety, help with filing of tax returns through AARP Tax-Aide, travel at reduced cost, and many other discounted products and services. In addition, it offers medical insurance plans to supplement private insurance and Medicare and the choice to become a volunteer advocate for improved health care, long-term care, consumer protection, financial and retirement security, transportation, housing, and other areas (Lanner, April 7, 2010, personal communication).

Peck's second stage of old age is body transcendence versus body preoccupation. Physical decline, along with a

marked decline in recuperative powers and increased body aches and pains, occurs in many elders in this stage. To those who especially value physical well-being, this may be the most difficult period of adjustment. For some elders, this adjustment means a growing preoccupation with their bodily functions. However, others have learned to define comfort and happiness in human relationships or creative mental activities. For them, only complete physical destruction can deter these feelings.

The third stage is ego transcendence versus ego preoccupation. With this stage of old age comes the certain prospect of death. Successful adaptation is not compatible with passive resignation or ego denial. It requires deep, active effort on the part of the elder to make life more secure, meaningful, and happy for those who will live after the elder's death. These elders experience a gratifying absorption in the future and are interested in doing all that is possible to make the world better for familial or cultural descendants. In practice COTAs may work with elders to do life review activities, such as developing a video to leave for future generations.

Exchange Theory

In clinical practice the OT practitioner may find it more rewarding to work with an elder who is motivated and has a "fun" personality than with an elder who does not relate well with others. COTAs may observe that the client who displays a winning personality receives more attention from everyone. This is an example of exchange theory.

Exchange theory, as originally developed by Homans,[49] assumes that people attempt to maximize their rewards and minimize their costs in interactions with others. The major attempts to use exchange theory in work with elders are attributed to Dowd.[50,51] Elders are viewed from the perspective of their ongoing interactions with a number of persons. Continuing interaction is based on what the elder perceives as rewarding or costly. Elders tend to continue with interactions that are beneficial and withdraw from those perceived as having no benefit. Rewards may be defined in material or nonmaterial terms and could include such components as assistance, money, information, affection, approval, property, skill, respect, compliance, and conformity. Costs are defined as an expenditure of any of these.

In American culture, more emphasis is often placed on resources a person is assumed to have rather than on the actual exchange resources. The concept of ageism includes assumptions about elders, such as that elders have less current information, outdated skills, and inadequate physical strength or endurance. If elders are perceived as having few resources to contribute to a relationship, an issue over power can result, with the elder at a distinct disadvantage. Elders may be seen as powerless actors who are forced into a position of compliance and dependence because they have nothing of value to withhold to get better intervention.[29,38] Many elders accept the validity of these assumptions and fear dependency on others more than death.[52]

Thriving: A Holistic Life Span Theory

For several years, gerontologists have become concerned with failure to thrive in elders, which is a sharp decline for no real physical or illness-related reason. A nursing research group was brought together to explore the phenomenon. The group broadened its vision from the syndrome failure to thrive to a more holistic life span concept called *thriving*. This theory seems quite applicable to our OT approach because we profess to view our clients holistically. This theory considers three interacting factors in a continuum: the person, the human environment, and the nonhuman environment. Critical to thriving are "social connectedness, ability to find meaning in life and to attach to one's environment, adaptation to physical patterns, and positive cognitive/affective function" (p. 22).[53]

■ CHAPTER REVIEW QUESTIONS

1 Scenario one: Ethel Shanas, a very famous gerontologist, once said that if you want to live a long time, you should choose your grandparents carefully. Which aging theory or theories support Dr. Shanas' suggestion?

2 Scenario two: Megan, the COTA introduced at the beginning of this chapter, decided to include reminiscence and life review as part of her therapeutic interventions with elders in the nursing home. Which aging theory supports the selection of these activities?

3 Scenario three: The family of one of Megan's elderly clients is upset because the elder insists on planning her own funeral and asking for specific clothes in which to be buried. In addition, she has made a list of all of her furniture and other property and has designated which of her children or grandchildren is to inherit these items. Although this client has accepted her terminal illness, her family has not. Which aging theory would Megan use to explain to the family what is happening with their relative?

4 Scenario four: Margaret's children decide to move her away from her current home town to a new assisted living facility in the town where they reside. Since the move Margaret seems more depressed and is having difficulty adapting to her new living arrangements. What aging theory explains her behavior?

5 The risk for having cancer increases significantly as people grow older. Use an aging theory to explain a possible reason for this.

6 Dr. Alex Comfort, a famous gerontologist, suggested that 2 weeks is about the ideal time to retire. What does he mean by this statement? Discuss the theory that supports your suggestion.

7 Some older adults may become extremely depressed once they retire. What could you suggest, other than antidepressant medications that may improve their outlook on life? Discuss the theory that supports your suggestion.

8 An 80-year-old man recently made headlines because he entered the Boston marathon. Why did this make the news? How do cultural age norms influence the persistence of ageism?

9 An 85-year-old woman with severe Parkinson's disease has requested that during her activities of daily living session the COTA help her dress herself and put on makeup. The woman's doctor has suggested that she is "too old for rehab" and is thinking of discontinuing her OT. Justify her intervention with a theory, and then explain how you would convince the doctor that it is important.

10 According to the exchange theory, why does an elder feel dependent on his or her relatives?

11 Give an example of the disengagement theory.

12 Give an example of the activity theory.

REFERENCES

1. Bengtson, V.L., Silverstein, M., Putney, N., Gans, D., 2009. Theorizing about age and aging. In: Bengtson, V.L. (Ed.), Handbook of Theories of Aging, 2nd ed. Springer, New York.
2. Medvedev, Z.A., 1990. An attempt at a rational classification of theories of ageing. Biological Reviews of the Cambridge Philosophical Society 65, 375-398.
3. Abrams, W., Beers, M., Berkow, R., 1995. The Merck Manual of Geriatrics. Merck Research Laboratories, Whitehouse Station, NJ.
4. Beers, M.H., Berkow, R., Bogin, R.M., Fletcher, A.J., Rahman, M.I., 2000. The Merck Manual of Geriatrics, 3rd ed. Merck Research Laboratories, Whitehouse Station, NJ.
5. Hayflick, L., 1987. Biological theories of aging. In: Maddox, G. (Ed.), The Encyclopedia of Aging. Springer, New York.
6. Hayflick, L., Moorhead, P., 1961. The serial cultivation of human diploid cell strains. Experimental Cell Research 25, 585-621.
7. Kirkwood, T.B.L., 1999. Time of Our Lives: The Science of Human Aging. Oxford University Press, Oxford.
8. Kirkwood, T.B.L., 2005. Understanding the odd science of aging. Cell 120, 437-447.
9. Campisi, J., d'Adda, D.F., 2007. Cellular senescence: When bad things happen to good cells. Nature Reviews: Molecular Cell Biology 8, 729-740.
10. American Occupational Therapy Association, 2008. Occupational therapy practice framework: Domain and process, 2nd ed. American Journal of Occupational Therapy 62, 625-683.
11. Holliday, R., 2007. Aging: The Paradox of Life. Springer, Amsterdam.
12. Finkel, T., Serrano, M., Blasco, M.A., 2007. The common biology of cancer and ageing. Nature 448, 767-774.
13. Bird, A., 2007. Perceptions of epigenetics. Nature 447, 396-398.
14. Harman, D., 1956. Aging: A theory based on free radical and radiation chemistry. Journal of Gerontology 11, 298-300.
15. Shringarpure, R., Davies, K.J.A., 2009. Free radicals and oxidative stress in aging. In: Bengtson, V.L., Gans, D., Putney, N.M., et al. (Eds.), Handbook of Theories of Aging, 2nd ed. Springer, New York.

16. Muller, F.L., Lustgarten, M.S., Jang, Y., Richardson, A., Van Remmen, H., 2007. Trends in oxidative aging theories. Free Radical Biology & Medicine 43, 477-503.

17. Harman, D., 2006. Free radical theory of aging: An update. Increasing the functional life span. Annals of the New York Academy of Sciences 1067, 10-21.

18. Ames, B.N., 2004. Delaying the mitochondrial decay of aging. Annals of the New York Academy of Sciences 1019, 406-411.

19. Cristofalo, V., 1988. An overview of the theories of biological aging. In: Birren, J., Bengtson, V. (Eds.), Emergent Theories of Aging. Springer, New York.

20. Finch, C.E., Ruvkun, G., 2001. The genetics of aging. Annual Review of Genomics & Human Genetics 2, 435-462.

21. Moody, H.R., 2010. Aging: Concepts and Controversies, 6th ed. Pine Forge Press, Thousand Oaks, CA.

22. Fraga, M.F., Ballestar, E., Paz, M.F., Ropero, S., Setien, F., Ballestar, M.L., et al., 2005. Epigenetic differences arise during the lifetime of monozygotic twins. Proceedings of the National Academy of Sciences of the United States of America 102, 10604-10609.

23. Bank, L., Jarvik, L., 1978. A longitudinal study of aging human twins. In: Schneider, E. (Ed.), The Genetics of Aging. Plenum Press, New York.

24. Franklin, N.C., Tate, C.A., 2009. Lifestyle and successful aging: An overview. American Journal of Lifestyle Medicine 3 (1), 6-11.

25. Mabry, B.J., Bengtson, V.L., 2005. Disengagement theory. In: Palmore, E.B., Branch, L.G., Harris, D.K. (Eds.), Encyclopedia of Ageism. Haworth Press, Binghamton, NY.

26. Cumming, E., Henry, W., 1961. Growing Old. Basic Books, New York.

27. Streib, G., Schneider, C., 1971. Retirement in American Society. Cornell University Press, Ithaca, NY.

28. Troll, L., 1971. The family of later life. Journal of Marriage and the Family 33, 263.

29. Atchley, R., Barusch, A.S., 2004. Social Forces and Aging: An Introduction to Social Gerontology, 10th ed. Wadsworth/Thomson Learning, Belmont, CA.

30. Havighurst, R., Neugarten, B., Tobin, S., 1963. Disengagement, personality, and life satisfaction. In: Hansen, P. (Ed.), Age with a Future. Munksgaard, Copenhagen.

31. Hochschild, A.R., 1975. Disengagement theory: A critique and proposal. American Sociological Review 40, 553-569.

32. Menec, V.H., 2003. The relation between everyday activities and successful aging: A 6-year longitudinal study. The Journals of Gerontology: Series B 58 (2), 74-82.

33. Bonder, B.R., Dal Bello-Haas, V., 2009. Functional Performance in Older Adults, 3rd ed. FA Davis, Philadelphia.

34. Bonder, B., Wagner, M., 2001. Functional Performance in Older Adults. FA Davis, Philadelphia.

35. Rowles, G., 1991. Beyond performance: Being in place as a component of occupational therapy. American Journal of Occupational Therapy 45, 265-271.

36. Cohler, B., 1982. Person narrative and life course. In: Baltes, P., Brim, O. (Eds.), Life Span Development and Behavior. Academic Press, New York.

37. Atchley, R., 1999. Continuity and Adaptation in Old Age. Johns Hopkins University Press, Baltimore.

38. Atchley, R., 1991. Social Forces and Aging. Wadsworth, Belmont, CA.

39. Law, M., 2005. Canadian Occupational Performance Measure, 4th ed. CAOT Publications ACE, Ottawa, Canada.

40. Kielhofner, G., 2007. A Model of Human Occupation: Theory and Application, 4th ed. Lippincott Williams & Wilkins, Baltimore.

41. Elder, G.H., Johnson, M.K., Crosnoe, R., 2004. The emergence and development of life course theory. In: Mortimer, J.T., Shanahan, M.J. (Eds.), Handbook of the Life Course. Springer, New York.

42. Erikson, E., 1985. Childhood and Society. WW Norton, New York.

43. Erikson, J.M., 1997. The ninth stage. In: Erikson, E.H., Erikson, J.M. (Eds.), The Life Cycle Completed. WW Norton, New York.

44. Brown, C., Lowis, M.J., 2003. Psychosocial development in the elderly: An investigation into Erikson's ninth stage. Journal of Aging Studies 17, 415-426.

45. Erikson, J.M., 1997. Gerotranscendence. In: Erikson, E.H., Erikson, J.M. (Eds.), The Life Cycle Completed. WW Norton, New York.

46. Stern, C., 1996. Who is old? Parade 21, 4.

47. Poon, L.W., Jazwinski, M., Green, R.C., Woodard J.L., Martin P., Rodgers W.L., et al., 2008. Methodological considerations in studying centenarians: Lessons learned from the Georgia centenarian studies. In: Poon, L.W., Perls, T.T. (Eds.), Annual Review of Gerontology and Geriatrics: Biopsychosocial Approaches to Longevity, Vol. 27. Springer, New York.

48. Peck, R., 1968. Psychological developments in the second half of life. In: Neugarten, B. (Ed.), Middle Age and Aging. University of Chicago Press, Chicago, pp. 88-92.

49. Homans, G., 1961. Social Behavior: Its Elementary Forms. Harcourt Brace Jovanovich, New York.

50. Dowd, J., 1975. Aging as exchange: A preface to theory. Journal of Gerontology 30 (5), 584-594.

51. Dowd, J., 1980. Exchange rates and old people. Journal of Gerontology 35 (4), 596-602.

52. Aitken, M., 1982. Self concept and functional independence in the hospitalized elderly. American Journal of Occupational Therapy 36 (4), 243-250.

53. Haight, B., Barba, B., Tesh, A., Courts N.F., 2002. Thriving: A life span theory. Journal of Gerontological Nursing 28 (3), 14-22.

3

The Aging Process

MIRTHA MONTEJO WHALEY AND DANIELLE LANCASTER BARBER

KEY TERMS

primary aging, secondary aging, successful aging, function,
occupational performance, environment

CHAPTER OBJECTIVES

1. Describe the aging process.
2. Explore the concepts of successful, primary, and secondary aging.
3. Discuss usual and pathological aging within the context of age-related physiological changes in the integumentary,

cardiopulmonary, musculoskeletal, neurological, and sensory systems.
4. Explore how normal and abnormal changes present in elder clinical case studies.

The process of aging is complex, multidirectional, and influenced by multiple contexts or environments.[1,2] Aging is a universal event that is inherent in the individual and occurs within biological and genetic parameters. We all age regardless of race, gender, ethnicity, or geographic location. The variability of the aging process among individuals, however, is not only dependent on our biological and genetic blueprint, but also is highly influenced by other factors such as (1) our lifestyle choices and behaviors over the life span; (2) our proximal contexts or environments (i.e., family, friends, community, culture, etc.), which impact our development, maturation, and function; and (3) the distal contexts (i.e., the historical period within which we develop and the public policies and decisions), which indirectly impact the opportunities afforded us to participate in occupation or the barriers that keep us from reaching our maximum potential. These factors can determine whether we are able to attain an education, engage in valued occupations, including employment, enjoy adequate and safe living conditions, have access to nutritious foods, be healthy, and have access to adequate health care.

AGING

The fact that we all age attests to the biological nature of aging, but although aging itself is universal, the process of aging, that is, the rate at which we age, varies both across individuals and even organ systems within the individual.[1,3] That we age differently explains the impact that environments, contexts, and lifestyle behaviors exert on each individual.[1,2] Aging is the sum total of our genetic and biological makeup combined with all of the lifestyle

decisions, events, and exposures (whether by choice or otherwise), which we experience throughout the life span. Despite arbitrary determinations as to when we become old, aging is really a lifelong process. In fact, aging is a chronic, progressive, and terminal event that begins at the moment of conception. Some authorities, however, would argue that aging begins at age 30 with the onset of decrements in physiological function and efficiency and that changes that occur through childhood and young adulthood are the result of maturation and development, rather than aging. Baltes,[4] as early as 1987, and Hayflick[3] in 2000 cautioned against that type of differentiation, which has been long adopted by scholars and researchers, because of its implications as to the perceived potential of older individuals of continuing to grow and develop throughout the life span.

Although through time there have been individuals who lived long past the life expectancy of their times, the increased life span of entire cohorts is a more recent occurrence, resulting from advances in public health and medicine during the 20th century.[5] This increased longevity has created a growing interest in aging, propelling aging research, theories of aging, and a variety of new aging fields. As health care professionals, learning about the process of aging has implications on several levels. On a personal level, the more we know about aging, the better equipped we are to make lifestyle decisions that have a bearing on our own aging process. On another level, enhancing our knowledge of aging can provide us with useful tools to assist our loved ones through their own aging process, given that most of us are or will be involved as family caregivers of aging parents.

Last, as a result of the changing demographics and the growing numbers of aging consumers of health services, COTAs are likely to provide services to elders. As such, there are several key issues to be aware of regarding services to an aging population:

1. The Institute of Medicine (IOM), in its report on the state of the health care workforce, identified serious gaps in knowledge of the aging process that potentially compromise the care provided to older persons. The IOM's report, Retooling for an Aging America: Building the Health Care Workforce, calls for actions to prepare competent health care practitioners to meet the health care needs of an aging population and improve the way in which care is delivered to the aging.[6]

2. The Centers for Disease Control and Prevention's Healthy People 2010 and Healthy People 2020 established goals for the health of the nation and identified health indicators to track progress toward these goals. These include improving the health and wellness of the aging population, preventing injuries, reducing disabilities, and addressing health disparities.

3. The American Occupational Therapy Association, through the Occupational Therapy Practice Framework, second edition,[7] provided the blueprint for the delivery of occupational therapy services. These are the principles and procedures that guide our interventions by delineating the domains and process of occupational therapy practice.[7]

These key issues are important because occupational therapy is but one component of a large ecological system that is inextricably connected to the public's health. As a profession and as individual practitioners, we must understand that the impact of our services and the outcomes we achieve extend beyond the clinical environment or in patients' homes. While we must be accountable to third-party payers and responsive to the fiscal requirements of our employers, we must also be cognizant that the extent and appropriateness of the services we deliver have a significant bearing on the health and functional status of not just our patients, but also on the health of our communities and our nation.

Successful, Primary, and Secondary Aging

Definitions and categories of aging abound in the literature and can be confusing, misleading, and even discriminatory in nature. Rowe and Kahn[8] proposed a definition of successful aging as an optimal state that could be attained by avoiding disease and disability, maintaining high cognitive and physical functioning, and continuing to be actively engaged with life. Despite its popularity and the substantial amount of research based on the concept of successful aging, that definition has been called to question by a number of researchers.

Some of the criticisms are based on research findings that indicate that "successful aging," as defined by Rowe

and Kahn[8] in their earlier work, describes the aging experience of a very narrow segment of the population. Others have objected to the use of a strictly quantitative research methodology in published studies because it fails to take into account individuals' constructions of successful aging. Still others propose that the aging experience cannot be understood through the individual alone, but that it must take into account the effect of contexts and environments on aging.[9] Labeling optimal or healthy aging as "successful" risks devaluing disabled individuals, institutionalized elders, and those with chronic illnesses who by default age otherwise "unsuccessfully."

The concepts of primary and secondary aging define the aging process from a different perspective. Primary aging describes the normal, gradual changes in organ systems that, although annoying, are inevitable, experienced by everyone and not associated with disease, impairment, or disability.[1] Some changes eventually become visible, as with the loss of moisture and elasticity of the skin that gives it a sagging, tired, and wrinkled appearance; or the changes in texture and color and even the loss of aging hair (Figure 3-1). Others, such as changes in visual and auditory acuity, slowed mobility, and decline in strength[1] may only be noticeable by the way in which an individual performs daily routines and/or the use of assistive devices such as eyeglasses and canes. Although primary aging changes manifest themselves later in life, they actually begin to take place much earlier, and it is estimated that organ systems begin to gradually lose function and efficiency at a rate of 1% per year after age 30.[1] Secondary

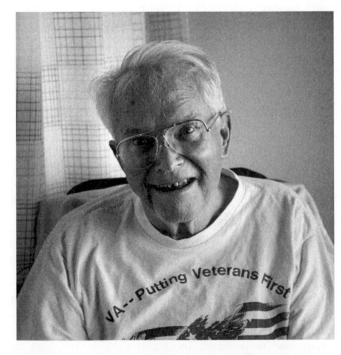

FIGURE 3-1 With aging hair tends to grow in a sparser pattern.

aging changes are neither normal nor usual, are experienced by some individuals but not all, are associated with disease, injury, dysfunction, and impairment, and are frequently preventable through lifestyle changes.[2]

What is certain is that whether primary or secondary, normal or pathological, aging brings about changes. Baltes,[4] in his Life Span Perspective, proposed that aging is marked by a series of gains and losses requiring adaptation through a process of selection, compensation, and optimization. That is, as we age and experience changes in our ability to engage in valued occupations, we select domains of function and activities that are important to us and compensate for the losses by changing the task, changing the environment in which we perform the task, or changing the manner in which we perform it. Selection and compensation allow us to optimize our engagement in life through involvement in valued roles and occupations.[2] Optimal aging can then be viewed in terms of our successful adaptation and continued participation in life, a premise that Pizzi and Smith[10] propose is at the very core of occupational therapy: "Successful aging … is having the physical, emotional, social and spiritual resources, combined with an ability to adapt to life changes, in order to engage in meaningful and important self-selected occupations of life as one ages."

AGING CHANGES

The aging are not a homogeneous group or wrinkled versions of their younger selves. Aging is marked by physiological, cognitive, and psychosocial changes that impact a person's occupational performance and quality of life. It stands to reason that, if aging is the sum total of all we have experienced, consumed, and/or engaged in throughout our lives, individuals who through their lifestyles have built a physiological and cognitive reserve capacity will fare better as they age than will individuals who age with limited reserves.

Having knowledge of the aging process allows COTAs to discriminate between changes that are a normal part of the process and between those that may be a sign of pathology. This knowledge is basic to designing and implementing appropriate and client-centered occupational therapy interventions. Additionally, given the time constraints and demands imposed on practitioners today, there is a risk of becoming so focused on the diagnosis and presenting problem as to exclude signs and symptoms that should not be ignored. There is also the risk of allowing stereotypes of aging to interfere with sound clinical reasoning. Being able to discriminate between what is usual or normal and what may be a manifestation of pathology allows the practitioner to design appropriate interventions, as well as to identify a potential problem and alert the appropriate health care professional(s) (i.e., the OTR, nurse, elder's physician, etc.), so that the issue can be addressed before it becomes a serious threat to the elder's well-being and quality of life.

INTEGUMENTARY SYSTEM

The integumentary system, consisting of the skin, hair, nails, sebaceous (oil), and sweats glands, has a protective and regulatory function and, indirectly, an aesthetic one as well. Smooth, healthy, and vibrant skin, hair, and nails are appreciated, sought after, and rewarded in our society. For the individual, the integrity and appearance of the integument have important implications in terms of self-appraisal, self-esteem, and self-confidence.

There are noticeable changes associated with primary aging. As we age, there is a decrease in the number of hair follicles, a slowing in the rate of growth of the follicles that remain, and a decrease in the production of melanin. These changes contribute to the loss, but, because hair also shields the scalp from the effects of the sun, the loss and thinning of hair also impair its protective function against exposure to sunlight.[11]

As the largest organ in the human body, the skin protects internal organs and serves as a barrier to infectious organisms and to noxious and injury-producing agents. The skin also prevents dehydration from the loss of water and is an important part of the immune system.[11,12] Through sensory receptors in the skin, we are able to detect temperature, pain, touch, and pressure. Through sweat glands and superficial blood vessels, the skin is able to cool the body and regulate its internal temperature.[12,13]

Loss of collagen and elastin, proteins that help the skin maintain its elasticity and tone, contribute to the thinning, sagging, and wrinkling of the skin, which we recognize as signs of aging. In primary aging, normal thinning of the epidermis combined with fragile capillaries and loss of fatty tissue increase the risk of bruising in older adults. These normal changes are further exacerbated in the presence of chronic conditions, such as diabetes, and the use of medications to treat these conditions. Changes precipitated by chronic conditions and medications are not normally experienced by all individuals and are associated with secondary aging.[14] These physiological and structural changes in the integumentary system make aging skin more vulnerable to injury and can increase the risk of adverse health outcomes for aging persons. As an example, fatty tissue, which normally cushions the skin, becomes thinner as we age. Aesthetically, this accounts for the structural changes in the face and the aged appearance of hands and feet (Figure 3-2). Physiologically, the loss of fatty tissue increases the risk of injury to the skin and, combined with a decrease in sweat production, interferes with the skin's ability to effectively regulate the body's internal temperature. Functionally, the loss of padding in the feet can cause pain and discomfort while walking[13] and can have implications as to the elder's tolerance for footwear and even his or her activity level.

The sluggish replacement of epidermal cells and a decline in the production of melanin decrease the skin's ability to protect against exposure to the sun's ultraviolet

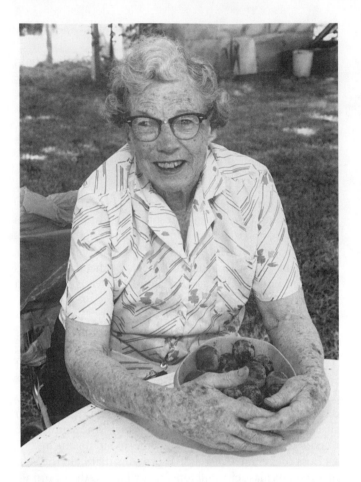

FIGURE 3-2   As people age, changes in skin, such as wrinkles and bruises, become evident.

rays and increase the risk of sunburn and skin cancer in elders.[11] Blood supply to the skin, also reduced as we age, impairs wound healing and interferes with what we recognize as signs of inflammation, such as redness and swelling, which is the body's way to alert us of an infection or injury. Injuries to the skin caused by infection or sunburn may go unnoticed in elders and treatment delayed or not provided.

Inefficient temperature regulation as a result of the reduction in sweat glands and loss of fatty tissue increases the risk of heat stroke in the aged.[11] Loss of sensory receptors in the skin affects sensitivity to touch, temperature, and pain, making the elder more susceptible to cuts, abrasions, and burns. These changes in sensory receptors are also responsible for an increase in pain threshold and impaired pain localization in elders and, as in the case of injury to the skin, can preclude prompt intervention and treatment.

Nutrition and hydration play an important part in maintaining the integrity of the skin and other components of the integumentary system. The frailty and decreased resilience of aging skin are further compromised by the use of prescription and over-the-counter medications that make it more susceptible to the effects of sun exposure, more prone to bleeding, and less able to heal. COTAs need to be particularly cautious when working on transfers with elders to prevent skin injuries. Avoiding and addressing pressure areas from splints and braces, from prolonged sitting and improper seating equipment, or from confinement to bed can prevent complications from wounds that endanger the health and well-being of elders.

NEUROMUSCULOSKELETAL SYSTEM

Aging of the nervous system is characterized by morphological and biological changes, which have an effect on the integrity and function of other systems as well. Aging brains undergo atrophic changes, decreased weight, and enlargement of the ventricles with loss of adjacent white and gray matter, which affect the normal activity of nerve cells and their processes. Loss of neurons and dendritic changes and impaired nerve conduction velocity affect the neuron's ability to communicate with other nerve cells.[15]

This biochemical, structural, and metabolic alterations in the aging nervous system have an effect on sensory and motor function, coordination, reaction time, gait, and proprioception. However, despite their potential effect, research has not been able to clearly establish an association between these aging changes and specific declines in functional performance. One explanation that has been offered is that the aged respond to nervous system changes in individual ways, so that changes that would precipitate functional decline and even dementia in some will not have the same effect on others. Another explanation is that of neuroplasticity, the ability of the brain to reorganize and form new pathways to compensate for atrophic changes and neuronal losses so that functional performance is maintained. Yet another explanation has been that changes in the nervous system may not have implications for the functional performance of daily activities of young-old adults (75 years of age and younger) but that the effect is more significant in those age 75 and older.[15]

SKELETAL SYSTEM

Skeletal system changes resulting from primary aging are responsible for a decline in bone density, lowered skeletal resistance to stress, and loss of skeletal flexibility and mobility. While both men and women experience age-related changes in bone density, the change is most pronounced in women following menopause and is associated with a decrease in estrogen.[16] Structural and physiological changes in muscles contribute to a loss in strength. Weak postural muscles and loss of bone density and cartilage in the vertebrae are responsible for the "shortening" and stooped and round-shouldered posture (kyphosis) often seen in elderly individuals.

While some skeletal changes result from the wear and tear caused by normal aging, others are the result of disease processes or trauma. Degenerative changes in the joints are frequently caused by osteoarthritis (OA), a condition that affects about 50% of the population age 65 years and older. Although OA generally involves weight-bearing joints such as the vertebrae, hips, and knees, it can also affect joints in the elbows, hands, and wrists. Osteoarthritic changes can cause pain and limited range of motion and consequently may have an impact on quality of life, but they are not life threatening and can be treated with medication, joint protection, surgery, therapy, and exercise.[15] Rheumatoid arthritis (RA) is a progressive autoimmune disease with onset in young adulthood or midlife. RA initially presents with inflammation and pain in the metacarpophalangeal and interphalangeal joints of the hands and eventually progresses to other organs. Signs and symptoms include inflammation, pain, joint deformities, fatigue, and weight loss. RA severely impairs functional performance and quality of life.

Osteoporosis is a disease that causes bone to become more porous and brittle and more prone to fracture. Although the disease affects both genders, it is more prevalent in women and is associated with drops in estrogen levels experienced with menopause. The risk of osteoporosis is lessened by building up a reserve starting in young adulthood through a diet rich in calcium and vitamins and exercise that includes weight-bearing activities, which are essential for maintaining bone density.[2,17] Occupational therapy interventions have shown promise in helping adults with osteoporosis maintain physical health and engagement in valued activities.[18]

Hundreds of thousands of fibers (muscle cells) make up each of approximately 350 skeletal muscles in the human body. These muscle fibers and the branches of motor nerves that innervate them form motor units (MUs) of varying sizes, depending on the work required of the muscle. At about age 30 we begin to experience declines in physical strength, speed, and control that continue gradually at an estimated rate of 10% to 15% per decade of life.[19] The rate of decline increases around our mid-fifties and, compared to young adults, may be as high as 50% for persons in their seventies and eighties.[19] This decline in strength, which depending on the muscle can range from 12% to 60%, is mainly due to physiological changes affecting muscle mass.[20] This age-associated loss of muscle mass (sarcopenia) involves decrements in both the number of muscle fibers and the size of the fibers, which affect the strength of the muscle contraction. However, research suggests it is the decrease in the number of fibers, rather than a change in their size, that accounts for the decline in strength.[21] Additionally, as MUs are lost, remaining units provide compensatory innervations, but these result in altered firing patterns that contribute to deficiencies in speed, motor control, and strength.[21]

Sarcopenia is responsible for functional declines in older persons[22,23] and is associated with physiological changes that increase the risk of disease in this population.

Physiologically, as muscle mass declines there is an increase in the deposition of fatty tissue (adiposity) in and around the muscle with a subsequent decline in basal metabolism, which increases the risk for obesity, malnutrition, and diabetes.[24] Functionally, changes in strength, motor control, and fatigability contribute to difficulties with balance, activities of daily living (ADL), and instrumental activities of daily living (IADL) performance in elders. Research conducted by McGee and Mathiowetz[25] found an association between the strength of shoulder abductors and external rotators on IADL function and elbow extensors on the ability to shop for groceries. Sarcopenia, unaddressed, increases the risk for falls and fractures, frailty, loss of independence, and can lead to a less than optimal quality of life.[26]

Elders naturally compensate for changes in strength and functional capacity by avoiding tasks that require high levels of force and by performing tasks at a slower pace. Compensation can be observed in gait patterns as well, with elders typically taking shorter steps and walking at a slower pace, maintaining a smaller heel-to-ground angle while walking and exhibiting a wider stance. The key in working with elders is to encourage and maintain a reasonable level of activity and prevent hypokinesis because inactivity can accelerate the loss of strength and endurance and further compromise mobility, ADL, and IADL performance.

Improving muscle strength and endurance in elders is crucial, and research indicates that exercise can reduce and even reverse the effects of sarcopenia.[21,27] COTAs working with elders should ensure that exercise programs take into account cultural, gender, and individual factors and preferences and incorporate functional activities because there is evidence of the sustained benefits of functional task exercise programs to improve daily function.[28] Community dwelling elders should be encouraged to participate in personally valued occupations that incorporate physical activity such as gardening, grocery shopping, golfing, mall walking, and so on. COTAs should also take advantage of opportunities to educate elders and their caregivers on the importance of proper nutrition and hydration in maintaining muscle strength, endurance, and overall health.

CARDIOPULMONARY SYSTEM

With age, the inner lining of the heart (endocardium) becomes fibrotic (more rigid and thicker), fatty tissue builds up in the heart and surrounding area, and there is a decline in the number of pacemaker cells that regulate the rhythm of the cardiac contraction.[11] Changes in the elastin of the arterial walls cause the walls to become thicker, more rigid, dilated, elongated, and twisted.[29] These arteriosclerotic changes have been associated with the development of systolic hypertension, which increases the risk of cardiovascular disease, disability, and mortality in individuals age 60 years and older.[30,31] Loss of elasticity in the heart valves can cause disruptions in the normal rhythm of the flow and may lead to the development of heart murmurs.[29] Structural and physiological changes in the heart and cardiovascular system reduce the efficiency of the cardiac muscle and its ability to respond to sympathetic stimulation. As a result, the stroke volume, maximum heart rate, and cardiac output decrease. These changes, which seem to not have a significant effect on the organism at rest, are noticeably altered in response to external stress, as when the organism is challenged during physical exertion. As a result, and compared to younger adults, the elderly have less endurance, tire more quickly, and experience shortness of breath in response to exercise.[11] Practitioners should take these changes into account when designing therapeutic interventions for older patients to ensure that exercises and activities meet specific goals and avoid unnecessary exertion.

In the pulmonary system, effective gas exchange is compromised by a decrease in lung volume associated with the loss of elasticity in the lungs and in the medium and small airways. Pulmonary function is further affected by neuromuscular and musculoskeletal changes that increase the effort required to breathe. These changes include weakened respiratory and postural muscles, changes in the costovertebral joints, and increased kyphosis, which affect the flexibility of the thoracic cage and prevent the normal movement of the chest wall, reducing the efficiency of the pulmonary system.[32,33,34]

IMMUNE SYSTEM

Immunosenescence is a term that refers to the changes in immune function that contribute to the increased susceptibility to disease in elders. Recent research suggests that immunosenescence is not likely the result of primary aging,[35,36] but rather is due to secondary changes caused by environmental and lifestyle factors, even in healthy elders free of chronic illnesses. Nutrition, exercise, and even medications taken over the life span can influence immune function as we age. Over time, the epithelial barriers of the skin, lungs, and digestive tract break down, making us more susceptible to pathogens.[37] On a cellular level, immune cells such as T cells and B cells behave differently in the aging body. The ability of these cells to respond to the threat of foreign bodies is diminished, increasing the risk of acquiring infections such as influenza and pneumonia.[38] Immunosenescence not only affects the immune system's ability to protect against disease, but also has a suppressant effect on vaccines, making them less effective in the aging. Elders should consult with their physicians and keep their influenza and pneumonia vaccinations up to date.[39] As a way of counteracting the effects of immunosenescence, physicians may recommend proper nutrition, vitamin and nutritional supplements, hormone therapy, or the administration of multiple doses of vaccines to boost their effectiveness.[39]

Given the effect of the aging immune system on its ability to protect against infections, COTAs should be aware of other factors that increase the risk of infection in older individuals. Hospitalized and institutionalized elders are at risk of acquiring serious and sometimes fatal iatrogenic (caused by medical treatment) and nosocomial (facility acquired) infections such as methicillin resistant *Staphylococcus aureus* (MRSA), Clostridium difficile (C-Diff), and vancomycin resistant *Enterococcus* (VRE). COTAs should observe universal precautions with elders and be alert for signs of possible infection and report them to the nurse, nurse practitioner, or physician so that proper assessment and treatment can be provided and preventable and life-threatening complications avoided.

COGNITION

As with the effect of aging on other bodily systems and physical abilities, the effect of aging on cognitive abilities is influenced by both personal and environmental factors. Cognition is influenced by our genetic makeup, lifestyle choices, health status, and by the external environments that have either provided opportunities for optimal development throughout our life span or have precluded us from achieving our optimal capacity. Just as reserve capacity in muscular strength varies across individuals based on their habitual level and types of activity, maintaining good intellectual functioning has been associated with factors such as achieving a high level of education and employment, having an intact family, engaging in activities that enhance cognitive abilities, enjoying good health, and having good sensory function.

In terms of age-related changes, research studies indicate that elders experience a slowing in information processing and psychomotor speed, deficits in tasks requiring abstraction, set-shifting, and divided attention, and declines in fluid intelligence. The latter, contingent on the health of the central nervous system (CNS), reflects intellectual processes that impact numerical reasoning and logic. Fluid intelligence allows us to solve novel problems and "think on our feet" when presented with new situations. It represents intelligence that is not a product of learning and is not influenced by social or cultural factors. In contrast is crystallized intelligence, the knowledge accumulated through the life span.[40]

For elders, executive function is crucial in setting and managing doctors' appointments, anticipating medication refills, anticipating and identifying hazards, and problem-solving their way out of situations, including those that may be potentially dangerous. Fluid abilities play an important part when faced with new situations, such as those patients often encounter in rehabilitation when they have to learn novel ways of doing routine activities, manage new medical and dietary regimes, or apply safety precautions.

Studies also indicate that factors such as physical illness, chronic conditions, depression, neurological damage, medication side effects, drug interactions, and the effects of surgery and anesthesia may also cause varying degrees of cognitive impairment.[41-43] Impairment of cognitive function is known to affect treatment and rehabilitation outcomes for elders and increases their likelihood of institutionalization.

Differentiating between normal age-related alterations in cognition and abnormal changes in cognitive function is crucial in geriatric rehabilitation. Screening/assessing the cognitive status of elders in occupational therapy is useful in establishing treatment plans based on ability to function, determining the type and extent of assistance needed, and addressing safety issues. Identification of cognitive impairment can lead to referrals for further evaluation, allow for treatment of reversible conditions, provide early intervention in cases of progressive decline, and assist with caregiver education.

Suitable screening and assessment instruments should be standardized, valid, and reliable, and explore the individual's capacity to problem-solve, shift, and divide attention. Conversing with a patient and/or observing the individual perform a familiar ADL can be misleading because people frequently retain social skills in the presence of a cognitive impairment, and ADL are overlearned activities and therefore not a good measure of ability to problem-solve, learn, and safely engage in ADL and IADL.

SENSORY SYSTEM

In our later years, almost every aspect of our sensory systems experiences a change in functioning. These changes can negatively impact social participation, occupational engagement, physical health, and overall quality of life.[44,45] When designing and implementing treatment activities for elders, occupational therapy professionals should understand the nature and consequences of age-related sensory changes and how elders typically respond to such changes.

Olfactory and Gustatory

It is estimated that almost a quarter of adults age 50 years and older experience impaired olfaction, and that the prevalence of this sensory impairment increases with age, as the number of olfactory receptor neurons and supporting cells in the olfactory epithelium decrease.[46] It is unclear whether anatomical changes in the taste system are to blame for changes in taste sensation, but it has been suggested that there may be a loss of taste buds or age-related changes to the taste cell membranes.[46] It is difficult to differentiate between primary and secondary changes to olfaction and taste. Like many other age-related changes, factors such as age, gender, and lifestyle are most commonly linked to chemosensory changes. Medical conditions, including neurological disorders such as Alzheimer's disease, endocrine disorders, nutritional deficiencies, cancer, and viruses, as well as medications taken, can all be contributors to alterations in taste and smell function.[46,47]

Age-related changes in the chemical senses of smell and taste are less apparent than many other sensory changes and therefore are typically less likely to be addressed. Impairment of chemical senses is really an issue of safety. Proper olfactory function alerts us to noxious odors that may themselves be detrimental to health or may indicate the presence of harmful gases such as methane. If the olfactory sense is impaired, an older adult may not realize that he or she has failed to turn off a gas stove or may not notice the smell of smoke. Impairment in taste may also pose a safety threat because an elder with diminished taste may not realize when food is spoiled. Because these changes are not reversible, it is important that elders learn to compensate for impairment of these senses.

Beyond concern for safety, changes in smell and taste function can impact quality of life.[47] Some studies have found that elders with chemosensory impairments report changes in mood, functional impairments such as difficulties with cooking and preparing foods, and lowered enjoyment in other areas of life.[44,46] Additionally, changes in taste and smell can negatively impact social participation. In many cultures, occupations of preparing food and sharing meals are central and profoundly influence quality of life. Chemosensory impairments can lead to decreased engagement or enjoyment of such activities. Impairments in olfaction may also be a source of uncertainty or vulnerability for elders because they may not be aware of personal body odor or the presence of dangerous fumes.[44]

Perhaps the most important issue regarding impairment in chemosensory functioning is the impact on physical health. Alterations in taste and smell have been found to be associated with decreased food intake and nutritional status.[46-48] The literature refers to this phenomenon as the "anorexia of aging." Many elders experience a loss of appetite,[44,46-48] perhaps because it is the enticing aroma of food that stimulates hunger or because a decreased intake of food leads to decreases in the need for food or, as some research suggests, because elders may experience changes in the digestive system that make them feel satiated sooner.[47,48] The issue of excessive weight gain or loss is also of concern for elders. Changes of taste and smell have been linked to a reduction in the consumption of nutrient-rich foods and overconsumption of foods high in fat, sugar, and salt.[46] Anorexia of aging has been linked to protein deficiencies that may contribute to impaired muscle function, impaired cognition, decreased bone mass, immune dysfunction, anemia, poor wound healing, and generally increased morbidity and mortality.[49]

There are several ways that COTAs can help remediate the negative consequences of olfactory and gustatory sensory impairments. The first is to educate elders about proper nutrition and appropriate food intake. The next is to make adaptations to food by adding flavorings that enhance taste without excessive salt, sugar, or fat or by designing meals that provide a variety of flavors, textures, and temperatures.[46] Collaborating with nutritionists and speech therapists whenever possible is recommended to address nutritional needs of elders. Last, because the social and temporal contexts in which meals take place can influence food intake, encouraging elders to consume meals with others and by creating a socially enriching environment for mealtime, COTAs may be able to ensure adequate nutritional intake.

Somatosensory and Kinesthetic

Proprioception is the sense that makes us aware of our body's position in space and gives us information about the static position as well as the kinesthetic movement of our joints.[50] Somatosensory and kinesthetic senses are clinically tested through passive movement to determine whether individuals are able to detect changes in joint position.

Proprioceptive function in the lower extremities has been extensively researched and found to decline with age and to affect elders sensorimotor performance, particularly balance. Problems with balance not only increase elders' risks for falling, but also may lead to restricted activity in response to a fear of falling and ultimately contribute to further decline. Less research has been conducted on the effect of aging on upper extremity somatosensory and kinesthetic function, but there is evidence of an age-related decline that contributes to decreased coordination during tasks involving the upper extremities. Research also suggests that declines in kinesthetic memory, the ability to perceive and remember movement patterns, may contribute to difficulty in learning new motor tasks.[51]

Studies indicate that, compared to younger subjects, elders experience more difficulty sensing joint movement and that this may result from the combined effect of changes in the peripheral nervous system and in central processing abilities.[50] There are also indications that age-related somatosensory and kinesthetic changes progress from distal to proximal joints. Exercises such as Tai Chi, with its slow and deliberate movements and a constant focus on monitoring motion, have been successful in improving position sense in elders.[50]

As with other declines in function, elders appear to compensate for these somatosensory changes by reducing the amplitude and the speed of their movements to maintain balance.[52] This type of compensation, mediated by the CNS, allows older individuals to remain functional. Conversely, changes leading to the loss of integrity of the CNS interfere with this integrative function, leading to disability.[52]

SUMMARY

Aging is marked by physiological, sensory, cognitive, and psychosocial changes that impact a person's occupational performance and quality of life. The process of aging is universal in that we all experience age-related changes; however, the rate at which we age varies both across individuals and even organ systems within the individual.

Aging is the product of our genetic and biological makeup, our life's experiences, our lifestyle decisions and choices, and the effect of the contexts or environments of which we have been a part. Therefore, it stands to reason that individuals who, through their lifestyles, have built physiological and cognitive reserve capacity will fare better as they age than individuals who age with limited reserves.

This chapter explored two major categories of aging—primary aging, the normal gradual changes in organ systems experienced by everyone and not associated with disease, impairment, or disability; and secondary aging, changes that are experienced by some individuals but not all, are associated with disease, injury, dysfunction, and impairment, and are frequently preventable through lifestyle changes.

Baltes' Life Span Perspective[4] proposes that aging is marked by a series of gains and losses (multidirectionality) requiring adaptation through a process of selection, compensation, and optimization. That is, as we experience changes in our ability to engage in valued occupations, we select domains of function and activities that are important to us and compensate for the losses by changing the task, changing the environment in which we perform the task, or changing the manner in which we perform it. Selection and compensation allow us to optimize our engagement in life through involvement in valued roles and occupations. Elders compensate for changes in strength and functional capacity by avoiding tasks that require high levels of force and performing tasks at a slower pace. Compensation can be observed in gait patterns as well, that is, shorter steps, slower pace, and maintaining a wider stance when walking.

Having knowledge of the aging process allows OTRs and COTAs to discriminate between changes that are a normal part of the process and those that may be a sign of pathology. This knowledge is basic to designing and implementing appropriate and client-centered occupational therapy interventions and proactively identifying abnormal conditions that may require treatment or referral to other professionals.

Musculoskeletal changes affect our strength and predispose us to conditions such as osteoporosis and osteoarthritis. Sensory changes affect our ability to receive and process sensory stimulus and can lead to isolation, depression, and impaired quality of life. Cardiovascular and pulmonary changes, which seem to not have a significant effect on the organism at rest, are noticeably altered during physical exertion. As a result, and compared to younger adults, the elderly have less endurance, tire more quickly, and experience shortness of breath in response to exercise. Practitioners should take these changes into account when designing therapeutic interventions for older patients to ensure that exercises and activities meet specific goals and avoid unnecessary exertion.

Immunosenescence not only affects the immune system's ability to protect against disease, but also has a suppressant effect on vaccines, making them less effective in the aging. Given the effect of aging on the immune system's ability to protect against infections, COTAs should be aware of other factors that increase the risk of infection in older individuals, observe universal precautions with all of their patients and residents, and be alert for signs of possible infection and report them to the nurse, nurse practitioner, or physician so that proper assessment and treatment can be provided and preventable and life-threatening complications avoided.

Information processing and psychomotor speed slow down with aging, and we experience deficits with tasks requiring abstraction, set-shifting, and divided attention. Fluid intelligence has an important function in dealing with new situations, such as those patients often encounter in rehabilitation when they have to learn novel ways of doing routine activities, manage new medical and dietary regimes, or apply safety precautions. Whereas fluid intelligence declines with normal aging, crystallized intelligence, the knowledge we accumulate, increases throughout the life span.

Age-related changes affecting smell and taste are less apparent and frequently not addressed. Taste and smell have a safety function in that they allow us to identify spoiled food and smell leaking gas or smoke. In terms of quality of life, they are important for food consumption, cooking, and social participation. Ultimately, these sensory impairments affect nutritional status, may lead to anorexia, and impact physical health.

Practitioners working with elders should provide client-centered, occupation-based interventions. The key in working with elders is to promote engagement in valued roles and occupations. Elders should be encouraged to remain active and prevent hypokinesis because inactivity can accelerate the loss of strength and endurance and further compromise mobility, ADL and IADL performance, and increase the risk of falling.

CASE STUDY

Shirley is a 68-year-old married woman admitted to a skilled nursing facility (SNF) after a 5-day hospital stay for a left hip replacement secondary to a fall in her home. Tasha is the COTA working with Shirley. On reviewing Shirley's OT evaluation, Tasha noted that Shirley had been diagnosed with multiple sclerosis (MS) approximately 20 years earlier, had a history of osteoporosis and panic disorder, and had recently experienced several falls. At the time of evaluation, Shirley required moderate assistance with ADL and mobility.

Over the course of Shirley's 15-day stay at the SNF, Tasha found a client-centered approach to be helpful, especially in helping Shirley manage her increased anxiety and feelings of loss of control within the environment. Because Shirley's MS was affecting her ability to remember new information, Tasha included Shirley's husband when providing patient/caregiver education. Tasha also suggested placing a cue card on the front-wheeled walker listing the steps for incorporating total hip precautions during mobility, as a memory aid for Shirley. Based

on Shirley's goals to be more independent in ADL, Tasha instructed her and her husband in the use of adaptive equipment for the lower extremities and provided them with information on the senior citizens group that furnished loaner durable medical equipment for the bathroom. Shirley called to arrange for a shower seat and bedside commode to be delivered to her home before discharge. In addition, Shirley also pursued ordering the adaptive equipment that Tasha had recommended through a local vendor and had the items sent to the SNF. As part of Shirley's plan of care to improve IADL performance, Tasha established a home exercise program to increase upper extremity strength and instructed both Shirley and her husband to promote compliance and safety.

In terms of IADL, Tasha also spent several sessions focusing on Shirley's goal of improving function with simple meal preparation and laundry tasks. Tasha incorporated total hip precautions and energy conservation/work simplification techniques with the IADL tasks to prevent fatigue and reduce the risk of falling. Responding to Shirley's concerns about being able to manage safely at home, Tasha recommended a home visit to assess home safety. On her discharge from the facility, Shirley's anxiety and low frustration level had markedly diminished. Involving Shirley in the treatment plan allowed her to become independent in performing occupations that she valued. Use of the recommended adaptive and durable medical equipment facilitated her post-surgical recovery and improved her functional status while preventing undue fatigue and decreasing her risk for falls.

■ CASE STUDY REVIEW QUESTIONS

1 List the strategies used by the COTA to compensate for the primary and secondary aging process changes exhibited by the patients.
2 Identify possible negative outcomes if there had been no OT intervention.
3 What are the positive outcomes that were achieved?
4 Discuss the influence of a client-centered approach with the case study.

■ CHAPTER REVIEW QUESTIONS

1 Explain the differences between primary and secondary aging.
2 Summarize primary and secondary changes, and describe possible functional implications of these changes for each of the following: cognitive, integumentary, cardiopulmonary, skeletal, muscular, neurological, and sensory systems.
3 Discuss why COTAs should have knowledge of sensory and physiological changes in elders.

REFERENCES

1. Erber, J., 2005. Aging and Older Adulthood. Thomson Learning, Belmont, CA.
2. Kail, R., Cavanaugh, J., 2007. Human Development: A Lifespan View, 4th ed. Thomson Learning, Belmont, CA.
3. Hayflick, L., 2000. The future of aging. Nature 408, 267-269.
4. Baltes, P., 1987. Theoretical propositions of life-span developmental psychology: On the dynamics of growth and decline. Developmental Psychology 23 (5), 611-626.

5. Ferrucci, L., Giallauria, F., Guralnik, J., 2008. Epidemiology of aging. Radiologic Clinics of North America 46 (4), 643.

6. Institute of Medicine, Retooling for an aging America: Building the health care workforce. Retrieved from www.iom.edu/Reports/2008/Retooling-for-an-Aging-America-Building-the-Health-Care-Workforce.aspx.

7. AOTA Commission on Practice, 2008. Occupational therapy practice framework: Domain and process, 2nd ed. American Journal of Occupational Therapy 62 (6), 625-683.

8. Bonder, B., 2009. Growing old in today's world. In: Bonder, B. (Ed.), Functional Performance in Older Adults. FA Davis, Philadelphia.

9. McLaughlin, S., Connell, C., Heeringa, S., Li, L., Roberts, R., 2009. Successful aging in the United States: Prevalence estimates from a national sample of older adults. Journal of Gerontology: Social Sciences Dec, 1-11.

10. Pizzi, M., Smith, T., 2010. Promoting successful aging through occupation. In: Scaffa, M., Reita, T., Pizzi, M. (Eds.), Occupational Therapy in the Promotion of Health and Wellness. FA Davis, Philadelphia.

11. Sandmire, D., 1999. The physiology and pathology of aging. In: Chop, W.C., Robnett, R.H. (Eds.), Gerontology for the Health Care Professional. FA Davis, Philadelphia.

12. Boelsma, E., Hendricks, H., Roza, L., 2001. Nutritional skin care: Health effects of micronutrients and fatty acids. American Journal of Clinical Nutrition 73 (5), 853-864.

13. Framgen, B., Frucht, S., 2005. Medical Terminology: A Living Language, 3rd ed. Pearson, Upper Saddle River, NJ.

14. Mosqueda, L., Burnight, K., Liao, S., 2005. The life cycle of bruises in older adults. Journal of the American Geriatrics Society 53, 1339-1343.

15. Dal Bello-Haas, V., 2009. Neuromusculoskeletal and movement function. In: Bonder, B.R., Dal Bello-Haas, V. (Eds.), Functional Performance in Older Adults. FA Davis, Philadelphia, pp. 130-176.

16. Warming, L., Hassager, C., Christiansen, C., 2002. Changes in bone mineral density with age in men and women: A longitudinal study. Osteoporosis International 13, 105-112.

17. Yee, B., Williams, B., 2002. Medication management and appropriate substance use for elderly individuals. In: Lewis C.B. (Ed.), Aging: The Health-Care Challenge. FA Davis, Philadelphia, pp. 243-274.

18. Randles, N., Randolph, E., Schell, B., Grant, S., 2003. The impact of occupational therapy intervention on adults with osteoporosis: A pilot study. Physical & Occupational Therapy in Geriatrics 22 (2), 43-56. doi:10.1300/J148v22n02_04.

19. Rice, C., 2000. Muscle function at the motor unit level: Consequences of aging. Topics in Geriatric Rehabilitation 15 (3), 70-82.

20. Frontera, W., Hughes, V., Fielding, R., Fiatarone, M., Evans, W., Roubenoff, R., 2000. Aging of skeletal muscle: A 12-year longitudinal study. Journal of Applied Physiology 88 (4), 1321-1326. doi:8750-7587/00.

21. Williams, G., Higgins, M., Lewek, M., 2002. Aging skeletal muscle: Physiological changes and the effects of training. Physical Therapy 82 (1), 62-68.

22. Kamel, H., 2003. Sarcopenia and aging. Nutrition Review 61 (5), 157-167. doi:10.131/nr.2003.may.157-167.

23. Lauretani, F., Russo, R., Bandinelli, S., Bartali, B., Cavazzini, C., Di Iorio, A., et al., 2003. Age-associated changes in skeletal muscles and their effect on mobility: An operational diagnosis of sarcopenia. Journal of Applied Physiology 95, 1851-1860.

24. Jaaffe, D., Marcus, R., 2000. Musculoskeletal health and the older adult. Journal of Rehabilitation Research and Development 37 (2), 245-254.

25. McGee, C., Mathiowetz, V., 2003. The relationship between upper extremity strength and instrumental activities of daily living performance among elderly women. OTJR: Occupation, Participation, and Health 23 (4), 143-154.

26. Faulkner, J., Brooks, S., 2006. Skeletal muscle. In: Schulz, R., Naelker, L., Rockwood, K., Sprott, R. (Eds.), The Encyclopedia of Aging. Springer, New York, pp. 107-1077.

27. Larsson, L., Ramamurthy, B., 2000. Age-related changes in skeletal muscle: Mechanisms and interventions. Drugs and Aging 17 (4), 303-316. doi:1170-229X/00/0010-0303.

28. De Vreede, P., Samsom, M., Meeteren, N., Duursma, S., Verhaar, H., 2005. Functional-task exercise vs. resistance strength exercise to improve daily function in older women: A randomized controlled trial. Journal of the American Geriatrics Society 53 (1), 2-10.

29. White, H., Sullivan, R., 2006. Cardiovascular aging. In: Schulz, R., Noelker, L., Rockwood, K., Sprott, R. (Eds.), The Encyclopedia of Aging. Springer, New York.

30. McEviery, C., Yasmin, Hall, I., Qasem, A., Wilkinson, I., Cockroft, R., 2005. Normal vascular aging: Differential effects on wave reflection and aortic pulse wave velocity: The Anglo-Cardiff Collaborative Trial (ACCT). Journal of American Cardiology 46, 1753-1760.

31. Najjar, S., Scuteri, A., Lakatta, E., 2005. Arterial aging: Is it an immutable cardiovascular risk factor? Hypertension 46, 454-462.

32. Dean, E., DeAndrade, A.D., 2009. Cardiovascular and pulmonary function. In: Bonder, B.R., DalBello-Haas, V. (Eds.), Functional Performance in Older Adults. FA Davis, Philadelphia.

33. Ekstrum, J., Black, L., Paschal, K., 2009. Effects of a thoracic mobility and respiratory exercise program on pulmonary function and functional capacity in older adults. Physical and Occupational Therapy in Geriatrics 27 (4), 310-327.

34. Gonzalez, J., Coast, J.R., Lawler, J.M., Welch, H.G., 1999. A chest wall restrictor to study effects on pulmonary function and exercise. Respiration 66 (2), 188-194.

35. Ahluwalia, N., 2004. Aging, nutrition, and immune function. Journal of Nutrition, Health, and Aging 8 (1), 2-6.

36. Drela, N., Kozdron, E., Szczypiorski, P., 2004. Moderate exercise may attenuate some aspects of immunosenescence. BMC Geriatrics 29, 4-8.

37. Gomez, C., Boehmer, E., Kovacs, E., 2005. The aging innate immune system. Current Opinion in Immunology 17, 457-462.

38. Hodes, R., 2005. Aging and the immune system. Current Opinion in Immunology 17, 455-456.

39. Kumar, R., Burns, E., 2008. Age-related decline in immunity: Implications for vaccine responsiveness. Expert Review of Vaccines 7 (4), 467-479.

40. Perez-Riley, K., 2009. Mental function. In: Bonder, B.R., Dal Bello-Haas, V. (Eds.), Functional Performance in Older Adults. FA Davis, Philadelphia.

41. Cohen-Zion, M., Stepnowsky, C., Johnson, S., et al., 2004. Cognitive changes and sleep disordered breathing in the elderly: Differences in race. Journal of Psychosomatic Research 56 (5), 549-553.

42. Cohendy, R., Brougere, A., Cuvillon, P., 2005. Anesthesia in older patients. Current Opinion in Clinical Nutrition and Metabolic Care 8 (17), 17-21.

43. Raz, N., Rodrigue, K., Acker, J., 2003. Hypertension and the brain: Vulnerability of the prefrontal regions and executive function. Behavioral Neuroscience 117 (6), 1169-1180.

44. Hummel, T., Nordin, S., 2005. Olfactory disorders and their consequences for quality of life. Acta Oto-Laryngologica 125 (2), 116-121.

45. Teitelman, J., Copolillo, A., 2005. Psychosocial issues in older adults' adjustment to vision loss: Findings from qualitative interviews and focus groups. American Journal of Occupational Therapy 59, 409-417.

46. Seiberling, K., Conley, D., 2004. Aging and olfactory and taste function. Otolaryngologic Clinics of North America 37, 1209-1228.

47. Donini, L., Savina, C., Cannella, C., 2003. Eating habits and appetite control in the elderly: The anorexia of aging. International Psychogeriatrics 15 (1), 73-87.

48. Chapman, I., 2007. The anorexia of aging. Clinics in Geriatric Medicine 23, 735-756.

49. Harris, C., Fraser, C., 2004. Malnutrition in institutionalized elders: The effects on wound healing. Ostomy Wound Management 50 (10), 54-63.

50. Goble, D., Coxon, J., Wenderoth, N., Van Impe, A., Swinnen, S., 2009. Proprioceptive sensibility in the elderly: Degeneration, functional consequences, and plastic-adaptive processes. Neuroscience and Biobehavioral Reviews 3, 271-278.

51. Fry-Welch, D., Campbell, J., Foltz, B., et al., 2009. Age-related changes in upper extremity kinesthetics. Physical and Occupational Therapy in Geriatrics 20 (3), 137-154.

52. Paquette, C., Paquet, N., Fung, J., 2006. Aging affects coordination of rapid head motions with trunk and pelvic movements during standing and walking. Gait and Posture 24, 62-69.

4

Psychological Aspects of Aging

YOLANDA GRIFFITHS AND ANDREA THINNES

KEY TERMS

stressors, loss, coping skills, adaptations, learned helplessness, occupational shifts

CHAPTER OBJECTIVES

1. Identify myths and facts about psychological aspects of aging.
2. Identify common stressors, changes, and losses to which elders must adapt.
3. Discuss common emotional problems that may accompany losses.
4. Discuss coping skills and interventions that promote healthy transition with age.

Physical milestones measure a person's age in years, but indications of mental aging are less clear. Learning about the psychological aspects of aging enhances the certified occupational therapy assistant's (COTA's) ability to deal effectively and empathetically with elders. This chapter explores key concepts about the psychology of aging that assist in understanding elders and enhancing empathy when working with elders.

MYTHS AND FACTS ABOUT AGING

The way elders are perceived significantly affects the way they are treated. Stereotypes are rigid concepts, exaggerated images, and inaccurate judgments used to make generalizations about groups of people. Positive and negative stereotypes create false images of aging. Western culture often perpetuates negative views of aging. Both positive and negative stereotypes can affect elders. In fact, some elders are empowered by positive stereotypes, and others are motivated to be an example of an active elder and dispel the negative stereotypes. "Seniors who are well educated, maintain a high level of health, and live in a city environment that welcomes seniors may result in individuals who are more resistant to negative characterizations. Such seniors may be the best antidote to negative stereotypes.[1]

Buying into the erroneous beliefs and myths of aging produces a biased negative perception of elders and colors objectivity when working with elders. "Stereotypes about aging and the old, both negative and positive, have significant influence upon the older people themselves."[2] This is a form of ageism and can deter from a realistic approach in working with elders. "Negative aging stereotypes have the power to influence reactions toward older people, creating assumptions in the midst of others about

their limited or poor abilities, judgment, and behaviors."[2] Clarifying misperceptions about elders is the first step in developing effective rapport when working with this population. Consider the following myths about the psychological aspects of aging.

Myth 1: Chronological Age Determines the Way an Elder Acts and Feels

Melissa, a COTA, receives a referral to see Simone who is 89 years of age. Melissa has images of an elderly, cranky woman sitting in a chair with her head bowed, responding in a belligerent way about receiving treatment. Melissa enters the room of the assistive living center that Simone shares with her roommate Julia. The room is filled with sports mementos, photos, and awards from both of their respective grandchildren. Julia taps Melissa's shoulder and says, "If you're looking for Simone, she's in the sun room teaching dance lessons. You have to get up pretty early to catch up with Simone or she'll leave you in the dust!"

The aging process varies with each individual, and each person has different perceptions about it. Some elders do believe that their minds will deteriorate along with their bodies. Personality, lived experiences, natural responses to actual losses, expected reactions to one's own aging process and death, and predictable emotional reactions to physical illness are separate aspects of aging. The truth is that elders are in a time of transition. Persons who are elderly should be treated as individuals and within their particular contexts, history, and circumstances. Refrain from generalizing that all elders approach aging in the same way.

For example, the stereotype that elders should avoid engaging in any strenuous exercise because their organs will fail or bones will break is a myth. Exercise is beneficial for most and dangerous for a few elders only (Figure 4-1).

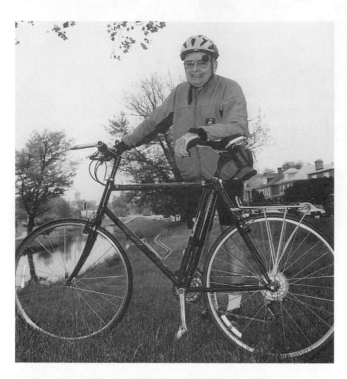

FIGURE 4-1 This elder remains physically active by regularly competing in races. *(Courtesy of Truby La Garde.)*

One study concluded that in "general elderly populations, moderate or high physical activity, compared with no physical activity, is independently associated with a lower risk of developing incident cognitive impairment after two years of follow-up."[3] Elders should check with their physician before they begin an exercise program for any limitations and recognize that the body does change in terms of stamina and flexibility in aging. It is not uncommon for elders to start exercising in later life even if they have been inactive for years.[4] From a therapeutic perspective, the elder should:

- Be aware of the safety concerns of beginning to exercise
- Set realistic goals and expectations
- Warm up and stretch before exercising and cool down and stretch following exercise
- Gradually progress to add more time or slightly more difficulty to the exercise routine
- Consider strengthening as well as aerobic activity as exercise

COTAs should encourage elders to take brisk walks, consider new activities such as Tai Chi or water aerobics, and enjoy life. Increased mobility, strength, and flexibility may lead to better overall health, a decrease in fall risk, and may hold off the need for long-term care.

Myth 2: You Can't Teach an Old Dog New Tricks

The applause is thunderous as the graduates walk across the stage. It is a very special day for both Emily and Eugenia Meyer as they receive their Bachelor of Science degrees in accounting. Eugenia Meyer is 68 years of age. Emily is her 24-year-old granddaughter. Eugenia experienced a heart attack and her granddaughter was her caregiver during her rehabilitation. Eugenia often expressed regret about not finishing college. Emily encouraged Eugenia to follow her dreams of furthering her education.

The potential of an elder should not be underestimated. One delightful example of the passion for lifelong learning can be found in Douglas's story. Douglas, 74 years old, was married to his wife for 53 years when she passed away. He moved to a retirement community after his wife's death. After recovering from his wife's death, Douglas desired a new challenge. He decided to go back to school and earn a master's degree in theology. He was concerned about the pace of school, the technology, and the way others would view him, but the concerns did not stop him from diving in. He first took a computer course for older adults and practiced his skills with his new friends at the retirement community. In his theology courses, he found that his younger colleagues valued his stories and life experiences he shared.

Douglas is not out of the norm of the capabilities of the typically aging brain. The ability to learn does not decline with age. In fact, the current number of persons older than age 55 years in noncredit continuing education courses is continuing to grow. According to Williamson,[5] the desire to learn is an uppermost priority for elders. Learning strategies and preferences may differ for elderly students and their younger classmates; however, the richness in experience that elders bring to the classroom can be beneficial to all learners—"Many older adults want to participate in a learning process and become actively engaged in that process when it is interesting, relevant, and recognizes the experience they bring to the education context."[6]

Crystallized and fluid intelligence must be considered in an elder learning environment. Crystallized intelligence comes from lived experiences, from which elders can tap into the wisdom gained. Fluid intelligence is new learning on the spot, such as in a classroom setting when learning a new concept. There may be increased time needed by the elder to grasp a new concept, technique, or skill. The COTA should remember that age-related changes in learning should be considered in the context that they occur and with regard to each individual, within a classroom setting, but also within the context of education when the elder is a client of occupational therapy services and must be educated on a variety of things. Education materials and presentation of the information must be modified to reflect the needs of the elder learner.

Biological changes also may affect learning. For example, elders may be unable to sit for long periods because of back or hip problems. Elders may tire quickly and demonstrate decreased physical stamina. With increased use of computers, good ergonomics with regard to the computer station will decrease fatigue and neck or back stiffness associated with sustained computer use.

As a result of poor vision or hearing skills, elders may not accurately process all sensory information. Elders may need additional time to organize and process new information. People may quickly assume that an elder is confused when the information recalled seems jumbled or inaccurate. Although there may be some cognitive decline with aging because of particular medical conditions, in many ways elders may be better learners.[4] Elders can integrate life experience and a broader perspective with new knowledge that younger persons often do not consider. The COTA can make an outstanding contribution in preserving the skills and fully using the lived experiences of elders. COTAs can assist by adjusting the environment or technique of completing a task to the capacities of the elder.

Elders who feel threatened by new situations may have poor self-confidence in learning situations. New situations require decision making and risk taking. Elders may avoid learning opportunities that may result in embarrassment, frustration, or conflict. In times of stress, elders may be less flexible in problem solving and rely on set ways and habits of dealing with situations. Ultimately, the elder must want to learn, be willing to recognize any limitations, and explore other learning techniques such as keeping the brain exercised with problem-solving tasks, crossword puzzles, board games, and "neurobic" exercises (see Chapter 3 for more information on cognitive changes with aging).

Myth 3: As You Age, You Naturally Become Older and Wiser

It was most disturbing to Jerry that he could not remember what he was doing sometimes. After all, Jerry was a former professor of chemistry and retired from teaching only last year. Now his body seemed slower and his mind so forgetful. His forgetfulness started with little things like losing his keys and progressed to forgetting the road home after driving to the store. Finally, one day Jerry became upset and confused in the grocery store parking lot, unable to recall the kind of car he owned. What was happening? His daughter feared that Jerry was experiencing early stages of Alzheimer's disease. Neither Jerry nor his daughter could understand why this was happening, especially because Jerry had always been so active and was only 63 years of age. Jerry has been an accomplished author and teacher and prided himself on his intellectual abilities.

Positive stereotyping can be as detrimental as negative stereotyping. Unrealistic expectations that elders can and should continue to perform as they did when they were younger may cause an elder to feel like a failure. Stating that all elders will be wiser or that all elders will become senile is not true. These contradictory statements prove that elders should not be lumped into one homogeneous group.

Intelligence does not decline with age. Studies done in the 1920s by Bayley and Bradway[7] indicate that intelligence

quotient (IQ) scores increase until the twenties, then level off and remain unchanged until late in life. Continued intellectual stimulation promotes successful aging. Staying active socially and engaged in activities make an elderly person less vulnerable to psychosocial situations.[8] With aging, it is important to determine which behaviors are caused by medical conditions versus personality traits or natural aging processes.[9]

Myth 4: Elders Are Not Productive, Especially at Work

Initially, all the young employees at the local burger place called the new employment program "adopt a geezer." Paul, the manager and owner of a thriving fast food restaurant located across from the high school, often came home and complained to his wife about the unreliability of many of the youth he hired to fill the shifts. Paul said that "it was as if the kids just wanted the paycheck and had no real concern about the quality of their work."

Paul's wife, Michelle, a COTA who worked 3 days a week at the senior citizen center, suggested a mutually beneficial program that would financially help elders who were interested and capable of fulfilling a part-time position. Paul would be able to fill shifts open during the school day with steady, reliable help.

To the amazement of the young employees, the elder employees were efficient and demonstrated stamina. In fact, the young employees often remarked, "They're cool!"

The opportunity for young employees to work beside their older counterparts will continue to increase. Between 2000 and 2015, the number of workers age 55 years and older will increase by 72%.[10] Work is not only a social or leisure pursuit of elders, but also a necessity to maintain a lifestyle they desire. The psychological adaptation to the new role of retiree can be either dreaded or embraced. For some elders, retirement is anticipated as a withdrawal from traditional, stressful workday events. They are capable of learning new skills and effectively solving problems in new situations. Upon retiring, many elders engage in social activities, community service or volunteer work, or become employed in a different line of work on a part-time basis to feel productive. According to the American Association of Retired Persons Work and Career Study, 60% of older persons plan to work in some capacity during their retirement years.[11] The study also indicates that elderly workers feel undervalued at work and want the opportunity to use their skills and talents (Figure 4-2). With challenges in the economy about job security and possible discrimination against elders in the workplace, older workers may feel vulnerable. After retirement, elders often seek new areas of employment. They are capable of learning new skills and effectively solving problems in new situations. COTAs can promote integration and participation of an older worker into the job successfully by looking at adaptations to the environment, supplies, and training required to fulfill the job description.

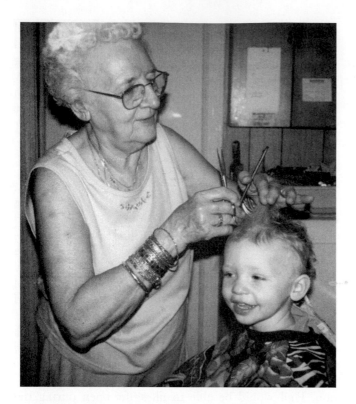

FIGURE 4-2 Some elders remain productive by using their talent and skills at work.

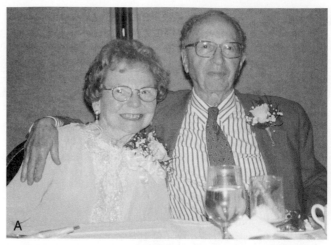

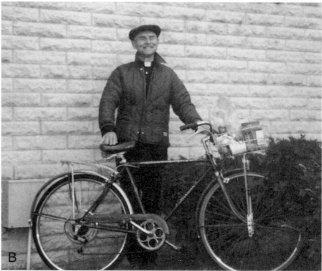

FIGURE 4-3 A, With added leisure hours elders must consider a new plan for managing time. B, This retired priest volunteers in the community while remaining physically fit.

For example, an elder who would like to work in the reception area of an office may answer phones and greet customers but may need additional time and training in computer data entry needed for the job.

Retirement is sometimes a paradox when elders may have time and energy but lack financial means to be active. Conversely, when elders have the financial means and have retired from their jobs, they may desire socialization or interesting activities. According to Kielhofner (2008),[23] elders may be challenged in their activity choices by lack of transportation, finances, companions, or self-limiting fears. Finch and Robinson[12] believe "training older adults in how to use technology can help reduce some of the fears that limit them from adopting technologies, including assistive technology in the workplace."[13] COTAs can help retired elders create a plan for managing added leisure hours (Figure 4-3, A). Productive engagement can help elders continue to be involved in their communities. Volunteerism in the community can be a wonderful channel for leadership and organizational skills gained over a career lifetime and can be an economic and social contribution to society (Figure 4-3, B).[14]

Myth 5: Elders Become More Conservative as They Age

Organizing a neighborhood petition to get an overpass built over the busy street next to the elementary school was the last thing Elena thought she would be doing on her 80th birthday. But here she was in the midst of neighbors and community workers stacking flyers, affixing petition forms to clipboards, and filling out a shift schedule. For years, Elena had observed many close calls when children crossing the street were almost hit by automobiles. She thought, "I could never forgive myself if one of those kids got hurt and I just sat here and watched from my front window."

Contrary to myth, many elders are receptive to new ideas and accept fresh roles. In fact, many elders become more politically active and even seek political office to initiate social change (Figure 4-4). According to the continuity theory, adults learn continuously from their life experiences and may pursue new interests and goals.[15] Even though habits and preferences contribute to a consistency in personality, developmental psychologists note that personality may be influenced as individuals deal with crisis points in each phase of life and add to their

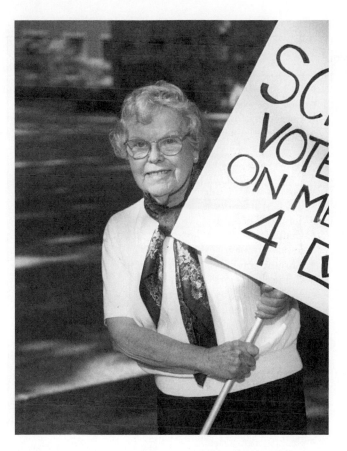

FIGURE 4-4 Many elders become politically active to initiate social change.

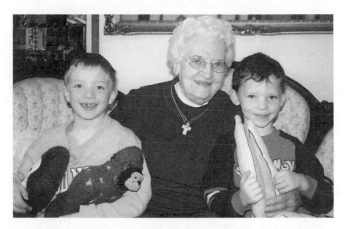

FIGURE 4-5 Activity levels can increase dramatically when elders live in their children's home.

repertoires of adaptive skills. According to Canja,[16] it is untrue that elders do not want to be active, contributing members of society and that the later years of life should be reserved for idleness.

Myth 6: Elders Prefer Quiet and Tranquil Daily Lives

Jose looked around the reception area of Applewood Manor on his first day of work as a COTA. Only the sounds of a television murmuring the chant of a daily game show and the shuffling of residents down the hall broke the silence. The head nurse, Mrs. Kessler, walked up to Jose and said, "Isn't it wonderful how quiet and peaceful it is here? We work very hard to preserve a sense of tranquility in the sunset years of one's life."

Jose interviewed all of the residents during the week to determine activities he could develop based on their interests. Not surprisingly, more than half of the residents wanted less sedentary activities than they currently were experiencing. Some even wanted organized sports like tennis. Other residents wanted a piano and perhaps a jazz hour scheduled.

Another incorrect generalization is that all elders prefer a sedentary lifestyle. An elder who has experienced a rather staid and uneventful life before retirement will not

necessarily continue that type of lifestyle. Elders often move in with their children's families, and their lives may become rather frenzied (Figure 4-5). Some pursue totally new interests that they may not have had time for earlier because of career and family demands. Many elders continue with vibrant lifestyles and do not sit awaiting death. Staying active is a key to healthy psychological aging.

Myth 7: All Elders Become Senile

The expression "senior moment" infers to an idea that as one ages, memory lapses become commonplace. Harry has always been a proud, independent man. He was decorated twice during his participation in World War II. After experiencing a heart attack, Harry adjusted to the many lifestyle changes that were suggested by the health care team. Today Harry sighed as he walked with multiple pieces of paper toward the receptionist in the Occupational Therapy department. This was the third stop in a confusing, mazelike journey inside the Veterans' Administration Hospital. The hospital was under reorganization again, and procedures for appointments had changed. Previously, Harry always called for an appointment, showed up characteristically 10 minutes early, and cheerfully greeted the young COTA who assisted with the treatments. Today a young man at the front desk rattled off multiple instructions about the new procedures and handed Harry a photocopied map of the building along with a stack of new forms to be completed. Harry was still trying to understand the map when he asked the young man to slowly repeat the instructions. The young man repeated himself in a louder tone and pointed Harry in the direction of the elevators. The young man muttered, "These senile old guys."

When elders appear confused or require more time to understand directions, misunderstandings often result. Getting older is not synonymous with feeble-mindedness or imbecility. Brain damage may be evident as a result of physical illness. However, senility is a label often used inaccurately to describe specific psychosocial disorders that elders may be dealing with, such as depression, grief, anxiety, or dementia. People age at different rates. Evidence points to the connection between engagement in physical exercise, a leisure time activity, and the overall health of older adults."[17]

STRESSORS, LOSSES, AND EMOTIONS ASSOCIATED WITH AGING

Elders often must deal with major life crises such as retirement, loss of spouse, economic changes, residence relocation, physical illness, loss of friends, and the reality of mortality. There are predictable shifts that occur in occupational patterns across the life span in regard to developmental processes and life stages.[18] The significant occupational shifts or changes in meaningful activities, associated with aging may include dealing with financial burden, emotional losses, variance in roles, adapting to different routines and habits, diminishing physical and mental performance, and challenges to adaptation.[18,19,20] Lieberman and Tobin[21] found that "events that lead to loss and require a major disruption to customary modes of behavior seem to be the most stressful for elders." Hayslip[22] identified the following personal factors that may influence stressors: flexibility, recognition of personal needs and limits, internal locus of control, perceived family support, and willingness to acknowledge feelings about death and dying (Box 4-1). More recent studies have attempted to measure other aspects of life events and stress levels. COTA s must consider the ways various life events affect elders to understand what motivates certain behaviors.

According to Kielhofner,[23] role changes can sometimes be involuntary, such as the unexpected death of a loved one, and elders struggle with the loss or diminishment of accompanying roles. Elders may need to adapt to shifts in occupational patterns possibly related to atypical or unpredictable life events and developmental aging. For example, unexpected economic demise of a company may lead to the unforeseen loss of a job and retirement funds. This significantly impacts a person's occupation, inherent roles, and habits.

NEED FOR SOCIAL SUPPORT

Pivotal to the ability of an elder to cope with a major life change is the social support of family, friends, church members, and neighbors. Although stressors may not be avoided, social support can help elders deal with losses.

The support an elder receives with the death of a loved one often diminishes to a large extent after the funeral or mourning period. The reality of the loss may not occur until later, when the elder is alone. The survivor may grieve over the loss of finances and possible change in residence, social status, or role associated with the death of the loved one. COTAs can assist the surviving spouse in adjusting to new roles, habits, and routines, as well as developing a strong network of social support.

BOX 4-1

Stressors that Affect Elders

- Social stressors
- Death of a loved one
- Caregiving for an ill spouse
- Family members moving away
- Moving to live with family members
- Retirement
- Relocation to a nursing home because of illness
- Loss of worker role
- Physical stressors
- Serious illness
- Cumulative sensory losses
- Sexual problems
- Chronic conditions that reduce mobility or self-care
- Cultural stressors
- Negative stereotyping of elders
- Health care policy management
- Personal stressors
- Diminished finances
- Grief
- Loneliness
- Anger
- Guilt
- Depression
- Anxiety
- Reality of own death

Data from MacDonald, K., & Davis, L. (1988). Psychopathology and aging. In L. Davis & M. Kirkland (Eds.). ROTE: The Role of Occupational Therapy with the Elderly. Rockville, MD: American Occupational Therapy Association.

Loneliness is a form of emotional isolation. Elders may experience increased social isolation with retirement, as family members relocate or as friends move or die. Social interactions with pets, weekly church services, grocery shopping trips, or occasional visits from family members may not be emotionally fulfilling enough for an elder. COTAs can assist in exploring and structuring more frequent or new areas of social interaction in the community. Community centers offer a variety of activities such as cooking and art classes, trips to local attractions, and classes specifically designed for grandparents and grandchildren to attend together.

Elders may become reclusive and socially paralyzed with anxiety as a result of increasing neighborhood violence. Intensifying anger is a common emotional problem experienced by many elders as they feel a loss of control over their lives. Elders may be viewed as cantankerous or verbally aggressive when in fact they may be using angry words to express feelings of helplessness. This anger also may be founded on fear and sadness over losses.

Other changes in environment such as new living arrangements, whether imposed or by choice, also may be a challenge for elders. According to Kielhofner,[23] elders develop habits sustained over a long period often in a stable environment; when the environment changes, demands to shift habits are stressful. Or the physical or mental ability to sustain previous habits in a new environment also may be diminished.

PHYSICAL ILLNESS

Elders may need to cope with a chronic disease or a serious physical illness. A serious physical illness with a sudden onset may be more debilitating to the elder in terms of independence and self-care. A chronic illness is no less stressful; however, the elder may have adapted to the illness more gradually. Box 4-2 lists stressors associated with common physical illnesses of elders.

Petra, an 81-year-old woman, who was legally blind, was receiving occupational therapy services in her home. She lived by herself in a cozy one-bedroom apartment. Petra was known to the home health care team to be quite rude; in fact, she had "fired" several home health nurses and therapists that had come to provide services for her in her home. The occupational therapist asked the COTA to see Petra one Saturday for her. Petra was on Rodney's caseload. Almost immediately after Rodney introduced himself, Petra told him she never met a health care worker that could think for themselves. She continued to insult his profession and his coworkers. Rodney tried to understand more about Petra and to find out reasons for her behavior. He learned from her past medical history that Petra's blindness has become progressively worse. In fact, she stopped leaving her home all together because she was embarrassed that she could not fix her hair and makeup the way she used to. Rodney took the time to speak to her about this and to offer suggestions for how he could assist her in being able to do those again. He was the first person to look beyond her sarcastic remarks and rude exterior

BOX 4-2

Stressors Associated with Physical Illness Common to Elders
■ Threat to life ■ Loss of body integrity ■ Change in self-concept ■ Threat to future plans ■ Change in social roles ■ Change in routine activities ■ Loss of autonomy ■ Need to rapidly make critical decisions ■ Loss of emotional equilibrium ■ Physical discomfort ■ Monotony and boredom ■ Fear of medical procedures

Adapted from Davis, L. (1988). Coping with illness. In L. Davis L & M. Kirkland (Eds.). ROTE: The Role of Occupational Therapy with the Elderly. Rockville, MD: American Occupational Therapy Association.

and notice that she was really scared and confronting her own mortality. Rodney continued to see Petra and work with her on coming to terms with her blindness and need for assistance. He felt that he made a difference in her life. He shared his experience with other members of the health care team so that they, too, could better understand Petra.

An elder person copes with physical illness through a psychosocial process. A negative perception of the situation and a hopeless attitude will adversely affect the way a person deals with the illness. Cohen and Larazus[24] pointed out that those elders who view a physical illness as a challenge cope better than those who view it as a punishment.

A grief process in dealing with any illness is to be expected. Five stages to the grief process originally identified by Kubler-Ross[25] continue to help health professionals better understand and help their clients: denial, anger, depression, bargaining, and acceptance.[26] This grief process may not be linear—that is, the elder may become depressed and then become angry or deny the situation again before accepting the illness.

An elder's ability to adapt is contingent on physical health, personality, life experiences, and level of social support.[9,27,28] To successfully deal with a chronic condition, an elder should adopt the following important concepts:
- Recognize permanent changes such as diet, lifestyle, work habits, or exercise that may promote recovery
- Mentally deal with losses caused by the illness
- Accept a new self-image
- Identify and express feelings such as anger, fear, and guilt
- Seek out and maintain social support from family and friends

COTAs can help an elder deal with a chronic illness in the following ways:
- Reduce fears about the illness through education
- Listen and be sensitive to the feelings expressed verbally and nonverbally
- Provide encouragement
- Assist in the development of creative yet realistic ways for elders to gain more control over their illnesses or losses associated with an illness
- Identify ways to reduce stress and to promote social support
- Surround the elder who has moved to a nursing care facility as a result of the illness with familiar objects, which may help maintain a sense of continuity, provide comfort and security, and aid memory

LEARNED HELPLESSNESS

When elders perceive that they have no control over a particular outcome or multiple stresses in their life, they may give up hope and become dependent on others to fulfill their needs.[29] A person with an external locus of control frequently feels powerless over decisions and actions, and the more this belief is reinforced, the more likely that learned helplessness occurs. Elders who experience loss of control also experience diminishing coping skills and are at risk for illness.[19,20] Health care workers and family members often contribute to this state of learned helplessness in the following ways:

- Expecting elders to be unable to do for themselves and completing tasks for them, thereby promoting dependence
- Imposing routines on elders for the sake of convenience, such as giving them a bath at 2:00 P.M.
- Showing a negative attitude by making condescending remarks about physical appearance or behaviors
- Perpetuating the sick or institutional role by validating somatic complaints or disapproving decisions

Learned helplessness often results when the elder believes a situation is permanent, and then depression and a marked lack of self-esteem follow. COTAs can encourage independence and self-care activities. As elders regain a feeling of competence, learned helplessness can be reversed. Robnett and Chop[9] suggest giving choices and options as much as possible and to challenge the client to work at a greater level than currently functioning. The concept of the client advocating for herself or himself enhances personal control in everyday life and should be integrated into daily therapy. COTAs can empower elders by creative problem solving to assist the elder in being as independent as possible.

Sena is an 88-year-old woman who is in a skilled nursing facility after falling at home. Shannon, the COTA, works with her daily and is aware of what Sena can and cannot do physically by herself. She continues to be fed because she is just too tired. Shannon knows that she can feed herself, and may well be tired, but does not oblige her request. While documenting later that afternoon, Shannon sees Sena's son eating dinner with her, and he is feeding her with a spoon. The COTA observes the interaction but does not say anything to Sena's son. The next evening Shannon observes the same scenario and decides to address the situation with Sena's son and explain to him that his mother is able to feed herself. Shannon is respectful of him but talks to him about learned helplessness and what he can do to help his mother. The COTA must relinquish some of the power and control as a health care advocate and empower the elder and their family members to engage in independent problem solving. One of the key concepts in preventing learned helplessness is for the COTA to be aware of his or her own beliefs about aging and mortality and to consider stereotypes that may bias attitudes toward working with elders.

CONCLUSION

Old age can be a time of self-reflection and exploration of new interests. It also can be a time of dealing with great losses and severe stress. Changes occur throughout the life span, and the way a person copes with changes and adapts to transitions ultimately determines his or her ability to psychologically cope with aging. Keeping active can help minimize the effects of the aging process. By clarifying assumptions and myths about aging, gaining awareness of the different stressors and losses associated with aging, and understanding the ways elders cope with serious illnesses, COTAs can help elders enhance their quality of life as they experience aging.

CASE STUDY

Margaret, 79 years of age, sits in the sun porch clutching a pot of orchids. This is the last day she will enjoy this scene because today Margaret is moving to an assisted living facility in a town 260 miles away, which is close to her son John. Margaret had lived in this home for almost 35 years with her husband Phillip. When Phillip died 2 years ago of pancreatic cancer, it was a shock almost too great for Margaret to bear. Phillip had been her rock. Margaret had been Phillip's primary caretaker while he was ill. During their 40-year marriage, Margaret and Phillip had traveled all over the world and shared lifelong interests, including cooking, golf, and cultivating orchids in their custom built greenhouse. Margaret had been a volunteer with the children at the homeless shelter downtown until Phillip required her full-time care. The walls in their den were covered with awards and letters of appreciation for her work with the children. Now the house has been sold and many of her mementos have been packed up, sold, or given away.

Margaret had been an energetic high school history teacher and Phillip had been a chemist. They had two children, John and Karen. Karen is married and lives in London with her two daughters. Margaret and Phillip loved to travel to London to visit their grandchildren. John is recently divorced and is busy managing his new safety consulting company. Margaret has a beloved 9-year-old Labrador retriever named Henry, but she is unable to take Henry with her to the assistive living facility.

In the last 3 years, Margaret has been diagnosed with arthritis, vertigo, and early stages of dementia. Margaret fell 6 months ago and fractured her hip. She had begun to forget things such as paying bills, which caused her electricity to be turned off; leaving the stove on, which caused a small fire; and not remembering to take her medication regularly. John and Karen decided it was time to move their mother into a safer, more supervised environment. Margaret became depressed and less active after the decision was made. It seemed as if Margaret resigned herself to a situation beyond her control physically and socially. Margaret spent much of her time sleeping or sitting in the sun porch staring out the picture window. Moving to the new town meant saying goodbye to friends, relatives, and her beloved pet, as well as Phillip.

■ CASE STUDY REVIEW QUESTIONS

1 Identify the losses Margaret has experienced.
2 Describe the stressors or emotional problems that may be related to these losses. What impact would this have on her

occupations? Describe shifts in occupational patterns that are linked to the changes in her life. Consider changes in roles, habits, routines, relationships, work, and leisure interests and activities.

3 Discuss what the COTA could do to help Margaret deal with these losses in terms of attitude, education, and activities.

EXERCISES

The following are a few activities to help the COTA gain empathy and rapport with the elderly.

INTO AGING

"Into Aging" is a commercially available game that focuses on building empathy for those who are growing old. The manual describes the game as a way for players to increase awareness of elders' problems by simulating experiences with similar problems, such as loss, isolation, powerlessness, dependency on others, and ageism. This game is available through Slack, Inc. (Thorofare, NJ).

ROLE PLAYING

Role playing is a useful activity for groups to understand aging-related issues. In preparation for the activity, each of the myths of aging discussed in the chapter should be written on index cards. Each small group will be given a set of index cards. Members of each group then enact some of the myths and stereotypes associated with the psychological aspects of aging. Each example should be followed with a discussion of feelings and thoughts about the stereotype or myth. What misconceptions did you have about aging before the activity that was subsequently clarified? What concept or concern is still puzzling or needs further exploration? How can you use the information learned in the role play in occupational therapy practice?

STEREOTYPE EXERCISE

Each member of a group should list the first six or seven images that immediately come to mind with the word *elder*. Group members should think about advertisements, movies, and personal experiences that influence their perceptions of elders. Each member should share the images with the group and explain the reasons the images are so vivid. All group members should discuss whether the images are realistic or stereotypical. Discuss how these stereotypes may bias the way a COTA would approach treatment with elders or with caregivers. Group members should brainstorm different ways to change stereotypical images to make them more realistic.

FIELD TRIP IMAGERY

Place yourself comfortably in a quiet room. You may sit in a comfortable chair or lie down. Take three deep breaths. As you exhale, clear your mind of any concerns and concentrate on the directions. Give yourself permission to use the next 10 to 15 minutes to explore what it would feel like to be 75 years old.

Pretend that you are looking into a large mirror. Imagine your physical appearance at age 75 years. What physical changes have taken place? Do you need any assistance with self-care? What emotions are you experiencing as a result of these changes?

What changes have occurred in your living arrangements? Do you live alone? Identify any changes in lifestyle as a result of finances.

What have you accomplished in your life thus far? Do you regret any events? Do you regret not achieving certain goals? Are you satisfied with your life?

Remember what you have just experienced with the visual imagery. Now slowly count to 10. As you get closer to 10, you will become more awake and tuned to the sounds of the room you are in. When you reach 10, gently open your eyes.

Free write for the next 5 minutes. It may be poetry, prose, or just phrases of what you remember of your visual imagery trip to age 75. Reflect on what key concepts of aging were apparent in the imagery. Describe your feelings.

RESOURCES

Older adult resources for mental health and wellness are available through Wellness Reproductions & Publishing, LLC (a Guidance Channel Company). This is a wonderful compilation of books, music cassettes, games, products, and tools to help those who work with the elderly deal with stress, aging, caregiving, and other challenges of older adults.

CHAPTER REVIEW QUESTIONS

1 Does chronological aging determine psychological aging? Discuss your position.
2 Identify aspects of aging that may affect learning for elders.
3 Coping with a serious illness can be especially stressful for an elder. Discuss any resulting occupational shifts and what a COTA can do to help elders understand change.
4 What is learned helplessness, and what can COTAs do to help elders vulnerable to learned helplessness?

REFERENCES

1. Horton, S., Baker, J., Pearce, W., Deakin, J., 2010. Immunity to popular stereotypes of aging? Seniors and stereotype threat. Educational Gerontology 36 (5), 353-371.
2. Bennett, T., Gaines, J., 2010. Believing what you hear: The impact of aging stereotypes upon the old. Educational Gerontology 35, 435-445.
3. Etgen, T., Sander, D., Huntgeburth, U., Poppert, H., Förstl, H., Bickel, H., 2010. Physical activity and incident cognitive impairment in elderly persons. Archives of Internal Medicine 170 (2), 186-193.

4. Tufts University, 2002. You can't teach an old dog new tricks and other myths about the aging process. Tufts University Health & Nutrition Letter 20, 1-3.

5. Williamson, A., 2000. Gender issues in older adults' participation on learning: Viewpoints and experiences of learners in the University of the Third Age (U3A). Educational Gerontology 26, 49-66.

6. Bonder, B.R., Dal Bello-Haas, V., 2009. Functional Performance in Older Adults, 3rd ed. FA Davis, Philadelphia.

7. Teichner, G., Wagner, M., 2009. The Test of Memory Malingering (TOMM): Normative data from cognitively intact, cognitively impaired, and elderly patients with dementia. Archives of Clinical Neuropsychology 24 (3), 455-464.

8. Bergua, V., Fabrigoule, C., Barberger-Gateau, P., Dartigues, JF., Swendsen, J., Bouisson, J., 2006. Preferences for routines in older people: Associations with cognitive and psychological vulnerability. International Journal of Geriatric Psychiatry 21 (10), 990-998.

9. Robnett, R., Chop, W., 2010. Gerontology for the Health Care Professional, 2nd ed. Jones and Bartlett, Sudbury, MA.

10. Dohm, A., Shniper, L., 2007. Occupational employment projections to 2016. Monthly Labor Review. Retrieved June 10, 2010, from http://www.bls.gov/opub/mlr/2007/11/art5full.pdf.

11. American Association of Retired Persons, 2003. Staying ahead of the curve: The AARP work and career study [WWW page]. URL http://research.aarp.org/econ/multiwork.html.

12. Finch, J., Robinson, M., 2003. Aging and late-onset disability: Addressing workplace accommodations. Journal of Rehabilitation 69 (2), 38-42.

13. Gupta, J., Sabata, D., 2010. Maximizing occupational performance of older workers. OT Practice 15 (7), CE 1-8.

14. Gonzalez, E., Morrow-Howell, N., 2009. Productive engagement in aging-friendly communities. Journal of the American Society on Aging 33 (2), 51-58.

15. Atchley, R., 1999. Continuity and Adaptation in Aging: Creating Positive Experiences. Johns Hopkins University Press, Baltimore.

16. Canja, E., 2001. Aging in the 21st century: Myths and challenges. Executive Speeches, 16, 24-27.

17. Simone, P., Haas, A., 2009. Cognition and leisure time activities of older adults. Osher Lifelong Learning Institute 22-28.

18. Royeen, C., 1995. The human life cycle: Paradigmatic shifts in occupation. In: Royeen, C. (Ed.), The Practice of the Future: Putting Occupation Back into Therapy. American Occupational Therapy Association, Bethesda, MD.

19. Hays, P., Bernstein, I., 2001. The Hayes and Lohse Depression Scale: Validity evidence. Clinical Gerontologist 24 (1-2), 39-54.

20. Metcalfe, J,, 2010. Metacognition of agency across the lifespan. Cognition 116 (2), 267-282.

21. Lieberman, M.A., Tobin, S.S., 1983. The Experience of Old Age. Basic Books, New York.

22. Hayslip, B., 1983. The Aged Patient: A Sourcebook for the Allied Health Professional. Mosby, St. Louis.

23. Kielhofner, G., 2008. A Model of Human Occupation: Theory and Application, 4th ed. Lippincott Williams & Wilkins, Baltimore.

24. Davis, L., 1988. Coping with illness. In: Davis, L., Kirkland, M. (Eds.), ROTE: The Role of Occupational Therapy with the Elderly. The American Occupational Therapy Association, Rockville, MD.

25. Kubler-Ross, E., 1969. On Death and Dying. Macmillan, New York.

26. Kubler-Ross, E., Kessler, D., 2007. On Grief and Grieving: Finding Meaning of Grief Through the Five Stages of Loss. Scribner, New York.

27. Higgins, L., Mansell, J., 2009. Quality of life in group homes and older persons homes. British Journal of Learning Disabilities 37 (3), 207-212.

28. Taylor, M., 2003. Involvement in occupations among older adults with physical and functional impairments is influenced by positive belief and a sense of hope. Australian Occupational Therapy Journal 50 (2), 111-122.

29. Punwar, A., 2000. Elder care. In: Punwar, A.J., Peloquin, S.M. (Eds.), Occupational Therapy Principles and Practice, 3rd ed. Lippincott Williams & Wilkins, Philadelphia.

5

Aging Well: Health Promotion and Disease Prevention

CLAUDIA GAYE PEYTON AND YAN-HUA HUANG

KEY TERMS

health, occupation, occupational deprivation, occupational alienation, occupational imbalance, successful aging, wellness, health promotion, occupational form, occupational performance, disuse syndrome, prevention, primary prevention, secondary prevention, health and risk screening, tertiary prevention, nutrition/overweight/obesity, rest

CHAPTER OBJECTIVES

1. Discuss how occupational therapy (OT) practitioners—registered occupational therapist (OTR) and certified occupational therapy assistant (COTA)—can influence health through programs and services for individuals, organizations, communities, and populations.
2. Identify methods of screening and assessment used in promoting health and well-being among elders.
3. Describe **health promotion** activities that can be incorporated into practice with elders.
4. Describe theoretical models that emphasize the importance of participation in meaningful occupations to decrease the negative effects of **occupational imbalance, alienation and deprivation,** and the promotion and the integration of healthy life patterns and routines.

5. Explain how the *Healthy People 2010*[1] goals of increasing quality of life and reducing health disparities may be carried out through OT practitioner services and programs.
6. Discuss the ways in which poor health practices, inadequate nutrition, and lack of self-care contribute to the incidence and prevalence of preventable diseases and disabilities common to elderly populations.
7. Identify factors that contribute most to influencing elders to participate in wellness-focused activities.
8. Describe factors that contribute to poor nutrition and obesity in elderly populations.
9. Name several lifestyle patterns that contribute to the development of preventable diseases in elderly populations.

Grow young along with me!
Grow young along with me
The best is yet to be,
The last of life for which
The first is made.

(Adapted from Robert Browning by Ashley Montagu[2])

Al is an 87-year-old man who hopes to live to be 100 years old. His wife Irene is 77 years of age and is content to have a few quiet hours each day to read and write letters. Al and Irene have been married for 56 years and have three adult children. They moved into a planned retirement community last year to ensure a safe living arrangement for whoever of the two lives longer. Al and Irene moved from their home of more than 40 years to this new environment with the help of a family friend.

After moving into their new home, Al and Irene often complained of feeling tired because of the demands of adaptation to their new environment. During the next few months, they organized their lives in their new setting. They laughed and talked about the process of getting to know some of their new neighbors. Overall, the move went well, and Al and Irene experienced the usual trials of adaptation to a change in most aspects of their lives: new home, changes in daily habits, patterns of time use and routines, adjusting to a different climate and learning about their neighbors, and availability and access to community services.

Al and Irene are among America's fortunate well elderly. However, they are not without challenges. Al has been totally blind since he was 22 years of age. He has survived a cranial subdural hematoma, which was removed from the left side of his brain, and was recently treated with radiation therapy for prostate cancer. Irene has experienced many surgeries during the past 15 years, including a heart double bypass, cataract surgery, a hip replacement, a rotator cuff repair, and gallbladder removal.

These two elders enjoy a remarkable level of independence given their ages and medical histories. Some of this level of independence and relatively good health is a result of genetic endowment. In addition, lifestyle changes or other factors contribute to their good health such as regular exercise and a balanced, low-fat diet have influenced independence. Historically, they have not lived without health risk. Al and Irene smoked for some time but eventually quit at ages 55 and 52 years, respectively. They agreed to adjust their diets on the basis of some research that Al had read in his Braille health journals about the positive effects of reducing fat, sodium, and refined sugar intake. Their dietary habits changed approximately 28 years ago. About that same time, Al began walking regularly. Initially, he experienced pain from angina, which required him to stop walking, rest, and take nitroglycerin tablets prescribed by his doctor. After several weeks of daily walking and taking the prescribed medication, Al could finally complete a trip around the block without interruption. He increased the daily walks to eventually complete 2 miles each day, which he continues to maintain. At age 84 years he went to guide dog training school for 3 weeks to be suited with a new guide dog because his previous dog died. His new guide dog, Chelsea, helps Al stay independent and mobile. Irene often accompanies Al and Chelsea on their daily walk (Figure 5-1).

This scenario about Al and Irene's transition from working to living in a retirement community offers many opportunities to consider how OT practitioners might help elders experience the richness of continued health and well-being with interventions and advocacy aimed at the person in context at the individual, organizational, community, and political levels. Al and Irene are well elders going through an adaptive process involving considerable demand and risk to their health because of the many stressors associated with movement from a familiar surrounding

to the unknown of a retirement community situated in a different state. During their transition, the services of an OT practitioner would have been instrumental in facilitating adaptation to this new and unfamiliar community. The stress on Al to learn to navigate in his new home and neighborhood required considerable assistance in orienting his guide dog and familiarizing Al with new routes for his daily walks. Initially, Irene accompanied Al to offer support and guidance and to ensure his safety. Services offered through collaboration with OT practitioners would have been helpful and reduced health risks. To better understand the needs of elders experiencing similar circumstances, OT practitioners should consider evaluating the individual, the organization, and community to formulate a broad public health approach to interventions.

Since Al and Irene moved to a planned retirement community designed specifically to meet the needs of aging clients over age 55 years, some of the architectural and community adaptations needed to encourage and support occupational participation were included in the design of their home and neighborhood. Yet, in their case, little had been considered to accommodate the needs of blind and partially sighted elder residents. The community center and recreational group activities were not accommodating to a person without vision. Al did experience an increased sense of isolation when sighted retirees were unwilling to include him in card games at the community center because playing cards had been a source of pleasure and weekly socialization in his life before retirement. In this case, OT services and advocacy could be very instrumental in easing the transition through evaluation and interventions provided at the levels of person, community, and organization.

Health and well-being are intrinsically linked to participation in occupations that are meaningful. The risk of decline in health in this population emerges when barriers to participation exist. The outcome of occupational imbalance, alienation, or disruption in important life habits, patterns, and routines often lead to a sedentary lifestyle. A shift to sedentary living for well elderly can increase health risks associated with falling, limitations in mobility, increased likelihood of respiratory illness, and increased incidence of depression.

Al and Irene were able to overcome the barriers and challenges presented in their new environment despite increased stress associated with many adaptations. Services from OT practitioners in consultation with this planned retirement community would have improved the ease of their transition and reduced the risk to their health associated with such high demands on this elderly couple. OT practitioners play a vital role in support of elders and can serve as advocates in the development of policy and legislation to enhance life satisfaction and reduction of risk by creating systematic solutions to daily living challenges. Retirement communities designed to meet the needs of elderly populations have many

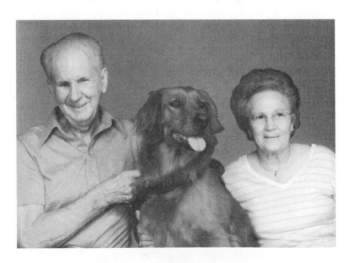

FIGURE 5-1   Al, Chelsea, and Irene.

necessary adaptations and safety devices in housing and neighborhood configuration but may lack services that help at-risk elderly continue to thrive once relocated.

This story could be about anyone. The later episodes of a life story itself depend, to some extent, on the self-care choices people make along the way. As health care providers, COTAs and OTRs can offer important health information and propose alternative lifestyle choices to elders. Society will increasingly look to health care providers for guidance and for models of healthful ways of living. This chapter describes the rationale for health promotion and disease or disability prevention programs that can be effective tools for use by COTAs working with elders.

CONCEPTS OF HEALTH PROMOTION AND WELLNESS IN OCCUPATIONAL THERAPY PRACTICE

The historical roots of OT philosophy and practice demonstrate the profession's long-standing belief in the value of occupation in promoting health and preventing functional loss caused by disease. Nelson and Stucky[3] reviewed important OT values over the decades and wrote, "The potency of occupation in promoting health has long been recognized; this recognition is the basis for the existence of the profession of occupational therapy" (p. 22). Since the inception of OT as a profession in 1917, its premise has been to promote a healthy balance of activities for those persons who seek intervention. Activities perceived by an individual to be meaningful occupations are believed to influence the state of actual or possible health and well-being. Gilfoyle[4] stated, "The therapeutic use of occupation to promote fullness of life is the basic value at the heart of our (professional) culture" (p. 400). The concepts of health and occupation are interrelated. Despite the various definitions and societal influences, the concept of occupation has remained centered on the value of activity

to maintain enthusiasm about living. In essence, humans find meaning in what they do.[4]

The value of occupation and the meaning of health are explicitly interrelated.[3,5-14] Nelson and Stucky[3] described "activation of function (occupation) as a main method of health promotion and disease prevention" (p. 21). Yerxa[14] further described this relationship between occupation and health in her working definition of occupation:

Occupations are units of activity which are classified and named by the culture according to the purposes they serve in enabling people to meet environmental challenges successfully. Some essential characteristics of occupation are that it is self-initiated, goal directed (even if the goal is fun or pleasure), experiential as well as behavioral, socially valued or recognized, constructed of adaptive skills or repertoires,[13] organized, essential to the quality of life experienced, and possesses the capacity to influence health. (p. 5)

Richard[15] suggested that health might be defined as "the ability to live and function effectively in society and to exercise self-reliance and autonomy to the maximum extent feasible, but not necessarily as total freedom from disease" (p. 79). Wilcox[11] defined health from an occupational perspective as "the absence of illness, but not necessarily disability; a balance of physical, mental, and social well-being attained through socially valued and individually meaningful occupation; enhancement of capacities and opportunities to strive for individual potential; community cohesion opportunities; and social integration, support, and justice, all within and as a part of sustainable ecology" (p. 110). Wilcox[12] advanced our perspective of the relationship between occupation and health by asserting that "occupation is clearly a pre-requisite to health" (p. 195), and that major risk factors to health include problems in occupational performance such as "occupational imbalance," "occupational deprivation," and "occupational alienation" (Table 5-1).

TABLE 5-1

Health Risk Factors

Health risk factors	Wilcox	Brownson and Scaffa
Occupational imbalance	Occurs when people engage in too much of the same type of activity, limiting the exercise of their various capacities (p. 195)	A lack of balance among work, rest, self-care, play, and leisure that fails to meet an individual's unique needs, thereby resulting in decreased health, well-being, or both (p. 657)
Occupational deprivation	When factors beyond them limit an individual's choice or opportunity (p. 195)	Prompted by conditions such as poor health, disability, lack of transportation, isolation, unemployment, homelessness, poverty, and so forth (p. 657)
Occupational alienation	When people are unable to meet basic occupational needs or use their particular capacities because of intervening sociocultural factors (p. 195)	A sense of estrangement and lack of satisfaction in one's occupations. Tasks or work perceived as stressful, meaningless, or boring may result in occupational alienation (p. 657).

Data from Wilcox, A. A. (1999). The Doris Sym Memorial Lecture: Developing a philosophy of occupation for health. *British Journal of Occupational Therapy, 62*(5), 191-198; and Brownson, C. A., & Scaffa, M. E. (2001). Occupational therapy in the promotion of health and the prevention of disease and disability statement. *American Journal of Occupational Therapy, 55*(6), 656-660.

Occupational engagement can have a profound and positive effect on the lives of elders who are well and living in the community and can improve life satisfaction among frail elders living in skilled nursing or assisted living environments. Habitual activities, those which are performed with consistency, can have a profound influence on health. "What people do is so much a part of the ordinary fabric of life that it is taken for granted and its health benefits are largely ignored" (p. 194).[12] Regular participation in a balance of meaningful daily occupations can prevent the development, occurrence, and progression of most disabling conditions. However, many elders have been typecast by society and health care professionals as being unable to improve their health status. This myth is detrimental to the health and well-being of older adults and dampens motivation to try to make small changes that could provide health improvements with small investments of time and effort.

Only in recent years has the literature associated with aging focused on healthy aging and long-term survival and moved away from medically oriented disease management. Recent literature suggests changing societal views of health and longevity. Promotion of "successful aging" (p. 107)[5] will likely replace past views of disease remediation and control. "Shifting the focus from disease management and survival to health through disease prevention, health maintenance, and health promotion provides great promise for occupational therapy practitioners" (p. 10).[16] The prevailing diseases contributing to morbidity and mortality among elderly people can be prevented through lifestyle changes.

Although leading causes of death or mortality, these diseases are also leading causes of morbidity or illness (Table 5-2). Morbidity can cause great suffering, occupational disruption, alienation, and cost. OT practitioners can educate clients about how to prevent or to control the long-range and deleterious effects of prevalent hazards to health and well-being. Nutrition, exercise, balance, and decreased stress, along with environmental adjustment for safety and management of medications, are a few examples of minor changes that can make long-range differences in health status. Regardless of age, unhealthy habits and patterns of living can be changed to improve health and to enhance life satisfaction.

Carlson and colleagues[5] asserted that "potentially controllable lifestyle factors play a crucial role in enabling people to experience healthy and satisfying lives well into old age" (p. 107). These authors proposed that an operational definition of aging in the future may in fact be the "disappearance of health" because careful living has such great potential to promote "successful aging" over a lifetime (p. 108).[5] Research conducted by Carlson and colleagues[5] provides insight into factors that lead to "successful aging" (p. 109) (Box 5-1). The concept that

BOX 5-1

Factors Contributing to Successful Aging

- Experiencing a sense of control over one's life
- Practicing healthy habits
- Achieving continuity with one's past
- Performing happy activities
- Participating in a social network of family and friends
- Exercising regularly
- Engaging one's mind in complex cognitive activities
- Stopping smoking
- Maintaining a healthy diet
- Consuming fewer calories
- Receiving preventive medical treatment
- Taking aspirin and antioxidant vitamins

Adapted from Carlson, M., Clark, F., & Young, B. (1998). Practical contributions of occupational science to the art of successful aging: How to sculpt a meaningful life in older adulthood. *Journal of Occupational Science, 5*(30), 107-118.

TABLE 5-2

Leading Causes of Death by Age Group by Percentage of the Total Number of Deaths: United States in 2002

Causes of Death by Age	55-64 Years	65-74 Years	75-84 Years	85+ Years
Cardiovascular disease	32.2%	35.4%	42.3%	51.7%
Malignant neoplasm	37.0%	34.0%	23.6%	11.7%
Chronic lower respiratory	4.5%	7.1%	6.8%	4.2%
Diabetes mellitus	3.8%	3.8%	3.2%	2.1%
Influenza and pneumonia	1.2%	1.6%	2.8%	4.8%
Alzheimer's disease	0.2%	0.8%	2.5%	4.3%
Motor vehicle accidents	1.5%	0.7%	0.5%	0.2%
Renal failure	1.3%	1.6%	1.7%	1.8%
Septicemia	1.2%	2.0%	1.4%	1.4%

Note: Adapted from the National Statistics Report, Volume 50, No. 15, September 16, 2002, responding to "Of the total number of deaths for all ages in each 'Cause of Death' what percentage was attributed to each age group?"

occupational therapy practitioners can "positively enhance lifestyle" (p. 299)[17] is in line with the projected goals of the U.S. Department of Health and Human Services (DHHS) for a healthy population as established in *Healthy People 2010*.[1] All OT personnel need to be aware of the major public health initiatives set forth in *Healthy People 2010*. The goals established in this document emphasize the need for increasing the quality of life of all people and prioritizing efforts leading to the achievement of a longer and healthier life for all citizens. Priority goals call for the elimination of health disparities on the basis of sex, race, ethnicity, disability, sexual orientation, education, income, or residence in a rural or urban setting.[1] These goals fit well with the needs of the current elder population. As discussed in this document, the first goal of *Healthy People 2010* is to increase the quality as well as the years of healthy life.[1] Here the emphasis is on the health status and nature of life, not just longevity. The emphasis on functional capacity and the satisfying productive life of our citizens parallels occupational therapy's focus on enabling engagement in a meaningful occupation, which supports and leads to productive and satisfying participation in life.[18]

OT practitioners have a responsibility and an opportunity to influence change in the quality of the lives of elders at the individual and also at the population levels by the implementation of health-promoting and wellness-centered programs. The 21st century is the time for needed health care reform, prompted by the urgency to reduce cost for care, and the time to return the responsibility for "successful aging" to the individual. Therapists should demonstrate leadership in helping individuals and communities plan health-promoting engagement in meaningful occupations as the path to a long and healthy life. "The organizing promise of occupational therapy emphasizes the important role of everyday activities or occupations in establishing routines and infusing meaning in daily life" (p. 13).[19]

Society is now better prepared to move toward health-centered, cost-effective approaches to prevention and wellness. Wellness has been defined as "a dynamic way of life that involves actions, values, and attitudes that support or improve both health and quality of life" (p. 656).[18] An important projected outcome of health promotion is personal wellness.

Assisting people at all ages to actively participate in taking responsibility for improving the quality of their health is not unique to OT, but it has been a prominent value held by OT personnel since the inception of the profession. Health can be enhanced, and disease can be prevented through occupation. Occupational therapy interventions are provided at the institutional, legislative, and personal level of care, thus encouraging health at the environmental and personal levels. OT practitioners can be instrumental in creating healthy environments through consultation with state, city, and institutional levels of care. Political, economic, and practice environments need health professionals who understand the essential relation between occupation and health. As Mary Reilly[20] stated in her Eleanor Clark Slagle Lecture of 1961, "Man through the use of his hands as energized by mind and will, can influence the state of his own health" (p. 2). Wilcox[12] further elaborated this association between occupation and health status stating, "Ultimately, health is created and lived by people within the settings of everyday life; where they learn, work, play, and love" (p. 195).

Health Risks and Their Effects on Occupational Engagement and Participation

Substantial research evidence supports the need for increased health promotion and disease prevention activities for elders. Hickey and Stilwell[21] maintain that the primary goal of health promotion programs for elders should be focused on prevention of "the progression of disease and the risks of disability and death that health promotion should be designed to help older persons maintain their functional independence and autonomy for as long as possible" (p. 828). Brownson and Scaffa[18] define health promotion as "any planned combination of educational, political, regulatory, environmental, and organizational supports for actions and conditions of living conducive to the health of persons, groups, or communities, or—more simply—the process of enabling people to increase control over and to improve their health" (p. 657). Health promotion is focused on preventive efforts. The promotion of health must be considered in the contexts in which people live and relate to others. OT practitioners contribute to health promotion by first identifying those factors at the individual, group, organizational, community, and policy levels that interfere with occupational engagement. Wilcox[13] suggests:

> *What people can do, be, and strive to become is the primary concern and that health is a by-product. A varied and full occupational lifestyle will coincidentally maintain and improve health and well-being if it enables people to be creative and adventurous physically, mentally, and socially. (p. 315)*

As described by Fidler and Fidler,[22] humans develop through "doing" and through "doing" become individuals. Through occupations, people adapt in both healthy and unhealthy ways. At times people learn maladaptive ways of living through occupational patterns. In daily practice settings, OT practitioners meet elders who can benefit from assistance in making positive choices to improve the quality of their health. Some elders do not recognize that the quality of their lives can change with even minor adjustments in their lifestyles. During daily therapeutic interactions, OT practitioners have an opportunity to influence their clients' considerations of healthy lifestyles and assist them in improving the quality of their lives. Encouraging exploration of health-promoting activities and providing educational information to elders and their families may help motivate them to take actions that promote health and limit the potential for occupational deprivation, alienation, or imbalance associated with current habits (see Table 5-1). Elders are frequently uninformed or believe that changes later in life may offer few benefits. Helping elders understand the tremendous potential for healthy outcomes associated with small changes in daily routines can make the difference between future independence and debilitating dependence.

Nelson and Stucky[3] suggest that "one's occupational patterns of self-care and interests comprise ... occupational situations (occupational forms) that are health promoting and disease preventing" (p. 22). The occupational form to which Nelson and Stucky refer includes the environmental context of the individual's life. The context is composed of physical and sociocultural characteristics that stimulate the individual to choose an occupational performance. For example, an elder who lives in a retirement village may choose to play golf (occupational form) because there is a golf course on the grounds (physical characteristic), and this is where most people at that village socialize (sociocultural characteristic). The value that the person places on the occupational form gives meaning and purpose to the individual's choice of actions. This sense of purposefulness is the motivator or stimulus that results in participation in activities such as playing golf. Playing golf on Thursday mornings may involve habituation of many occupational performance skills such as socialization, preparation of refreshments for guests, and the actual performance of playing golf. This involves motor performance, cognition, and other complex functions. Activation of an interest in and performance of a cherished occupation help the person establish a positive and continuous cycle or habit pattern. Fidler and Fidler[22] theorize that imagery is linked with purpose. They perceive that actions related to achievement are a result of conceptualizing an image before taking action. Thus, mental imagery adds purpose to occupations. Mental images are constructed before taking action and facilitate the person's participation (Figure 5-2).

The actual enjoyment of participation in chosen occupations or activities is referred to as *intrinsic motivation*.[23] Baking a pie, walking a dog, and gardening are intrinsically motivated occupations. Actions taken toward a goal provide feedback that, if positive, may inspire continued participation in the activity or similar activities. Feedback may take the form of wonderful tomatoes from a well-nurtured garden or excitement from the completion of a small but meaningful project. Recognition from meaningful others can serve as a source of encouragement, and their enjoyment may motivate continued occupational engagement. Each interaction sets up the potential for additional involvement in occupations that ultimately contribute to growth, development, self-confidence, and improved self-esteem. Conversely, negative feedback or

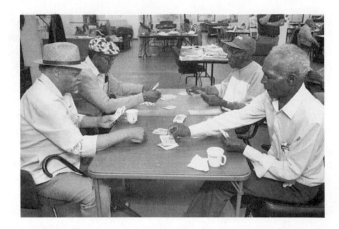

FIGURE 5-2 Purposefulness stimulates participation in activities such as the hobby of playing cards.

experiences may result in a cycle of feelings of fear, helplessness, humiliation, and failure.[3]

The outcome of an effective health promotion program is the enhancement or maintenance of function in activities of daily living (ADL), instrumental activities of daily living (IADL), and overall life satisfaction. The need for elders to maintain functional capacity, interests, and participation in meaningful occupations has been demonstrated by research findings suggesting that losses occur in the ability to perform ADL functions as a result of the disabling effects of disuse syndrome, a common sequel to physical and cognitive disabilities. Approximately 14.2% of elders living in the community experience difficulty completing one or more ADL because of health-related problems. Approximately 21.6% of elders report difficulties with IADL.[24] Research shows that the need for assistance in the completion of ADL and IADL increases with age.[1] Recently the U.S. Surgeon General and the Centers for Disease Control and Prevention have reported that limitations in ADL and IADL functions are key indicators of declining health and wellness.[25] These authors go on to suggest that OT practitioners' "prevention-oriented interventions" should include a public health focus by including evaluation data on population health. OT service should reflect population level services and describe population limitations, such as in the area of ADL, by measuring numbers of limits experienced in ADL as reflected in a simple scale of "no problem," "1-3" difficulties, or "3 or more" difficulties. Measures of this type can be collected and data banked to large scale and multi-site studies reflecting indicators of population health.

McMurdo and Rennie[26] report that elders in nursing homes who participated in a seated exercise group for 8 weeks showed significant improvement in grip strength, chair-to-stand time, and function in ADL, and they also experienced decreased feelings of depression. "Even very elderly residents of nursing homes can benefit from

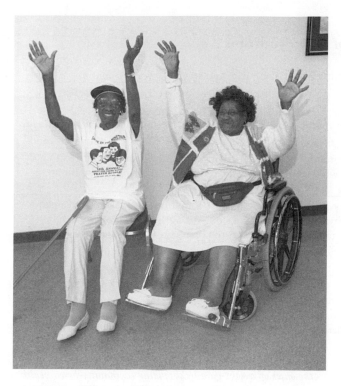

FIGURE 5-3   Elders can benefit from regular seated exercise.

TABLE 5-3

Nutritional Standards Based on the Modified Food Pyramid for 70+ Adults

	Original pyramid	Modified pyramid
Calcium, vitamin D, and vitamin B$_{12}$ supplements	Not included	Daily
Fats, oils, and sweets	Use sparingly	Use sparingly
Milk, yogurt, and cheese groups	2-3 servings	3 servings
Meat, poultry, fish, dry beans, eggs, and nut groups	2-3 servings	≥2 servings
Vegetable group	3-5 servings	≥3 servings
Fruit group	2-4 servings	≥2 servings
Bread, cereal, rice, and pasta group	6-11 servings	≥6 servings
Water	Not included	8 servings

Note: Food pyramids compared to show differences in nutritional standards for adults and older adults of 70+ years.

Data from Functional performance in older adults. (2009). In B. R. Bonder & V. Dal Bello-Haas (Eds.). *Cardiovascular and Pulmonary Function*. Philadelphia: FA Davis; and Russell, R. M., Rasmussen, H., & Lichtenstein, A. H. (1999). Modified guide food pyramid for people over seventy years of age. *Journal of Nutrition, 129,* 751-753.

participation in regular seated exercise and can improve in functional capacity" (p. 12) (Figure 5-3).[26] Unfortunately, research literature indicates that "despite the known importance of and preponderance of media attention to exercise, more than 60% of women over the age of 60 participate in little or no sustained physical activity of at least moderate intensity" (p. 602).[27] Studies further indicate a correlation between fear of falling and a loss of physical endurance and strength. Nuessel and Van Stewart[28] found that "35% of community dwelling elderly avoided doing things they wanted to do because they were afraid of falling" (p. 4). The fear of falling impaired choices of occupation and life satisfaction. Evidence supports that exercise programs can reduce falls by increasing endurance, improving balance, and improving confidence. Rubenstein and colleagues[29] concluded:

A simple program of progressive resistance exercises, walking, and balance training can improve muscle endurance and functional mobility in elderly men with chronic impairments and risk factors for falls. In addition, this study provides new evidence on the complex relationship between physical activity and falls: exercise participants significantly increased their physical activity, yet experienced fewer falls per unit of activity. (p. 319)

Exercise has an effect on the mind and the body. As the body grows stronger, the individual's self-confidence increases, and with positive changes come greater options for engagement in meaningful occupations.

Nutrition and Overweight or Underweight Elders

Balanced nutrition is essential to health maintenance and prevention of disease, obesity, and malnutrition in elders. OT practitioners can provide elders with important information and encouragement to ensure a balanced intake of foods high in nutrients and low in saturated fats, refined sugars, and sodium (Table 5-3). IADL include the activities of shopping and meal preparation. Selection and preparation of foods with high nutritional value, high fiber content, and portion control contribute to the maintenance of a healthy weight. The intake of a balanced diet can prevent or slow the progression of serious conditions, including diabetes, hypertension, and cardiovascular disease.

Table 5-3 provides a contrast of two food pyramids showing a recommended adjustment in the number of servings and balance of food groups for younger adults in contrast to recommendations for persons age 70 years and older. This table highlights the importance of adequate fluid intake and vitamin regimes to support healthy aging for persons 70+ years.

OT practitioner assessment of personal factors associated with nutrition and weight is important in intervening in cases of underweight or overweight. Issues that may impact eating and thus contribute to poor nutrition and underweight status include loss of teeth, low tolerance for

TABLE 5-4

Possible Causes of Poor Nutrition

Changes in senses	Appetite may diminish because of decline in the senses of taste and smell.
Effects of medications	Medications may change appetite or cause discomfort because of nausea or other medication effects.
Poor dental health	Loss of teeth, sore tongue or lips, chewing endurance, or poor fitting dentures may make eating difficult.
Financial burden	Reduced grocery expenses and living on a fixed income may limit the ability to pay for nutritious foods.
Lack of transportation	Lack of available private or public transportation, hazardous driving conditions, and winter road conditions coupled with fears of falling while entering and navigating shopping areas may limit access to nutritional foods.
Physical difficulty	Seniors may become frail as they age, especially when dealing with conditions such as fibromyalgia, arthritis, vertigo (dizziness), and disability. Physical pain and poor strength can make even simple tasks (opening a can, peeling fruit, and standing long enough to cook a meal) excessively challenging.
Forgetfulness	May limit food variations in food choices or reduce intake of adequate amounts of food due to confusion and memory loss associated with Alzheimer's disease or other cognitive losses.
Depression	Loss or decrease in appetite can be due to feelings of loneliness, apathy, or as a result of losses of physical capacity or the death of loved ones.

Adapted from Beattie, L., & Nichols, N. (2010). Nutrition and the elderly. Retrieved January 4, 2010, from www.resources/nutrition-articles. asp?id=869.

textured foods, jaw pain when chewing, and medication side effects such as nausea, dry mouth, and fear of choking. Other issues that contribute to undereating can include impaired cognition and forgetfulness, loss of physical stamina and sufficient endurance to prepare a simple meal, depression and limited vision, or pain due to arthritis. At the environmental level, limited access to a grocery store, lack of transportation either public or private, and limited or declining finances may reduce nutritional intake and cause loss of weight (Table 5-4). OT intervention strategies can be instrumental in helping seniors overcome barriers to adequate nutritional intake through client-centered intervention plans.

Obesity is another nutrition-related health problem experienced by many older adults and "the leading modifiable risk factor contributing to early mortality" (p. 680).[30] High levels of dietary fats, carbohydrates, sugars, and sodium are most associated with the development of obesity. A reported 65% of adults are overweight secondary to diet and a sedentary lifestyle.[24,31] Obesity has a significant negative effect on quality of life, self-concept and self-esteem, health, and longevity. Among adults who experience a high rate of obesity are African American women at 53%, followed by Hispanic women at 51%, and Caucasian women at 39%.[32] Health conditions that occur as a result of obesity include diabetes, cardiac and peripheral vascular disease, hypertension, and stroke. The sequel of such diseases creates added disability and occupational imbalance as a result of conditions such as peripheral neuropathy, retinopathy, joint pain and weakness, and reduced endurance.

OT practitioners can be vital to interventions at the primary, secondary, and tertiary levels of care. OT practitioners can provide primary prevention of

the onset of weight gain by providing community-based health education and wellness programs. Secondary prevention combines health education with progressive and graded energy expenditure required to perform meaningful occupations (e.g., caloric expenditure during routine activities of daily living) and, at the level of tertiary prevention when the OT practitioner focuses on the occupational needs of the client once the condition becomes chronic.[33] (p. 64)

Interventions might include assisting the client in formulating weekly nutritionally balanced menus, shopping for food and encouraging planning of meals that incorporate socialization, pleasant food aromas, and meaningful rituals.

Poorly balanced nutritional intake can contribute to the development of many preventable conditions that affect health and quality of living. As suggested previously, careful assessment of areas of OT practice associated with nutrition can lead to the prevention of serious diseases and limit the progression of existing diseases. Obesity and malnutrition can be addressed through the careful assessment of client factors and environmental contexts.

The benefit of health promotion and disease prevention programs may be best understood by considering the most common risks to the health of elders. Physical and psychological risks to health and well-being, which are common to elders after retirement, are numerous. The DHHS has identified the following chronic conditions as those that most frequently "contribute to difficulty in independently performing activities of daily living (ADL) and instrumental activities of daily living (IADL) functions: arthritis, hypertension, hearing impairment, heart disease, cataracts, diabetes, orthopedic impairments, tinnitus, and diabetes" (p. 12).[24]

Other authors suggest that the decline seen in aging may not be caused by age but by a condition referred to as *disuse syndrome*. This term alludes to the detrimental effects of sedentary living and the limited use of capabilities in the development of chronic and debilitating conditions. Approximately 50% of symptoms currently associated with aging, such as increases in body fat and decreases in endurance, lean body mass, and strength and flexibility, are actually a result of hypokinesia, a disease of disuse.[34-37] Experimental immobilization has been noted to cause decreases in musculoskeletal, cardiovascular, and metabolic functions similar to those seen with aging. Thus, a portion of the loss of physiological integrity in elders may be attributable to disuse syndrome.[38] According to Nied and Franklin,[39] "Muscle strength declines by 15% per decade after age 50 and 30 percent per decade after age 70; however, resistance training can result in 25 to 100% strength gains in older people" (p. 421). Jett and Branch[40] conducted The Framingham Study of Disability and found that 45% of elderly women age 65 years and older and 65% of women older than age 75 years cannot lift 10 pounds. Loss of strength and endurance among the elderly is most often an outcome of disuse or inactivity and is a serious impediment to daily living function and increased potential for falls. Results of this study identified numerous risk factors and lifestyle habits, which now have

led researchers to study how genes contribute to common metabolic disorders such as obesity, hypertension, diabetes, and even Alzheimer's disease.

PREVENTION AND HEALTH PROMOTION AMONG ELDERS

COTAs working with elders should be familiar with categories of prevention used by public health agencies. Many health problems of elders are especially suited for prevention planning. Impaired mobility, injury from falls, sensory loss, adverse medication reactions, disuse syndrome, depression, malnutrition, alcohol abuse, hypertension, and osteoporosis are serious problems of the elderly that can be prevented or postponed through prevention-focused health education efforts.[41] Brownson and Scaffa[18] assert that "occupational therapy practitioners provide health promotion services, which typically involve 'lifestyle redesign' or the development of supports for healthy engagement in occupations as a means of preventing the unhealthy effects of inactivity" (p. 656).

Prevention and health promotion strategies are generally organized into three categories: primary, secondary, and tertiary (Table 5-5). Primary prevention focuses on reducing the risk for disease before its onset. Primary

TABLE 5-5

	Roles of OT Practitioners in Prevention and Primary Health Promotion	
	Prevention	**Health promotion**
Primary	"Education or health promotion strategies designed to help people avoid the onset and reduce the incidence of unhealthy conditions, diseases, or injuries. Primary prevention attempts to identify and eliminate risk factors for disease injury and disability (e.g., fall prevention programs for community dwelling seniors)."[43]	"Activities that target the well population and aim to prevent ill health and disability through, for example, health education (often targeting lifestyles and behavioral change) and for legislation (such as smoking policies)."[13]
Secondary	"Early detection and intervention after disease have occurred and is designed to prevent or disrupt the disability process (e.g., education and training regarding eating habits, activity levels, and prevention of disabilities secondary to obesity)."[43]	"Directed at individuals and groups in order to change health damaging habits and/or to prevent ill health moving to a chronic or irreversible stage and, where possible, to restore people to their former state of health. Health promotion practices at this level might involve empowering individuals to take more control of their health and/or community development approaches that encourage structural and environmental changes."[13]
Tertiary	"Refers to treatment and services designed to arrest the progression of a condition, prevent further disability, and promote social opportunity (Patrick, Richardson, Starks, Rose, & Kinne [1997]) (e.g., "groups for older adults with dementia to prevent depression, enhance socialization, and improve quality of life)."[43]	"Takes place with individuals who have chronic conditions and/or are disabled and is concerned with making the most of their potential for healthy living. This might include client-centered approaches, such as those used in rehabilitation or the management of chronic disease programmes."[13]

Note: The variation in definitions of prevention and health promotion definitions as adapted from Scriven, A., & Atwal, A. (2004). Occupational therapists as primary health promoters: Opportunities and barriers. *British Journal of Occupational Therapy*, 67(10), 425; and Scaffa, M. E., Van Slyke, N., & Brownson, C. A. (2008). Occupational therapy services for the promotion of health and the prevention of disease and disability. *American Journal of Occupational Therapy*, 62(6), 695.

preventive efforts with elders may consist of facilitation of lifestyle changes and the use of necessary medications to reduce the development of life-threatening conditions such as cardiovascular disease and stroke. Primary prevention programs include immunization, accident prevention, exercise, nutritional counseling, and smoking and alcohol cessation.[41] A critical primary prevention effort should be focused on the prevention of falls in elders because accidents are the sixth leading cause of death among people older than 65 years.[42]

Primary Prevention

OT practitioners may represent the first line of primary prevention for well, homebound, or institutionalized elders. *Primary* prevention is defined as "education or health promotion strategies designed to help people avoid the onset and reduce the incidence of unhealthy conditions, diseases, or injuries. Primary prevention attempts to identify and eliminate risk factors for disease injury and disability" (p. 696).[43] Primary prevention might include fall prevention programs for community dwelling seniors. In this capacity, COTAs have an opportunity to influence change in elders' awareness of health risks. By assisting elders to develop or to return to interests that stimulate increased activity and mobility, COTAs may help reduce ill effects of a sedentary lifestyle or disuse syndrome. Many disabilities of elders start with disuse and are preventable. Studies have demonstrated the long-reaching effects of regular exercise in the prevention of weakness and fatigue, which interfere with independence in ADL functions.[26,29,36,38,44-46] Exercise also has helped prevent obesity, thus reducing consequent hypertension and diabetes. A daily or three times weekly exercise program or regular participation in an activity such as walking or chair aerobics can significantly reduce the potentials for falls,[29] which is a serious threat to the health and well-being of elder clients. In addition, exercise is related to improvements in elders' psychological well-being.[47]

Noteworthy outcomes exist between clients involved in rote exercise and those participating in personally meaningful occupations. Rote exercise involves the repetition of a particular movement, such as lifting a 10-lb dumbbell 10 times to develop strength, endurance, or skill. Personally meaningful occupations are intrinsically motivated—that is, characteristic of activities that have a purpose in and of themselves, such as picking up a 10-lb infant. Yoder and colleagues[48] found that elderly women engaged in significantly more exercise repetitions with intrinsic activities such as food preparation than with a rote exercise program. Riccio and colleagues[8] later found that the use of imagery as a cue facilitated more exercise repetitions than a rote exercise program. In this study, elders imagined that they were using first the right and then the left arm to pick apples and place them in a basket.[8] In a study of elder women performing a kicking task, Thomas[49] found that the subjects who did the task with the actual

balloon performed better than those doing rote exercise or those using imagery. He concludes that using actual tasks that have meaning might result in a better performance. A number of other studies have investigated the effects of a purposeful use of materials to facilitate movement beyond the benefits of rote exercise.[48,50-56] These studies validate OT beliefs regarding the health-enhancing value of participation in actual occupation and point to the limited effects of simulated activities. Meaningful activities important to the client help generate motivation and excitement that rote exercise cannot. Thus, clients gain more from exercises that are "embedded in meaningful, purposeful occupations" (p. 19)[3] than from a rote regimen of exercise, unless such regimen is part of a meaningful daily routine.[57,58]

Fall prevention is another critical aspect of primary prevention practices that OT practitioners can facilitate. A home or an institutional environmental assessment may identify many fall hazards for elders (see Chapter 14). A Matter of Balance is a well-researched fall prevention program that COTAs can implement in practice. The program uses a multi-model approach that addresses physical, social, and cognitive factors affecting a fear of falling.[59] The use of the Fall Risk Factor Screening Checklist[60] can contribute significant information to fall prevention.

Secondary Prevention

Secondary prevention efforts consist of "identification and treatment of persons with early, minimally symptomatic diseases to improve outcomes and maintain health" (p. 299).[61] Secondary prevention emphasizes "early detection and intervention after disease has occurred and is designed to prevent or disrupt the disability process" (p. 696).[43] An example of secondary prevention with elderly might include education and training regarding eating habits, activity levels, and the prevention of disabilities secondary to obesity. Early detection of hypertension and cancers may prevent early disability and mortality. Vision and hearing deficits are also preventable at times if detected early, as are breast and cervical cancers and depressive or substance use disorders. COTAs can contribute to early detection of serious conditions that contribute to disability and interfere with ADL and IADL functions by reminding elders of the importance of annual examinations, such as the mammogram and Papanicolaou (Pap) test. Recommendations for health and risk screening of elder populations can be different in some cases. For example, the DHHS does not provide specific suggestions for upper age limits of Pap testing but suggests recommending discontinuation after age 65 if the woman's previous regular screenings were consistently normal.[62]

Minority group and non-ambulatory elderly women are at a greater risk for serious health conditions, including increased incidence of cervical cancer and cervical cancer mortality. "Women age 35 years or older, who are racial or ethnic minorities and low income, are at increased risk for invasive cervical cancer due to lower likelihood of Pap smear screen test" (p. 1).[63] Reduced access to health care and to culturally appropriate health care messages has increased the risk for cervical cancers in both Hispanic and Vietnamese women in the United States. "Cervical cancer occurs most often among minority women, particularly Asian American (Vietnamese and Korean), Alaska Native and Hispanic" (p. 2).[64]

Analysis of invasive cervical cancer incidences by age and stage at diagnosis indicated that, except for women aged 20-29 years, incidences for Hispanic women were significantly higher than those for non-Hispanic women, the incidence for Hispanic women was second only to that of Vietnamese women, which was more than twice the incidence for Hispanics. For Hispanic and non-Hispanic women, approximately 30% of all new invasive cervical cancers diagnosed among women ages <50 years were at an advanced stage; among women who were aged 50> years, advanced stage cervical cancer represented 52% of new diagnoses.[65] (p. 1068)

Iezzoni and colleagues[66] found that women with lower extremity mobility difficulties are significantly less likely than other women to receive screening and preventive services such as mammograms and Pap smears. Because of the multiple and complex factors that contribute to health disparities among elderly, disabled, and minorities, health care providers at all levels should have an awareness of and a concern for the overall health of their clients. All health care providers should assume responsibility for encouraging and reminding elderly clients to schedule regular physical examinations.

Careful observation of functional capabilities may facilitate early detection of changes in elders' capabilities. OT practitioners can monitor loss or change of sensory capacity during routine interactions with elders (see Chapters 15 and 16). COTAs also may be instrumental in educating family members to monitor elders for changes in mood or cognitive functioning that may influence independence in ADL and IADL. Changes in mood or cognition can be associated with poor nutrition or dehydration, which can be prevented or remediated (see Chapter 21). Changes also may indicate reactions to or side effects of medications or more serious physiological changes that require medical evaluation and attention (see Chapter 13).

Tertiary Prevention

Tertiary prevention refers to preventing the progression of existing conditions (see Table 5-5). It "relates to functional assessment and rehabilitation both to reverse and to prevent progression of the burden of illness" (p. 3).[41] Brownson and Scaffa[18] have defined *tertiary* prevention as "treatment and service designed to arrest the progression of a condition, prevent further disability, and promote social opportunity" (p. 656). An example of tertiary prevention initiated by the OT practitioner could be the intervention of a homebound elder who is experiencing limitations because of the pain of arthritis. The COTA would provide education about self-care activities such as joint protection and energy conservation to prevent further deterioration of arthritic joints. In addition, joint mobility can be facilitated through regular participation in a hobby within the elder's range of tolerance. Performing energy conservation activities also may assist the elder in feeling in control of his or her daily routine. Control of pain and implementation of environmental adaptations and work simplification could assist the elder and encourage greater involvement in meaningful occupations and engagement with others.

ROLE OF THE CERTIFIED OCCUPATIONAL THERAPY ASSISTANT IN WELLNESS AND HEALTH PROMOTION

OT practitioners play a critical role in promotion of health and prevention of disease among elders. Health education facilitates health promotion, disability reduction, and illness prevention.[67,68] Chronic illnesses that affect ADL and IADL functions are more often related to lifestyle, genetic predisposition, and environmental exposure than to age alone. Frequently, elders must change behaviors to prevent disability from developing or progressing. Professional evaluation, intervention, and educational programs implemented by COTAs can foster such life-enhancing changes. A health behavior questionnaire can determine the need for intervention through health education activities (Box 5-2). Hickey and Stilwell[21] stated, "The overall goal of health promotion in the elderly should be to prevent the progression of disease and the risks of disability and death" (p. 823). Health promotion should also help elders maintain functional autonomy as long as possible. Glantz and Richman[45] proposed guidelines for the development of wellness programs for elders who emphasize goals of "optimum achievement and maintenance of competence and independence" (Box 5-3).

Hettinger[69] developed the following ABCs of the wellness model in OT, which may assist COTAs in encouraging their elder clients to learn to improve and maintain their health:

- Attitude that includes actively pursuing wellness and ADL that promote satisfaction and quality of life.
- Balancing productive activity, positive social support, emotional expression, and environmental interactions.
- Controlling health through education about behaviors that lead to wellness.
- This model encourages COTAs to serve as mentors, coaches, and educators.

The American Occupational Therapy Association (AOTA) published a position statement entitled "Occupational Therapy Services in the Promotion of Health and

BOX 5-2

Prevention Behavior Questionnaire

1. Name some behaviors in your life that you believe endanger or compromise your health.
2. How much control do you have to change them? (circle one)
   a. some b. little c. none
3. Do you participate in some form of physical activity on a regular basis? (circle one)
   a. yes b. no
4. What activities do you participate in? (circle all that apply)
   a. walking b. swimming c. gardening d. other
5. How often in a week do you engage in these activities? (circle one)
   a. daily b. twice c. three times d. other
6. How much time do you devote to these activities? (circle one)
   a. less than 30 minutes b. 1 hour c. 2 hours d. other
7. Rate the level of stress in your life. (circle one)
   a. very high b. high c. moderate d. occasional
   e. very low
8. What do you do to relieve stress in your life? (circle all that apply)
   a. hobbies b. exercise c. drink alcohol d. smoke
   e. other(s)
9. How many meals do you eat each day? (circle one)
   a. three b. two c. one d. less than one
10. Do you usually eat alone or with others? (circle one)
    a. alone b. with others
11. What do you consider your weight to be? (circle one)
    a. too high b. average c. too low
12. Do you monitor your daily fat intake? (circle one)
    a. yes b. no
13. How many servings do you have each day from the following food groups? (circle your answers)

a. bread and cereal	1	2	3	4	more
b. fruits and vegetables	1	2	3	4	more
c. meat	1	2	3	4	more
d. beans, peas, tofu	1	2	3	4	more
e. milk	1	2	3	4	more
f. dairy products	1	2	3	4	more

14. Is it necessary for you to monitor your blood cholesterol level? (circle one)
    a. yes b. no

15. Do you monitor your sodium intake? (circle one)
    a. yes b. no
16. Have you fallen recently? (circle one)
    a. in the past week   b. in the past month
    c. in the past 3 months   d. in the past 6 months
    e. in the past 9 months   f. in the past year
    g. in the past 18 months
17. If so, how many times have you fallen? (circle one)
    a. 1 b. 2 c. 3 d. other
18. Have you scalded or burned yourself recently? (circle one)
    a. in the past week   b. in the past month
    c. in the past 3 months   d. in the past 6 months
    e. in the past year   f. in the past 18 months
19. Do you have arthritis? (circle one)
    a. yes b. no
20. Do you have a heart disease? (circle one)
    a. yes b. no
21. Do you have cancer? (circle one)
    a. yes b. no
22. Do you have difficulty catching your breath
    a. when walking? (circle one)   yes   no
    b. when climbing stairs? (circle one) yes   no
    c. when sitting? (circle one)   yes   no
23. Do you have asthma or emphysema? (circle one)
    a. yes b. no
24. Do you have difficulty
    a. bending over to remove items from   yes   no
       low cabinets? (circle one)
    b. going up or down stairs? (circle one) yes   no
    c. getting up from a bed or chair?   yes   no
       (circle one)
25. Do you need assistance to walk? (circle one)
    a. yes b. no
26. What distance can you safely walk without assistance or stopping? (circle one)
    a. less than 1 block   b. 1 block   c. 1/4 mile
    d. 1/2 mile   e. 1 mile   f. other
27. What would you like to change about your health?

Adapted from Lohman, H., & Peyton-Runyon, C. (1991). Intergenerational experiences for occupational therapy students. *Physical Occupational Therapy in Geriatrics*, 2(10), 17.

the Prevention of Disease and Disability."[43] This statement calls on OT practitioners to be involved with health promotion and disease prevention. Three main roles have been outlined: (1) Promoting healthy lifestyles, (2) Emphasizing occupation as an essential element of health promotion strategies, and (3) providing interventions not only with individuals, but also with populations (p. 696).[43]

The Well Elderly Study, conducted at the University of Southern California, illustrates a successful model for OT wellness programming.[6,70-72] Indications of this well-designed study validate that the lives of elders living in an urban community can be enhanced through reactivation of interests and participation in meaningful occupations. The content of the program, based on elders' input,

Wellness Program for Elders

Program goals
- Enhance awareness of the positive effect of wellness on health at any age
- Promote awareness of the sensory changes that occur as aging progresses
- Improve knowledge of food consumption and effects on health
- Improve decision-making skills
- Encourage self-responsibility for health
- Encourage independence and environmental mastery
- Maximize a positive focus
- Heighten awareness of behaviors that inhibit health and perpetuate disease
- Encourage independence in self-care

Possible topics
- Personal nutrition
- Exercise: sitting, standing, low-impact aerobics
- Planning of health screenings, including annual screening for cancer
- Smoking cessation
- Activities: exploring interests
- Stress and effects on the heart
- Relaxation
- Responsibility for health
- Sensory loss and safety: eliminating hazards

Adapted from Glantz, C. H., & Richman, N. (1996). The wellness model in long-term care facilities. *Quest*, 7, 7.

provided detailed instructions about areas such as transportation, safety, social relationships, and finances. Interventions through education and self-discovery processes were offered in both individual and group contexts. A key outcome of this study was demonstrating the importance and health-enhancing effects of reengaging elderly participants in meaningful occupations. Elderly participants assigned to a group facilitated by occupational therapists had better outcomes than those participants assigned to the control group or those participants of the group facilitated by a volunteer nonprofessional.[6] Overall, this prevention program found that occupational therapist-led groups offered a significant benefit to positive outcomes measures, and that therapy helped the elders improve health and functional ability necessary for community living.[72] The results of this program have been sustained over time.[70]

Health education empowers elders to take increasing responsibility for their health. COTAs have many opportunities across practice domains to provide health education programs for elders. Health promotion can occur through individual or group education efforts.[70] COTAs can rely on their knowledge of group skills to facilitate discussion of materials and to encourage group development and cohesion. Generally, health-related topics include awareness building activities to heighten elder valuing and understanding of the benefits of exercise, cardiac risk reduction, methods of management of arthritis, stroke prevention, immunization, osteoporosis, cancer, early detection, home safety, assistive devices, and sensory changes that occur with aging.[73] Discussion topics educate elders about leading causes of functional limitation, disability, and death, thereby facilitating the potential to change behaviors and improve quality of life.

In their research of effects of an exercise program for older adults, Hickey and Stilwell[21] pointed out evidence to inspire OT practitioners to provide health-promoting activities. "The older adult responds to exercise training in the same manner as a young adult, with a 10% to 20% increase in cardiovascular fitness and strength gain of between 50% and 174%, depending on the extent of reconditioning" (p. 823). Such research shows that it is never too late to begin exercising.

CONCLUSION

The United States is moving into an era of health care reform that focuses on improving the quality of life for the lowest cost. The OT practitioner's role in this reform is to promote personal responsibility for health through facilitation of self-discovery activities that can enhance interest and participation in meaningful occupations. In addition, the belief that small adaptive changes can improve the quality of a person's life regardless of age or disability must be encouraged. As Ashley Montagu[2] wrote in *Growing Young*, "The youth of the chronologically young is a gift; growing young into what others call 'old age' is an achievement, a work of art: It takes time to grow young" (p. 194).

▮ CHAPTER REVIEW QUESTIONS

1 Give examples of primary, secondary, and tertiary prevention functions of certified occupational therapy assistants (COTAs) working with elders.
2 Name two activity groups that could be used with each classification of prevention and health promotion.
3 Explain how health and occupation are interrelated.
4 How do occupational imbalance, deprivation, and alienation contribute to the development of disease and disability?
5 How can occupation be characterized as health promoting?
6 Describe the role of OT practitioners in wellness and health promotion program implementation.
7 How can COTAs assist elderly in preventing or overcoming occupational imbalance, occupational deprivation, and occupational alienation?

REFERENCES

1. U.S. Department of Health and Human Services, 2000. Healthy People 2010: Understanding and Improving Health. U.S. Government Printing Office, Washington, DC.
2. Montagu, A., 1981. Growing Young. McGraw-Hill, New York.
3. Nelson, D.L., Stucky, C., 1992. The roles of occupational therapy in preventing further disability of elderly persons in long-term care facilities. In: Levine, R.A., Rothman, J. (Eds.), Prevention Practice: Strategies for Physical Therapy and Occupational Therapy. WB Saunders, Philadelphia.
4. Gilfoyle, E.M., 1986. The future of occupational therapy: An environment of opportunity. In: Ryan, S.E. (Ed.), The Certified Occupational Therapy Assistant. Slack Inc, Thorofare, NJ.
5. Carlson, M., Clark, F., Young, B., 1998. Practical contributions of occupational science to the art of successful aging: How to sculpt a meaningful life in older adulthood. Journal of Occupational Science 5 (30), 107-118.
6. Jackson, J., Carlson, M., Mandel, D., Zemke, R., Clark, F., 1998. Occupation in lifestyle redesign: The well elderly study occupational therapy program. American Journal of Occupational Therapy 52 (5), 326-334.
7. Johnson, J.A., 1986. Wellness: A Context for Living. Slack Inc, Thorofare, NJ.
8. Riccio, C.M., Nelson, D.L., Bush, M.A., 1990. Adding purpose to the repetitive exercise of elderly women through imagery. American Journal of Occupational Therapy 44, 714-717.
9. Scaffa, M.E., Reitz, S.M., Pizzi, M.A., 2010. Occupational Therapy in the Promotion of Health and Wellness. FA Davis, Philadelphia.
10. Speake, D.L., 1987. Health promotion activity in the well elderly. Health Values 11, 6-25.
11. Wilcox, A.A., 1998. Occupation for health. British Journal of Occupational Therapy 61 (8), 340-345.
12. Wilcox, A.A., 1999. The Doris Sym Memorial Lecture: Developing a philosophy of occupation for health. British Journal of Occupational Therapy 62 (5), 191-198.
13. Wilcox, A.A., 2006. An Occupational Perspective of Health, 2nd ed. Slack Inc, Thorofare, NJ.
14. Yerxa, E.J., 1993. Occupational science: A new source of power for participants in occupational therapy. Journal of Occupational Science 1, 1-3.
15. Richard, B., 1991. Workplace literacy technology for nursing assistants. Journal of Health Occupations Education 6 (1), 73-85.
16. Hanft, B., 2002. Promoting health: Historical roots-renewed vision. OT Practice 2, 10-15.
17. Richards, S.E., 1998. The Carson Memorial Lecture 1998: Occupation for health—and wealth? British Journal of Occupational Therapy 61 (7), 294-300.
18. Brownson, C.A., Scaffa, M.E., 2001. Occupational therapy in the promotion of health and the prevention of disease and disability statement. American Journal of Occupational Therapy 55 (6), 656-660.
19. Scott, A.H., Butin, D.N., Tewfik, D., Burkhardt, M.A., Mandel, D., Nelson, L., 2001. Occupational therapy as a means to wellness with the elderly. Physical & Occupational Therapy in Geriatrics 18 (4), 3-22.
20. Reilly, M., 1962. Occupational therapy can be one of the great ideas of 20th century medicine: Eleanor Clarke Slagle lecture. American Journal of Occupational Therapy 16, 1-9.
21. Hickey, T., Stilwell, D.L., 1991. Health promotion for older people: All is not well. Gerontologist 31 (6), 822-828.
22. Fidler, G.S., Fidler, J.W., 1978. Doing and becoming: Purposeful action and self-actualization. American Journal of Occupational Therapy 32 (5), 305-310.
23. Florey, L., 1976. Development through play. In: Schaefer, C. (Ed.), The Therapeutic Use of Child's Play. Jason Aronson, New York.
24. U.S. Department of Health and Human Services, 2001. A profile of older Americans [WWW page]. URL http://www.hhs.gov.
25. Mallinson, T., Fischer, H., Rogers, J.C., Ehrlich-Jones, L., Chang, R., 2009. The Issue Is—Human occupation for public health promotion: New directions for occupational therapy practice with persons with arthritis. American Journal of Occupational Therapy 63, 220-226.
26. McMurdo, M.E., Rennie, L., 1993. A controlled trial of exercise by residents of old peoples' homes. Age-Ageing 22 (1), 11-15.
27. Caserta, M.S., Gillett, P.A., 1998. Older women feelings about exercise and their adherence to an aerobic regimen over time. Gerontologist 38 (5), 602-609.
28. Nuessel, F., Van Stewart, A., 1999. Literary exemplars of illness: A strategy for personalizing geriatric case histories in clinical settings. Physical and Occupational Therapy in Geriatric Medicine 16, 33-46.
29. Rubenstein, L.Z., Josephson, K.R., Trueblood, P.R., Loy, S., Harker, J.O., Pietruszka, F.M., et al., 2000. Effects of a group exercise program on strength, mobility, and falls among fall-prone elderly men. Journal of Gerontology Series A, Biological Sciences and Medical Sciences 55A (6), M317-M321.
30. American Occupational Therapy Association, 2006. AOTA's statement on obesity. American Journal of Occupational Therapy 60 (6), 680.
31. U.S. Department of Health and Human Services, 2006. Nutrition and overweight. Retrieved December 29, 2009, from www.healthypeople.gov/Document/HTML/Volume2/19NUtrition.htm.
32. Centers for Disease Control and Prevention, 2008. Prevalence of obesity in adults. Retrieved December 28, 2009, from http://www.cdc.gov/nchs/data/databriefs/db01.pdf.
33. Blanchard, S.A., 2010. Variables associated with obesity among African-American women in Omaha. American Journal of Occupational Therapy 63 (1), 58-68.
34. Drinkwater, B.L., 1988. Exercise and aging: The female master athlete. In: Journal of Public Health, Brown, C., Voy, R.O. (Eds.), Sports Science Perspectives for Women: Proceedings from the Women and Sports Conference. Human Kinetics, Chicago.
35. Hjort, P.F., 2000. Physical activity and health in elderly—walk on. Tidsskr Nor Laegeforen 120 (24), 2915-2918.
36. Schuster, C., Petrosa, R., Petrosa, S., 1995. Using social cognitive theory to predict intentional exercise in post-retirement adults. Journal of Health Education 26, 1-14.
37. Smith, M.T., 1995. Implementing annual cancer screening for elderly women. Journal of Gerontological Nursing 2 (7), 12-17.
38. Fiatarone, M.A., Evans, J.E., 1990. Exercise in the oldest old. Topics in Geriatric Rehabilitation 5 (2), 63-77.
39. Nied, R.J., Franklin, B., 2002. Promoting and prescribing exercise for the elderly. American Family Physician 65, 419-426.
40. Jett, A.M., Branch, L.G., 1981. The Farmington Disability Study: ii. Physical disability among the aging. American Journal of Public Health 71, 1211-1216.
41. Webster, J.R., 1992. Prevention, technology, and aging in the decade ahead. Topics in Geriatric Rehabilitation 7, 4.
42. Centers for Disease Control and Prevention (CDC), 2002. Deaths: Final data for 2000. National Vital Statistics Reports 50 (15), 1-120.
43. Scaffa, M.E., Reitz, S.M., Pizzi, M.A., 2010. Occupational therapy in the promotion of health and wellness. Philadelphia, PA: F. A. Davis.
44. Butler, R.N., Davis, R., Lewis, C.B., Nelson, M.E., Strauss, E., 1998. Physical fitness: How to help older patients live strong and longer. Geriatrics 53 (9), 26-28, 31, 32, 39, 40.
45. Glantz, C.H., Richman, N., 1996. The wellness model in long-term care facilities. Quest 7, 7-11.

46. Lohman, H., Givens, D., 1999. Balance and falls with elders: Application of clinical reasoning. Physical and Occupational Therapy in Geriatrics 16, 17-32.

47. Stewart, A.L., Mills, K.M., Sepsis, P.G., King, A.C., McLelland, B.Y., Roitz, K., et al., 1998. Evaluation of CHAMPS: A physical activity program for older adults. Annals of Behavior and Medicine 19 (4), 353-361.

48. Yoder, R.M., Nelson, D.L., Smith, D.A., 1989. Added-purpose versus rote exercise in female nursing home residents. American Journal of Occupational Therapy 43, 581-586.

49. Thomas, J.J., 1996. Materials based, imagery based, and rote exercise and occupational forms: Effects on repetitions, heart rate, duration of performance, and self-perceived rest periods in well elderly women. American Journal of Occupational Therapy 50 (10), 783-789.

50. Bloch, M.W., Smith, D.A., Nelson, D.L., 1989. Heart rate, activity, duration, and effect in added purpose versus single-purpose jumping activity. American Journal of Occupational Therapy 43, 25-30.

51. Heck, S.H., 1988. The effect of purposeful activity on pain tolerance. American Journal of Occupational Therapy 42, 577-581.

52. Kircher, M.A., 1984. Motivation as a factor of perceived exertion in purposeful versus nonpurposeful activity. American Journal of Occupational Therapy 38, 165-170.

53. Miller, L., Nelson, D.L., 1987. Dual purpose activity versus single purpose in terms of duration on task, exertion level, and affect. Occupational Therapy in Mental Health 7, 55-67.

54. Sakemiller, L.M., Nelson, D.L., 1998. Eliciting functional extension through the use of a game. American Journal of Occupational Therapy 52 (2), 150-157.

55. Schmidt, C.L., Nelson, D.L., 1996. A comparison of three occupational forms in rehabilitation patients receiving upper extremity strengthening. Occupational Therapy Journal of Research 16 (3), 200-215.

56. Thomas, J.J., Rice, M.S., 2002. Perceived risk and its effect on quality of movement in occupational performance of well-elderly individuals. Occupational Therapy Journal of Research 22 (3), 104-110.

57. Wagstaf, S., 2005. Supports and barriers for exercise participation for well elders: Implications for occupational therapy. Physical and Occupational Therapy in Geriatrics 24 (2), 19-33.

58. Fredman, L., Bertrand, R., Martire, L., Hochberg, M., Harris, E., 2006. Leisure-time exercise and overall physical activity in older women caregivers and non-caregivers from the Caregiver-SOF study. Preventive Medicine 43 (3), 226-229.

59. Boston University Center for the Enhancement of Late-Life Function, 2000. Fear of falling: An emerging health problem. Roybal Program Brief, pp. 1-6. Retrieved December 22, 2003, from http://www.applied-gerontology.org/BUBrief.pdf.

60. Carlson, A., 1996. Fall prevention in Hilo, Hawaii. OT Week 10 (36), 14, 15.

61. Garner, D.J., Young, A.A. (Eds.), 1993. Women and Healthy Aging: Living Productively in Spite of It All. Haworth Press, New York.

62. Centers for Disease Control and Prevention (CDC), 2002b. Cervical cancer and Pap test information. The National Breast and Cervical Cancer Detection Program [WWW page]. URL http://www.cdc.gov/cancer/nbccedp/info-cc.htm.

63. Washington State Department of Health., 2002. Early cervical cancer detection important for women of color and women living in rural areas [WWW page]. URL http://www.doh.wa.gov/Publicat/2002_News/02-06.htm.

64. Agency for Healthcare Research and Quality, 2003. Breast and cervical cancer research highlights [WWW page]. URL http://www.ahcpr.gov/research/breastca.htm.

65. Centers for Disease Control and Prevention (CDC), 2002. Invasive cervical cancer among Hispanic and non-Hispanic women—United States, 1992-1999. Morbidity and Mortality Weekly Report 51 (47), 1067-1070.

66. Iezzoni, L.I., McCarthy, E.P., Davis, R.B., 2001. Use of screening and prevention services among women with disabilities. American Journal of Medical Quality 16 (4), 135-144.

67. Pinch, W.J., 1993. Health promotion and the elderly. NSNA/Imprint 40 (2), 83-86.

68. Poland, B., Krupa, G., McCall, D., 2009. Settings for health promotion: An analytic framework to guide intervention design and implementation. Health Promotion Practice 10 (4), 505-516.

69. Hettinger, J., 1996. The wellness connection. OT Week 10, 12, 13.

70. Clark, F., Azen, S.P., Carlson, M., Mandel, D., LaBree, L., Hay, J., et al., 2001. Embedding health promoting changes into the daily lives of independent-living older adults: Long-term follow-up of occupational therapy intervention. Journals of Gerontology-Series B: Psychological Sciences and Social Sciences 56B (1), P60-P63.

71. Clark, F., Azen, S.P., Zemke, R., Jackson, J., Carlson, M., Mandel, D., et al., 1997. Occupational therapy for independent-living older adults: A randomized control trial. Journal of the American Medical Association 278 (16), 1321-1326.

72. Mandel, D.R., Jackson, J.M., Zemke, R., Nelson, L., Clark, F.A., 1999. Lifestyle Redesign: Implementing the Well Elderly Program. The American Occupational Therapy Association, Bethesda, MD.

73. Mount, J., 1991. Evaluation of a health promotion program provided at senior centers by physical therapy students. Physical and Occupational Therapy in Geriatrics 10 (1), 15-25.

6

The Regulation of Public Policy for Elders

HELENE L. LOHMAN, CORALIE H. GLANTZ, AND NANCY RICHMAN

KEY TERMS

advocacy, care planning, Inpatient Rehabilitation Facility Patient Assessment
Instrument (IRF-PAI), managed care, Medicare, Medicaid, Medicare Administrative
Contractures (MACs), Minimum Data Set (MDS), Older Americans Act, Outcome and
Assessment Information Set (OASIS), Omnibus Budget Reconciliation Act of 1987,
prospective payment system, skilled services/unskilled services

CHAPTER OBJECTIVES

1. Describe payment systems that influence practice developed as a result of public policy.
2. Clearly define the role of the certified occupational therapy assistant (COTA) within the Omnibus Budget Reconciliation Act (OBRA) regulations.
3. Describe the prospective payment system and COTA practice in different practice settings.
4. Learn ways that input of the COTA into the various screening measurements and care plans is valuable for an integrated team approach.
5. Learn the importance of advocacy for the occupational therapy (OT) profession.
6. Understand how COTAs can become more aware of public policy trends and changes that impact practice.

Marie is a COTA who was invited to speak to a class of occupational therapy assistant (OTA) students about public policy. Marie began her lecture by stating, "Today we are going to discuss the influence of public policies such as Medicare and Medicaid on occupational therapy practice." Marie scanned the faces of the students. They appeared to look disinterested. She observed students gazing out of the window, using their laptops to access the Internet, and a few stifling yawns. "Okay," Marie slowly stated as she reorganized her thoughts, "I have decided to first share my story. In 1998 I was working for a rehabilitation company that contracted at several skilled nursing facilities in the area. I was making a very high salary—over $50,000 a year for a COTA just out of school! I didn't think to question where that salary came from. Later I realized that to pay my salary the contract company must have been getting money from somewhere and that money possibly came from charging large amounts to Medicare for patient interventions. You see, Medicare was paid retrospectively based on what was charged after interventions. Today, as you will learn, cost measures have been established called 'prospective payment,' or payments paid ahead of time based on preestablished amounts. Anyway, one day your instructor Sally brought the OTA students

to observe patients at the facility where I was employed. During a free moment Sally asked me if I had considered the impact of the Balanced Budget Act on my practice. 'No,' I responded. 'I assume that my contract company will take care of me.' You see, I never paid much attention to public policy. I found that subject far removed from my life, and, frankly, I was not interested. I was only interested in my patient interventions. My ignorance about public policy ended up affecting me personally, as in 1999, soon after the new law became instituted in skilled nursing facilities, I lost my job. The contract company reorganized because of the changes and I was among several rehabilitation personnel who lost their jobs. In a blink of an eye I went from earning $50,000 a year to being on unemployment, which was difficult as a single mother." Marie paused and looked around the classroom and observed a group of attentive students gazing back at her. Marie continued, "I found myself reflecting about my career. What was I going to do? Should I enter another area of practice? The more I thought about it I realized that my passion was in working with elders. So I did a huge amount of networking and within 3 months I was lucky to be hired by a skilled nursing facility as an in-house staff therapist. Practice changed so I had to learn the prospective payment system. It was difficult at first but, eventually, I adjusted.

Now I pay close attention to policy trends, I have become involved in the state and national occupational therapy organizations, and I try to influence change by writing letters and making phone calls to the senators and congress people from this district. I even visited my representative while attending a conference in Washington, D. C. I never again want to be uninformed about public policy and its impact on practice. Practice will change again with any health reforms. I urge you to think beyond the classroom to how public policy can impact your lives as citizens and your professional practice." As Marie continued with her lecture, the class was attentive.

As Susan, a member of the class, listened to the lecture she felt overwhelmed. She was thinking, *How can I ever learn all this material so I can apply it in practice? How can I become more aware of changes in public policy that impact practice?* These concerns bothered her so much that she asked Marie about them. Marie answered "I am glad that you asked those questions. Pay close attention now and review what I teach. In a year from now when you are out in practice, this information will fall into place. Be sure to learn how documentation and billing is done in your practice setting and don't be shy about asking any clarification questions. Also, for those of you going into practice settings that receive Medicare payment be aware of the Centers for Medicare & Medicaid Services (CMS) website, which is a good resource, and there are many other resources online that can help you." A year later Susan is employed as a COTA at a skilled nursing facility (SNF). She is very excited and feels prepared to work with the residents. As she overviews what she will do, she remembers the questions she had asked Marie and decides to review her course notes, study the policy and procedural manual at the facility, and question anything she needs further clarification about.

INTRODUCTORY CONCEPTS

Public policy develops from legislation at the federal and state levels and represents society's values. (MacClain, 1996, personal communication) For example, the Medicare Act, which resulted in a national health insurance plan for elders, was enacted in 1965. Medicaid, a combined federal and state insurance program that addresses the health care needs of the indigent, was enacted in 1966. Both measures were enacted at a time when civil rights was valued by society and was reflected in many government acts that passed around that time such as the Developmental Disabilities Act and the Vocational Rehabilitation Act. The language of public policies is meant to be general. The specifics about each public policy are in its regulations, which COTAs need to comprehend because they directly impact OT practice. COTAs working in an SNF should understand the Omnibus Budget Reconciliation Act (OBRA) of 1987 and the prospective payment system

(PPS) resulting from the Balanced Budget Act (BBA) of 1997 to provide appropriate care and be effective treatment team members. COTAs also must have a direct understanding of how Medicare and Medicaid is regulated in any setting to ensure that intervention they provide is reimbursed by third-party payers.

In this chapter, COTAs will overview key payment sources and related public policies that they will work with in practice settings. Medicare, Medicaid, OBRA, and the Older Americans Act (OAA) are examples of such public policies. The intent of this chapter is to provide an introduction and overview of these key public policies that influence therapy practice and how they are regulated. New policies are enacted, such as for health reform, and policies can also change with amendments and regulations. Therefore, not every specific detail of changes will be or can be included. For example, in 2010 a new Minimum Data Set (MDS) 3.0 and Resource Utilization Groups (RUG-IV) in SNFs was instituted and newer versions will come out in the future. With each version there are changes. One change with the MDS 3.0 was making it more client centered.[1] With the chapter readers will get a strong foundation for practice and then will need to keep updated with changes through resources provided in the chapter. The chapter begins by discussing health care trends in the United States and then goes into specifics about federal public policies that influence OT practice and overviews health reform and Medicare. The chapter concludes with suggestions for COTAs on ways to keep up with public policy trends as well as promote changes with public policy through advocacy.

HEALTH CARE TRENDS IN THE UNITED STATES

Health care in the United States is transforming rapidly as a result of a quickly changing society. A knowledge of these health care trends helps with understanding policies that develop. Previously, the family physician was the sole provider of health care. The physician knew individuals throughout their lives and treated them as whole people rather than as illnesses or diseases. Recently, the health care industry has undergone an extensive period of fragmented approaches to service delivery. The current trend, especially for elders, is toward comprehensive, cost-effective health care. Consumers want simplified access to a range of services with predictable costs. This has led to the emergence and growth of various public and private sources of health coverage. With health care reform systems will become even more integrated, and there will be a strong focus on quality, cost-efficient care. Electronic records as a result of public policy (e.g., the HITECH Act [P.L.111-5][2]) will become a reality. Because health care is a large part of the gross national product and costs have been consistently increasing along with a growing aged population, ways to monitor costs with the major programs such as Medicare, Medicaid, and Social Security will be

TABLE 6-1

Parts	Part A	Part B	Part C	Part D
	Hospital insurance	Medical insurance (voluntary benefit)	Medicare advantage	Prescription drug coverage
Facilities covered				Individual Voluntary Coverage
Acute care hospital	X	X	X	
Hospice	X	X	X	
Long-term care hospital	X	X	X	
Inpatient rehabilitation facility	X	X	X	
Skilled nursing facility	X	X	X	
Home health agency	X	X	X	
Hospital outpatient		X	X	
Comprehensive outpatient rehabilitation facility		X	X	
Rehabilitation agency		X	X	
Partial hospitalization in hospital or community mental health center		X	X	
Inpatient psychiatric facility	X		X	
Physician's office		X	X	
Payment	Prospective Payment System (PPS) instituted differently in many of the listed systems	Medicare physician fee schedule		

Adapted from AOTA, 2008. Reimbursement and Regulatory Policy Fact Sheet: Medicare basics. American Occupational Therapy Association, Bethesda, MD. www.aota.org/Practitioners/Reimb/Pay/Medicare/ FactSheets/37788.aspx

continually evaluated and discussed on the national agenda. The following sections describe public regulated sources.

Public Regulated Sources

Public regulated sources include Medicare, Medicaid, federal and state employee health plans, the military, and the Veterans Administration. Medicare and Medicaid are often accessed by the elder clients whom COTAs treat and are discussed in the following sections. Please refer to Table 6-1 for an overview of the Medicare system that COTAs may work with.

Medicare

Medicare, or Title 18 of the Social Security Act, was first implemented in 1966. As part of the Social Security Amendment of 1965, the Medicare program was created to establish a health insurance program to supplement retirement, survivors, and disability insurance benefits. Originally, Medicare covered most people age 65 years and older. However, since then the program policy has expanded to cover other groups of people, including those entitled to disability benefits for at least 24 months, those with end-stage renal disease, and those who elect to buy into the program.[3] Medicare is the largest entitlement program in the United States, and other insurance companies often follow the same standards as set up by Medicare.

Parts of the medicare program and occupational therapy practice Medicare is divided into four parts (A, B, C, and D).[3] Parts A, B, and C directly influence OT practice. Part A refers to hospital insurance. It covers "inpatient care in hospitals, including critical access hospitals, and skilled nursing facilities (not custodial or long-term care). It also helps cover hospice care and some home health care. Beneficiaries must meet certain conditions to get these benefits."[4] OT practitioners (registered occupational therapists [OTRs] and COTAs) follow Medicare beneficiaries under Part A in many settings both inpatient and outpatient (see Table 6-1). In most settings, therapy is reimbursed under a PPS. PPS are rates established in advance, based on the anticipated resource usage by the Medicare beneficiary and are "a pre-determined fixed amount."[5] These rates can be based by time, such as a per diem amount provided per case or per episode. Rates can also be established by a patient classification system such as with the diagnostic-related groups (DRGs) used in inpatient hospitals or the resource utilization groups (RUGs) used in SNFs.[6]

Medicare Reimbursement under Part A as a PPS system was first instituted in inpatient acute hospital settings in 1983 based on a DRG patient classification system, and this system continues today.[7] PPS in each system (e.g., hospital, home health, SNF) is instituted differently, so

TABLE 6-2

Screening Tools and Payment Specifics for Home Health, Inpatient Rehabilitation Facilities, and Skilled Nursing Facilities (Medicare Part A)

	Home health	Inpatient rehabilitation facilities	Skilled nursing facilities
Screening tool	Home Health: Outcome and Assessment Information Set (OASIS)	Inpatient Rehabilitation Facilities: Inpatient Rehabilitation Facility Patient Assessment Instrument (IRF-PAI)	Skilled Nursing Facilities: Minimum Data Set (MDS 3.0)
Payment system	Prospective Payment System (PPS) based on Home Health Resource Groups (HHRGs)	PPS based on Case Mix Group (CMGs)	PPS based on Resource Utilization Categories (RUGs)

Adapted from AOTA. (2008).

COTAS will need to understand the specific system they work in. For example, in inpatient hospitals costs are bundled into the PPS rate. Some of the systems have a specific screening tool, such as the minimum data set (MDS) in SNFs. For an overview of screening tools and payment systems for Part A in home health, inpatient rehabilitation facilities, and SNFs, refer to Table 6-2.

Medicare Part B is the medical insurance that covers "doctors' services and outpatient care. It also covers some other medical services that Part A doesn't cover, such as some of the services of physical and occupational therapists, and some home health care."[8] Part B is a voluntary benefit, which is paid for by monthly premiums. The cost of this premium continues to increase. It is important for COTAs to be aware that Medicare beneficiaries pay 20% of their Part B costs unless they have purchased supplemental insurance.

Therapists can provide therapy and bill under Part B in many outpatient settings, including physicians' offices, outpatient, home health services, assisted living, SNFs, and comprehensive outpatient rehabilitation.[7] Certain regulations are required to be followed with Part B, such as getting physician certification and a plan for therapy that is approved by the physician. Therapy services are billed under a physician's fee schedule using the Physician's Current Procedural Terminology (CPT) codes. CPT codes are revised annually, and the amount of reimbursement is calculated on the basis of a number of factors. COTAs in collaboration with the OTR decide how to code delivered intervention. Codes describe outcomes. They may be service codes that are billed only once per day regardless of the amount of time spent in delivering the procedure. Service codes include evaluation, reevaluation, splint application, and most modalities. Timed codes are the majority of the codes applicable to intervention provided by the COTA. Multiple units of timed codes can be delivered during a day of intervention. They are based on 15-minute units, and Medicare regulations guide how to calculate the units. For example, to count as 1 unit therapists follow a client between 8 and 22 minutes. This is also known as the *8-minute rule*, and Medicare requires

that time be accurately recorded for timed codes. (Please refer to CMS Internet manual 100.4, Chapter 5, Section 20.2. for more information.)

HCPCS Level II are another type of coding used for "products, supplies, and services not included in the CPT codes, such as ambulance services and durable medical equipment, prosthetics, orthotics, and supplies."[9] CMS has also instituted for Part B claims national coding methodologies to avoid misuse of billing procedures based on a policy called the Correct Coding Initiative (CCI).[10,11] The purpose of these edits is "to prevent improper payment when incorrect code combinations are reported."[10]

Currently Medicare beneficiaries who purchase Part B coverage have a *therapy cap*, or set financial amount, per year that they can use for all of their outpatient rehabilitation costs (occupational therapy, physical therapy, and speech therapy), except for hospital outpatient costs, which is exempt from the therapy cap. Over the years, the American Occupational Therapy Association (AOTA)[12] has advocated for adding an exception process to extend coverage for certain conditions that may warrant more therapy, and AOTA is working on a permanent fix for the therapy cap. (More information on therapy caps can be found in IOM 100-04, Chapter 5, Section 10.2.)

Part C "are health plans offered by private companies approved by Medicare."[13] Part C includes the basic services covered by parts A and B and is covered by a variety of payment types such as managed care, fee for service, and medical savings accounts. Some plans have offered more benefits than the traditional Medicare plans. Medicare Part D is the outpatient prescription drug coverage, an optional benefit. Although this part of the law does not directly influence occupational therapy practice, therapists may want to read more about it on the CMS website.

GENERAL GUIDELINES FOR OT PAYMENT AND INTERVENTION

Table 6-3 overviews examples of justifiable therapy service. Professional therapy intervention should be developed according to client needs relative to the complexity and intensity of required intervention. Intervention plans

TABLE 6-3

Justification for Professional Therapy Service	
Patient example	**Justification**
Hilde was admitted into an SNF to recuperate from hip replacement surgery. In addition, she was to learn to ambulate with a walker and independently perform ADL functions, particularly her own dressing. Once Hilde learned these skills, she might return to her retirement home apartment and receive home health care to ensure her continued progress and safety.	The immediate or short-term potential for progress toward a less intensive or lesser skilled service area exists.
Hilde was depressed and the COTA primarily treated her for depression rather than the total hip replacement. However, intervention may be considered skilled if the COTA could demonstrate that the intervention was directly related to motivating the client to safely perform ADL functions.	The philosophy and plan of intervention must realistically focus on achievement of outcomes for the specific phase of rehabilitation, such as being an inpatient in a skilled facility.
The COTA focuses on Hilde's intervention on going home with safety considerations.	Intervention also must focus on the plan for the next expected phase such as outpatient or home care.
During intervention, the COTA should address short-term deficits in safely performing ADL functions. The OT intervention should also take into account the performance component of the client's difficulty	Intervention is expected to address the type and degree of deficits and effects of other problems in relation to the short-term or interim goals with problem solving.
The COTA would thoroughly document changes in Hilde's status and her motivational level.	The therapist must emphasize variances in the elder's response to intervention and new developments.

ADL, activities of daily living; COTA, certified occupational therapy assistant; OT, occupational therapy; SNF, skilled nursing facility.

should be based on function and must integrate the plan of care. Intervention should be reinforced by other disciplines, such as skilled nursing. The client's prior level of function, mobility, and safety in addition to self-care deficits are primary and essential indicators for professional intervention and must be reflected in assessments.[14] COTAs should understand and follow specific guidelines to receive payment and not have a claim denied, such as receiving a denial for not having the physician sign off on the plan of care.

Refer to the Medicare Benefit Policy Manual 100-02[15] for specifics about occupational therapy coverage. Also refer to the personnel qualifications for occupational therapy assistants, which are discussed in the 2008 Physician Fee Schedule.[16] See the Federal Register of November 27, 2007,[17] for the full text. See also the correction notice for this rule, published in the Federal Register on January 15, 2008.[18]

SKILLED AND UNSKILLED THERAPY

The concept of skilled and unskilled therapy must be understood to obtain reimbursement from Medicare for OT intervention. Skilled care involves specific guidelines. For example, in SNFs care is covered if performed under the supervision of a professional and ordered by a physician and provided on a daily basis. Care "must be reasonable and necessary for the treatment of a patient's illness or injury" and "reasonable in terms of duration and quality."[19] Examples of unskilled services would be exercises that are repetitive in nature, or passive exercises

to maintain range of motion or strength that do not require the involvement of skilled rehabilitation. Usage of heat as a "palliative and comfort measure" and routine assistance in dressing, eating, or going to the toilet, and positioning in bed should be considered as unskilled services (Table 6-4).[19]

Although a client's diagnosis is a valid factor in deciding the need for skilled services, it should never be the only factor considered. The key issue is whether the skills of a therapist are needed for the required services. Skilled therapy services cannot be denied on the basis of diagnosis. This was clarified in a CMS Program Memorandum as it relates to therapy services needed by individuals with a diagnosis of Alzheimer's disease or other dementias.[20] Before this memorandum, there had been many denials on the basis of having the diagnosis of Alzheimer's disease. (Refer to the Internet Medicare Benefit Policy Manual[19] for more information about skilled and unskilled services.)

MEDICARE ADMINISTRATIVE CONTRACTURES

Since the inception of Medicare, the Centers for Medicare and Medicaid Services (CMS) has contracted out vital program operational functions (claims processing, provider and beneficiary services, appeals, etc.) to a set of contractors known as Medicare Fiscal Intermediaries (FIs) and Carriers. Currently, with contract reform throughout the United States, Medicare claim review and payment are monitored by Medicare Administrative Contractors (MACs). MACs determine local coverage determinations

TABLE 6-4

Skilled Occupational Therapy Services	
Patient example	**Justification**
Linferd: An 89-year-old client who recently had a stroke. Prior level of function was independent living at home. Because of hemianopsia and problem-solving difficulties, Linferd requires moderate assistance with ADL functions that require use of upper and lower extremities. He is motivated to do OT intervention.	Recent condition Identifiable functional deficits in performance areas with requiring moderate assistance with dressing and grooming upper and lower extremity
Gertrude: A 72-year-old client who recently had a total hip replacement. She is unable to safely dress and requires education in hip safety precautions. The COTA provides instructions for lower extremity dressing and other ADL functions. Intervention includes teaching safety precautions.	Recent condition (hip surgery) Safety concerns Identifiable functional deficit in lower extremity dressing
Fred: A 92-year-old client who recently sustained a right wrist fracture. He is right hand dominant. The client was independently performing ADL functions before his wrist was fractured. He now requires moderate assistance with ADL functions because of decreased ROM in the right upper extremity. The COTA provides a home ROM program and instruction in ADL functions.	Recent injury Functional deficits with ADL (dressing, feeding, and grooming) caused by difficulty with the performance component of ROM Prior level of independence Skilled expertise of the COTA needed to teach home ROM program

ADL, activities of daily living; COTA, certified occupational therapy assistant; OT, occupational therapy; ROM, range of motion.

(LCDs). "An LCD is a decision by a Medicare administrative contractor (MAC) whether to cover a particular service."[21] Payment coverage from each MAC can vary, so it is important for COTAs to become familiar with their area MAC and pay attention to LCDs. COTAs can go to their MAC website to determine claims processing information, educational options, and any regulation changes.

WORKING WITH MEDICARE AND RELATED REGULATIONS IN DIFFERENT PAYMENT SYSTEMS

COTAs work with Medicare beneficiaries in many different systems, including SNFs, home health, inpatient rehabilitation facility, hospital outpatient, comprehensive outpatient rehabilitation facility (CORF), rehabilitation agency, occupational therapy private practice, partial hospitalization programs, inpatient psychiatric facilities, and physician's offices. In each setting therapy coverage will be different and "therapists need to conform to the requirements of the PPS" if that is part of the system.[22] In this section COTAs will be provided with resources to help them best understand the systems that they end up working in. In addition, some key aspects of a few of the systems that they may practice in (SNFs, home health, and inpatient rehabilitation) will be overviewed.

The best resources for COTAs to understand practice in different systems reimbursed by Medicare is to overview the Internet resources on the CMS website. As stated earlier, regulations change and COTAs need to stay current. The online CMS Manual System is organized by functional areas (e.g., eligibility, entitlement, claims processing, benefit policy, program integrity). The

Internet-only manuals address coverage in many systems and are most up to date. It is especially helpful to refer to The CMS, Benefit Policy Manual, Publication, 100-02, Chapter 15 (Covered Medical and other Health Services), Sections 220-230.[22] The outpatient regulations in this manual form the basis of coverage for all therapy services. Specific policies may differ by setting. Different policies concerning therapy services are found in other manuals. When a therapy service policy is specific to a setting, it takes precedence over these general outpatient policies. Finally, keep in mind that all Medicare regulations are periodically reviewed and updated. The most current Medicare regulations will always prevail.[22] Table 6-5 overviews Medicare resources that COTAS can go to understand different systems they may work in.

WORKING IN SKILLED NURSING FACILITIES

As of 2006 the largest employer of COTAs has been in SNFs.[12] Practice in SNFs is primarily influenced by the public policies of OBRA, Medicare, and Medicaid.

OBRA, a landmark act of Congress, is not influenced by budgetary concerns. This act focuses on elders' rights, quality of care, and quality of life in the nursing home setting. OBRA went into effect in October 1990 and was revised with final rules published in 1995.[23,24] Compliance with the OBRA regulation is necessary for a nursing facility to receive reimbursement from Medicare or Medicaid. This discrepancy between what is required for good care, rehabilitation, and dignity and what is funded can cause ethical and moral dilemmas for COTAs. Knowledge of the regulations that govern care can help the COTA advocate for the services the patients need.

TABLE 6-5

Medicare Resources Online	
Resources	**Information covered**
100-01: Medicare General Information, Eligibility, and Entitlement Manual	Provides general information on program requirements
RAI Manual	This manual provides information on how to code therapy sections for the RUGs IV and provides a lot of information about what is included in sections of the MDS 3.0
100-02: Medicare Benefit Policy Manuals	General coverage criteria and guidelines for various Medicare settings
100-03 Medicare National Coverage Determinations (NCD) Manuals	Describes whether specific medical items, services, treatment procedures, or technologies can be paid for under Medicare
100-04 Medicare Claims Processing Manual	Provides all of the billing and claims processing information

MINIMUM DATA SET

The OBRA law was the impetus for developing the screening tool of the MDS, as it "called for the development of a comprehensive assessment tool to provide the foundation for planning and delivering care to nursing home residents."[25] Working in SNFs, COTAS need to be aware of the MDS because this screening tool identifies strengths and deficits that are recognized for further assessment. Many sections of the MDS address areas within the scope of OT practice. For example, COTAs might be able to add input to the cognitive patterns section among others. Data from OT practitioners contribute to the section on physical functioning (Figure 6-1). The MDS has been revised, and, with the MDS 3.0, the resident is involved in the assessment process and changes have been made in how data are collected for therapy.[26,27]

Under the regulations for the PPS, a system that regulates Part A payments in SNFs, the MDS is also used to determine Medicare payment for those residents who meet the eligibility qualifications. OT intervention influences that payment system, and COTAs may be responsible for tracking minutes of intervention for sections of the MDS. Even if no intervention has taken place, the data collection and resident interview may help COTAs give the necessary information to others on the interdisciplinary team. If COTAs complete any portion of the MDS assessment, they must certify accuracy of the section(s) they complete by noting their credentials and the date and indicating the portion of the assessment completed. The signature of a registered nurse is required to certify completion of the assessment.

THE PROSPECTIVE PAYMENT SYSTEM IN SKILLED NURSING FACILITIES

COTAs need to be aware of the PPS in SNFs. The PPS was established by the Balanced Budget Act (BBA) of 1997.[28] These regulations were created to control the increasing costs of health care with Medicare A in SNFs. Reimbursement occurs prospectively on the basis of a level of care or an anticipated level of care rather than

retrospectively on the basis of what was charged. The final rule governing PPS was published in July 1999.[29] Under this rule there were significant reimbursement changes in SNFs, and the impact on the delivery of therapy services was monumental. One of the big changes impacting practice was the organization of patients into RUGs. RUGs are determined by the number of therapies providing intervention (physical occupational or speech), therapy minutes that the Medicare beneficiary has used in the first 7-day reference period or is expected to use, need for services (e.g., respiratory therapy), specific medical conditions (e.g., pneumonia), and ADL score based on an index.[30] RUGs categories for therapy vary from a low to ultra high categories and can be combined with extensive services (refer to the RAI manual listed in Table 6-5). As regulations change and to learn more about the specifics, COTAs need to refer to the aforementioned Medicare coverage manuals in Table 6-5. Box 6-1 provides some hints for operating in an SNF under a PPS system.

Medicare Coverage for Home Health

The BBA of 1997,[28] as amended by the Omnibus Consolidated and Emergency Supplemental Appropriations Act of 1999,[31] called for the development and implementation of a PPS for Medicare home health services. The following discussion overviews the Medicare regulations for the home health system.

Eligibility for Medicare Part A home health services does not require a 3-day hospital stay as is required for Part A eligibility in skilled nursing homes. However, the elder must be homebound, have a physician's referral, and require skilled services. Homebound means that it is not recommended that the person leave the home and leaving the home requires considerable effort and help.[32] The elder does not have to be bedridden.[33] Visiting a physician is an example of a legitimate reason to leave the home. With revisions of the law home health eligibility has broadened to include "participating in therapeutic, psychosocial, or medical intervention in an adult day-care program and occasional absences from the home for

Resident _____   Identifier _____   Date _____

Section G   Functional Status

G0110. Activities of Daily Living (ADL) Assistance
Refer to the ADL flow chart in the RAI manual to facilitate accurate coding

Instructions for Rule of 3
! When an activity occurs three times at any one given level, code that level."
! "When an activity occurs three times at multiple levels, code the most dependent, exceptions are total dependence (4), activity must require full assist every time, and activity did not occur (8), activity must not have occurred at all. Example, three times extensive assistance (3) and three times limited assistance (2), code extensive assistance (3)."
! When an activity occurs at various levels, but not three times at any given level, apply the following:"
　# When there is a combination of full staff performance, and extensive assistance, code extensive assistance."
　# When there is a combination of full staff performance, weight bearing assistance and/or non-weight bearing assistance code limited assistance (2)."
If none of the above are met, code supervision.

1. ADL Self-Performance
　Code for **resident's performance** over all shifts - not including setup. If the ADL activity occurred 3 or more times at various levels of assistance, code the most dependent - except for total dependence, which requires full staff performance every time

Coding:
　　Activity Occurred 3 or More Times
　0. **Independent** - no help or staff oversight at any time
　1. **Supervision** - oversight, encouragement or cueing
　2. **Limited assistance** - resident highly involved in activity; staff provide guided maneuvering of limbs or other non-weight-bearing assistance
　3. **Extensive assistance** - resident involved in activity, staff provide weight-bearing support
　4. **Total dependence** - full staff performance every time during entire 7-day period
　　Activity Occurred 2 or Fewer Times
　7. **Activity occurred only once or twice** - activity did occur but only once or twice
　8. **Activity did not occur** - activity (or any part of the ADL) was not performed by resident or staff at all over the entire 7-day period

2. ADL Support Provided
　Code for **most support provided** over all shifts; code regardless of resident's self-performance classification

Coding:
　0. **No** setup or physical help from staff
　1. **Setup** help only
　2. **One** person physical assist
　3. **Two+** persons physical assist
　8. ADL activity itself **did not occur** during entire period

	1. Self-Performance	2. Support
	↓ Enter Codes in Boxes ↓	
A. Bed mobility - how resident moves to and from lying position, turns side to side, and positions body while in bed or alternate sleep furniture		
B. Transfer - how resident moves between surfaces including to or from: bed, chair, wheelchair, standing position (**excludes** to/from bath/toilet)		
C. Walk in room - how resident walks between locations in his/her room		
D. Walk in corridor - how resident walks in corridor on unit		
E. Locomotion on unit - how resident moves between locations in his/her room and adjacent corridor on same floor. If in wheelchair, self-sufficiency once in chair		
F. Locomotion off unit - how resident moves to and returns from off-unit locations (e.g., areas set aside for dining, activities or treatments). **If facility has only one floor**, how resident moves to and from distant areas on the floor. If in wheelchair, self-sufficiency once in chair		
G. Dressing - how resident puts on, fastens and takes off all items of clothing, including donning/removing a prosthesis or TED hose. Dressing includes putting on and changing pajamas and housedresses		
H. Eating - how resident eats and drinks, regardless of skill. Do not include eating/drinking during medication pass. Includes intake of nourishment by other means (e.g., tube feeding, total parenteral nutrition, IV fluids administered for nutrition or hydration)		
I. Toilet use - how resident uses the toilet room, commode, bedpan, or urinal; transfers on/off toilet; cleanses self after elimination; changes pad; manages ostomy or catheter; and adjusts clothes. Do not include emptying of bedpan, urinal, bedside commode, catheter bag or ostomy bag		
J. Personal hygiene - how resident maintains personal hygiene, including combing hair, brushing teeth, shaving, applying makeup, washing/drying face and hands (**excludes** baths and showers)		

FIGURE 6-1   Example of the Physical Functioning and Structural Problems Section G of the Minimum Data Set 3.0.

Resident _____ Identifier _____ Date _____

Section G	Functional Status

G0120. Bathing

How resident takes full-body bath/shower, sponge bath, and transfers in/out of tub/shower (**excludes** washing of back and hair). Code for **most dependent** in self-performance and support

Enter Code	A. Self-performance
	0. **Independent** - no help provided
	1. **Supervision** - oversight help only
	2. **Physical help limited to transfer only**
	3. **Physical help in part of bathing activity**
	4. **Total dependence**
	8. **Activity itself did not occur** during the entire period

Enter Code	B. Support provided
	(Bathing support codes are as defined in item **G0110 column 2, ADL Support Provided**, above)

G0300. Balance During Transitions and Walking

After observing the resident, **code the following walking and transition items for most dependent**

Coding:
- 0. **Steady at all times**
- 1. **Not steady, but able to stabilize without human assistance**
- 2. **Not steady, only able to stabilize with human assistance**
- 8. **Activity did not occur**

↓ **Enter Codes in Boxes**

	A. **Moving from seated to standing position**
	B. **Walking** (with assistive device if used)
	C. **Turning around** and facing the opposite direction while walking
	D. **Moving on and off toilet**
	E. **Surface-to-surface transfer** (transfer between bed and chair or wheelchair)

G0400. Functional Limitation in Range of Motion

Code for limitation that interfered with daily functions or placed resident at risk of injury

Coding:
- 0. **No impairment**
- 1. **Impairment on one side**
- 2. **Impairment on both sides**

↓ **Enter Codes in Boxes**

	A. **Upper extremity** (shoulder, elbow, wrist, hand)
	B. **Lower extremity** (hip, knee, ankle, foot)

G0600. Mobility Devices

↓ **Check all that were normally used**

☐	A. **Cane/crutch**
☐	B. **Walker**
☐	C. **Wheelchair** (manual or electric)
☐	D. **Limb prosthesis**
☐	Z. **None of the above** were used

G0900. Functional Rehabilitation Potential
Complete only if A0310A = 01

Enter Code	A. **Resident believes he or she is capable of increased independence** in at least some ADLs
	0. **No**
	1. **Yes**
	2. **Unable to determine**

Enter Code	B. **Direct care staff believe resident is capable of increased independence** in at least some ADLs
	0. **No**
	1. **Yes**

FIGURE 6-1

BOX 6-1

Operational Hints for Working in a Prospective Payment System (PPS) in a Skilled Nursing Facility (SNF)

- Communicate well with other members of the interprofessional team to coordinate care.
- Know guidelines for PPS and the Resources Utilization Groups (RUGs).
- Know approximately how many minutes of intervention are needed to generate desired outcomes and for type of therapy you are providing (individual, concurrent, or group).
- Recognize that timing of therapy is critical for working effectively within this system.
- Obtain therapy orders before admission for effective planning.
- Prioritize care by dividing therapy minutes based on resident needs and desired outcomes.
- Begin therapy with treatment minutes as soon as possible using good judgment based on the resident's health status.
- Be organized and track time accurately to the minute. If the number of qualifying minutes is not achieved, the resident's status with the RUGs will default to a lower category.
- Document accurately intervention minutes daily.

Adapted from Flanagan, J. (2009 & 2010). *Guide to Prospective Payment System*; Linda Spurrell, July 26, 2010, personal communication.

nonmedical purposes, for example, an occasional trip to the barber, a walk around the block or a drive, attendance at a family reunion, funeral, graduation, or other infrequent or unique event."[33] A client does not qualify for Part A home health services based solely on the need for OT. Nursing, physical therapy, or speech-language pathology must first open the case. However, OT may be introduced along with these other services and may continue after the other services have ended.[34] The legislative attempts to change these qualification regulations continue but have been unsuccessful so far.

The regulations for HHAs are, of course, quite extensive. With assessment, the Outcome and Assessment Information Set (OASIS) is a key component of Medicare's partnership with the home care industry to foster and monitor improved home health care outcomes. It represents core items of a comprehensive assessment for an adult home care patient and forms the basis for measuring patient outcomes for purposes of outcome-based quality improvement. Most data items in the OASIS were developed as systems of outcome measures for home health care. The items have use for outcome monitoring, clinical assessment, care planning, and other internal agency-level applications. OASIS data items encompass sociodemographic, environmental, support system, health status, and functional status attributes of adult patients. In addition, selected attributes of health service use are included. Refer to the Medicare online manuals listed in Table 6-5 for more information about current regulations on the CMS website.

Medicare in Inpatient Rehabilitation Facilities

COTAs employed in inpatient rehabilitation facilities (IRFs) will need to be informed about how the system works because there are very unique regulations for this area of practice. An admission regulation is called the "75% rule."[35] Although still called this, legislative changes now require that 60% of the admitted patients have one of 13 diagnoses. Examples of diagnoses are stroke and amputations.[35] Similar to other settings, IRFs follow a PPS system for Medicare Part A beneficiaries. This PPS system establishes residents in one of numerous case mix groups (CMG) based on a screening tool called the Inpatient Rehabilitation Facility Patient Assessment Instrument (IRF-PAI) and a customized Functional Independence Measure (FIM). The customized FIM evaluates the client and assigns the client to a CMG. The IRF-PAI is used to establish client categories.[11] COTAs can contribute functional information to the assessment process. As in other health care settings (SNFs and inpatient hospitals), there are time limitations that influence therapy. In IRFs, COTAs and OTRs provide intensive rehabilitation in 3-hour time blocks per day along with physical therapists and speech therapists. Patients need to be able to tolerate this level of intensive therapy.[35]

Medicaid

Medicaid is a health insurance "for low-income individuals and families who fit into an eligibility group that is recognized by federal and state law."[36] Because such a large portion of Medicaid dollars goes toward financing long-term care coverage,[37] COTAs should become aware of this important public policy. States must provide basic health services, including inpatient and outpatient hospital services, laboratory and x-ray examinations, nursing facility services, physician and nurse practitioner services, and family planning services. State administrations can choose to cover any of 30 or more optional services, including OT. States also have been required to ensure that descriptions of their services meet federal guidelines and that all Medicaid recipients are treated equally.[38]

In many states the Medicaid program is administered as a managed care plan. Medicaid pays a high percentage of nursing care expenditures in the nursing home industry. Because of funding restrictions, Medicaid places an emphasis on institutional care rather than on other options that might permit elders to remain in their communities. However, the degree of emphasis varies among states because some have waiver programs and demonstration projects that involve broader funding for innovative programs and nontraditional care management. As

Evashwick[39] states, "An extremely important feature of the public long-term care system is the lead role that state governments have in shaping the characteristics of local financing and delivery systems for long-term care services." Thus, the Medicaid program varies considerably from state to state and within each state over time. Because of these variances, the COTA must have access to local information and be an advocate for OT on local and national levels. In addition, COTAs should become aware of major changes that may occur with the health reform law, including expanded Medicaid coverage to populations under age 65[37] and other demonstration projects that may influence care of their elder clients.

Managed Care

Elders may be in a managed care plan whether in Medicaid or Medicare Part C. Managed care organizations manage the care given to consumers and often involve the entire range of utilization control tools applied to manage the practice of physicians and others, regardless of practice setting. With Medicare Part C, care may be managed through a health maintenance organization (HMO) or preferred provider organization (PPO). Reimbursement rates to managed care providers are capitated, meaning that a set rate is provided either per intervention or per condition. This payment may sometimes not be enough to include extensive therapy. The OTR/COTA team needs to familiarize itself with the type of managed care services their clients may be receiving, emphasize in documentations the functional intervention they provide, and advocate for services if there are any issues.

Older Americans Act

In 1965 the Older Americans Act (OAA)[40] was enacted to provide services for elders. The premise of OAA was that services provided to elders at least 60 years of age would enable them to remain in their homes and communities. Funding was established for nutrition programs, senior centers, transportation, housing, ombudsman, and legal services. Differences in these programs exist among states because administration is at the state level. In addition, more opportunity for OT involvement exists in some regions than in others. The original OAA was designed to foster independence, but rehabilitative services were not included. The act established the Administration on Aging, an agency specifically responsible for developing new social services for elders. COTAs should pay attention to the OAA when it is reauthorized because some of the changes may help their clients. It is also beneficial for COTAs to become aware of services offered by their local office on aging because many of these services can help their clients.

TRENDS WITH FEDERAL HEALTH CARE POLICIES: HEALTH CARE REFORM

As of this writing the Patient Protection and Affordable Care Act,[41] as amended by the Health Care Education Reconciliation Act of 2010,[42] will result in sweeping changes in our health care system as it is gradually instituted between 2010 and 2020. Parts of the law related to Medicare directly influence the provision of health care of elders. With health care reform the basic benefit package of Medicare will remain unchanged. Medicare beneficiaries will continue to receive their health insurance and physicians and hospitals will continue to be reimbursed per procedure.[43] However, new changes with the law involve adding provisions to help elders manage their health care. Examples of these changes are gradually closing up in Medicare Part D, the voluntary prescription drug program that was known as the "donut hole." The donut hole referred to a coverage gap in which elders had to pay out of pocket for their prescription medications. Another change with health reform is that subsidies will be offered for people with low income for Part D (prescription drug coverage). Preventive services in medical areas, such as Medicare financing annual physicals and regular colon screens will become covered benefits. With Medicare Part C (Medicare Advantage plans), reforms include restructuring and reducing payments and providing bonuses for quality programs. There will be many other cost savings provisions, which are predicted to save the Medicare program billions of dollars. Delivery reforms such as reducing hospital payments linked with needless readmissions or hospital-acquired infections[44] will hopefully improve quality of care and decrease unnecessary spending. It is believed that the changes to Medicare will extend the solvency of the Hospital Insurance Trust Fund for Part A in the next 10 years.[44]

A voluntary long-term care insurance program, or the Community Living and Assistance Services and Support Program (CLASS), will help citizens finance long-term care services and supports.[45] It is also important to be aware of pilot programs because they may eventually influence practice. One such pilot program is bundling the costs for delivery of post-acute care for Medicare beneficiaries. Finally this historical legislation is yet to be settled and more changes may occur as the makeup of Congress fluctuates.

ADVOCACY FOR ELDERS

Health care is always in a state of flux that directly affects OT practice. To deal with constant changes advocacy is important to any profession. Eleanor Roosevelt once stated, "Every person owes a portion of his time and talent to the up building of a profession to which he/she belongs."[46]

Involvement of COTAs in advocacy for elders and the OT profession can make a difference. Advocacy is clearly discussed in the Occupational Therapy Code of Ethics and Ethics Standards.[47] As stated in Principle 4 Part D of the Occupational Therapy Code of Ethics, therapists should "advocate for just and fair intervention for all patients, clients, employees, and colleagues, and

TABLE 6-6

Nonskilled Occupational Therapy Services	
Example	**Justification**
Gwendolyn: A 69-year-old client diagnosed with right cerebral vascular accident. Previously, she performed all ADL functions independently. On initial evaluation, Gwendolyn was able to perform ADL functions independently but slowly. Her status on initial evaluation was independent with ADL, although performance was slow.	Slow performance with ADL functions is not significant enough to require the intervention of a skilled practitioner. The client will likely improve on her own over time without intervention.
Sebastian: A 75-year-old client diagnosed with rheumatoid arthritis. OT was ordered to provide an adapted pencil gripper to assist with writing. The COTA provided the gripper.	Intervention does not require the skilled expertise of the COTA. Anyone could provide an adapted pencil gripper.
Bob: A 74-year-old client diagnosed with Alzheimer's disease. He is dependent in feeding. The COTA monitors feeding three times a week for 2 weeks.	The client's condition is chronic and has not shown significant improvement. Intervention is routine therefore not requiring the skilled expertise of the COTA.

ADL, activities of daily living; COTA, certified occupational therapy assistant; OT, occupational therapy; ROM, range of motion.

encourage employers and colleagues to abide by the highest standards of social justice and the ethical standards set forth by the occupational therapy profession."[47] Part E states that therapists should "make efforts to advocate for recipients of occupational therapy services to obtain needed services through available means."[47]

Every COTA and OTR must encourage the benefits of OT and establish the role of the profession within society. COTAs must stay informed about all government decisions regarding health care (Table 6-6). The rapidly changing face of today's health care economy demands innovative and progressive responses from individuals. OTRs and COTAs must be strong advocates for their profession and the clients that benefit from OT intervention by adjusting to change and adapting to new ways to deliver intervention. An example of a direct benefit of advocacy with CMS was the successful effort to get clarification of coverage for patients with the diagnosis of Alzheimer's disease.[48] Box 6-2 provides suggestions for ways that COTAs can become more involved with public policy and advocacy.

KEEPING UP WITH CHANGES

Let us return to Susan the COTA discussed in the opening scenario. On the first day of her job she meets with her boss Sonya. After reviewing some of the documentation and billing aspects of the job, Sonya asks Susan how she will keep updated with the frequent changes in regulations related to payment provision. Sonya challenges Susan to research that question and come up with ideas the next day when they meet. That evening Susan researches the CMS website and the AOTA website. She learns about and plans to follow postings on the CMS website called *transmittals*, which are used "to communicate new or

BOX 6-2

Ways for Certified Occupational Therapy Assistants to Become Involved with Public Policy and to Advocate

- Be able and ready to articulate a clear definition of occupational therapy (OT) for the public; be visible.
- Regularly access the American Occupational Therapy Association (AOTA) website, the Centers for Medicare & Medicaid Services (CMS) website, and their Medicare Administrative Contracture (MAC) website to keep abreast of public policy trends.
- Serve on OT task forces and committees on a state or national level.
- Become involved in advocacy groups in other associations related to therapy practice with elders, such as the AARP and the Alzheimer's Association.
- Read public (Web-based) and OT literature as much as possible to keep up on trends. Write and submit articles to professional and consumer publications about OT practice and public policy.
- Find a mentor who understands public policy.
- Write letters or visit people involved with public policy such as legislators, managed care and corporate executives, third-party payers, and case managers.
- Learn the legislative process in your state and testify for relevant issues at public hearings.
- If questions or concerns cannot be answered or addressed on a local level, network with the legislative division of AOTA.

changed policies, and/or procedures that are being incorporated into specific Centers for Medicare & Medicaid Services (CMS) program manual."[49] She finds manuals on the site that overview different Medicare regulations. Then she goes to the AOTA website. There in the *Issues and Advocacy* section she finds many resources to keep abreast with policy trends as well as practical suggestions for advocacy. She also finds the MAC site for her area and reads about regulation changes and looks at the LCDs. She searches further on the Internet and finds the AARP website that overviews extensive background related to public policy and advocacy. The next day when they meet again Sonya is pleased to learn about Susan's efforts and states, "I hope that you make initiative to keep current from now on at least about this area of practice. In this rapidly changing health care environment I expect all my employees to be pro-active. I like to have monthly meetings where along with our practice discussions we educate and share about current health care changes and public policy."

CHAPTER REVIEW QUESTIONS

1 Name and describe the four parts of Medicare and those directly related to occupational therapy practice.
2 How is Medicare billed under Part B?
3 What is a Medicare Administrative Contracture (MAC), and how can it help inform practice?
4 Describe the prospective payment system used in skilled nursing facilities and how it influences therapy practice.
5 What is a resource utilization group?
6 What is Medicaid, and is OT a required or optional benefit?
7 What is home-bound status for clients in a home health care setting under Medicare Part A and allowable reasons for leaving the home?
8 What is the current assessment system used in home health care?
9 What is the current assessment system used in inpatient rehabilitation settings?
10 How can COTAs access the Older Americans Act (OAA) for their clients?
11 How might health reform influence practice?
12 How can COTAs be advocates for the OT profession?
13 How can COTAs stay aware of public policy changes that influence practice?

REFERENCES

1. MDS 3.0 for Nursing Homes and Swing Bed Providers. Centers for Medicare & Medicaid Services. https://www.cms.gov/NursingHomeQualityInits/30_NHQIMDS30Technical Information.asp#TopOfPage.
2. Health Information Technology for Economic and Clinical Health Act, 2009. Pub. L. No. 111-5, 123 Stat. 226, 467.
3. "What is Medicare?" Centers for Medicare & Medicaid Services, April 2008. www.medicare.gov/Publications/Pubs/pdf/11306.pdf.
4. "Medicare Part A." In Medicare Program: General Information. Centers for Medicare & Medicaid Services. www.cms.gov/MedicareGenInfo/02_Part%20A.asp.
5. "Prospective payment systems: General information." Centers for Medicare & Medicaid Services. www.cms.gov/ProspMedicareFeeSvcPmtGen/.
6. Robinson, M., Bogenrief, J., 2009. Introduction to reimbursement and documentation for the new graduate. Retrieved from http://www.aota.org/documentvault/conference/reimbursement.aspx.
7. AOTA, 2008. Reimbursement and Regulatory Policy Fact Sheet: Medicare basics. American Occupational Therapy Association, Bethesda, MD. www.aota.org/Practitioners/Reimb/Pay/Medicare/FactSheets/37788.aspx.
8. "Medicare Part B." In Medicare Program: General Information. Centers for Medicare & Medicaid Services. www.cms.gov/MedicareGenInfo/03_Part%20B.asp#TopOfPage%20Part%20B.
9. "Healthcare common procedure coding system level II coding procedures." Centers for Medicare & Medicaid Services. www.cms.gov/MedHCPCSGenInfo/Downloads/LevelIICodingProcedures.pdf.
10. "National correct coding initiatives edits." In Centers for Medicare & Medicaid Services. www.cms.gov/NationalCorrectCodiNitEd/01_overview.asp.
11. Robinson, M., 2007. Medicare 101: Understanding the basics. OT Practice, 12 (2), CE-1-7.
12. 2006 Occupational therapy compensation and workforce report, 2006. American Occupational Therapy Association, Bethesda, MD.
13. Medicare.gov. (n.d). Medicare advantage: Part C. Retrieved from http://www.medicare.gov/navigation/medicare-basics/medicare-benefits/part-c.aspx.
14. Lubarsky, M., Swerwan, J.R., Schroeder, E.L., Duffy, J.L., 1995. Medicare resource manual: A guide through the critical steps Life Services Network of Illinois.
15. "Practice of occupational therapy." Section 230.2, Chapter 15: Covered Medical and Other Health Services. In: Centers for Medicare & Medicaid Services: Medicare Benefit Policy Manual. https://www.cms.gov/manuals/Downloads/bp102c15.pdf.
16. Centers for Medicare & Medicaid Services (CMS), 2008. Physician Fee Schedule. Retrieved from http://www.cms.gov/apps/physician-fee-schedule/search/search-criteria.aspx.
17. "Medicare Program; Revisions to Payment Policies Under the Physician Fee Schedule, and Other Part B Payment Policies for CY 2008; Revisions to the Payment Policies of Ambulance Services Under the Ambulance Fee Schedule for CY 2008; and the Amendment of the E-Prescribing Exemption for Computer-Generated Facsimile Transmissions." Federal Register 72 (27 November 2007):66222-66578. http://edocket.access.gpo.gov/2007/pdf/07-5506.pdf.
18. "Medicare Program; Revisions to Payment Policies Under the Physician Fee Schedule, and Other Part B Payment Policies for CY 2008; Revisions to the Payment Policies of Ambulance Services Under the Ambulance Fee Schedule for CY 2008; and the Amendment of the E-Prescribing Exemption for Computer-Generated Facsimile Transmissions; Corrections; Final Rule." Federal Register 73 (15 January 2008): 2567-2710. http://edocket.access.gpo.gov/2008/pdf/07-6308.pdf.
19. "Chapter 8: Coverage of extended care (SNF) services under hospital insurance." In Centers for Medicare & Medicaid Services: Medicare Benefit Policy Manual. www.cms.gov/manuals/Downloads/bp102c08.pdf.
20. "Program memorandum intermediaries/carriers: Medical review of services for patients with dementia." Centers for Medicare &

Medicaid Services: Transmittal AB-01-135. www.cms.gov/Transmittals/downloads/AB-01-135.pdf.

21. "Chapter 13: Local coverage determinations." In Centers for Medicare & Medicaid Services: Medicare Program Integrity Manual. www.cms.gov/manuals/downloads/pim83c13.pdf.

22. "Chapter 15: Covered medical and other health services." In: Centers for Medicare & Medicaid Services: Medicare Benefit Policy Manual. www.cms.gov/manuals/Downloads/bp102c15.pdf.

23. Omnibus Budget Reconciliation Act, 1987. Pub. L. No. 100-20, 101 Stat. 1330.

24. Medicare and Medicaid Programs; Survey, Certification and Enforcement of Skilled Nursing Facilities and Nursing Facilities, 60 Fed. Reg. 50115 (Sept. 28, 1995)

25. "MDS long-term care." Continuity of Care Task Group. http://continuityofcaretaskgroup.pbworks.com/MDS%20Long%20Term%20Care.

26. "MDS 3.0 for nursing homes and swing bed providers." In Nursing Home Quality Initiatives. Centers for Medicare & Medicaid Services. www.cms.gov/NursingHomeQualityInits/25_NHQIMDS30.asp.

27. Keane Care, July 2010. Preparing for MDS 3.0. Retrieved from http://www.keanecare.com/products/pdf/mds30-flyer.pdf.

28. Balanced Budget Act of 1997, Pub. L. 105-133, 111 Stat. 329.

29. "Medicare program; prospective payment system and consolidated billing for skilled nursing facilities—Update; final rule." Federal Register, 64(31 July 2001), 39562-39607.

30. Medpac, 2008. Skilled nursing facilities services payment section: Payment basics. Retrieved from http://www.medpac.gov/documents/MedPAC_Payment_Basics_08_SNF.pdf.

31. Omnibus Consolidated and Emergency Supplemental Appropriations Act of 1999.

32. "Medicare and home health care." Centers for Medicare & Medicaid Services. http://www.medicare.gov/publications/pubs/pdf/10969.pdf.

33. "Chapter 7: Home health services." In Centers for Medicare & Medicaid Services: Medicare Benefit Policy Manual. www.cms.gov/manuals/Downloads/bp102c07.pdf.

34. Youngstrom, J.J., 1995. Reimbursement for home health services: Guidelines for occupational therapy in home health. Commission on Practice Home Health Task Force, Bethesda, MD.

35. "Coverage of inpatient rehabilitation services." Medical Learning Network, Centers for Medicare & Medicaid Services. www.cms.gov/MLNMattersArticles/downloads/MM6699.pdf.

36. "Medicaid program: General information." Centers for Medicare & Medicaid Services. www.cms.gov/MedicaidGenInfo/.

37. The Kaiser Commission on Medicaid and the Uninsured, 2010. Medicaid: A primer. Retrieved from http://www.kff.org/medicaid/upload/7334-04.pdf.

38. Sommers, F.P., Browne, S., Carter, M.E., 1996. Medicaid: Current law and issues in reform proposals. American Occupational Therapy Association, Bethesda, MD.

39. Evashwick, C.J., 1996. The Continuum of Long-Term Care. Delmar, Albany, NY.

40. The Older Americans Act of 1965, Pub. L. 89-73, 79 Stat. 218.

41. Patient Protection and Affordable Care Act, 2010. Pub. L. 111-148, 124 Stat. 119.

42. The Health Care and Education Reconciliation Act of 2010, Pub.L. 111-152, 124 Stat. 1029

43. Tumulty, K., Pickert, K., Park, A., 2010. America's new prescription: Will it work? Time, 175 (13), 24-32.

44. Kaiser Family Foundation, 2010. Medicare: A primer. Retrieved from http://www.kff.org/medicare/upload/7615-03.pdf.

45. Kaiser Family Foundation, 2010. Health care reform and the CLASS Act. Retrieved from http://www.kff.org/healthreform/upload/8069.pdf.

46. Scott, S.J., Acquaviva, J.D., 1985. Lobbying for healthcare. Government and Legal Affairs Division, American Occupational Therapy Association, Rockville, MD.

47. Occupational Therapy Code of Ethics and Ethics Standards, 2010. American Occupational Therapy Association, Bethesda, MD. www.aota.org/Practitioners/Ethics/Docs/Standards/38527.aspx.

48. Centers for Medicare & Medicaid Services (CMS), 2002b. Statement of Tom Scully, administrator centers for Medicare & Medicaid services on therapy coverage of Alzheimer's disease patients [WWW page]. URL http://www.hcanys.org/dementia/AlzheimerScully4-1.PDF.

49. "Transmittals." Centers for Medicare & Medicaid Services. www.cms.gov/Transmittals/.

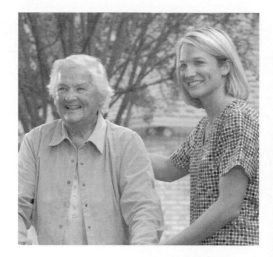

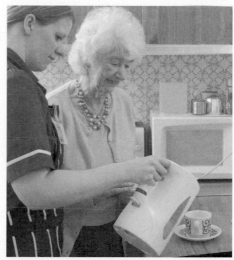

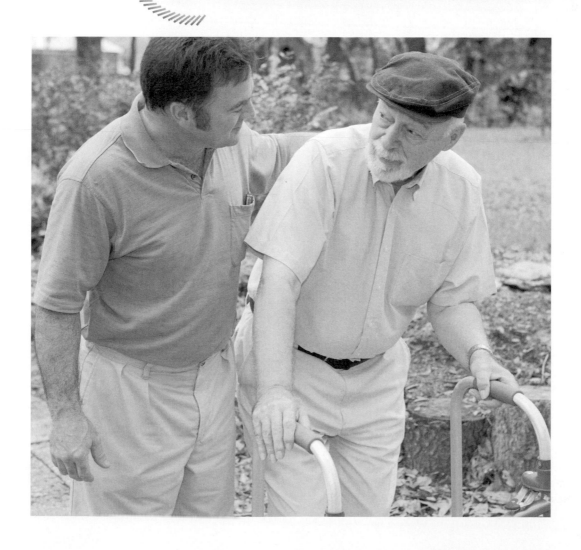

Occupational Therapy Practice Models

RENÉ PADILLA

KEY TERMS

clinical practice models, values, dysfunction, skills, occupation, function, assessment, task, roles, performance, culture, environment, self-care, work, play and leisure, intervention, context, cognition, maturation, motor action, subsystem, habits

CHAPTER OBJECTIVES

1. Explain the importance and use of practice models in occupational therapy intervention with elders.
2. Briefly summarize the Occupational Therapy Practice Framework (2nd edition) and three occupational therapy practice models as they relate to aging, including Facilitating Growth and Development, Cognitive Disabilities, and the Model of Human Occupation.
3. Demonstrate the ways certified occupational therapy assistants can incorporate theoretical principles into practice with elders.

Deepak was admitted to the rehabilitation center with a severe infection in the left knee that had been replaced just 3 months earlier. Deepak had been looking forward to his recent retirement. As an executive for a large firm, he and his family had lived in 10 different countries around the world. Now that all of his children had graduated from college, he was planning a peaceful life in a small town by the ocean where he and his wife could play golf every day, attend cultural events in a nearby city, and occasionally go deep-sea fishing. A few days after he was admitted to the rehabilitation center he received news that his wife had fallen and fractured a hip. While preparing her for surgery at a different hospital, the doctors had discovered that she had a very aggressive cancer that had metastasized throughout her body. There was no hope for recovery, and she was discharged home under the care of her daughter and a hospice service. Deepak spoke to his wife on the telephone twice a day, and often was tearful during his conversations with her. The purpose of Deepak's hospitalization was that he become independent in his self-care and in his mobility while not bearing any weight on his left leg. The weight-bearing restrictions were expected to be necessary for at least 10 weeks while his infection cleared and his knee was replaced again.

Martha is a small, frail woman in her late sixties who has been living in a skilled nursing facility for more than a year. When she was in her late twenties her automobile had been hit by a train and she sustained a head injury that resulted in her inability to speak and left hemiplegia. She had regained the ability to do her self-care and to walk without assistance, although over the years she had suffered many falls because of poor balance. For more than 40 years she had lived with her sister. When her sister died, Martha attempted to live on her own for some time but became ill with pneumonia. Her relatives insisted she live at a skilled nursing facility because they were not able to care for her. Because of another bout with pneumonia, Martha is very weak and is unable to bathe and dress herself without assistance. She is also not able to walk.

Ursula was recently referred to an adult day care center in the downtown area of a large city. Her Alzheimer's disease has progressed to the point where she needs supervision 24 hours a day. Ursula's husband has been working at a local bookstore to make some money to supplement his retirement income. Ursula and her husband were prisoners in a Nazi concentration camp in their youth, and in the last month Ursula has seemed to be reliving that experience, often becoming quite agitated and isolated at the center.

Carlos immigrated to the United States from Cuba nearly 30 years ago. Although he is in his late sixties, he continued to work running a family-owned restaurant until 5 days ago when he had a stroke. Because of his stroke, Carlos seems unable to understand and speak in English and continually repeats the same two lines of a Spanish song whenever he does speak. He also is unable to hold himself in midline and does not seem aware of one side of his body. Nearly every day his room in the acute care hospital has been full of relatives and friends, many of whom bring food. Carlos has a fever, and the doctors suspect he is having difficulty swallowing.

Deepak, Martha, Carlos, and Ursula represent the diversity of people who seek occupational therapy (OT) intervention because they are not able to carry out the activities that are important to them in their daily lives. The certified occupational therapy assistant (COTA) needs tools to address all of these unique needs according to basic OT philosophy and theoretical principles. The OT programs for these individuals must not consider only the physical and cognitive limitations that affect their ability to care for themselves. These programs must also take into account the whole history of these individuals and the adjustments that are needed because of dramatic changes in their environments. Deepak's wife is dying, and his children no longer live at home. Martha has been moved against her will from her familiar home to a skilled nursing facility where she knows no one. Carlos has gone from spending nearly all of his waking hours at his business to a hospital room, and Ursula's mind has gradually replaced her physical surroundings for dreadful ones that reside in her memory. Although these OT programs must maintain a common thread that identifies them as "occupational therapy," they also should be flexible enough to provide individual meaning for each client. OT clinical practice models are intended to connect professional philosophy and theory with daily practice.

OVERVIEW OF PRACTICE MODELS

This chapter provides an overview of several conceptual models in which occupation is described as the principal feature of any OT intervention. First, the Occupational Therapy Practice Framework[1] is reviewed, which articulates the general domain and process of intervention of the OT profession and gives the broadest look at how we might go about understanding Deepak's life and current needs. Second, an overview of Llorens's[2] Facilitating Growth and Development model is provided, which, although published nearly 3 decades ago, is still the only conceptual model that emphasizes a developmental perspective in the practice of OT with adult clients. This model can help us understand how to consider Martha's stage in life. Third, the Cognitive Disabilities Model[3,4,5] is described, which helps us understand how cognitive process affects the performance of occupation and will be particularly useful in working with elders such as Ursula, although it certainly also has applications for Deepak, Martha, and Carlos. Finally, the Model of Human Occupation[6] is discussed as a model that makes an effort to assist practitioners to consider clients holistically. This model will help us understand elders like Carlos as people with dynamic abilities and needs who actively interact with their environments.

The common link among all forms of OT intervention cannot be overemphasized. The philosophy of OT practice includes values, beliefs, truths, and principles that should guide the general practice of the profession. One tenet of this philosophy is that the human being is inherently active and can influence self-development, health, and environment with purposeful activity. Thus, the

human is able to adapt to life's demands and become self-actualized. Dysfunction occurs when the human being's ability to adapt is impaired in some way. OT intervention seeks to prevent and remediate dysfunction and facilitate maximal adaptation through the use of purposeful activities.[7] The use of meaningful and purposeful activity, or occupation, is the common thread for every OT intervention.

Since the OT profession began, the term *occupation* has described the individual's active participation in self-care, work, and leisure,[8] which constitute the ordinary, familiar things people do every day.[7] The person must use combinations of sensorimotor, cognitive, psychological, and psychosocial skills to perform these occupations.[9] Specific environments and different stages of life influence these occupations. Kielhofner[10] defined occupation as "doing culturally meaningful work, play or living tasks in the stream of time and in the contexts of one's physical and social world."

To understand the concepts of occupations and use them to facilitate function and adaptation, COTAs must have broad knowledge of the biological, social, and medical sciences in addition to OT theoretical premises. OT practice models provide organized frameworks for that knowledge, which allow the therapist to apply pertinent information to a specific client's problem. Thus, practice models guide the therapist in creating individual intervention programs that are culturally meaningful and age-related and that facilitate development of sensorimotor, cognitive, psychological, and psychosocial skills. By using a practice model for guidance, the four COTAs assisting the patients discussed earlier can ensure professional intervention programs that are tailored to meet the needs of each client.

Theorists have articulated many practice models or approaches. Those presented here are certainly not the only ones that can provide guidance for OT intervention with elders. For example, the Kinesiological Model,[11,12] also referred to as the *Biomechanical Approach*, provides insight into how elders move based on mechanical principles of range of motion, muscle strength, and physical endurance. Concepts of this approach help us restore movement to an elder after a stroke or apply hip precautions during participation in occupation after a hip replacement (refer to Chapters 19 and 22 for examples of applications of this approach). Another example is the Sensory Integration Model,[13,14] which addresses dysfunctions that make it difficult for the brain to modulate sensory stimulation. Intervention guided by this model provides strategic sensory stimulation designed to organize the central nervous system and promote adaptive responses according to the person's neurological needs (refer to Chapter 20 for an understanding of intervention guided by this model).

OT practice models do not offer concrete plans for improvement of function. Instead, these models suggest

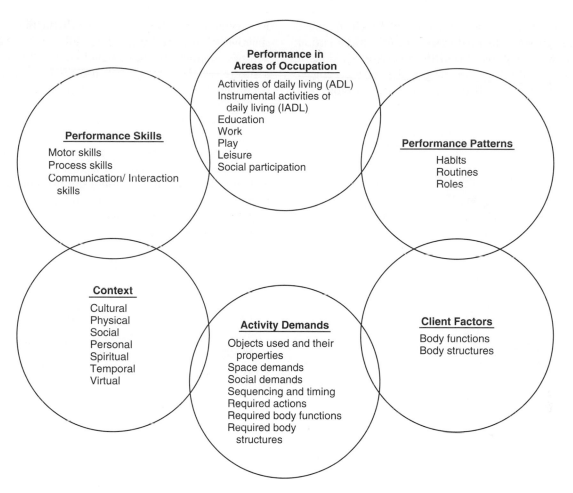

FIGURE 7-1 Domain of occupational therapy. *(Adapted from American Occupational Therapy Association. (2008). Occupational therapy practice framework: Domain and processes, 2nd ed.* American Journal of Occupational Therapy, *62, 625-683.)*

the use of various graded occupations that demand the development of performance abilities, thereby improving function. COTAs may use the information in the practice models to formulate questions to assess the client's needs, interests, and meanings; select assessment tools; and accordingly design a unique intervention strategy. COTAs should be familiar with several practice models because each model usually has a specific focus and does not address all dimensions of occupational functioning.

Occupational Therapy Practice Framework

The Occupational Therapy Practice Framework: Domain and Processes (subsequently referred to as "the Framework"[1]) represents the latest effort of the AOTA to articulate language with which to describe the profession's focus. As such, the Framework is intended to help occupational therapy practitioners analyze their current practice and consider new applications in emerging areas. In addition, the Framework was developed to help the external audience (physicians, payers, community groups, and others) understand the profession's emphasis on function and participation in social life.

The domain of concern of a profession refers to the areas of human experience in which practitioners of the profession help others (Figure 7-1). According to the Framework, the focus of the OT profession is "the promotion of health and participation of people, organizations, and populations through engagement in occupation."[1] For OT, the breadth of meaningful everyday life activities is captured in the notion of "occupation." OT practitioners help people perform meaningful occupations that affect their health, well-being, and life satisfaction. These occupations and activities permit desired or needed participation in home, school, workplace, and community life. Notably, personal meaning is emphasized as the central characteristic of occupation. The degree to which personal meaningfulness is decreased may render a therapeutic intervention as merely purposeful (i.e., achieving a goal a client understands but in which he is not particularly invested) or simply inconsequential.

According to the Framework, meaningfulness of occupation is tightly intertwined with the contexts in which the person lives. The Framework recognizes that "occupational engagement occurs individually or with others."[1]

Thus, the many types of occupations in which the client might engage should be addressed in OT intervention. The Framework has organized the many occupations in which an individual, group, or population may engage into broad categories called *areas of occupation* (Table 7-1).

TABLE 7-1

Areas of Occupation	
Areas	**Types of occupations**
Activities of daily living	Bathing/showering Bowel and bladder management Dressing Eating Feeding Functional mobility Personal device care Personal hygiene and grooming Sexual activity Toilet hygiene
Instrumental activities of daily living	Care of others Care of pets Child rearing Communication device use Community mobility Financial management Health management and maintenance Home establishment and management Meal preparation and cleanup Religious observance Safety and emergency maintenance Shopping
Rest and sleep	Rest Sleep Sleep preparation Sleep participation
Education	Formal educational participation Informal personal educational needs or interests exploration (beyond formal education) Informal personal education participation
Work	Employment interest and pursuits Employment seeking and acquisition Job performance Retirement preparation and adjustment Volunteer exploration Volunteer participation
Play	Play exploration Play participation
Leisure	Leisure exploration Leisure participation
Social participation	Community Family Peer, friend

Adapted from American Occupational Therapy Association. (2008). *Occupational therapy practice framework: Domain and processes*, 2nd ed. *American Journal of Occupational Therapy, 62*, 625-683.

Engagement in these areas depends on the client's perspective, needs, and interests as well as his or her specific abilities, characteristics, or beliefs, which the Framework identifies as *client factors* because they reside within the client. For example, to tie one's shoes (a dressing activity within the ADL area of occupation) one must, among many things, possess sufficient body functions supported by body structures and performance skills to maintain an erect posture while bending and reaching one's foot, and then one must manipulate the laces and pull on them with sufficient force to tighten them but not enough to break them (all examples of motor and praxis skills). This sequence of actions is carried out by one's ability to plan and sequence events (examples of cognitive skills). A fascinating feature of human occupation is that many combinations of performance skills (Table 7-2) are integrated

TABLE 7-2

Performance Skills	
Skill*	**Examples**
Motor and praxis	Bending and reaching Pacing Coordinating Maintaining balance Anticipating or adjusting posture and body position Manipulating
Sensory-perceptual	Positioning the body Hearing and locating Visually determining Locating by touch Timing Discerning flavors
Emotional regulation	Responding to feelings of others Persisting despite frustration Controlling anger Recovering from disappointment Displaying emotion Utilizing coping strategies
Cognitive	Judging Selecting Sequencing Organizing Prioritizing Creating Multitasking
Communication and social	Looking Gesturing Maintaining acceptable space Initiating and answering Taking turns Acknowledging

*Skills listed as verbs to denote they imply action.

Adapted from American Occupational Therapy Association. (2008). *Occupational therapy practice framework: Domain and processes*, 2nd ed. *American Journal of Occupational Therapy, 62*, 625-683.

and choreographed into automatic or semiautomatic patterns that enable one to function on a daily basis without demanding undue attention. After one has tied his or her shoe laces with sufficient frequency, he or she can often do it without thinking or looking at the laces because it has become a habit. Broader habits can be said to become organized into routines (e.g., one might dress in a certain way and take a particular route to get to work), and frequently routines correspond to the variety of roles in which one functions (e.g., because one is the supervisor of an office, one might routinely meet with employees each morning at a certain time). The Framework notes that "when practitioners consider the client's patterns of performance, they are better able to understand the frequency and manner in which performance skills and occupations are integrated into the client's life."[1]

As stated earlier, the Framework emphasizes the importance of considering the environments and contexts in which a person engages in occupation. *Environments* are the external physical and social surroundings in which the client's daily life occupations take place. *Contexts* refer to the "variety of interrelated conditions that are within and surrounding the client."[1] Contexts, therefore, can be cultural (customs, beliefs, activity patterns, behavior standards, and expectations), personal (age, gender, socioeconomic, and educational level), temporal (stage of life, time of day/year, duration, rhythm of activity, or history), and virtual (simulated interactions absent of physical contact). These contexts offer opportunities for occupational engagement, but at the same time they restrict it; for example, a theater may offer an elder the opportunity to watch a theatrical performance but not to swim or ride a horse, whereas a swimming pool may offer the opportunity to swim but not to watch a theatrical performance.

Two other elements may affect how a person engages in occupation. A person may not be able to meet the demands inherent in an activity (e.g., without a fair amount of conditioning, an elder might not be able to climb up a mountain), or the person may find the demands too low (e.g., a champion chess player may find it quite boring to play Tic Tac Toe). Activity demands include such things as the objects used in the activity and the characteristics of these objects, space and social demands, required actions, and required body functions and structures. For example, the activity of playing golf requires balls and golf irons; takes place on a golf course; is often played with others and therefore requires taking turns; involves a sequence of tasks from placing the ball, hitting it, and then locating it in the distance; and requires the bodily functions of joint mobility and muscle power to swing the iron while not letting the iron fly away and harming someone standing nearby. Furthermore, playing golf involves the person's cardiovascular system while walking, vestibular functions while turning one's trunk and following through with the swing, and a variety of other body structures and

functions. Interestingly, engagement in occupation is not only affected by these functions and structures, but also it may affect them in turn; for example, an elder's cardiovascular and neuromuscular functions become conditioned while gradually increasing the time spent walking in a golf course.

The Framework describes the OT process as consisting of three dynamic and interactive phases: evaluation, intervention, and outcome.[1] Evaluation consists of the initial step of obtaining the client's occupational profile and a second step of analysis of the client's occupational performance. The occupational profile is focused on the person's history, experiences, daily living patterns, values, needs, beliefs, and so on. The profile consists, essentially, of understanding what the person finds important and meaningful and, therefore, of high priority. Although obtaining contextual information is important throughout the whole intervention process, it is particularly essential at this stage because it will provide the foundation for specific evaluation of occupational performance and certainly for the selection of intervention strategies later in the OT process. For example, if an elder who has had a mild stroke states that he has assembled and collected fishing flies during his whole life, a detailed assessment of fine motor skills may be indicated to ascertain whether he has the necessary motor skills to manipulate the small pieces used in this meaningful occupation. Likewise, an analysis of any other areas of occupational performance that may negatively influence the person's engagement in meaningful occupation should be performed. Notably, barriers to participation in occupation may not necessarily reside in the client but may be located in the client's context. For example, although an elder may like to tie fishing flies, his family may not make the materials available to him because they cannot imagine him going fishing any time soon. In this case, they may not understand the meaningfulness of the occupation of fly tying and therefore create a barrier for his participation in the occupation.

The occupational profile and analysis of occupational performance guide the identification of OT intervention goals and strategies. Thus, the intervention phase is centered around what the client finds most meaningful in life and of greatest priority. An intervention plan will include strategies to address performance skills, patterns, contexts, activity demands, and client factors that may be hindering performance. An ongoing collaboration among the OTR, COTA, and client is indispensable to assure that goals, intervention strategies, and progress are continually evaluated and adapted to meet the client's priorities.

According to the Occupational Therapy Practice Framework, OTRs and COTAs "determine the client's success in achieving health and participation in life through engagement in occupation."[1] This means that it is the responsibility of OT practitioners to assure that their interventions lead to actual participation in life situations and not simply to improvement in performance skills. In the earlier example of the elder who found tying fishing flies meaningful, it is not sufficient to help him develop the motor skills necessary to maintain this interest. The ultimate goal of OT is for the elder to actually engage in fly tying in the most natural context possible. Thus, instructing the elder to exercise his fingers with elastic bands may contribute to his skills but cannot be the limit of OT intervention. Likewise, using fly fishing to develop dexterity can be considered insufficient intervention if the elder never has the opportunity to use the product of his hands in a meaningful way.

Deepak: The Framework in use

The Framework can help us understand Deepak's life situation and plan intervention that best supports his participation in all areas of life. According to the Framework, the initial phase of evaluation should involve obtaining an occupational profile. By asking Deepak about his current concerns related to engaging in occupations and daily life activities, as well as about his work history, life experiences, family traditions, and other personal facts, we find out that he has relied heavily on his wife to help with the family's transition from country to country. Deepak now has a great sense of debt toward her and some guilt for having spent much time working away from home. The physician has recommended that Deepak not put any weight on his left leg for 6 weeks. Deepak's main concern is that, because of his left knee infection, he will not be able to be of any assistance to his wife in her last weeks of life.

Understanding Deepak's main concern will help us establish a collaborative relationship with him while we evaluate his skills and environment. If, for example, we had proceeded to evaluate his ability to dress and bathe himself and assessed his endurance and joint range of motion without knowing about his concerns, we might have further reinforced his sense of uselessness and limited potential for social participation. Instead, we can now identify which activities he believes would be the most important for him to be able to do to convey caring for his wife. For Deepak, these include being able to help her move in bed, get in and out of a bed and a chair, run errands for her and, if necessary, help her eat. Thus, we can proceed by evaluating his endurance, balance, and strength, all needed to help his wife move in bed or get in and out of a chair. We can help adapt the environment and teach him body mechanics to have the maximum leverage while moving his wife. We can further evaluate his ability to complete activities of daily living (ADL) because he will need to be dressed to run errands outside of the home.

Naturally, there are many other areas for assessment and intervention with Deepak. However, the previous illustrates how the central concern for him is related to an area of occupation rather than to a body structure. OT intervention can still be organized to address many client factors, but the intervention is not likely to seem meaningful unless Deepak is able to understand that it contributes to his main concern.

Facilitating Growth and Development

The Facilitating Growth and Development Model views the OT practitioner's role as one "concerned with facilitating or promoting optimal growth and development in all ages of man."[2] An individual's growth and development may be threatened by disease, injury, disability, or trauma. The OT practitioner may be required to assist the individual in coping with illness, trauma, or disability, or to help with rehabilitation. The OT practitioner also may seek to prevent maladaptation and promote health maintenance.

This model requires the OT practitioner to understand the developmental tasks and adaptive skills that are usually mastered at different ages. The model describes the belief that the human being "develops simultaneously in the areas of neurophysiological, physical, psychosocial and psychodynamic growth, and in the development of social language, daily living, sociocultural, and intellectual skills during the life span."[2] The way the individual integrates and organizes these areas of development to perform in work, education, play, self-care, and leisure activities during each stage of life is of primary concern to OT. In addition to understanding the individual's development, the OT practitioner must understand the ways illness, disease, trauma, and disability may threaten that development. Finally, OT addresses the environmental variables necessary to support the development and maintenance of the important adaptive skills cited by Llorens.[2]

The Facilitating Growth and Development Model synthesizes the work of numerous authors who have contributed to the understanding of human maturation.[2] The model includes descriptions of the adaptive skills mentioned during each life stage, including infancy to age 2 years, ages 2 to 3 years, ages 3 to 6 years, ages 6 to 11 years, adolescence, young adulthood, adulthood, and maturity. Each stage is built on the foundation of the stages that the person has completed (Table 7-3). This text, however, focuses on the last stage.

During the OT process, the OTR and COTA assess the client's development and determine potential disruptions in each adaptive skill area. The OTR and COTA analyze this information to determine the effects on age-appropriate occupational performance in the areas of work, education, self-care, and play and leisure. The OTR and COTA may then devise intervention strategies that facilitate development of a specific skill needed for successful occupational performance (Table 7-4). Matching the client's needs with the right therapeutic activities requires careful analysis of inherent requirements of each activity.

Depending on the client's needs, selected activities may include sensory, developmental, symbolic, and daily life tasks. These activities are combined with the social

TABLE 7-3

Characteristics of Maturity	
Neurophysiological and physical development	Possible alterations in sensory functions (visual, auditory, tactile, kinesthetic, gustatory, and olfactory), motor behavior (coordination of extremities), information processing (higher level integration, including conceptualization and memory), and physical endurance
Psychosocial—ego integrity and maturity	Acceptance of life experiences and the life cycle
Psychodynamic	Coping with continued growth after middle age, decision making regarding growth or death (giving up on life), dealing with insincerity of friends and acquaintances, inner life trends toward survival, possible decrease in efforts to maintain false pride, often a reduction in defenses, more suspiciousness, and necessity of dealing with psychological deterioration
Sociocultural	Group affiliation: family, social, interest, civic
Social language development	Predominantly verbal use, some use of nonverbal behavior to communicate
Activities of daily living and developmental tasks	Adjustment to decreasing physical strength and health, adjustment to retirement and reduced income, adjustment to death of spouse, adjustment to one's own impending death, establishment of affiliations with own age group, and meeting of social obligations
Ego-adaptive skills	Ability to function independently; ability to control drives and select appropriate objects; ability to organize stimuli, plan, and execute purposeful motion; ability to obtain, organize, and use knowledge; ability to participate in primary group; ability to participate in a variety of relationships; ability to experience self as a holistic, acceptable object; ability to participate in mutually satisfying relationships oriented to sexual needs
Intellectual development	Possible neurophysiological and physical development alteration and return of egocentrism

Adapted from Llorens, L. A. (1976). *Application of a Developmental Theory for Health and Rehabilitation.* Rockville, MD: American Occupational Therapy Association.

interaction that is most beneficial for the client. Sensory activities are those that primarily influence the senses through human action, such as touching, rocking, running, and listening to sounds. Developmental activities involve the use of objects such as crafts and puzzles in play, learning, and skill development situations. The client develops specific performance skills by engaging in these types of activities. Symbolic activities are designed to help the client satisfy needs and elicit and cope with emotional responses. Examples include gouging wood and kneading clay, which may release muscle tension and help process anger. Another example of a symbolic activity is leading a group in a task. This activity may satisfy the client's need to be heard and feel competent. The emotional response from leading a group may be improved self-esteem. Daily life tasks, also called activities of daily living, include tasks such as brushing teeth, getting dressed, cooking, and cleaning. Finally, social interaction includes participation in dyads with the therapist or another person and groups. These activities encourage the development of sociocultural competence and language and intellectual skills.

According to the Facilitating Growth and Development Model, OT intervention should continue until the client reaches sufficient competence in performing the skills and activities described as developmentally appropriate. The OTR and COTA continually monitor and reevaluate the client's progress in improving, maintaining, or restoring areas of occupational performance and therefore clearly know when the client no longer requires specialized OT services.

Martha: The model in use

Llorens's[2] developmental model can help give us a more complete picture of Martha's life and occupational needs. She has lived for more than half her life with the disability that resulted from her head injury. However, she has been relatively healthy and independent. She now is facing the neurophysiological and physical alterations that are normal with maturity but that seem to compound the occupational performance challenges brought by her disability. Her bouts with pneumonia have left her debilitated, and she has been moved to a skilled nursing facility.

According to Llorens's developmental model,[2] a life priority for Martha is to accept life experiences and the life cycle, not to distinguish which of her problems are caused by her age and which by her head injury. Of great importance will be for her to continue developing coping skills to deal with both her limitations in function and the changes in her environment now that she no longer lives with her sister. She has the opportunity to participate in a variety of relationships with fellow patients and staff. Finally, of great importance will be to stimulate her

TABLE 7-4

Activity Analysis	
Sensory aspects	How much touch and movement does the activity require?
	To what extent are visual perception skills used in the activity?
	Does the activity require auditory perception and discrimination?
	Are perception and discrimination of smells and taste involved in the activity?
Physical aspects	How much does the activity require bilateral movements of arms and legs?
	Does the activity require the use of both hands at the same time?
	Can the activity be completed with one hand?
	How much muscle strength and joint range of motion does the activity require?
	How much sitting, standing, and variability in position is necessary to complete the activity?
	Does the physical performance require much thought organization?
	Which fine and gross motor movements does the activity require?
	How much eye–hand coordination is needed for the activity?
	How much time, and what equipment is needed for the activity?
Psychodynamic aspects	Does the activity permit expression of feelings, thoughts, original ideas, and creativity?
	Is there opportunity for the constructive expression of hostility, aggression, expansiveness, organization, control, narcissism, expiation of guilt, dependence, and independence?
	How does the activity permit or require sex role identification?
Social aspects	How much contact and guidance from others are required to complete the activity?
	How much does the activity require the person to work alone or with others?
	How much socialization does the activity permit?
Attention and skill aspects	How much initiative and self-reliance does the activity require?
	Does the activity require technical skills?
	Are manipulative and creative abilities needed?
	Does the activity require persistence to complete?
	How much repeated motion is needed?
Practical aspects	How much noise and dirt are created during the activity?
	What materials and equipment are used, and what are their costs?
	Can waste or scrap material be used?

Data from Llorens, L. A. (1976). Application of a developmental theory for health and rehabilitation. Rockville, MD: American Occupational Therapy Association.

continued intellectual development. Although her ability to bathe and dress herself independently is important, that need should not overshadow the other needs she has as a developing human being.

Cognitive Disabilities

As its name indicates, the Cognitive Disabilities Model is concerned with OT services that are designed for clients with cognitive impairments. These impairments may be the result of psychiatric illness, medical diseases, brain traumas, or developmental disorders. Psychiatric illnesses such as depression and schizophrenia have associated cognitive impairments. Alzheimer's dementia and cerebrovascular accidents are examples of medical conditions that result in cognitive impairments, and closed head injuries are an example of trauma to the brain that can also result in a brain disorder. Brain dysfunction also may result from use of prescribed medications or other drugs. The cognitive impairment that results from these conditions may be short-term or long lasting.

Assertions of the Cognitive Disabilities Model are based on information from neuroscience, biology, psychology, and traditional OT theory.[5] According to this model, occupation is synonymous with voluntary motor action. Observing voluntary motor actions such as dressing, completing a craft, or preparing a simple meal is of primary interest to the OT practitioner because of the inferences that can be made about brain function. Voluntary motor actions are "behavioral responses to a sensory cue that are guided by the mind."[3] That is, voluntary motor actions occur as a consequence of the relation among the external physical environment of matter, which provides sensory cues; the internal mind, which provides purpose; and the body, which produces behavior in the form of motor activity. Observing a person's voluntary motor action gives the OT practitioner insight into the relation among these three domains. Each domain is further described by subclassifications.

Based on extensive research, the Cognitive Disabilities Model proposes a categorization of six cognitive levels that describe the way an individual relates matter, behavior, and mind as demonstrated in performance of voluntary motor actions (Table 7-5).[3,5] Level 1 represents the greatest degree of impairment, and level 6 represents normal performance. As this model has evolved, each cognitive level has been expanded to include several

TABLE 7-5

Allen Cognitive Levels

		Level 1	Level 2	Level 3	Level 4	Level 5	Level 6
Matter	Sensory cues	Automatic actions	Postural actions	Manual actions	Goal-directed actions	Exploratory actions	Planned actions
		Awareness is at threshold of consciousness	Responds to proprioceptive cues	Responds to tactile cues	Follows visible cues	Follows related cues	Follows symbolic cues
	Perceptibility	Attends to cues that penetrate subliminal state	Aware of own body and objects that come into contact with it	Aware of immediate external surfaces	Aware of concepts of color and shape of objects	Aware of concepts of space and depth	Aware of intangible concepts
	Setting	Mainly internal	Within range of motion	Within arm's reach	Within visual field	Restricted to task environment	Expanded to potential task environments
	Sample	Responds to alerting stimuli	Copies demonstrated body action	Identifies material objects	Makes exact match of sample	Conceives tangible possibilities of variations	Conceives hypothetic ideas
Behavior	Motor actions	Actions are habitual and automatic and have little thought	Spontaneous actions are postural (bending and stretching)	Hands are used to manipulate material objects repetitively	Actions are goal directed but restricted to tangible environment	Possibilities are explored through motor action that causes a visible effect	Actions are preceded by pause to think and plan
	Tool use	Needs stimulation to use body parts in habitual tasks	Uses body parts spontaneously	Uses found objects by chance; success is accidental	Uses hand tools as a means to a concrete end	Uses hand tools to vary means and end	Creates tools; uses power tools

Continued

93

TABLE 7-5

Allen Cognitive Levels—cont'd

		Level 1	Level 2	Level 3	Level 4	Level 5	Level 6
		Automatic actions	Postural actions	Manual actions	Goal-directed actions	Exploratory actions	Planned actions
	Number	Completes one action at a time	Completes one action at a time	Completes one action at a time	Completes task one step at a time	Completes several steps at a time	Completes indefinite steps
	People	Attends to those who shout or touch	Attends to those who move	Attends to the object manipulation of others	Shares goals with others	Shares exploration with others	Shares plans and recognizes autonomy
	Directions	Understands single verbs; physical contact is needed for action	Understands pronouns and names of parts; gross motor and guided movements	Understands names of material objects and actions on an object	Understands adjectives and adverbs; must see each step in a series	Understands prepositions and explanations; each step and potential errors must be demonstrated	Understands conjunction and conjectures; demonstration is not necessary
Mind	*Attention*	Attention is focused on subliminal cues; external attention is very transient	Attends to proprioceptive cues, to own body, and to movement	Attends to tactile cues, focuses attention on the immediate effects of own actions	Attends to clearly visible cues; focuses attention to complete a task, end product sustains attention	Attends to related visual cues; may seek novelty through variation, but must see effects first	Attends to symbolic cues, thinks before testing results
	Goal attainment	Is awake; completes very habitual behaviors (eating and drinking)	Chance body movement creates interesting results that may be repeated	Chance movement creates visible results that are repeated many times	Uses several movement schemes to achieve an end goal	Becomes aware of problems when they become visible; uses trial and error approach	Problems are solved covertly; images are used to test solutions
	Time	Attention is maintained for seconds at a time	Attention is directed for minutes at a time	Attention is directed for half an hour at a time	Attention is maintained for an hour at a time	Attention is maintained and goals are remembered for weeks at a time	Sense of past, present, and future is maintained

Data from Allen, C. (1985). *Occupational Therapy for Psychiatric Diseases: Measurement and Management of Psychiatric Diseases.* Boston: Little, Brown.

subcategories or *modes*. Only the global characteristics of each level are described in this text. This practice model may be used to describe client performance and to guide selection of activities or tasks that permit the client to function consistently at the greatest possible level. (Other chapters in this text describe conditions associated with elders for whom the application of the cognitive disabilities model may be appropriate, including the aging process in Chapter 3; side effects of medication in Chapter 13; malnutrition and dehydration in Chapter 18; strokes in Chapter 19; Alzheimer's dementia in Chapter 20; depression, schizophrenia, and drug addiction in Chapter 21; and brain tumors in Chapter 25.)

Observing clients perform activities and tasks that are part of their daily routines is ideal during assessment because these activities are usually important to the client and caregivers. These activities also allow the OTR and COTA team to separate issues related to learning a new activity, which might not accurately convey the client's current cognitive performance. Consequently, task assessment should be preceded by information obtained from the client and caregivers regarding the client's most familiar tasks. After observing the client, the OTR and COTA team can compare the performance with the characteristic behaviors for each cognitive level. The OTR and COTA must remember that a client may function at a variety of levels depending on familiarity with the task and the time of day. Knowledge of the client's optimal functional level helps the OTR and COTA team design intervention strategies that maximize the client's abilities.

Several standardized tests may be used to determine cognitive level, including the Expanded Routine Task Inventory (RTI)[3,15] and the Allen Cognitive Levels (ACL) Test.[5,16] The RTI evaluates the individual's ability at each of the six levels to complete a variety of routine tasks along a physical scale, such as grooming, dressing, bathing, walking, exercising, feeding, toileting, taking medication, and using adaptive equipment; a community scale, such as housekeeping, obtaining and preparing food, spending money, doing laundry, traveling, shopping, telephoning, and taking care of a child; a communication scale, such as listening, talking, reading, and writing; and an employment scale, such as maintaining pace and schedule, following instructions, performing simple and complex tasks, getting along with coworkers, following safety precautions and responding to emergencies, and supervising and planning work. The ACL test helps determine cognitive level by assessing the response to verbal instructions and problem-solving techniques when a client is presented with a leather lacing project.[3] The large ACL was developed to compensate for visual loss in the elder population, and the Cognitive Performance Test was developed to provide a standardized, ADL-based instrument for the assessment of functional level in Alzheimer's dementia.

Once the client's cognitive level has been determined, the OT intervention goals must be considered.[4] Allen states that participation in an occupation does not necessarily mean the client will improve.[3] This assumption fails to recognize other possible reasons for recovery, including that the client may recover spontaneously without any intervention. Consequently, the purpose of OT intervention should be to document alterations and improvements in functional abilities, sustain current performance, and reduce pain and distress associated with the symptoms. Goals are not intended to improve cognitive level but to ensure consistency of performance at the safest and least restrictive level. The case of Ray illustrates this point. Ray is a 70-year-old man with Alzheimer's dementia. An OTR and COTA team determined that he is currently functioning at cognitive level 4. This means that Ray can spontaneously complete tasks when cues are clearly visible. A goal for Ray to live independently would not be appropriate because he does not deal with cues that are not within his field of vision and consequently can easily place himself in danger. Appropriate OT goals for Ray according to this model may include consistent initiation of daily self-care routines, initiation of laundry washing, consistent monitoring of Ray in unfamiliar environments, and provision by his caregivers of appropriate cues to maximize his performance.

Once the client's goals have been determined, the COTA may select a variety of activities that match the characteristics of the matter, mind, and behavior domains appropriate to the client's cognitive level. The COTA must be adept at analyzing a task to know precisely the way it requires matter, mind, and behavior to interact for the client to successfully perform a voluntary motor action. Tasks are selected by the degree of demand on the client to perform consistently at a particular cognitive level. The OTR and COTA team evaluated Ray and determined he was at cognitive level 4. Consequently, he can understand basic goals of activities, can purposefully use objects placed within his field of vision, and is able to match examples of tasks demonstrated to him. To reinforce his ability to maintain a sense of accomplishment, the COTA may select a simple woodworking project for Ray. The COTA can place all materials for this project on a table in front of Ray and instruct him to sand the wooden pieces. Telling him to pick up the sandpaper, hold it so the grain comes in contact with the wood, and rub it against the wood is unnecessary. These steps would be obvious to Ray because the materials are in his field of vision. Once Ray completes the sanding, the COTA may instruct him in a similar way to glue the pieces together as shown in the sample, stain the stool, and varnish it. Ray lacks the foresight to plan for potential problems; consequently, the COTA should demonstrate the amount of glue, stain, and varnish needed in addition to the application procedures.

Once the client is performing at a level that most consistently demonstrates remaining task abilities and the environment has been structured to compensate for the client's limitations, skilled OT services should be discontinued. Discharge considerations are made from the beginning of OT intervention. The cognitive disabilities model specifically focuses on preparing the client for discharge to the least restrictive environment.[5] Therefore, the COTA must observe voluntary motor actions to understand the way each client interacts with the environment. The COTA and OTR should recommend that the client be discharged to the setting that best supports the client's task abilities.

Ursula: The model in use

Ursula's Alzheimer's disease has progressed to the point where there is a clear cognitive deficit. Therefore, the Cognitive Disabilities Model is ideal to help us develop a suitable intervention plan. The first step is to determine the cognitive level at which Ursula is functioning. During the RTI, Ursula shows that she performs at cognitive level 4. This is consistent with her husband's report, who states that at home Ursula follows his visible cues and seems to pay attention to only objects within her immediate visual field. He notes that she does not seem able to find items she needs even though they are in plain view in the room. However, once she finds the item, she is able to use it correctly.

The OT program for Ursula should consist of activities at level 4 that encourage her to complete steps of repetitive tasks after they have been demonstrated for her. For her safety, the environment should be structured so that all of the items she needs are in plain view in front of her. She should be given one instruction at a time, and instructions should focus on the motor actions rather than on the abstract goal of projects. Examples of suitable projects include simple printing or painting tasks, woodworking kits with few and large pieces, and simple food preparation tasks that do not require use of a stove or other potentially dangerous appliances. For her safety, Ursula should never be left alone or unattended.

Model of Human Occupation

The Model of Human Occupation was designed for use with any individual experiencing difficulties in performing an occupation. This model evolved from earlier research by Reilly[17] on occupational behavior. Using concepts from General Systems Theory, Open Systems Theory, and Dynamical Systems Theory, this model gives an explanation for the way occupation is motivated, organized, and performed, thereby emphasizing the human system's spontaneous, purposeful, tension-seeking properties and acknowledging its creative properties.[6] In addition, this model provides a view of the degree of intimacy between the environment and the performance of occupation.

Human beings maintain constant interaction with the environment and receive many types of input such as olfactory and sensory stimulation and behavior expectations. The individual uses that input in many ways (e.g., food becomes energy; sensory stimulation may translate to touch, pain, or temperature; and words are interpreted). This process is known as throughput. Part of the result of the process of input and throughput is that a behavior, or output, is produced. Finally, as the person performs the behavior, the experience of doing it and any results from it form the process of feedback, which becomes a new source of input into the system. The Model of Human Occupation explains occupation as the cumulative and highly dynamic expression of this process. For example, in meal preparation, the cook sees the food items (input), considers what recipe to use (throughput), prepares the food items (output), feels arm movement, and sees the result of the preparation (feedback). While seeing that feedback, the cook notices that the food is beginning to turn brown (input), decides it is burning (throughput), removes the pan from the stove (output), and experiences moving the pan until it is off of the stove (feedback). To further explain this dynamic interaction between the individual and the environment from which the occupation arises, the Model of Human Occupation describes external and internal environments of the human being as composed of several subsystems.

According to this model, the external environment offers opportunities for certain behaviors while requiring others. For example, the institution of school offers the teacher a room in which to walk around, speak, write on the chalkboard, and sit in a chair. At the same time, the school requires from the teacher the behavior of instructing the students. The teacher will be fired if those requirements are not met. Providing opportunity and requiring behavior is a complementary relationship. The influence of this relationship comes from several sources in the environment, including the physical realm, such as objects and built or natural structures; the social realm, which includes the tasks deemed appropriate and desirable and the social groups sanctioning the behavior; the settings or spaces in which occupation occurs, such as home, neighborhood, school, workplace, and gathering, recreation, and resource sites; and the overall culture, such as values, norms, and customs, which affect the individual's life. In addition, political forces and socioeconomic conditions of the society in which a person lives have an impact on the person's occupation by making resources available or restricting access to them. For example, a person in a wheelchair may not be able to access an entertainment venue if the society does not mandate the presence of cut curbs, ramps, and elevators in public spaces. However, the presence of adapted environments will not make much difference if the person lacks economic means to obtain a wheelchair in the first place (Figure 7-2).

The earlier example of meal preparation can be used to further elaborate on these external environment concepts. To perform this occupation, the cook requires several objects, including food ingredients and seasonings, a knife, some pans, and the stove. The processes of dicing, chopping, stirring, and frying the food are all tasks recognized as cooking. Because of health concerns, the cook may choose to prepare a meal consisting only of vegetables for his or her family (social group). The setting of the meal is the cook's home, where he or she can exercise creativity in preparing and seasoning the food and

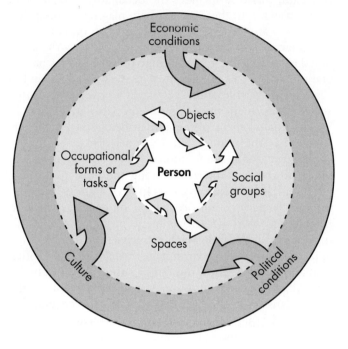

FIGURE 7-2 External environment layers.

presenting the meal. In addition, the choice of vegetables only may be influenced by a cultural value that an athletic body is preferable to an obese one. If the cook were performing the occupation of cooking as the main task of his or her job at a restaurant, however, the objects, tasks, social group, setting, and possibly cultural expectations may present completely different opportunities and behavior expectations. There he or she might use industrial-size knives and tools, prepare large amounts of fried fish, be part of a team of cooks, and work in a restaurant that specializes in ethnic food.

The Model of Human Occupation describes the individual's internal environment as composed of interrelated components (Figure 7-3). Volition is responsible for guiding the individual through occupation choices throughout the day. According to this model, occupation choice is influenced by the individual's disposition about expected outcome and by self-knowledge, or awareness of the self as an active participant in this world. Both of these influences determine the way the individual anticipates, chooses, and experiences occupation. These concepts are illustrated by George and Pam, an elder couple residing in a senior housing community. Every Saturday night they dress in their best clothes and walk to the common hall to play bridge with other members of their community. They choose to do this because they anticipate the pleasure of friends' company and because they believe they are capable bridge players. Helen, who lives in the same

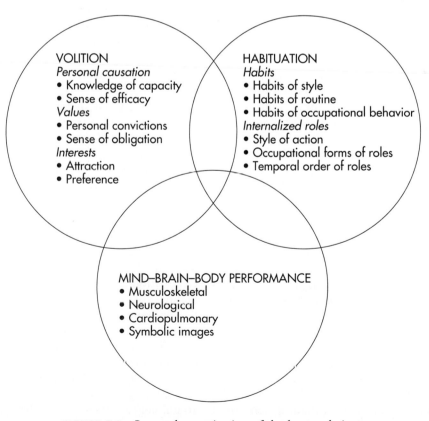

FIGURE 7-3 Internal organization of the human being.

community as George and Pam, chooses not to play bridge. Although she is a champion player, she anticipates feeling out of place because she is a widow and does not have a regular partner.

Volition is composed of personal causation, values, and interests. Personal causation refers to the awareness individuals have of their abilities (i.e., knowledge of capacity) and to individuals' perceptions that they have control over their behavior (i.e., sense of efficacy). An individual is more likely to engage in an occupation he or she feels capable of doing. Values refer to the convictions people have that help them assign significance and standards of performance to the occupations they perform. Each individual has values that form the individual's views of life. These values elicit a sense of obligation to do what the individual believes is right. Finally, interests refer to the desire to find pleasure, enjoyment, and satisfaction in certain occupations. Interests may also be attractions that people feel toward certain occupations and preferences regarding ways that occupations are performed. For example, George, Pam, and Helen each has a sense of themselves as good or effective bridge players (personal causation). This sense was developed through experience over time, so that after playing as partners for more than 30 years, George and Pam have a specific playing style (preference) and are attracted to the opportunity to play bridge on Saturday nights rather than staying home and watching television. Although Helen may have developed the same interest and personal causation, she believes that playing bridge is most meaningful with your spouse as your partner. Because she has no spouse, this value is sufficient to deter her from participating in the Saturday night games at the senior housing community.

In contrast to volition, which has to do with conscious choice and motivation of occupation, habituation has to do with the routine ADL. These routines require little deliberation because they are built on repetition. Habituation is composed of habits and internalized roles. Habits have to do with the typical way an individual performs a particular occupation and organizes it within a typical day or week and the unique style the individual brings to performance. For example, going to the common hall on Saturday night to play bridge is part of George and Pam's weekly routine. While playing bridge, both drink coffee. George typically puts one teaspoon of sugar in his cup before pouring in the coffee, and Pam pours her coffee first and then mixes in the sugar. During the game, George is talkative and Pam is quiet, but both break into song when they win the game.

Internalized roles refer to typical ways in which an individual relates to others. Roles are the identities and behaviors that people assume in various social situations. These roles are based on the individual's perceived expectations of others. Thus, roles involve obligations and rights of the individual in the various social contexts. According to the Model of Human Occupation, the specific occupational behaviors that encompass a role, the style in which actions in a role occur, and the way an individual's roles are prioritized are of particular interest to the OT practitioner. George, Pam, and Helen each have an image of the role of bridge player. For George and Pam, this role includes the occupations of dressing nicely, walking to the common hall, playing by the rules, and sitting around a table conversing with others. Helen may view the role in a similar way, but she has the additional sense that the role of bridge player requires having one's spouse as partner. Because she is a widow, Helen has abandoned the role of bridge player. Conversely, George and Pam routinely enter this role on Saturday nights.

The final element of the human being's internal environment is the mind–brain–body performance capacity component. As its name implies, this component represents the complex interplay among the musculoskeletal, neurological, perceptual, and cognitive abilities required to actually perform an occupation or enact a behavior. Interaction with the environment occurs through this subsystem. The individual perceives challenges and opportunities in the environment through the perceptual system and processes this information in the brain. According to the meaning ascribed to the perception, the brain plans an action, which is carried to the muscles, joints, and bones of the limbs that perform the action. Whereas an occupation's meaning is ascribed by volition and the social context is determined by habituation, the related actions are enabled though the person's performance capacity. George and Pam like to play bridge (volition subsystem) and do so every Saturday night (habituation subsystem). During the bridge game, George and Pam keep in mind the rules and play accordingly. They sit with others around a table and maintain a grasp on the cards (performance subsystem). The complex interplay between mind, brain, and body inherent in the performance of any occupation occurs through specific skills, including motor skills, process skills, and communication–interaction skills (Table 7-6). Performance capacity, however, entails more than simply possessing intact body structures and functions upon which the actions of occupation are built. The person's subjective experience or sense of being oneself in one's own body, significantly shapes what occupations are engaged in and the quality of such engagement. This involves knowing things, knowing how to do things, and then, finally, actually doing things. The Model of Human Occupation refers to this as *mid-body unity*, in which the bodily experience of doing is intricately intertwined with the embodied mind.

A strength of the Model of Human Occupation is the holistic view that it provides of any dysfunction. Traditional health practice often focuses on one or two particular traits of a dysfunction rather than on all of the contributing factors. All of the effects of dysfunction on an individual's life are rarely fully explored.[6] This lack of understanding the whole situation may be particularly

TABLE 7-6

	Performance Skills	
Motor domains and skills	Posture	Stabilizes
		Aligns
		Positions
	Mobility	Walks
		Reaches
		Bends
	Coordination	Coordinates body parts
		Manipulates
		Uses fluent movements
	Strength and effort	Moves objects
		Transports objects
		Lifts objects
		Calibrates force, speed, and movement
	Energy	Endures
		Paces work
Communication and interaction domains and skills	Physicality	Gestures
		Gazes
		Approximates body appropriately
		Postures
		Contacts
	Language	Articulates
		Speaks
		Focuses speech
		Manages
		Modulates
	Relations	Engages
		Relates
		Respects
		Collaborates
	Information exchange	Asks
		Expresses
		Shares
		Asserts
Process domains and skills	Energy	Paces
		Attends
	Knowledge	Chooses tools and materials
		Uses tools and materials appropriately
		Handles tools and materials appropriately
		Heeds directions
		Inquires for directions
	Temporal organization	Initiates
		Continues
		Sequences
		Terminates
	Organization	Searches and locates
		Gathers
		Organizes
		Restores
		Navigates
	Adaptation	Notices and responds
		Accommodates
		Adjusts
		Benefits

Continued

TABLE 7-6

Performance Skills—cont'd		
Social interaction domains and skills	Acknowledging	Turns body or face toward others
		Looks at partner
		Confirms understanding
		Touches others appropriately
	Sending	Greets
		Answers
		Questions
		Complies
		Encourages
		Extends
		Clarifies
		Sets limits
		Thanks
	Timing	Times response
		Speaks fluently
		Takes turns
		Times duration
		Completes
	Coordinating	Approaches
		Places self at appropriate distance
		Assumes position
		Matches language
		Disclosure
		Expresses emotion

detrimental to the elder. For example, Calvin is a 78-year-old man recently admitted to the hospital after falling and fracturing his left femur. On admission, an x-ray examination was done, Calvin was taken to surgery, and an open reduction of the fracture was performed. A cast was put on Calvin's leg, and he was referred to physical and OT for a brief rehabilitation course. The physical therapist focused rehabilitation on getting in and out of bed and walking with the reduced weight-bearing guidelines recommended by the physician. The OTR evaluated Calvin and identified difficulties in dressing and toileting because of the cast and weight-bearing precautions. The OTR asked the COTA to train Calvin to dress and toilet with adaptive equipment, to which Calvin easily complied. Calvin was discharged to return home in 2 days, at which time the OTR and COTA team documented that Calvin was independent in dressing and toileting with necessary equipment and was aware of home modifications needed to avoid further falls. Unfortunately, nobody on the health team carefully investigated the reason that Calvin fell. Although he can care for himself, he finds living alone unbearably lonely. In addition, three of Calvin's lifelong friends died in the past year. Thus, Calvin has a deep sense of hopelessness. He occasionally tries to alleviate his feelings of loneliness and despair by drinking alcohol. He fell after one of these drinking episodes. When the admitting health worker at the hospital asked him if he consumed alcohol, Calvin responded truthfully that he did so only occasionally. During his hospital stay, Calvin appeared bright and friendly because he received much desired social contact. A more systematic evaluation of Calvin's life would have revealed a deeper problem related to his volition and habituation subsystems. Instead, the OTR and COTA team focused on the obvious performance subsystem problem, which actually was only a symptom of a more complex issue. The team's care also should have addressed Calvin's feelings of hopelessness (volition) and the reduced number of roles he has to help himself organize his days (habitation). Furthermore, the COTA and OTR should have helped Calvin explore community resources.

According to the Model of Human Occupation, any traditional OT tool is valid for assessment and intervention. Not one single assessment or intervention tool can completely address the complexity of the individual. Some suggested evaluation tools include the Assessment of Communication and Interaction Skills,[18] the Assessment of Motor and Process Skills,[19] the Assessment of Occupational Functioning,[20] the Occupational Case Analysis Interview and Rating Scale,[21] and the Occupational Performance History Interview.[22] Interest and role checklists, activity configurations, manual muscle tests, range-of-motion tests, and cognitive tests are among the many tools that may be used to evaluate each subsystem. Ultimately, data should be gathered regarding all subsystems of the individual's internal and external environments. Once problems are identified, intervention is prioritized according to all subsystems that are interdependent. In Calvin's case, if the volition and habituation issues had been identified, OT intervention could have focused on helping Calvin find other meaningful activities and resources for continued social contact, in addition to addressing his dressing and toileting needs.

Carlos: The model in use

Because Carlos is unable to speak, an observational assessment tool should be used to describe a baseline of occupational functioning. An Assessment of Motor and Process Skills[19] can help us see that although Carlos is unable to speak, he is able to perform fairly complicated motor tasks. As part of the Assessment of Motor and Process Skills, Carlos was asked to make a fruit salad. Carlos positioned his body appropriately for the task, stabilized all objects, including the fruit and knife, maintained a secure grasp on the objects, chose the right tools, sequenced the task correctly, and cleaned the workspace without being asked to do so. This demonstrated that Carlos continued to consider his role as cook as very important and that he was motivated to remain active. When tasting the fruit salad, there was no coughing, and it became apparent that part of his problem may have been that his family was feeding him while he was in bed. By making the fruit salad, Carlos demonstrated to his family that he was not an invalid and that he was motivated to be upright and active. This allowed the family to step back and encourage him to increase his level of activity rather than overprotect him as they had been doing. In 2 days Carlos's fever was gone and he was developing a system to communicate with his family members through gestures and pictures.

CONCLUSION

Building on the use occupation as a common thread for any OT intervention, each of the practice frameworks or models provides a unique way to organize and think about information regarding the individual's function. In addition, each model guides the selection of intervention strategies appropriate for the specific needs of the individual. Finally, the use of practice models assists the COTA in looking beyond the obvious functional deficits, thereby ensuring a more holistic approach to care of complexities of an elder's life.

▌ CHAPTER REVIEW QUESTIONS

1 Explain the meaning of occupation and why this concept should be at the core of any OT intervention.
2 Describe at least two ways in which a practice model can help the COTA work with elders.
3 Explain why it is important to consider context in an elder's occupational performance.

4 Considering Llorens's developmental model, explain the social interaction needs that an elder is likely to have when placed in a long-term care facility.
5 You have planned a task group for psychiatric clients during which you plan to carve pumpkins for Halloween. Using the Cognitive Disabilities Model, describe how you would modify the activity if the members of the group are functioning at a cognitive level 4.
6 Using the language of the Model of Human Occupation, explain how you would prioritize intervention for an elderly Native American elder who was admitted to the hospital after a car accident in which his wife and adult son died. He has severe fractures in all extremities, and there is the possibility of a mild head trauma. When you approach this gentleman, he refuses to speak and remains staring out the window.

REFERENCES

1. American Occupational Therapy Association, 2008. Occupational therapy practice framework: Domain and processes, 2nd ed. American Journal of Occupational Therapy 62, 625-683.
2. Llorens, L., 1976. Application of a Developmental Theory for Health and Rehabilitation. American Occupational Therapy Association, Rockville, MD.
3. Allen, C., 1985. Occupational Therapy for Psychiatric Diseases: Measurement and Management of Cognitive Disabilities. Little Brown, Boston.
4. Allen, C., Earhart, C., Blue, T., 1992. Occupational Therapy Treatment Goals for the Physically and Cognitively Disabled. American Occupational Therapy Association, Rockville, MD.
5. Allen, C., Earhart, C., Blue, T., 1995. Understanding cognitive performance modes. Allen Conferences, Ormond Beach, FL.
6. Kielhofner, G., 2007. A Model of Human Occupation: Theory and Application, 4th ed. Lippincott Williams & Wilkins, Baltimore.
7. American Occupational Therapy Association, 1995. The philosophical base of occupational therapy. American Journal of Occupational Therapy 49, 1026.
8. American Occupational Therapy Association, 1993. Position paper: Purposeful activity. American Journal of Occupational Therapy 47, 1081.
9. American Occupational Therapy Association, 1994. Uniform terminology for occupational therapy—3rd ed. American Journal of Occupational Therapy 48, 1047.
10. Kielhofner, G., 1995. A Model of Human Occupation: Theory and Application, 2nd ed. Lippincott Williams & Wilkins, Baltimore.
11. Trombly, C., 1995. Occupation: Purposefulness and meaningfulness as therapeutic mechanisms. Eleanor Clarke Slagle Lecture. American Journal of Occupational Therapy 49(10), 960-972.
12. Ma, H., Trombly, C., 2004. Effects of task complexity on reaction time and movement kinematics in elderly people. American Journal of Occupational Therapy 58(2), 150-158.
13. Ayres, A.J., 1991. Sensory Integration and Praxis Test. Western Psychological Services, Los Angeles.
14. Mountain, G., 2005. Occupational Therapy with Older People. Wiley, Hoboken, NJ.
15. Katz, N., 1989, unpublished. Routine Task Inventory: Expanded (RTI-E) manual, prepared, and elaborated on the basis of C. K.

Allen. Unpublished manuscript available at www.allen_cognitive_network.org.

16. Pollard, D., Olin, D.W., 2005. Allen's cognitive levels: Meeting the challenges of client-focused services. SELECTone Rehab, Monona, WI.

17. Reilly, M., 1962. Occupational therapy can be one of the great ideas of 20th century medicine. American Journal of Occupational Therapy 16, 1-9.

18. Salamy, M., Simon, S., Kielhofner, G., 1993. The Assessment of Communication and Interaction Skills (research version). University of Illinois, Chicago.

19. Fisher, G., 1999. Assessment of Motor and Process Skills, 3rd ed. Three Star Press, Ft. Collins, CO.

20. Watts, J., Newman, S., 2007. The assessment of occupational functioning. In: Hempill-Pearson, B. (Ed.), Assessments in Occupational Therapy in Mental Health, 2nd ed. Slack, Thorofare, NJ.

21. Kalplan, K., Kielhofner, G., 1989. The Occupational Case Analysis and Interview and Rating Scale. Slack, Thorofare, NJ.

22. Kielhofner, G., Mallinson, T., Crawford, C., Nowak, M., Rigby, M., Henry, A., et al., 1997. A user's guide to the Occupational Performance History Interview II (OPHI-II) (version 2.0). Model of Human Occupation Clearinghouse, Department of Occupational Therapy, College of Applied Health Sciences, University of Illinois at Chicago, Chicago.

Opportunities for Best Practice in Various Settings

STEVE PARK AND SUE BYERS-CONNON

KEY TERMS

client-centered practice, COTA/OTR partnership, occupational therapy practice framework, service competency, continued competency, geropsychiatric unit, inpatient rehabilitation, adult foster home, skilled nursing facility (SNF), assisted living, home health, adult day care, hospice, emerging practice

CHAPTER OBJECTIVES

1. Illustrate certified occupational therapy assistant (COTA) practice in traditional and emerging practice settings.
2. Become familiar with the Occupational Therapy Practice Framework (second edition) and the COTA's role during occupational therapy (OT) service delivery.
3. Understand the need for service competency for COTAs and continued competency for occupational therapy practitioners: COTA and registered occupational therapist (OTR).
4. Appreciate the COTA/OTR partnership.
5. Value the importance of a client-centered practice.

[T]he defining contribution of occupational therapy is the application of core values, knowledge, and skills to assist clients (people, organizations, and populations) to engage in everyday activities or occupations that they want and need to do in a manner that supports health and participation.[1]

Marta works with elders in a geropsychiatric unit, assisting elders and families to manage daily life activities on the ward and at home. Arianna works with elders in an adult foster home, helping the elders engage in leisure and social activities throughout their week. Rachel works in an inpatient rehabilitation unit, helping elders to regain their competence in basic activities of daily living (ADL). Jean works as a resident services coordinator at an assisted living facility, overseeing the delivery of services. Drew works with elders in an SNF, facilitating their ability to participate in basic and instrumental daily activities and regain former roles. Amanda works on-call for SNFs and is exploring the possibility of including OT services at the independently owned hospice where she volunteers. Manisha works in home health, helping elders engage in a routine of needed and desired daily life activities within their homes. Carlos works at an adult day care center, assisting elders engage in a routine of productive and leisure activities and achieve life satisfaction.

These COTAs attended a reunion for graduates from the Occupational Therapy Assistant (OTA) program at Blue Lake Community College, established 20 years ago. Of the 150 COTAs in attendance, the majority work with elders in one capacity or another, reflecting the U.S. national trends of 75% of COTAs working with rehabilitation/disability/productive aging populations and 50% working in SNFs.[2] Some COTAs work in more traditional settings, such as an SNF or geropsychiatric unit; others work in emerging practice settings, such as adult foster homes and assisted living facilities. Despite working in different settings, the common thread is that the COTAs are assisting elders engage in daily activities and meaningful occupation. Although the settings differ, the focus and process of delivering OT services are similar.

This chapter addresses the role of COTAs, emphasizing the similar focus and process of OT service delivery with elders across different practice settings, using the Occupational Therapy Practice Framework (hereafter known as the *Framework*)[1] as a guide.* Other initial concepts presented are the importance of the COTA/OTR partnership, service competency, continued competency, and practice issues during OT service delivery. A series of vignettes follow that describe COTAs' work with elders in specific settings and illustrate best practice for COTAs,

---

*Throughout this chapter, terms from the Occupational Therapy Practice Framework (2008) are identified in italics.

that is, when OT practitioners deliver services "based on knowledge and evidence that reflect the most current and innovative ideas available."[3]

OCCUPATIONAL THERAPY PRACTITIONERS: A COLLABORATIVE PARTNERSHIP

To support elders to achieve health, well-being, and life satisfaction through participation in a meaningful occupation, the COTA/OTR team provides valuable OT services. Even though OTRs are ultimately responsible for OT service delivery and for supervising COTAs, the delivery of occupational services occurs collaboratively between the two partners.[4] According to AOTA,[4] supervision is defined as "a cooperative process in which two or more people participate in a joint effort to establish, maintain, and/or elevate a level of competence and performance."[4] This supervisory relationship is necessary to ensure the safe and effective delivery of OT services and to promote the professional development of the COTA. Moreover, OT service provision is done in accordance with the Occupational Therapy Code of Ethics,[5] continuing competency and professional development guidelines, relevant workplace policies, and state laws and regulations.[4,6]

Together, the COTA/OTR partners should decide the type of contact (direct or indirect) and frequency of supervision[4] and then develop and document a supervisory plan that details what type of supervision is needed, what areas should be addressed, and how often to meet. For example, a COTA/OTR team works in an SNF and meets face-to-face (direct contact) once a week for an hour to review and discuss their clients' concerns and status. In addition, they discuss specific ways to foster the COTA's professional expertise, such as developing advanced therapeutic skills when working with elders experiencing depression and better ways to incorporate the learning–teaching process when working with an elder's family members, significant others, and caregivers. In other settings, such as home health, the COTA and OTR meet face-to-face several times a month for an hour; however, during the week, they keep in frequent contact through telephone calls and e-mail messages (indirect contact). Although these contacts focus primarily on service delivery for clients, they also discuss areas for professional development. The frequency, methods, and focus of supervision vary according to the skills of the COTA and OTR, the needs and complexity of clients, the service setting's needs and requirements, and state regulatory requirements.[4]

To establish a collaborative partnership and deliver quality services, the COTA and OTR need to value their common beliefs and skills and honor their different contributions during service delivery.[7] A respectful relationship occurs when partners communicate openly, trust each other, share each other's knowledge, and are willing to learn from each other.[8] Sue, a COTA, worked at a rehabilitation unit for 3 years when Steve, an OTR and recent graduate, joined the team. Steve appreciated Sue's expertise to identify, plan, and adapt therapeutic activities related to elders' specific interests and needs, particularly leisure, household, and community activities. Sue appreciated the way Steve fostered her understanding of elders' specific emotional, cognitive, and physical conditions and how to apply this knowledge during evaluation and intervention. Sue taught Steve new and different ways of engaging clients in activities while Steve modeled a client-centered approach when interacting with elders. Steve trusted Sue to carry out interventions, particularly those focusing on adaptation, and share her thoughts and professional opinion, and Sue felt comfortable asking Steve for additional supervision when needed. Sue and Steve were respectful of each other without their partnership being a hierarchical relationship.

Establishing a strong collaborative COTA/OTR partnership is an ongoing process that requires active participation by the COTA and OTR to identify the partnership's strengths and areas of improvement.[8] To assist with the process, COTAs and OTRs should identify each other's competencies, as well as the common knowledge and skills they share. This requires a comprehensive understanding of the role and responsibilities of COTAs and OTRs during the evaluation, intervention, and outcomes process of service delivery. To understand this, the second (and most recent) edition of the Framework[1] and its relation to the COTA/OTR team process is presented in the following section.

OCCUPATIONAL THERAPY PRACTICE FRAMEWORK

In 2002, AOTA introduced the Occupational Therapy Practice Framework: Domain and Process, a document designed to assist OTRs and COTAs to more clearly affirm and articulate OT's unique focus on occupation and daily life activities and to illustrate an intervention process that facilitates clients' engagement in occupation to support their participation in life.[9] Because the Framework is an official AOTA document, it is reviewed every 5 years; consequently, a second edition was published in 2008.[1] Following is a brief overview of the two major areas from the second edition—(1) Domain of Occupational Therapy and (2) Process of Occupational Therapy—that COTAs and OTRs should be familiar with when working with elders. Because the following sections focus on only highlights from the Framework, occupational therapy practitioners are encouraged to obtain the most recent edition for use in practice.

DOMAIN OF OCCUPATIONAL THERAPY

Occupational therapy practitioners assist "clients (people, organizations, and populations) to engage in everyday activities or occupations that they want and need to do in a manner that supports health and participation."[1]

Engagement in everyday occupation (the breadth and meaning of everyday activity) is the focus of occupational therapy, encompassing both subjective and objective aspects of engagement. Thus, the meaning and purpose of engaging in occupation is unique to each client.

In occupational therapy practice, the terms *occupation* and *activity* are used interchangeably, and in the Framework, the term *occupation* encompasses activity, making no real distinction between the two terms.[1] Some professionals, however, do differentiate occupation from activity.[10,11] For example, an elder enjoys creating wooden toys in his workshop for his granddaughter, deriving pride in his skill as a craftsman and from the pleasure the toys bring to his granddaughter. For another elder, that same activity may not hold the same meaning. In fact, some elders may view making wooden toys as a chore or childish. If so, then making wooden toys would be considered merely an activity, one without the meaning that would make it a personal, meaningful occupation.

Although the distinction between activity and occupation is not always clear, it can be helpful for occupational therapy practitioners to consider the distinction between activity and occupation when working with elders. If only an elder's occupation is considered, there may be important activities in the elder's life that are not adequately addressed during intervention. For example, when using the toilet, it may be important for an elder to assist to the best of his or her ability to reduce the physical and emotional stress on the caregiver. If an OT practitioner does not address toileting because the elder does not think it is important to become as independent as possible, then both the elder and the caregiver are at risk for physical injury and emotional distress. However, if an OT practitioner focuses solely on an elder's performance in activities and ignores the elder's engagement in meaningful occupation, an important contribution to the elder's health, well-being, and life satisfaction may be ignored. For example, focusing therapy on increasing an elder's independence in dressing when he or she does not find much personal meaning in this objective may not only damage the therapeutic relationship, but also the OT practitioner may miss an opportunity to enhance the elder's health, well-being, and life satisfaction through assisting the elder to engage in meaningful occupation. Enhancing the elder's engagement in occupation that has meaning to him or her, such as tending to tomato plants, walking the dog around the block twice a day, or washing the dishes after a meal his or her spouse has prepared, may be of greater benefit than achieving "independence" in dressing. The important aspect is that all activities and occupations addressed during OT intervention consider the contexts in which the elder lives, loves, works, and plays.

With a primary focus on a client's engagement in occupation, the Framework outlines six major elements that constitute the primary domain of OT (Table 8-1). No one element is considered more important than the other.

TABLE 8-1

Domain of Occupational Therapy

Performance in areas of occupation	Activities of daily living (ADL) Instrumental activities of daily living (IADL) Rest and sleep Education Work Play Leisure Social participation
Performance skills	Motor and praxis skills Sensory-perceptual skills Emotional regulation skills Cognitive skills Communication and social skills
Performance patterns	Habits Routines Rituals Roles
Organization and population	Routines Rituals Roles
Contexts and environments	Cultural Personal Temporal Virtual Physical Social
Activity demands	Objects and their properties Space demands Social demands Sequence and timing Required actions and performance skills Required body functions Required body structures
Client factors	Values, beliefs, and spirituality Body functions Body structures

Based on data from American Occupational Therapy Association (AOTA). (2008). Occupational therapy practice framework: Domain and process. *American Journal of Occupational Therapy*, 62(6), 625-683.

OT practitioners need to consider all elements when focusing on the targeted outcome of OT intervention: the client's health, participation in life, and engagement in occupation.[1]

The first element, areas of occupation, identifies the primary categories of occupation that OT practitioners consider when working with individuals, organizations, or populations.[1] These categories represent the primary focus of OT: a client's engagement in ADL, instrumental activities of daily living (IADL), rest and sleep, education, work, play, leisure, and social participation. Depending on the specific setting in which a COTA works, some areas may be emphasized more than others. For example, after an acute care hospitalization for pneumonia, it is important for elders to be able to manage their ADL when they return home. Although this may be a major area of concern for discharge, the Framework prompts occupational therapy practitioners to also address other potential areas, such as leisure and social participation, which may be equally important to an elder after discharge.

The second element, client factors, represents the underlying characteristics and capacities (i.e., values, beliefs, and spirituality; body functions; and body structures) specific to each client and that influence a client's performance in occupation.[1]

The third element, activity demands, signifies the particular features of an activity required to engage in that specific activity[1] and reflect a unique skill that occupational therapy practitioners possess: the ability to analyze activities.[12] Each activity "possesses" specific demands—some activities require a large outdoor physical environment, such as a lawn to play croquet, whereas other activities require a relatively quiet indoor environment that promotes conversation, such as a living room where coffee and pastries can be served for church members. Furthermore, each activity will demand more or less of a particular body function or structure—some activities require more fine motor coordination, such as needlepoint, whereas others require greater strength, such as vacuuming.

The fourth element, performance skills, is the "abilities clients demonstrate in the actions they perform"[1] and reflect the interaction of the underlying client factors. OT practitioners use their observation skills to identify those skills that are effective or ineffective when a person is engaging in occupation. For example, a COTA and an elder are in a pharmacy where the COTA is primarily interested in the elder's communication and social skills while picking up a prescription. Throughout the process, the COTA observes the elder's skill to project his voice to the pharmacist behind the counter and effectively ask questions about a medication's side effects.

The fifth element, performance patterns, reflects the configuration of habits, routines, rituals, and roles as clients engage in occupation.[1] An important factor for clients is the ability to engage in a series of activities over time that sustains engagement in occupation. For example, a COTA working with an elder experiencing mild memory loss might assist the elder to develop a consistent routine to safely prepare toast and coffee each morning.

The sixth (and final) element, context and environment, refers to the varied conditions and surroundings under which people engage in occupation. Engaging in occupation is influenced by cultural, personal, temporal, virtual, physical, and social conditions. For example, a cultural norm that a family values and follows may forbid female individuals from providing personal, intimate care for male elders, such as bathing, toileting, or dressing.

PROCESS OF OCCUPATIONAL THERAPY: EVALUATION, INTERVENTION, AND OUTCOME

OT practitioners view occupation as both the means and end of OT intervention.[13] With this in mind, service delivery begins with an evaluation of a client's occupational needs, problems, and concerns, continues with an intervention process that emphasizes the therapeutic use of occupations, and ends with a review of outcomes to identify whether the client's occupational needs, problems, and concerns were resolved.[1] The Framework contains three major elements that represent the process of delivering OT services.

The first element, evaluation, represents the first stage and focuses on understanding what the client wants and needs to do with respect to engaging in occupation and identifying the features that support or hinder the client's engagement in occupation.[1] To do so, OT practitioners must consider those elements identified in the Framework domain—client factors, activity demands, performance skills, performance patterns, and context and environment—and how they influence the client's concerns about engagement in occupation and performance of activities.

The evaluation process consists of two steps: (1) creating an occupational profile and (2) conducting an analysis of occupational performance. Using a client-centered approach, OT practitioners gather information to create an occupational profile that clarifies what is important and meaningful to a client, focusing on the client's occupational history and experiences, patterns of daily living, interests, values, and needs.[1] The process to create a client's occupational profile will vary, depending on the client and the setting, but the focus remains the same: What are the client's current priorities and problems relative to engaging in occupation? Information from the occupational profile guides the next stage in the evaluation process: analysis of occupational performance. This involves observing clients engage in activities and occupation and requires an understanding of the complex and dynamic interaction of the client's performance skills and patterns, the contexts and environments in which occupation needs to occur, the activity demands, and client factors. To analyze a client's performance, specific activities (and the contexts and environments in which they occur) are identified, and the client is observed performing the activities. During this process, the occupational therapy practitioner notes the effectiveness of the client's performance skills and patterns. Using other information gathered during the evaluation process, the OT practitioner then interprets the data to identify what supports and/

TABLE 8-2

Certified Occupational Therapy Assistant/Registered Occupational Therapist Responsibilities During Process of Occupational Therapy Service Delivery

	COTA	Framework	OTR
Evaluation	Contributes to evaluation process Shares information with OTR Administers specific assessments after establishing service competency	Occupational profile Analysis of occupational performance	Responsible for evaluation process, coordinating with COTA Initiates and completes the evaluation Interprets data with input from COTA
Intervention	Provides input to intervention plan	Intervention plan	Responsible for developing intervention plan collaboratively with clients, COTA, and other professionals
	Provides intervention appropriate to demonstrated competency Provides information to assist with intervention review	Intervention implementation Intervention review	Responsible for intervention, coordinating with COTA Responsible for intervention review and documentation, coordinating with COTA
Outcomes	Provides information to OTR related to outcome achievement	Evaluation of outcomes	Responsible for evaluation of outcomes, coordinating with COTA

COTA, certified occupational therapy assistant; OTR, occupational therapist.
Based on data from American Occupational Therapy Association (AOTA). (2009c). *Standards of Practice*. Bethesda, MD: American Occupational Therapy Association; and American Occupational Therapy Association (AOTA). (2008). Occupational therapy practice framework: Domain and practice. *American Journal of Occupational Therapy*, 62(6), 625-683.

or hinders the client's engagement in occupation. OTRs are ultimately responsible for initiating and completing the evaluation. COTAs, supervised by an OTR, assist during the evaluation process according to their skill level (Table 8-2).[1]

The second element, intervention, consists of three steps: (1) developing the plan, (2) intervention implementation, and (3) intervention review. Although OTRs are ultimately responsible for developing the intervention plan, COTAs may contribute during the plan's development.[1] The intervention plan, developed in collaboration with clients (and other professionals), focuses on OT approaches to create, promote, establish, restore, maintain, or modify clients' engagement in occupation or prevent future problems engaging in occupation. An essential element of the intervention plan is the collaboration between clients and OT practitioners to identify and set goals for intervention that focus on specific aspects of a client's occupation that could improve or be maintained over the course of intervention.

Interventions are then implemented to address the client factors, activity demands, performance skills, performance patterns, contexts, and environments that hinder the client's engagement in desired activities and occupations.[1] Again, this is a collaborative process between clients and OT practitioners and focuses on facilitating a change in the activity demands, the contexts and environments, client factors, and/or a client's performance skills and patterns that directly result in improved or maintained engagement in occupation. Throughout intervention implementation, the process is monitored for its effectiveness and progress toward the identified goals and is modified accordingly. Intervention implementation is when COTAs are most active in their role as OT practitioners, using their skills to promote engagement in occupation.[7]

The final element, outcomes, focuses on identifying the success of the intervention.[1] Did intervention foster an improvement with a client's engagement in occupation? Were future problems with a client's engagement prevented? Methods to evaluate outcomes should be used during the evaluation process and throughout intervention to identify what progress, if any, a client is making toward the goals and priorities identified at the beginning of OT intervention. As with evaluation and intervention, COTAs and OTRs work collaboratively to monitor intervention outcomes.

CERTIFIED OCCUPATIONAL THERAPY ASSISTANT/REGISTERED OCCUPATIONAL THERAPIST COMPETENCIES WITH EVALUATION, INTERVENTION, AND OUTCOME PROCESS

Continuing competence is a process by which OT practitioners "develop and maintain the knowledge, performance skills, interpersonal abilities, critical reasoning, and ethical reasoning skills necessary to perform current and future roles and responsibilities within the profession."[12] Demonstration of continuing competency is a requirement of most regulatory boards, employers, and accrediting bodies. The American Occupational Therapy Association[12] serves to ensure that OT practitioners are providing services based on current knowledge and skills. Establishing continuing competency is ongoing and may involve various methods, such as (a) professional service (e.g., volunteering, peer review, and mentoring), (b) completing workshops/courses/independent learning (e.g., attending seminars, lectures, and conferences; reading peer-reviewed journals and textbooks), (c) presenting (e.g., presenting at state, national, and international conferences; serving as adjunct faculty), (d) fieldwork supervision (e.g., Level I or II), and (e) publishing (e.g., journal articles and book chapters).[14] For example, Rachel attended a workshop specifically for COTAs that focused on incorporating a neurodevelopmental approach when providing OT services for elders with strokes. After returning to the rehabilitation center, she directly applied the knowledge and skills from the workshop with elders who had experienced a stroke (see Chapter 19). One elder, Elmer, liked to restore vintage cars and Rachel asked his wife to bring one of their cars to the rehabilitation center. While Elmer polished the car, Rachel worked with him and his wife so that Elmer could learn how to incorporate more normal movement patterns (performance skills) and inhibit muscle tone (client factors).

Establishing competence to practice begins after graduating from an accredited OTA program, successfully completing fieldwork, and passing a nationally recognized entry-level examination for OT assistants.[15] In the United States, OT assistants are initially certified by the National Board of Certification in Occupational Therapy (NBCOT).[14] Initial certification permits the use of the COTA credential for 3 years. After this period, COTAs may choose to recertify, a requirement to continue using the COTA credential after their name and identify themselves to the public as a certified occupational therapy assistant. Re-certification also requires the completion of professional development units, indicating continuing competency.[14]

A unique feature within the COTA/OTR partnership is the establishment of service competency for COTAs. Establishing service competency is the process by which a COTA collaborates with an OTR to demonstrate and document that the COTA's reasoning, judgment, and performance is satisfactory for specific evaluation and intervention methods.[4,7] For example, to establish service competency, an OTR may observe a COTA administer the Canadian Occupational Performance Measure (COPM)[16] several times with different elders. If the COTA consistently administers the COPM according to the manual's instructions and the OTR concurs that the results are accurate with each administration, then the COTA has demonstrated service competency to perform this specific assessment. After this time, the COTA may independently perform the assessment and share the results with the OTR, although the COTA may not interpret the results.[7] In essence, with the establishment of service competency, less direct supervision is required. Documentation of service competency is recommended and is required by many state regulatory agencies.[17]

When reentering the workforce or changing practice areas, the demonstration of continued competency is important and likely a statutory requirement.[17] For example, Drew had worked in a school setting for 1 year. He always had an interest in working with elders and accepted a job offer from an SNF. Before he began work, he attended a workshop to become familiar with Medicare guidelines and the prospective payment system (see Chapter 6). He also attended study groups with three other COTAs who worked in SNFs, where they focused on specific skills, such as transfer techniques, use of adaptive equipment, and application of hip precautions during ADL. In doing this, Drew was actively demonstrating continuing competency relevant to his new area of practice and meeting state regulatory requirements.

ISSUES RELATED TO CERTIFIED OCCUPATIONAL THERAPY ASSISTANT PRACTICE

Overuse and underuse of COTAs in the workplace may occur. COTAs may be underused when employers, as well as supervising OTRs, do not understand a COTA's degree of skill and knowledge. Restricting a COTA to tasks below his or her skill level, such as those performed by a restorative aide, does not allow COTAs to work to their greatest potential. Tasks such as transporting and scheduling patients, keeping inventory of bath equipment, and assisting patients to eat meals do not reflect the greater knowledge and skills that COTAs acquire during their education. COTAs are underused when they are not permitted to fully contribute when delivering OT services. COTAs are qualified to provide safe and effective OT services under the supervision of and in partnership with an OTR, including conducting assessments and reporting observations; selecting, implementing and modifying therapeutic interventions; and contributing to the transition/discharge process.[15]

Overuse may occur when COTAs are asked to contribute beyond the scope of their competency and qualifications. Accepting referrals, conducting initial OT evaluations, and interpreting data are examples of tasks that OTRs are required to complete.[15] In some instances, this may occur when COTAs are encouraged to take on tasks beyond the legal and ethical scope of practice. For example, an OTR may say "I don't have time to see the client. Why don't you start the initial evaluation?" In other instances, COTAs may be asked to perform these tasks when there is inadequate supervision or not enough practitioners to provide OT services.[18] For example, the facility administrator may ask the COTA to complete the discharge summaries because he or she wants to employ an OTR only 4 hours a week. In these cases, the COTA must advocate for proper use of COTAs and discuss the issues with the OTR and others who need to understand the legal, ethical, and professional responsibilities of a COTA/OTR partnership.

CERTIFIED OCCUPATIONAL THERAPY ASSISTANTS WORKING WITH ELDERS IN VARIOUS SETTINGS

During the class reunion, Chris Henson, the OTA instructor for the adulthood and aging course, invited graduates to share their work experiences with the OTA students during a series of class presentations. She was particularly interested in graduates who worked in traditional and emerging practice settings. A synopsis of each of the presentations is presented and integrates concepts from the Framework.[1]

Geropsychiatric Unit

Marta has worked at a 15-bed geropsychiatric unit in a small urban town for 7 years where she enjoys working with elders admitted with varied psychiatric diagnoses such as dementia, bipolar disorder, and schizophrenia. Although most elders are admitted directly from their homes, typically for behaviors with which their family members can no longer cope, such as aggression and confusion, Marta does not let these behaviors become the focus of her practice. Instead, she views each elder as a unique occupational being, focusing on those daily life activities and occupations of priority and concern to elders and their family members. Marta recently worked with one elder, José, a 62-year-old former migrant farm worker born and raised in Mexico who was admitted to the unit with suspected early-onset dementia. After she and Noel, the OTR with whom she collaborates, discussed the information from José's occupational profile, they realized that José no longer walked to and visited with friends within the local Hispanic community, one of his most meaningful occupations. José's family had become increasingly concerned about his memory loss and confusion and was afraid to let him leave the house for fear he would become lost or have an accident. Furthermore, they wanted to preserve José's dignity and did not want his friends and acquaintances to know about his increasing confusion and memory loss. Although José was admitted to the unit for suspected early-onset dementia, Marta viewed José as an occupational being who was experiencing the loss of meaningful occupations, rather than as a confused man who was becoming a burden to his family.

With Marta's 9 years of experience as a COTA, the staff relies on her judgment to identify those daily activities and occupations in which elder patients can successfully engage and which aspects of their daily routine present additional challenges and require support and assistance. Marta said that the elders "often look okay and say that they don't have any problems but the reality is they can get into trouble carrying out simple daily life tasks, if they chose to do them at all." To restore and maintain more successful engagement in routine activities, Marta relies on her skill to analyze an elder's performance of activities and occupations, identifying those factors that support or hinder the elder's successful engagement. Although Noel, the OTR, works with the elders during the morning, Marta works from 2:30 p.m. to 8:00 p.m. during the week, providing her with opportunities to observe elders during their early evening routine of eating dinner, undressing, bathing, toileting, and preparing for bed because performance patterns are important to support successful engagement in activities.[19-21] Marta works closely with families and staff to establish consistent routines and habits for elders on the ward, focusing on creating a physical and social environment that promotes success and decreases confusion. With José, she and Noel worked closely with his family so they could create a routine of activities and meaningful occupations when he returned home to help reduce José's confusion and his verbal outbursts.

Because Marta begins her workday at 2:30 p.m. and Noel ends his at 4:30 p.m., they have little scheduled time for consultation and supervision. Both agree, though, that this time is essential, not only to meet state regulatory requirements, but also to ensure that patients receive quality OT intervention. After her meeting with Noel, Marta leads group activities at 3:30 in the afternoon. Depending on the needs of the group of elders at any one time, Marta will lead groups that focus on life skills, such as craft and cooking groups. Because of the elders' short stay on the unit, often less than 2 weeks, Marta finds that engaging them in activities that are familiar and not too challenging helps them to make sense of their daily life in the unit. Marta particularly enjoys leading the reminiscence group activity where she engages elders with the use of familiar scents, pictures, and objects, encouraging them to interact and share their personal stories. The gardening group activity is particularly enjoyable because Marta can adjust the challenge of the activity to each elder's capability. For those elders who experience difficulty potting a plant on their own, Marta decreases the activity demands, such as asking an elder to help scoop dirt out of the bag or holding a pot while someone else scoops in the dirt. For others, merely sitting at the table and smelling the flowers is enough of a challenge. Those elders who are more able can choose what they would like to plant and carry out the process more independently, often sharing their own gardening expertise with Marta and other elders. No matter what capacity an elder may possess, Marta always ensures that all elders have a potted plant at the end of the group activity that they can give to a family member or friend during evening visits.

After leading groups in the afternoon and completing her notes on each elder's participation, Marta works with the unit staff during the evening dinner hour, observing each elder's ability to eat meals. Because Marta successfully achieved AOTA Specialty Certification in Feeding, Eating, and Swallowing,[22] and she and Noel have agreed she has achieved service competency to manage eating and feeding problems with elders on the unit, Marta is responsible for identifying successful strategies to encourage elders to eat their meals and conveys those strategies to staff members for all meals and snacks. As needed, she will suggest and monitor the use of adaptive equipment. Although it can be challenging at times, Marta also works to create a pleasant and supportive environment during the dinner hour in which elders can successfully interact with family members when they choose to visit.

Because Marta works a later shift, she is responsible for meeting with family members and educating them not only about their elder's diagnosis, but also about what level of care is currently required. She is particularly adept at identifying what aspects of activities each elder can do on his or her own and what aspects with which he or she requires assistance. Occasionally, family members may want to protect and help the elder too much and Marta works with them to preserve the elder's independence and dignity while teaching family members to provide the right amount of support.

Although Marta relies primarily on informal observation to gather important information about the elders, she occasionally administers the Allen Cognitive Level (ACL) screening tool[23] for which she has established service competency. Although Noel interprets the results, together they share the information with other team members. This information is useful because it provides insight into an elder's cognitive abilities and his or her capacities in specific tasks or groups. Most of the time, though, Marta relies on her skills to analyze an elder's performance of activities during groups and their evening routine. These informal observations provide her with the valuable information that she needs to help the elders and their family members plan to return to their own homes.

Inpatient Rehabilitation

After graduating from Blue Lake Community College 5 years ago, Rachel moved to a large metropolitan city and began full-time work at an inpatient rehabilitation facility. She and Beth, the OTR with whom she works, share a caseload of 12 patients, the majority of whom are elders who have experienced a cerebrovascular accident (CVA). Rachel, who does not consider herself a "morning" person, nonetheless arrives at work Monday through Friday at 7:30 a.m. She starts her day working with patients in their rooms, assisting them to achieve greater independence and satisfaction with their morning ADL, such as eating, grooming, dressing, toileting, and bathing (Figure 8-1). One of her favorite elders was Glen, with whom she worked after he experienced a CVA. When Rachel was assisting Glen in the mornings to get ready for the day, Glen would become frustrated because he could never

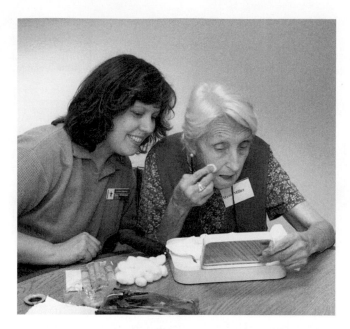

FIGURE 8-1 Certified occupational therapy assistants work with those personal activities of importance to the elder.

find his hearing aide. One day it would be in the drawer under his clothes and the next it would be under the bed sheets. Rachel communicated with the evening nursing staff to ensure that Glen always put his hearing aide in the top right drawer before he went to bed. Although this seemed like such a small thing to do, Glen was much happier each morning because he could easily locate his hearing aide. Rachel works extra hard to establish routines for elders on the ward, recognizing that establishing performance patterns is particularly important for elders when they are away from their usual home environment.

During the initial OT evaluation conducted by Beth, the OTR, Glen raised a concern that he did not want to be a burden on his wife when he returned home. During Glen's short 12-day admission, Rachel worked diligently to ensure that Glen's wife would be comfortable and safe assisting Glen at home. Thus, although independence with toileting, dressing, and bathing was not the ultimate goal, during Glen's morning routine Rachel and Beth focused on developing Glen's performance skills so it would be easier for both Glen and his wife when Glen returned home. Although Glen was not pulling up his pants on his own by discharge, Rachel had worked out a system whereby Glen was able to stand upright on his own and safely stabilize himself on a solid counter while his wife pulled up his pants and fastened them for him.

After morning ADL and during the remainder of the day, Rachel and Beth work together to help the elders reach their goals, collaborating to share the responsibility for gathering initial evaluation information, implementing intervention, and evaluating outcomes. During her level II fieldwork, Rachel had observed her supervisor administer the COPM,[16] although Rachel had never done it herself. Because the COPM is an open-ended interview requiring the OT practitioner to solicit the occupational performance issues of concern to the client, Rachel and Beth developed a plan for Rachel to become comfortable and achieve service competency to administer the COPM and other standardized assessments.

When Rachel interviewed Glen using the COPM,[16] Glen identified that he still wanted to be able to take care of his 5-year-old grandson Brandon because Glen and his wife provide child care 3 days a week. Because this was a priority for Glen, the afternoon OT sessions were devoted to help Glen develop the performance skills needed for Glen to play catch and read story books with Brandon. Rachel worked with Glen to develop the specific motor skills necessary to play catch, such as bending and reaching for a ball on the ground and grasping and lifting the ball with his affected arm and hand. Rachel also worked with Glen on skills necessary to read story books, such as manipulating the pages and coordinating his affected arm with his other arm to hold the book. On the basis of the occupational profile completed during the initial evaluation, Rachel knew that Glen enjoyed challenging physical activities because he considered himself a sportsman. She particularly enjoyed working with Glen to identify various physical activities, both within the OT department and outside of the hospital, which would further develop his motor skills to help him reach his personal goals. Rachel was able to draw on Glen's strengths, specifically his relatively good communication, social, and cognitive skills to help Glen improve his ability to perform daily life activities.

An important aspect of Rachel's work, although not her favorite, is documentation. To demonstrate the need for OT intervention, Rachel and Beth have worked together to develop their documentation skills. They have attended conference workshops and met with local insurance representatives to explain the focus of OT and to understand the insurance representative's point of view. Rachel and Beth share responsibility to write progress notes for their caseload. Although the OTR is ultimately responsible for documenting outcomes,[15] Rachel contributes to the process, sharing her understanding of what has occurred during intervention. Because Beth and Rachel agree it is important that clients also express their views regarding their progress, Rachel often readministers the COPM[16] before discharge. Although Glen did not make much progress with his morning ADL in terms of physical independence, the use of the COPM revealed that he was more satisfied with his performance because he believed that he was no longer as much of a burden to his wife. Although he did not believe he was entirely able to take care of his grandson, he felt he was far better than when admitted to the rehabilitation unit. By using a standardized assessment such as the COPM, Rachel and Beth have

more credible evidence to document an elder's progress and communicate the outcomes and benefit of OT services to help elders achieve their personal goals.

Adult Foster Home

After graduating 2 years ago, Arianna reflected about what aspects of OT practice she liked. She decided she liked working with elders and particularly enjoyed group activities. Because she had the opportunity during her professional education to explore settings that were not based on a medical model, Arianna also recognized that she preferred more nontraditional settings. During her course on adulthood and aging, she spent time at a local senior center where she helped with an exercise program for people with arthritis. Through this experience, she became a certified instructor in exercise and aquatics, which qualified her to teach exercise classes and swim classes.[24] Moreover, a portion of her fieldwork was spent at an assisted living center where she spent time running groups with the activity director. She was able to incorporate the skills and knowledge she learned in her OTA classes, such as designing and organizing groups, leadership strategies, group dynamics, and stages of group process, as well as meeting the individual needs of the group participants.[25]

She noticed an adult foster home in her neighborhood and approached the owners, Elizabeth and Danny, about providing group activities for the elders. Arianna knew, per state regulations where she lived, that adult foster homes are required to provide 6 hours of activities a week for each resident, not including television and movies. Because the state requires the activities to be of interest and meet each elder's abilities, her COTA skills to identify, adapt, and implement appropriate activities for elders were exactly what the owners needed. Arianna talked about her experience working with elders and her abilities to develop and lead group activities. She explained to the owners that, although she was a COTA, the services she would provide would not be considered OT. She would use expertise that did not require OTR supervision, such as making sure that elders were seated securely with their feet flat on the floor and using activities that incorporated full range of motion. Elizabeth and Danny were interested because they had been trying to provide activities without any outside help. After clarifying her intent with the state licensing board, Arianna began working, providing 2 half days of activity programming and consultation per week.

Most of the seven elders at the adult foster home were ambulatory; only one elder used a wheelchair. Anthony and Florence were legally blind, Maria had a severe hearing loss, Alfred used oxygen 24 hours a day for his chronic obstructive pulmonary disease, Herbert had Parkinson's disease, and Leona and Alfonso had mild dementia. Arianna met with each elder individually to get to know them and identify their interests. She used her COTA skills to develop a profile that noted each elder's interests and dislikes, as well as information related to medical needs, such as dietary restrictions, allergies, and "do not resuscitate" status. She also developed a form to document the type of group activity, the length of time each elder participated, the degree of participation, how each elder responded during the activity, and whether he or she declined to participate that day. This form was left at the adult foster home at the end of the month for the owners and served the purpose of documenting participation, as well as a time sheet for her hours worked. The owners employed other people so a payroll tax system was already in place. Because Arianna's husband's employer provided health insurance coverage for spouses, she was fortunate in not having to worry about this.

To provide a solid basis when designing group activities, Arianna organized and implemented a variety of activities, following Howe and Schwartzberg's[25] guidelines for group process. Arianna began each group with small talk, encouraging each resident to discuss current events. Arianna would then incorporate warm-up activities to encourage movement, such as telling a story with the elders acting out the movements. Activities such as marching in a parade or playing balloon volleyball were popular with the elders. Then the main activities would follow, focusing on those activities of interest to the elders, such as preparing the salad for the evening meal, planting herbs in pots, making place mats for holiday meals, and learning new card games. Each group activity closed, by asking the elders to help plan future activities.

As with well-designed groups, the elders would often direct the activities themselves. For example, while making strawberry shortcake, Leona began reminiscing about growing up in an area where there were many berry farms. She lamented that a community college and housing development now occupy the berry fields. Others joined in and talked about how they had to pick berries to earn money to buy their school clothes. Despite her memory loss, Leona shared her mother's favorite jam recipe and asked if the group could make the jam at the next meeting. During another activity, Florence shared how she used to enjoy playing Bingo but is currently not able to get out to games and cannot see the cards well enough to play. Arianna took note and another activity was designed where the elders made Bingo cards with large black numbers so that everyone could see and participate. Arianna also purchased poker chips to cover the numbers because Herbert had trouble picking up small disks. The elders' favorite activities, though, were ones that included cooking or baking. They took pride in preparing meals and inviting family members. Even Alfred, who "never cooked a meal in his life," participated and took pride in telling his daughter that he made the cornbread by himself (even though he did require some help!). During the majority of the time, Arianna planned activities for all residents to participate. She also made sure that when an elder did not want to participate in group activities, she would offer alternative solitary activities.

Not all of the activities were confined to the foster home. The owners had a van and would occasionally take the elders to eat at local restaurants because they enjoyed getting out and eating their favorite foods. On those occasions when Arianna accompanied them, she sat close to Florence and Anthony, both legally blind, and suggested that they orient the food on their plate like a clock. Elizabeth took note and followed through with this suggestion at home with the elders. She reported that both Florence and Anthony were much happier with not needing someone to hover over them during meals. Arianna also suggested a weighted cup for Herbert and provided the phone number of a local vendor. As Arianna became more familiar with the residents, she suggested other community outings such as a trip to a lilac garden, a drive to see Christmas lights, a picnic in the park, and attending local music events at the senior center.

After working at the foster home for 3 months, Arianna expanded her services to other local adult foster homes. The owners were happy with her services and passed along Arianna's business card to other adult foster home owners. Arianna now provides group activities to five foster homes and hopes to find another COTA who is interested in this work to expand the business. Moreover, with senior centers becoming an emerging practice setting for occupational therapy practitioners,[26] Arianna is considering approaching the local senior centers to discuss the development of educational programs. She wants to again contact her state licensing board, however, to understand the parameters under which she can provide health promotion services while also licensed as a COTA.

Skilled Nursing Facility

After graduating 1 year ago, Drew moved to a rural city of 30,000 people and now works full-time at an SNF. At the reunion, he shared that, although he is frustrated at times with the facility rules and insurance regulations, he enjoys working with family members to help elders return home as soon as possible. He shared, "It's tough working toward discharge right away, but then you realize most people's priorities are to get home as soon as they can." Drew primarily sees elders with CVA, as well as those with hip fractures and recent surgeries. Many have secondary health conditions, such as high blood pressure, diabetes, or pneumonia.

Drew particularly enjoys working with elders and their families to figure out the best way to manage ADL at home, including the need for adaptive equipment; thus, the primary intervention approaches he uses with elders are restore and modify. One of the most problematic issues for elders leaving the SNF is toileting and bathing at home. Drew particularly prides himself on his ability to analyze each elder's performance. When observing an elder on the ward, Drew recognizes that the elder's home environment may be very different from the accessible and well-equipped rooms at the SNF. For example, he recently worked with Clarence, an elder who was admitted with a severe case of pneumonia and long-standing arthritis. Clarence and his partner were concerned about Clarence still being able to get in and out of his bathtub and soak in the warm water to relieve his arthritic pain. As best he could in the OT bathroom, Drew re-created the layout of Clarence's bathroom at home. He then observed Clarence's partner assisting Clarence to get in and out of the tub. After they tried out different methods, Drew identified the safest and least painful transfer method, which they practiced until Clarence and his partner felt confident. Drew also identified which specific equipment would best meet their needs at home. This was particularly important because many elders may not start home health immediately after discharge from the SNF, and all necessary equipment needs to be in place before their departure.

Although a main focus of the SNF is promoting independence with ADL, Drew also addresses other roles that are important to the elder (Figure 8-2). Because Clarence was a retired veterinary technician, he was also concerned that he could not take care of his many birds at home. Drew worked with Clarence and his partner to figure how Clarence could safely stand and easily reach while feeding and watering the birds and cleaning the cages. Drew also arranged with the staff for Clarence to play with the resident dog and cat as often as possible when he was not scheduled for therapy. Because Clarence also sang in the church choir, Drew worked with Clarence and his partner to develop a plan so that Clarence could conserve enough energy to attend church twice a week.

In addition to his direct work with the elders, Drew has additional responsibilities. He participates in the weekly team meetings, sharing the reporting responsibilities with Sheryl. Drew and Sheryl also collaborate to leave clear instructions for Brooke, the COTA who works weekends.

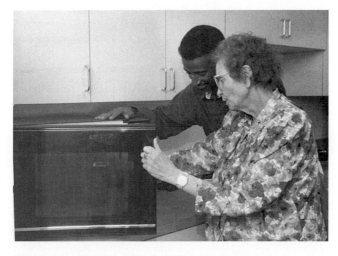

FIGURE 8-2 Instrumental activities of daily living are often important for elders for when they return home.

Drew also spends part of his time working with restorative aides, ensuring that they can follow through with intervention plans. Drew and Sheryl agree that he would assume the primary responsibility to be aware of current regulatory and reimbursement issues related to SNF (see Chapter 6) and share the information with Sheryl and Brooke.

Assisted Living Facility

Jean has been a COTA for 17 years. After graduating, she took a job at a local rehabilitation hospital and worked mainly with adults experiencing neurological disorders. She enjoyed the work, but, because of budgetary problems, her position was eliminated. She then worked at a large long-term care facility where her level of responsibilities increased over time. Having established service competency with the OT evaluation and intervention methods used at the facility, she worked fairly autonomously with occasional OTR supervision. Four years ago, Jean returned to school on a part-time basis to complete her bachelor's degree in health care administration. As Jean was learning management skills, she decided to apply for a position as the director of the OT department. Given her competency as a COTA and her current interest and skills in management, she was offered the position. Jean was now responsible for running the department, including scheduling therapy, coordinating the training and supervision of the employees, and maintaining communication between OT and the other services offered at the facility.

After graduation and the completion of her business degree, she began to seriously consider her future. She enjoyed the management skills that she had learned and developed over the past few years as OT director. She was not sure that remaining in her current position would allow her to grow further so she began looking at other possibilities. First, Jean compiled a list of her abilities that she could bring to the job. She tried to be as realistic as possible and asked for assistance from her husband, parents, and friends who knew her professionally. She felt that she had good supervisory, interpersonal, verbal, and written communication skills. Finally, she was familiar with health care and rehabilitation in particular. However, her challenges were that she had limited experience in marketing, operations management beyond the OT department, and budgeting.

At first, Jean looked for jobs related to OT, rehabilitation, and health care delivery and was discouraged by what she had found. Then, she expanded her search after talking with her neighbor, whose mother was living in an assisted living complex. Jean searched the Internet for information about assisted living facilities and found the website for a corporation that operated a number of facilities in her area. She learned that there were three categories of positions: activities coordinator, executive administrator, and resident services coordinator.

TABLE 8-3

Activities Coordinator Job Description	
Job position	Activities Coordinator
Primary purpose	This person is responsible for the development and coordination of individual activity programming for each resident. Responsibilities include planning and coordinating appropriate resident activities, day-to-day operations, supervising staff, and ensuring program quality.
Qualifications/ skills needed	Prefer an individual with a minimum of 2 years geriatric experience. Experience working with people with Alzheimer's disease/dementia is essential. Experience in staffing and managing the day-to-day operations is preferred. Must demonstrate good interpersonal skills and excellent written and verbal communication. Reports to resident services coordinator.

TABLE 8-4

Executive Administrator Job Description	
Job position	Executive Administrator
Primary purpose	This person is responsible for the creation of resident-focused work teams that support the philosophy of partnering with families. Responsibilities include staffing, training, program implementation, budgeting, sales, marketing, and community relations.
Qualifications/ skills needed	Prior experience managing senior resident services is required along with a bachelor's degree. Experience in marketing, operations management, and budgeting is essential. Strong leadership skills, including organization and interpersonal skills, are a must. Excellent verbal and written communication skills required, as well as computer experience. Occasional travel required.

Jean downloaded the three job descriptions and compared them to her list of abilities. The first job description that Jean reviewed was for activities coordinator (Table 8-3). Jean believed that this job was not challenging enough. Moreover, according to state regulations, if a perception existed that she was providing direct OT services, she would require OTR supervision. Besides, she felt this was not the type of job that interested her enough to leave her current position at the long-term care facility.

The next position that she reviewed was for executive administrator (Table 8-4). Jean compared the job expectations with her abilities and realized that she was lacking in several categories. Although she has had experience at managing a small department, she lacked the marketing, budgeting, and operational management background required for this position.

The final job description Jean reviewed was for services coordinator (Table 8-5). Jean studied the job description and compared it to her list of abilities. Because she believed that this was the right position, Jean contacted the assisted living corporation and requested an application. She applied and was contacted for an interview. Before the interview, Jean wanted to clarify that the services she would provide in this position were not those of a COTA requiring OTR supervision. She contacted her state's OT licensure board and asked them to review the job description. On careful review, the Board determined the

TABLE 8-5

Resident Services Coordinator Job Description	
Job position	Resident Services Coordinator
Primary purpose	This person is responsible for overseeing the delivery of resident services and supervising the resident assistant staff. As a member of the management team, responsibilities include supervising unit teams, staff development, and monitoring quality of resident service and staff recruitment. Reports to executive administrator.
Qualifications/ skills needed	Person should possess a bachelor's degree in a health-related field. Five years experience in senior resident services, including staff supervision, is required. Excellent organizational and interpersonal skills are a must. Strong verbal and written communication skills are essential. Computer proficiency is strongly preferred.

following: (1) Her status as a COTA in this position did not violate state laws and regulations; (2) although the position oversaw the coordination of programs, including OT, it did not require Jean to perform hands-on OT; and (3) Jean could use her COTA initials after her name (she had kept her NBCOT certification up to date) as long as it was understood that she could not provide any OT services without the supervision of an OTR.

Meanwhile, Jean prepared for the interview by identifying the major points she wanted to emphasize. First, she wanted to stress the importance of addressing the elders' needs, including physical, social, emotional, cognitive, and spiritual, and how this belief would guide staff recruitment and development. Second, she wanted to demonstrate how she would coordinate the services in a manner that supported the corporation's philosophy of partnering with families. Third, she wanted to show that her background as a COTA brought a unique perspective on quality of life for elders. She located information that identified that life satisfaction is multifaceted for elders[27] and that the manner in which elders occupy their time contributes to their health, well-being, and quality of life.[28,29]

During the interview, Jean did well and was offered the position. Since then, she has been working with the new executive administrator, assisting with recruitment and development of the resident service teams. One of the first tasks she undertook was to develop a screening tool to identify the physical, social, emotional, cognitive, and spiritual needs of the residents. Her goal was to match the services with the identified needs and eventually demonstrate how the residents' overall needs were being met.

Home Health Agency

Manisha recently changed jobs after working 9 years in an acute care hospital when she obtained a job at a home health agency within a major metropolitan city. Because Manisha used only public transportation before this job, she needed to purchase her first car, one that was spacious enough to carry needed equipment and supplies. Furthermore, Manisha needed to brush up on her map reading skills because her new supervisor emphasized that she would be traveling extensively, often up to 80 miles a day. Because this agency recently converted to a computer-based documentation system, Manisha signed up for a computer course at a local community college. An important issue emphasized during her interview was client confidentiality. Although Manisha was aware of this issue from her work in acute care, Manisha would be visiting many elders during the day, carrying the required documentation from house to house, and would need to take extra care to ensure that that information was kept confidential during her visits.

During her first few weeks on the job, she traveled with different team members, including nurses, physical therapists and physical therapist assistants, social workers,

nutritionists, and home health aides. During these visits, Manisha was surprised by how different things were in the elders' home environment than what she imagined when she worked in acute care. Sometimes, solutions that were proposed in the hospital (similar to those proposed by Manisha when she worked there) turned out to be impractical or the elders just did not want to use them. Recognizing this, Manisha was excited to be working with elders in their own homes where she could assist them to achieve their goals within their familiar home environment, focusing on practical solutions in context (Figure 8-3). Manisha looked forward to working with elders and their caregivers to achieve their goals, such as getting out in the back garden on their own, emptying the trash, getting the mail, operating the radio, or using the telephone to reorder prescription medications.

One elder, Irene, had lived by herself in a one-room apartment and was getting along fairly well despite her legal blindness. Irene recently broke her foot while getting off a high stool in her kitchen. After receiving the doctor's referral, Antonio, the OTR with whom Manisha worked, completed the initial evaluation. Antonio shared the initial evaluation results and developed the intervention plan with Manisha, stressing that her input was important to monitor the effectiveness of the plan. Manisha then

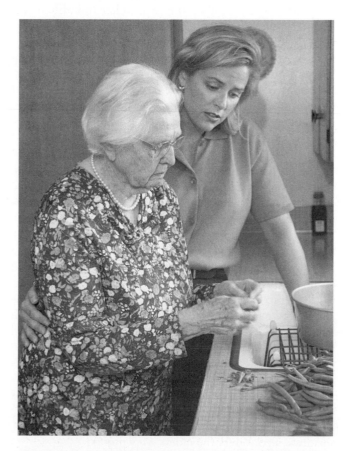

FIGURE 8-3 An elder's home provides many opportunities to work on practical solutions.

assumed primary responsibility for implementing the intervention plan and monitoring the achievement of outcomes. Although Manisha would be on her own visiting Irene over the next month, Manisha would consult as needed with Antonio when they were both in the office in the morning. Furthermore, she frequently communicated with him, as well as with Irene's social worker and physical therapist, through cell phone calls throughout the month.

One of Irene's first priorities was to prepare her own meals rather than rely on the Meals on Wheels initially organized by the social worker. Although it was important to Irene that she prepare her own meals, she did not want to spend a lot of time doing so. After Manisha's first visit, Irene searched for recipes that would be easy to prepare and nutritious and arranged for her neighbor to purchase the necessary ingredients. During the next visit, Manisha and Irene problem solved how to safely prepare simple meals that would not compromise her fractured foot, such as safely using a low chair and safely maneuvering within the kitchen. To make it easier to transport items, Manisha also arranged for Irene to purchase a basket for her walker and to practice safely carrying her recycling items and trash down the hallway.

Because Irene was a volunteer at the blind commission, it was important for her to be able to use public transportation as soon as possible to return to her monthly meetings. Although Irene's home visits would end as soon as she became more mobile, she and Manisha problem solved how best to manage her walker while using the bus. They practiced skills such as managing doors, stepping up and down different levels while using the walker, and folding up her walker once she was seated. Another priority of Irene's was to plan and be able to execute an emergency exit from her third-floor apartment. She and Manisha developed a plan with Irene's neighbors to deal with different types of emergencies. For some situations, a buddy system would be used; for other situations, Irene could make the necessary arrangements through a telephone call.

Because Irene's broken foot presented additional challenges to safely maneuver within her apartment, Manisha and she worked together to rearrange her living and dining room to make it easier and safer for her to listen to the radio and books on tape, as well as use her computer. Although Manisha works most of the time with individual elders, such as Irene, on occasion she is called in to an adult foster home to recommend environmental modifications. For example, she has recommended suitable bath and toilet equipment and more appropriate furniture arrangement to prevent falls. Manisha understands the significant meaning that home has for many elders,[30] and so when recommending environment modifications, she always considers the elders' viewpoints.

Manisha enjoys working in home health because it provides a lot of variety. She visits four to five people a day, the majority of whom are elders. Because she visits elders in their own homes, Manisha is particularly sensitive to being a guest, respecting the elders' privacy and following their lead to establish intervention priorities. This includes collaborating with elders and their families/caregivers as to the best approach to achieve their priorities. Many times this involves working closely with family members to provide education and training, emphasizing safety for not only the elders, but also for the caregiver (see Chapter 11). Because Manisha is skilled with body mechanics and safety concerns/issues, she is responsible for home health aide staff training, providing them with information and skills to safely assist elders (e.g., while toileting, dressing, and bathing).

One of the most important skills that Manisha brings to this particular job is that of observation. Because she has been the primary OT practitioner working with the elder, Manisha must provide accurate information to the OTR. Often, detailed information is required per regulatory and facility guidelines.[31] In Irene's case, to complete the discharge summary, Manisha needed to provide information to Antonio, not only about Irene's ADL status, but also such factors as Irene's ability to accurately express herself, whether any sanitation hazards were present in the home, which social supports she consistently relied on, and whether she was capable of making safe decisions.

Free Standing Hospice

When Amanda graduated from Blue Lake Community College 14 years ago, her children were toddlers. To balance her work and family life, she chose to work on-call 2 to 3 days a week at various local SNFs, which she continues to do. For the past 10 years, she has volunteered at Riverview House, an independently owned hospice that provides end-of-life care for individuals who cannot receive services at home. Amanda appreciates the approach at Riverview House where staff and volunteers focus on enhancing a person's quality of life, paying equal attention to the spiritual, emotional, and physical aspects of life. The pace at Riverview House is unhurried with an emphasis on quality time until death. Amanda finds great personal reward in her volunteer work.

Almost 2 years ago, Amanda faced the prospective of death in her own family. Her favorite aunt, Paula, was diagnosed with ovarian cancer and expressed a wish to stay at home. Amanda decided that she could help fulfill her aunt's wish. Her volunteer experience at Riverview House, as well as her COTA experience working in SNFs, provided her with the capacity to feel comfortable with terminally ill individuals and the ability to cope with loss. Moreover, having attended an in-service at Riverview Hospice that emphasized strategies to prevent burnout in hospice personnel,[32] Amanda knew that it was important to maintain her physical well-being, engage in hobbies and interests, take time away from her caregiving, talk with others, and engage in meaningful activities. Amanda arranged for her daughter and niece to provide respite care several times a week so she could spend time with her partner and friends and go to the gym. She and her partner also spent time each week engaged in contemplative activities, walking the labyrinth at a nearby Buddhist retreat and meditating at the local church.

Although Amanda previously experienced the challenges and responsibilities of caring for dying persons, she soon found herself physically and emotionally drained. She was distraught as her aunt experienced a loss of control, diminished ability to engage in her favored daily activities, and physical and emotional pain. As her aunt's condition worsened, home care hospice services were formally instituted. Although a substantial commitment, Amanda decided she wanted to continue as her aunt's primary, live-in caregiver, a usual requirement for home-based hospice services. She also decided to attend a caregivers' support group at the local hospital to help cope with such a challenging, emotional endeavor. Aunt Paula lived long enough to attend the college graduation of her great grandson and died at home with family by her side.

After her aunt died, Amanda spent time recuperating, re-engaging in projects she had put on hold during the 8 months she cared for her aunt and taking a month-long vacation with a close friend. When she returned, she contacted the director at Riverview Hospice to initiate discussions about the potential inclusion of OT services. Because the director was familiar with Amanda's volunteer work, she was happy to meet and discuss her ideas. Amanda shared how the philosophy and approach of hospice were very compatible with those of occupational therapy.[33] She then shared her vision of how OT services might further enhance hospice care.

Amanda emphasized the skills that OT practitioners possess to facilitate participation in daily activities that people find meaningful, such as cooking simple meals, engaging in art projects, and writing in journals. Amanda then shared one of her volunteer experiences. She was with Joe, an elder who previously enjoyed fishing and camping and who was complaining that there was nothing he could do now. Amanda gently suggested that Joe might consider barbecuing a trout for the staff at Riverview House; he agreed and contacted his wife to bring in his secret spices to prepare the trout. Meanwhile, Amanda made arrangements with staff to make it easier for Joe to safely use the backyard barbecue. Connecting to his love of fishing and camping through the simple preparation of a barbecued trout provided Joe with a sense of self, and connecting his current self to his past life.

Amanda went on to explain that occupational therapy practitioners work with individuals throughout the life span, death and dying being one phase among many. Amanda discussed her experience with Vivian, a lively woman with a sense of humor and quick wit. Vivian enjoyed being with others, especially her family. When

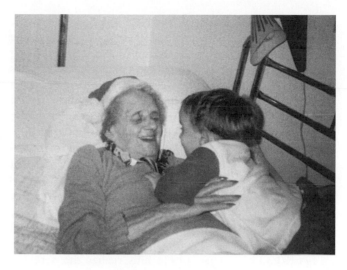

FIGURE 8-4 A special bond existed between Vivian and her 3-year-old great-grandson. *(Courtesy Sue Byers-Connon).*

she was diagnosed with terminal breast cancer, she decided to move from another state to be near her family of four generations. She would live at Riverview Hospice until her death, where her care could be provided without being a burden to her family, a point she was emphatic about. Vivian was thrilled to be near her 3-year-old great-grandson with whom she shared a special bond (Figure 8-4). She looked forward to his daily visits but soon found herself exhausted and in pain by the time he usually arrived in mid-afternoon. Amanda suggested whether it might be possible for Vivian's family to arrange for her great-grandson to arrive during lunch, where they could eat together and cuddle afterward during a nap. Moreover, Amanda suggested that Vivian listen to some relaxation tapes just before lunch to help alleviate her pain before her great-grandson arrived. Amanda explained that it was important to not only schedule rest periods, but also to consider when to schedule valued activities throughout the day.

Amanda went on to explain that OT practitioners are committed to facilitating the process of enhancing the quality of life of individuals and that they have particular expertise to modify a person's performance so that he or she can engage in desired activities. She shared the story of Cora, who was experiencing end-stage congestive heart failure and neuropathy in her fingers, making it difficult for her to hold eating utensils. Amanda knew that changing the silverware would make it easier for Cora to eat, but she also understood the enjoyment that eating meals with others can bring. The next week she brought in some silverware with sticky handgrips (which still looked normal) and asked if she could join Cora for lunch in her room. She showed the silverware to Cora and asked if she would like to give them a go. Cora agreed and found eating a bit easier; however, she still chose to eat in her room. A few weeks later, Amanda gently asked if Cora would join her in the dining room for lunch. Cora agreed, and when lunch was over, asked if Amanda would come back next week. When Amanda returned the following week, she discovered that Cora had been eating her meals in the dining room. Because Amanda gradually modified Cora's engagement, Cora was able to enjoy her meals, socializing with other residents and family members in the dining room.

The director was impressed with Amanda's understanding of the compatibility of OT with the practice of hospice and realized that other professional practitioners exist who bring important skills that support the hospice philosophy. Amanda and the director agreed to continue meeting and discuss the possibility of instituting formal OT services at Riverview House, including the need for an OTR/COTA partnership to fully realize the potential of OT services with elders at the end of life.

Adult Day Care

Carlos, who graduated 4 years ago, works at an adult day care center in an urban setting. This particular setting has a continuum of care that also includes assisted living, independent apartment living, and adult foster homes. The elders attend day care 5 days a week from 9:00 a.m. until 3:00 p.m., receiving lunch, health services, and activities in which to participate. Carlos has a dual role within this setting. His primary role is as an activities director, in that he identifies and plans individual and group activities for the day care participants throughout the week.[34] In his other role, he works with Sydney, an OTR, in providing OT services for all clients along the care continuum.

To determine whether an elder requires individual OT intervention, Sydney, the OTR, begins the initial evaluation with an occupational profile, identifying what is currently important and meaningful in regard to the elder's occupational needs. Mr. Kirov, a new day care attendee, had recently fractured his humerus and was having difficulty performing activities with only one arm and hand; consequently, Sydney conducted an initial evaluation. As a result, specific OT intervention was initiated to address his problems with performing activities. To identify which group and individual activities would be appropriate for each elder attending the day care center, Carlos (in his role as the activities director) meets with each elder (and the family, when possible). Carlos also met with Mr. Kirov who identified that he enjoyed using his hands to make things and that he liked to talk with people. From this, Carlos recommended that he participate in the craft activities and other activities that included discussion, such as current events and reminiscence. Note: In his role as the activities director, Carlos does not provide OT services.

Carlos starts off his day by attending a team meeting. At this center, the bus drivers, the chaplain, the custodial staff representative, and home health aides attend, as well as the more typical team members, such as nurses, social workers, physicians, and physical and OT practitioners.

Everyone contributes during the team meetings. Recently, the bus driver reported that Mrs. Chang experiences shortness of breath while getting on the bus, and a home health aide shared the progress that Millie has made with feeding her cat by herself. After the team meeting, Carlos divides his time—he provides one-on-one occupational therapy intervention under the supervision of Sydney and designs and implements group and individual activities for the day care attendees. Because social participation is integral to an elder's health and well-being,[35,36] Carlos uses his COTA background to plan and implement groups to ensure that the elders engage in culturally rich and sensitive social activities that they enjoy and find meaningful. One of the most popular groups is the Helping Hands group. The theme of this group is to provide the elders with a sense of contribution to the community. In the past, they have put together gift baskets for migrant workers, solicited grooming and hygiene products for military personnel, read to preschool children, and stuffed envelopes for a local school board election. Carlos enjoys this group because he knows that elders enjoy engaging in altruistic activities in which they help other people.[37,38] Other groups that Carlos plans and implements weekly and monthly are gardening, music, reminiscence, movement, and crafts. In addition, Carlos makes an extra effort to contact family members to discuss options for activities at home in which the elders can successfully engage and enjoy.

During one-on-one OT intervention, Carlos addresses specific concerns with performance of daily living activities and occupations. Recently, Carlos worked with Mrs. Chang after she began experiencing increased breathlessness caused by her chronic bronchitis. Mrs. Chang's family reported that during the weekends she wanted to help her daughter and son-in-law with household chores and would push herself too far and become breathless. Because Mrs. Chang valued her role as a family member, Carlos worked with her and her family to identify which activities she considered important and which activities her family felt comfortable allowing her to do. Carlos then worked with Mrs. Chang and her family to develop a routine, incorporating energy conservation techniques that would allow her to complete activities without becoming breathless and tired.[39] Within a month, Mrs. Chang's family reported that she was helping with household chores without getting tired and breathless. More importantly, she was extremely happy to be able to make a valuable contribution to the family and felt that her health, well-being, and life satisfaction was better than before. Because health promotion is a primary focus of the organization, Carlos also works with other team members to deliver a falls prevention program during which elders meet in small groups for 7 weeks.[40] Carlos is particularly proud that he is the team member responsible for the follow-up home visit to oversee the implementation of safety strategies by the group participants in their home environment. In doing so, Carlos can see first-hand the important role that COTAs can play to promote health for elders.

CONCLUSION

Over the next 3 to 4 decades, the population of elders will increase significantly, the number of elders with disabilities living in the community will expand sharply, and the percentage of elders (particularly those over age 85 years) residing in SNFs will rise dramatically.[41] Such trends suggest that COTAs will continue to work with elders in both traditional and emerging practice settings, focusing on daily life activities that are meaningful to elders. In doing so, COTAs will continue to provide a valuable contribution during the delivery of OT services.

After the series of presentations at Blue Lake Community College, the OTA students were excited and enthusiastic about the variety of opportunities waiting for them after graduation. Their instructor, Chris Henson, emphasized that their unique COTA skills and knowledge prepared them to work with elders in traditional settings such as SNFs, rehabilitation centers, geropsychiatric units, and home health. She went on to say that the job opportunities did not stop there. As Arianna and Jean had demonstrated, they used their COTA background to create new job opportunities in emerging practice areas. Chris Henson concluded that Carlos, who worked in adult day care, was a good example of a COTA who works in collaboration with an OTR to provide OT services but also can use his COTA background to assist elders in engaging in meaningful activities that do not require the direct supervision of an OTR. In all cases, whether in typical or emerging practice settings, the Blue Lake Community College graduates were engaged in opportunities that brought satisfaction to themselves and quality services for elders.

▌ CHAPTER REVIEW QUESTIONS

1 Discuss service competency and continued competency for COTAs and ways to establish each.
2 A COTA and OTR work together in a rehabilitation setting and have different ideas regarding intervention for elders. Suggest three ways that they can learn from each other and form a collaborative partnership.
3 A COTA who is a new graduate and an OTR who recently moved from another state are working to develop a supervision plan. Locate three resources to assist them, develop this plan, and explain what information they would seek from each resource.
4 Identify three activities that you consider meaningful (an occupation) and identify three that you consider merely an activity. Explain the differences.
5 Explain why it is important to focus on both occupations and activities to enhance an elder's health, well-being, and life satisfaction.

6 Why should COTAs consider the caregiver/significant other/spouse/family when collaborating to develop an intervention plan for an elder?
7 Three COTAs have been hired to work in an SNF. One is a new graduate, one has 5 years of experience working in a rehabilitation setting, and one previously worked in an outpatient adolescent psychiatric unit. Develop a continued competency plan for each COTA.
8 Identify three different potential emerging practice settings in which COTAs might consider working. List five skills for each setting that COTAs receive during their education that would be helpful to secure a position in that specific setting.
9 What previous experience should a COTA have before considering hospice work?

REFERENCES

1. American Occupational Therapy Association, 2008. Occupational therapy practice framework: Domain and practice. American Journal of Occupational Therapy 62 (6), 625-683.
2. National Certification Board for Certification in Occupational Therapy, 2009. Executive summary for the practice analysis study: Certified occupational therapy assistant, COTA. Author, Gaithersburg, MD.
3. Dunn, W., 2009. Best practice philosophy for community services for children and families. In: Dunn, W. (Ed.), Best Practice Occupational Therapy: In Community Service with Children and Families. Slack, Thorofare, NJ.
4. American Occupational Therapy Association, 2009. Guidelines for supervision, roles, and responsibilities during the delivery of occupational therapy services. American Journal of Occupational Therapy 63 (6), 797-803.
5. American Occupational Therapy Association, 2005. Occupational therapy code of ethics. American Journal of Occupational Therapy 59 (6), 639-642.
6. American Occupational Therapy Association, 2009. Scope of practice. American Occupational Therapy Association, Bethesda, MD.
7. Sands, M., 2003. The occupational therapist and occupational therapy assistant partnership. In: Crepeau, E.B., Cohn, E., Schell, B.A.B. (Eds.), Willard and Spackman's Occupational Therapy, 10th ed. Lippincott Williams & Wilkins, Philadelphia.
8. Dillon, T.H., 2001. Practitioner perspectives: Effective intraprofessional relationships in occupational therapy. Occupational Therapy in Health Care 14 (3-4), 1-15.
9. American Occupational Therapy Association, 2002. Occupational therapy practice framework: Domain and practice. American Journal of Occupational Therapy 56 (6), 609-639.
10. Christiansen, C., Townsend, E., 2000. An introduction to occupation. In: Christiansen, C.H., Townsend, E.A. (Eds.), Introduction to Occupation: The Art and Science of Living. Prentice Hall, Upper Saddle River, NJ.
11. Pierce, D., 2001. Untangling occupation and activity. American Journal of Occupational Therapy 55 (2), 138-146.
12. American Occupational Therapy Association, 2005. Standards for continuing competence. American Journal of Occupational Therapy 59 (6), 661-662.
13. Gray, J.M., 1998. Putting occupation into practice: Occupation as ends, occupations as means. American Journal of Occupational Therapy 52 (5), 354-364.

14. National Board for Certification in Occupational Therapy, 2010. Certification Renewal Handbook. Author, Gaithersburg, MD.

15. American Occupational Therapy Association, 2009. Standards of Practice. American Occupational Therapy Association, Bethesda, MD.

16. Law, M., Baptiste, S., Carswell, A., Polatajko, H., Pollock, N., 2005. Canadian Occupational Performance Measure, 4th ed. Canadian Association of Occupational Therapists, Toronto.

17. AOTA State Affairs Group, 2006. Occupational therapy assistant supervision requirements. American Occupational Therapy Association, Bethesda, MD.

18. Black, T., 1996. COTAs and OTRs as partners and teams. OT Practice 1 (3), 42-47.

19. Gitlin, L.N., Corcoran, M., Chee, Y.K., 2005. Occupational therapy and dementia care: The home environmental skill-building program for individuals and families. American Occupational Therapy Association, Bethesda, MD.

20. Rogers, J., 2000. Habits: Do we practice what we preach? Occupational Therapy Journal of Research 20 (Suppl 1), 119S-122S.

21. Rowles, G.D., 2000. Habituation and being in place. Occupational Therapy Journal of Research 20 (Suppl 1), 52S-67S.

22. American Occupational Therapy Association, 2010. Board and specialty certification. Retrieved July 12, 2010, from www.aota.org/Practitioners/ProfDev/Certification.aspx.

23. Allen, C.K., Austin, S.L., David, S.K., Earhart, C.A., McCraith, D.B., Riska-Williams, L., 2007. Allen Cognitive Level Screen-5 (ACLS-5) and Large Allen Cognitive Level Screen-5 (LACLS-5). ACLS and LACLS Committee, Camarillo, CA.

24. Arthritis Foundation, 2010. Offering life improvement series programs: Program instructors/leaders. Retrieved June 30, 2010, from www.arthritis.org/leaders-instructors.php.

25. Howe, M.C., Schwartzberg, S.L., 2001. A Functional Approach to Group Work in Occupational Therapy. Lippincott Williams & Wilkins, Philadelphia.

26. American Occupational Therapy Association, 2006. Occupational therapy's role in senior centers. American Occupational Therapy Association, Bethesda, MD.

27. McPhee, S.D., Johnson, T., 2000. Program planning for an assisted living community. Occupational Therapy in Health Care 12 (2-3), 1-17.

28. Horowitz, B.P., Vanner, E., 2010. Relationships among active engagement in life activities and quality of life for assisted-living residents. Journal of Housing for the Elderly 24 (2), 130-150.

29. McKenna, K., Broome, K., Liddle, J., 2007. What older people do: Time use and exploring the link between role participation and life satisfaction in people aged 65 years and over. Australian Occupational Therapy Journal 54 (4), 273-284.

30. Tanner, B., Tilse, C., de Jonge, D., 2008. Restoring and sustaining home: The impact of home modifications on the meaning of home for older people. Journal of Housing for the Elderly 22 (3), 195-215.

31. Glantz, C.H., Richman, N., 1997. OTR-COTA collaboration in home health: Roles and supervisory issues. American Journal of Occupational Therapy 51 (6), 446-452.

32. Swetz, K.M., Harrington, S.E., Matsuyama, R.K., Shanafelt, T.D, Lyckholm, L.T., 2009. Strategies for avoiding burnout in hospice and palliative medicine: Peer advice for physicians on achieving longevity and fulfillment. Journal of Palliative Medicine 12 (9), 773-777.

33. Cooper, J., 2006. Occupational Therapy in Oncology and Palliative Care. Wiley, Chichester, England; Hoboken, NJ.

34. Krawcyk, A., 1988. The certified occupational therapy assistant as an activity director. Occupational Therapy in Health Care 5 (2-3), 111-118.

35. Herzog, A.R., Ofstedal, M.B., Wheeler, L.M., 2002. Social engagement and its relationship to health. Clinics in Geriatric Medicine 18 (3), 593-609.

36. Martinez, I.L., Kim, K., Tanner, E., et al., 2009. Ethnic and class variations in promoting social activities among older adults. Activities, Adaptation & Aging 33 (2), 96-119.

37. Cipriani, J., 2007. Altruistic activities of older adults living in long-term care facilities: A literature review. Physical & Occupational Therapy in Geriatrics 26 (1), 19-28.

38. Williams, A.L., Haber, D., Weaver, G.D., Freeman, J.L., 1997. Altruistic activity: Does it make a difference in the senior center? Activities, Adaptation & Aging 22 (4), 31-39.

39. Dreiling, D., 2009. Energy conservation. Home Health Care Management and Practice 22 (1), 26-33.

40. Peterson, E.W., Clemson, L., 2008. Understanding the role of occupational therapy in fall prevention for community-dwelling older adults. OT Practice 13 (3), CE1-CE8.

41. Administration on Aging, 2009. Aging into the 21st century. Retrieved June 20, 2010, from www.aoa.gov/AoARoot/Aging_Statistics/future_growth/aging21/health.aspx.

Cultural Diversity of the Aging Population

RENÉ PADILLA

KEY TERMS

diversity, culture, values, beliefs, race, sex, age, ethnicity, sexual orientation, religion, ethnocentrism, assimilation, performance context, melting pot, conformity, bias, prejudice, discrimination, minority, cognitive style, associative, abstractive, truth, equality

CHAPTER OBJECTIVES

1. Explain the meaning of *diversity* and related terms.
2. Explore personal experiences, beliefs, values, and attitudes regarding diversity.
3. Discuss the need to accept the uniqueness of each individual and the importance of being sensitive to

issues of diversity in the practice of occupational therapy with elders.
4. Present strategies to facilitate interaction with elders of diverse backgrounds.

Today is Susan's first day at her first job as a certified occupational therapy assistant (COTA). She was hired to work as a member of the rehabilitation team in a small nursing home in the town where she grew up. Susan is excited because this job will permit her to stay close to her family and work with elders. When she arrives at the nursing home she and the registered occupational therapist (OTR) discuss the elders who are participating in the rehabilitation program. Susan is told about Mr. Chu, a Chinese gentleman who experienced a stroke and often refuses to get out of bed, and Mrs. Pardo, a Filipino woman who is constantly surrounded by family and consequently cannot get anything accomplished. The OTR also tells Susan about Mr. Cooper, an elderly man dying of acquired immunodeficiency disorder (AIDS); Mrs. Blanche, a retired university professor who is a quadriplegic; and Mr. Perez, who was a migrant farm worker until the accidental amputation of his left arm 4 weeks previously. Susan notes the distinct qualities of each of these elders.

OVERVIEW OF CULTURAL DIVERSITY

The cultural diversity of clients adds an exciting and challenging element to the practice of occupational therapy (OT). Each client comes from a cultural context with a unique blend of values and beliefs. This uniqueness affects all aspects of the client's life, including the occupational dimension. The ways in which a person chooses to do a task, interacts with family members, moves about in a community, looks to the future, and views health are in

many ways the result of past experiences and the expectations of the people with whom that person comes in contact. COTAs have an important role in supporting elders' health and participation in life through engagement in occupation.[1] Consequently, COTAs have to deal with many issues that arise from interactions with persons unlike themselves in terms of race, sex, age, ethnicity, physical ability, sexual orientation, family composition, place of birth, religion, level of education, and work experience (including retirement status) or professional status, among other factors.[2,3]

Culture, ethnocentrism, assimilation, and diversity are discussed to provide a framework for working with elders in a sensitive manner. This chapter includes general guidelines for assessment and intervention. The challenge for COTAs is to contribute to the creation of a therapeutic environment in which diversity and difference are valued and in which elders can work to reach their goals.

WHAT IS CULTURE?

The concept of culture has long been considered important in the practice of OT. For example, the official definition of *occupational therapy* for licensure states, "Occupational therapy is the use of purposeful activity with individuals who are limited by physical injury or illness, psychosocial dysfunction, developmental or learning disabilities, poverty and cultural differences, or the aging process in order to maximize independence, prevent disability, and maintain health."[4] Likewise, the *Accreditation Standards for and Educational Program for the Occupational Therapy*

Assistant,[5] the Code of Ethics,[6] and the Occupational Therapy Practice Framework: Domain and Process[1] all support the consideration of culture in intervention. However, the term *culture* has not been clearly defined or described in OT professional literature and has not been consistently considered in the assessment and intervention process.[7,8] Part of the reason for this lapse may be the breadth of complex concepts encompassed by this one term. The Occupational Therapy Practice Framework[1] identifies culture among the contexts that influence performance skills and performance patterns (observable behaviors of occupations). Culture is listed with physical, social, personal, temporal, and virtual factors that influence occupation within particular contexts and environments. In addition, values, beliefs and spirituality are considered client factors that arise from these contexts. The Occupational Therapy Practice Framework describes the cultural context as "customs, beliefs, activity patterns, behavior standards, and expectations accepted by the society of which the client is a member. Includes ethnicity and values as well as political aspects, such as laws that affect access to resources and affirm personal rights. Also includes opportunities for education, employment, and economic support" (p. 645).[1] The Occupational Therapy Practice Framework describes culture as existing "outside of the person but is internalized by the person, also sets expectations, beliefs, and customs that can affect how and when services may be delivered" (p. 646).[1] Kielhofner[9] also offered a broad perspective when he defined *culture* as the beliefs and perceptions, values and norms, and customs and behaviors that are shared by a group or society and are passed from one generation to the next through both formal and informal education.

This broad and consequently vague definition of *culture* is not unique to the OT profession. Entire books in other fields are devoted to describing culture, and authors have been unable to agree on a single definition. Most include concepts relating to observable patterns of behavior and rules that govern that behavior. They also emphasize the conscious and subconscious nature of culture in the way it is dynamically shared among people. Some of the commonalties in those definitions, including that culture is learned and shared with others, may be used as a basis for an understanding of culture.[7,8]

Culture is learned or acquired through socialization. Culture is not carried in a person's genetic makeup; rather, it is learned over the course of a lifetime. Obviously, then, the context and environment in which each person lives are central to his or her culture. A person's environment may demand or offer opportunities for some types of behaviors and restrict opportunities for other types. For example, individuals in the United States are offered the opportunity to choose the color of their clothing, but generally wearing dresses is culturally restricted to women. In the United States, persons are generally expected to drive on the right side of the street, pay taxes, and arrive at work according to schedule. Through interaction with the environment, individuals learn a variety of values and beliefs and eventually internalize them. Internalized values direct the interactions among people and with the environment. As a result, people assume that others have internalized the same values and beliefs and consequently behave in the same ways.[10,11] However, culture is the result of each person's unique experiences with his or her environment and thus is an ongoing learning process.

Another commonality in the various definitions of culture is that because it is learned from others, it is also shared. What is shared as culture, however, is very dynamic. Because culture is learned throughout one's lifetime, each person learns it at different points. On the basis of each person's status in learning culture, the person expects something from others and contributes to others' cultural education. In this way, each person learns and teaches something about culture that is unique. Over time, shared beliefs and values change. These changes in cultural beliefs and values may not be easily observed because the actual behaviors that express them seem to remain the same. However, over time, a periodic recommitment to the dynamic transmittal of beliefs and values has occurred.[12] For example, the attire of women in some regions of the Arabian Peninsula has changed very little in the past 200 years. Originally, the black gowns, robes, and veils were probably intended to guard the woman's modesty. Many women who wear these garments today, in addition to guarding modesty, do so as a symbol of resistance to westernization, a concern that was probably not common 200 years ago.[13,14]

Finally, culture is often subconscious.[15,16] Because learning of culture occurs formally and informally, a person is not usually aware, particularly at a young age, of learning it. Instead the person simply complies with the demands and restrictions of behavior set in particular environments and chooses behaviors from among those that are allowed. For example, when a child is not permitted to touch a frog found by a pond during a family outing, that child is being formally taught that frogs are dirty and therefore should not be touched, a value the child might internalize and then generalize to other animals. This value is informally reinforced when the child sees other people wince and make gestures of repulsion when they see certain types of animals. When the child sees a younger sibling attempting to touch a frog, the child might tell the sibling not to do so because touching it is "bad." In effect, the child internalized a value received from the culture of his or her family and passed it on to a sibling with the slight reinterpretation that it is bad to do the particular behavior. In a similar way, all persons continue to learn culture from each physical and social environment in which they participate. When elders enter a nursing home for a short-term or long-term stay, for example, some of the facility's rules of behavior are formally explained, whereas others are implied, including meal times (and consequently when elders must eat), visiting hours (and consequently when elders must and must not socialize), visiting room regulations (and consequently where and how elders may socialize), and "lights out" time (and consequently when elders must sleep). Elders also informally learn an entirely different set of rules. As they experience the daily routine in the nursing home, they also learn whether it is acceptable to question the professionals who work there, to decline participation in scheduled group activities, and even to express their thoughts, feelings, desires, and concerns. Staff members have likely not formally stated, "You are not permitted to state your feelings here." However, this value may be communicated informally by staff members if they cut off conversation when an elder begins to explain feelings or simply never take time to invite an expression of the elder's feelings. In this way, values and beliefs become sets of unspoken, implicit, and underlying assumptions that guide interactions with others and the environment.[17]

Culture is a set of beliefs and values that a particular group of people share and re-create constantly through interaction with each other and their environments. These beliefs and values may be conscious or unconscious, and they direct the opportunities, demands, and behavior restrictions that exist for members of a particular group. Essentially, every belief and value that humans acquire as members of society can be included in their culture, thus explaining the broadness of the concept of culture. Therefore, the beliefs and values on which we form our own understanding of elders' behaviors and the rules for these behaviors have also been socially constructed and form part of our own culture.

LEVELS OF CULTURE

Various levels of culture exist at which values and beliefs are shared. Many authors[18-20] have proposed that a multidimensional view of culture be adopted. In this view, culture can be defined in terms of the individual, the family, the community, and the region. At the individual level are the relational, one-to-one interactions through which people learn and express their unique representations of culture. Examples of this level of culture are each person's use of humor, definition of personal space, coping style, and role choices. Included at the level of the family are beliefs and values that are shared within a primary social group—the group in which most of the person's early socialization takes place. This level includes issues such as gender roles, family composition, and style of worship. Each family can be seen as a variation of the culture that is shared at the level of a community or neighborhood, in which economic factors, ethnicity, housing, and other factors may be considered. Communities may be seen as variations in the culture that is shared with a larger region, such as language, geography, and industry. Erez and Gati[18] noted that variation exists at each level and within each group.

Adopting a more relational framework helps overcome some of the difficulties inherent in viewing culture as synonymous with ethnicity. Ethnicity is the part of a person's identity that is derived from membership in a racial, religious, national, or linguistic group.[21] The viewing of culture as synonymous with ethnicity relies on generalizations about the people who belong to a particular group and can lead to mistaken assumptions about an individual's personality and beliefs. For example, the assumption that all persons of Hispanic ethnicity have brown skin and black hair is not true, because Hispanics of all racial backgrounds exist. Equally, people cannot assume that all white individuals are educated, that all Jews observe kosher practices, or that everyone who speaks English attaches the same meaning to the word *gay*.

Equating ethnicity with culture can lead to many misinterpretations.[22] In addition, this practice is often used to justify superiority of one group over another. The term *ethnocentricity* describes the belief held by members of a particular ethnic group that their expression of beliefs and values is superior to that of others, and consequently that all other groups should aspire to adopt their beliefs and values. In extreme cases of ethnocentricity, a particular ethnic group has attempted to destroy other ethnic groups, as in (Nazi) Germany, Bosnia, and the Sudan. Ethnocentrism can be and often is an underlying, subconscious belief that powerfully guides a person's behavior. An unexamined ethnocentric attitude may lead COTAs to place particular emphasis on certain areas of rehabilitation and disregard others that elders may consider essential for their recovery. OT itself can be viewed as a subculture with beliefs and values that guide practitioners toward independence, productivity, leisure, purposeful activity, and individuality. This bias may sometimes lead practitioners to ignore the client's wishes and impose their own values in the belief that they are more important and worthwhile.

THE ISSUE OF DIVERSITY

The variety of clients whom Susan, the COTA, introduced at the beginning of this chapter will work with underscores a well known fact about the United States: It is a country of immigrants, a conglomeration of diverse peoples. How is it possible that all of these groups live together? The metaphor of the "melting pot" has been used to describe the way in which distinct cultural groups in the United States "melt down" and how differences between groups that were once separate entities disappear. This process is the result of the continuous exposure of groups to one another.[23] Kimbro[24] described a process of conformity in which an individual or a cultural group forsakes values, beliefs, and customs to eliminate differences with another culture. In the United States, conformity may be demonstrated by people who Americanize their names, speak only English, abandon religious practices or social rituals, shed their ethnic dress, attend night school, and work hard to take part in the "American dream." Both conformity and the melting pot metaphor imply that new ethnic groups entering the United States will be judged by the degree to which their differences with the values and beliefs of the established American culture disappear. Some people accept the pressure to abandon their cultural identity as an inevitable or even desirable fact of life, whereas others avoid it at all costs.[23] This expectation can easily create bias, prejudice, and discrimination toward many individuals. The term *minority* is an outgrowth of these views. This term is used to designate not only smaller groups, but also groups that have less power and representation within an established culture despite their size.

The realization that some differences such as age, race, sex, and sexual orientation can never be eliminated, even with effort and education, has led many people to discern that they should also value the characteristics that make them unique, such as their cultural heritage and their religious practices. Cultural pluralism is a value system that recognizes this desire and focuses not on assimilation but on accepting and celebrating the differences that exist among people.[7] Persons who value cultural pluralism believe that these differences add richness to a society rather than detract from it.

Valuing Diversity

People in the United States are clearly diverse. Diversity is demonstrated through race, sex, age, ethnicity, sexual orientation, family composition, place of birth, religion, and level of education; in addition, people also differ from each other in physical ability or disability, intelligence, socioeconomic class, physical beauty, and personality type. In essence, any dimension of life can create identity groups or cohorts that may or may not be visible. Most people find that several of these dimensions have particular meaning for them.[25]

Ironically, diversity becomes an inclusive concept when we view it as that which makes us different from each other. This view of diversity embraces everyone because each person is in some way different from everyone else. At the same time, however, each person in some way is also similar to someone else. This viewpoint provides a framework for approaching the diversity that one encounters when working with elders: COTAs can recognize the ways in which they are both different from and similar to elders. These differences and similarities can be used during therapy to enrich the elder's life. A welcome side effect of this approach is that the COTA's life is often enriched as well.

Diversity of the Aged Population

A summary of statistical reports on the elder population is presented in Chapter 1. Each of these reports is an example of diversity. The following facts should also be taken into account when considering diversity among the rapidly growing elder population.

Persons older than age 65 years represent 12.8% of the U.S. population, or about 39 million people.[26] In 2008, 19.3% of elders belonged to minority populations, 8.3% were African Americans, and persons of Hispanic origin (who may be of any race) represented 6.6% of the older population. About 3.2% were Asian or Pacific Islander, and less than 1% were American Indian or Native Alaskan. In addition, 0.6% of persons age 65 and older identified themselves as being of two or more races. The overall number of minority elders is expected to grow to 25% by 2030.[27] A growth of 81% is expected in the white non-Hispanic elder population in that same period. The growth among Hispanic elders is projected to be the largest (328%), followed by Asian and Pacific Islander elders (285%), American Indian, Eskimo, and Aleut elders (147%), and African American elders (131%).[27] A breakdown of the U.S. racial and ethnic population is provided in Figure 9-1. Notably, these figures represent the numbers of elders who belong to broad categories only, not cultural distinctiveness. Each of the categories listed may include numerous cultures and subcultures. These numbers are used here simply to emphasize that the population served by OT practitioners will increasingly include elders from diverse backgrounds.

No reliable figures are available regarding the sexual preference of persons in the United States who are age 65 years or older. Mosher and colleagues[28] reported that 4.1% of men and women in the general population are homosexual or bisexual, and that the previous estimate of 10% was inflated because it included people who had reported a single homosexual experience in their lifetime. Studies suggest that these figures are consistent for elders older than 65 years.[29-31] If this is true, approximately 1.5 million elders are homosexual.

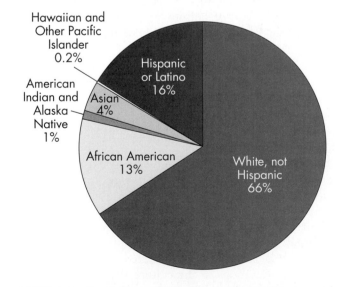

FIGURE 9-1 Breakdown of general population by race and ethnic origin. (*Data from Internet releases of the Census 2008 data by the U.S. Census Bureau.*)

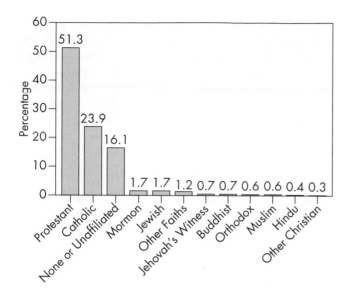

FIGURE 9-2 Distribution of faiths in the general population. *(From Pew Research Center's Forum on Religion and Public Life. (2008). U.S. religious landscape survey: Religious affiliation: Diverse and dynamic. Washington, DC: Pew Research Center.)*

The United States is one of the most diverse countries in the world in terms of religious affiliation. Approximately 83% of people in the United States claim to have a definite religious preference.[32] The trend toward increased religious diversity is fueled both by conversion and immigration. Since 1957, the Christian population (i.e., Catholics and Protestants) in the United States has decreased from 92% to 78.4% of the total population, whereas the number of practitioners of other religions, including Buddhism, Hinduism, and Islam, has increased from 1% to 4.7%. Information on the distribution of faiths of the general U.S. population is provided in Figure 9-2.

In 2008, the overall poverty rate in the United States grew to 13.5% (about 40 million people) in comparison to 12.5% in 2007.[33] The largest growth came for people ages 22 to 64. However, 9.7% of the elderly population, or 3.7 million persons, lived below the poverty line, and another 6.6%, or 2.5 million elderly, were classified as "near-poor" (income between the poverty level and 125% of this level). While there was no statistical difference between the percent reported 5 years earlier, an overall growth in numbers was experienced as the proportion of people age 65 and older in the U.S. population has grown steadily. These data are quite different when minority groups are considered individually. For example, 24% of elderly African Americans and 23% of elderly Hispanics were impoverished. More than half (51.3%, which is the highest poverty rate) of older Hispanic women who lived alone or with nonrelatives experienced poverty.[27]

Sensitivity to Culture and Diversity in Intervention

To be culturally sensitive, people must acknowledge their own prejudices and biases. COTAs should realize that prejudices are learned behaviors and can be unlearned through increased contact with and understanding of people of diverse cultural groups. Furthermore, communication always takes place between individuals not cultures. Gropper[34] suggests that in the clinical encounter the cultures of both the client and the clinician play important roles in successful outcomes. Gropper wrote that misunderstandings and miscommunication between clients and clinicians usually result from cultural differences, and that the clinician's responsibility is to adapt to the client's culture rather than demand that the client adapt to the clinician's culture. Rozak[3] proposed that in addition to the cultures of the client and the clinician, the culture of the institution in which the interaction takes place in many ways directs interaction between the client and clinician. In health care, institutional culture has strongly valued the biomedical approach to intervention, which places the control of health care with the physician rather than with the client. In addition, the U.S. medical system has placed little emphasis on the development of specific programs to address the needs of elders from culturally diverse groups.

Culture and diversity are extremely broad and complex concepts. Attempts to make generalizations about various groups would be useless because COTAs are certain to come across elders who do not fit into the expected behavior. Few persons are perfect representations of their culture. Generalizations may also limit the COTA's ability to see each client as a unique individual. Consequently, COTAs should be cognizant of general issues about culture that should be assessed and remembered at every step of the OT program. COTAs must realize that cultural sensitivity is an ongoing process. In addition, COTAs should not assume that by following the guidelines presented in the following sections, they have done everything necessary to provide culturally appropriate OT services. The COTA's responsibility is to develop ongoing strategies that allow the client to maintain personal integrity and be treated with respect as an individual.

The two most important strategies COTAs can use are asking questions and observing behavior carefully. The values and beliefs that encompass culture direct elders in their particular way of performing activities of daily living (ADL) functions and work and leisure occupations. Consequently, COTAs must be oriented to the elder's culture to provide relevant and meaningful intervention. This cultural orientation should include an understanding of the following: (1) the cognitive style of the elder, (2) what he or she accepts as evidence, and (3) the value system that forms the basis of the elder's behavior. A fourth and final area of understanding has to do with communication style. If elders are unable to answer questions regarding these areas for themselves, COTAs should attempt to obtain this information from the elder's family or friends. If this is not an option, the COTA should obtain information about the elder's culture from other sources, such as a coworker who is of the same national origin as the elder or from library materials. However, COTAs should remember that the more removed the information source is from the elder, the less likely that the information will apply to that particular elder.

Let us return briefly to Susan, the COTA starting a new job who was introduced at the beginning of the chapter. One of the elders with whom Susan would be working was Mr. Chu, a Chinese gentleman who refused to get out of bed. The OTR informed Susan that soon after Mr. Chu's admission several of the elders who had Alzheimer's disease and were disoriented had become agitated in Mr. Chu's presence because they associated him with World War II experiences. The nursing home staff did not want Mr. Chu to be offended by this behavior, so they moved him to a private room. When Susan entered Mr. Chu's room she said, "Hello! I'm from occupational therapy and I'm here to help you get out of bed and do your ADL." As anticipated, he signaled his refusal to cooperate by turning his head and closing his eyes. He remained silent whenever Susan spoke to him. When she attempted to put her hand behind his shoulder to help him sit up, he grabbed her wrist and pushed her arm away. Susan was perplexed. She called Jon, a therapist of Japanese descent whom she had met at an orientation session a week earlier, and asked him to provide any insight into Mr. Chu's behavior. Jon told Susan that, in general, Asians are very circumspect, preferring to be with members of their own group, and that Mr. Chu was probably reacting to Susan not being Asian. Jon suggested that a family member be called in to enlist Mr. Chu's cooperation. Susan contacted Mr. Chu's son, Edwin, who met her later that afternoon at Mr. Chu's bedside. After some discussion with his father, Edwin informed Susan that Mr. Chu refused to get out of bed because he believed he had been placed in a private room to isolate him because he was Chinese. He viewed being informed about OT intervention plans as further evidence that he was being treated differently. Susan explained the staff's concern that Mr. Chu would be offended by the comments and behavior of the other elders. Mr. Chu said he understood that such behavior was part of an illness. Susan facilitated Mr. Chu's move to a room with three other elders, and he began to participate daily in the OT program. Susan was careful to ask Mr. Chu what he wanted to accomplish in each session. Jon's report about Asians wanting to be with members of their own group was only partially true. Mr. Chu wished to be with other elders, not specifically other Chinese people. Susan was able to discover this with the help of only someone very familiar with Mr. Chu.

Cognitive Style

COTAs need to understand how elders organize information. This process does not refer to an assessment of cognitive functions that indicate the presence or absence of brain dysfunction.[35,36] Rather, cognitive style refers to the types of information a person ignores and accepts in everyday life. Because cognitive style is the result of habits, it tends to be automatic or subconscious. Studies of cognitive style suggest that people vary along a continuum of open-mindedness or closed-mindedness, and that cultural patterns are reflected in these styles.[37] Depending on the situation, people may vary along this continuum, and no one is likely to always operate from one of the poles. Open-minded persons seek out additional information before making decisions and tend to admit that they do not have all of the answers and need to learn more before reaching proper conclusions. Open-minded persons usually ask many questions, want to hear about alternatives, and often ask COTAs to make personal recommendations regarding alternatives. Closed-minded individuals, however, see only a narrow range of data and ignore additional information. These persons usually take this approach because they function under strict sets of rules about behavior. For example, a devout Hindu elder would likely be appalled at being served beef at a meal and would not be willing to consider the potential nutritional benefits of this meal. Similarly, the dietitian who offers this meal to a Hindu elder may do so on the basis of a closed-minded cognitive style, assuming that beef is the ideal and only source of the particular nutrients the elder needs. Both persons are functioning under rules of behavior, with the Hindu elder's rules dictated by religious practice and the dietitian's rules dictated by professional training. Other examples of a closed-minded cognitive style include the female elder who refuses to work with a male COTA during dressing training because she believes this is not proper, and the explosive retired executive who bellows that he does not wish to walk with a cane despite safety concerns. Both of these people have attended to only part of the data available—that is, the data contrary to the rules of behavior under which they function. Their cognitive styles have limited their abilities to consider the benefits of the alternatives. Studies show that most cultures produce closed-minded citizens.[37]

Another aspect of cognitive style is the way in which people process information, which can be divided into associative and abstractive processing styles. As with open-mindedness and closed-mindedness, people may vary along this continuum, and no one is likely to always operate from one of the styles. People who think associatively filter new data through the screen of personal experience—that is, these people tend to understand new information in terms of similar past experiences only. Conversely, abstractive thinkers deal with new information through imagination or by considering hypothetical situations. An example of an associative thinker is an elder who has had a stroke and wants the COTA to provide him with a set of weights because using weights was how he increased upper extremity strength when he was younger. An example of an abstractive thinker is an elderly woman who asks the COTA to write down the principles of joint protection and is able to apply that information to all situations in which she may find herself. When approaching an associative thinker with a new task, COTAs should point out the ways in which it is similar to other tasks that the elder has accomplished. Often elders who are associative thinkers need one or more demonstrations of the task and do best with small incremental increases in task complexity. Alternately, when approaching an abstractive thinker with a new task, COTAs should emphasize the desired outcome and permit the elder to think of ways in which to reach the goal. For example, when teaching an elder who thinks associatively to transfer to the toilet, COTAs should point out the ways in which this transfer is similar to the transfer of getting to the wheelchair from the bed. When teaching the elder who thinks abstractly to transfer to the toilet, COTAs should point out that the goal is to maintain alignment when standing, pivot on both legs, and sit by bending the knees.

What Is Accepted as Truth

When COTAs engage people in therapy, they assume the individuals will act in their own best interest. On the basis of this assumption, COTAs can ask the question: How do clients decide if it is in their best interest to learn the task presented to them? Or, in a broader sense, what is the truth? People from different cultures arrive at truth in different ways. These methods of arriving at truth can be separated into faith, fact, and feeling. The process of evaluating truth tends to be more conscious, in contrast to the automatic cognitive style discussed previously. Furthermore, most people use combinations of methods, but for reasons of clarity, these methods are explained separately in the chapter.

The person who acts on the basis of faith uses a belief system such as that derived from a religion or political ideology to determine what is good or bad. For example, many people believe in self-sufficiency and may decline to use a wheelchair or other adaptive equipment that would clearly help them reduce fatigue. Their belief in self-sufficiency operates independently of the fact that they are too fatigued to stay awake for more than an hour. Other examples of people who act on the basis of faith include the elder who refuses a blood transfusion because this procedure is explicitly prohibited by his or her religion, and the elder who calls on a priest, rabbi, pastor, or other spiritual advisor before making a decision about care. Before OT intervention is initiated, COTAs should always ask whether the elder wishes to observe any particular rules and should consider the elder's response when selecting therapeutic occupations.

Obviously, people who act on the basis of fact want to see evidence to support the COTA's recommendation or prioritization of a certain intervention. These people often want to know the benefits that a certain intervention has proven to give in the past. To make plans for their future, these people often wish to know the length and cost of required OT services. People who act on the basis of fact may stop participating in a particular activity if they do not see the exact results that they anticipated. COTAs may find it helpful to have these elders participate in some form of group intervention that allows them to directly observe results of OT intervention with other elders. In addition, written information about their conditions and about resources can be useful for these elders.

The most common group is people who arrive at truth on the basis of feelings.[37] Such people are those who "go with their gut instincts." When faced with a difficult decision they often choose the option that "feels right" over the one that seems most logical if this option makes them too uncomfortable. People who function on the basis of feelings often need to establish a comfortable rapport with the COTA before committing themselves wholeheartedly to working with the COTA. Building a relationship with these individuals may take a long time. However, once the relationship is established it is very strong. People who function on the basis of feeling will probably want the COTA to continue treating them after they are discharged from a facility if further services are needed; they place less importance on cost considerations than on continuing the relationship. As with any client, COTAs should consistently and periodically ask elders how they are feeling about their situations and permit them time to process these feelings as needed.

Value Systems

Each culture has a system for separating right from wrong or good from evil. A person's cognitive style and the way in which the person evaluates truth provide general clues about the values of that person's culture. However, more specific value systems exist that form the basis for behavior. Althen[38] identified eight values and assumptions that characterize dominant American culture, including the importance of individualism and privacy, the belief in the equality of all people, and informality in interactions with others. In addition, Althen[38] described emphasis on the future, change, progress, punctuality, materialism, and achievement as salient American values. In the chapter, the locus of decision making, sources of anxiety reduction, issues of equality and inequality, and use of time are discussed. Numerous other value systems also direct behavior, but these four systems are discussed here because they are more related than other systems to the concerns of OT.

Locus of decision making

Locus of decision making is related to the extent to which a culture prizes individualism as opposed to collectivism. Individualism refers to the degree to which a person considers only himself or herself when making a decision. Collectivism refers to the degree to which a person must abide with the consensus of the collective group. Pure individualism and collectivism are rare. In most countries, people consider others when making a

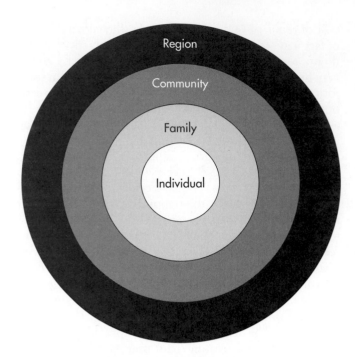

FIGURE 9-3   Levels of culture.

decision, but they are not bound by the desires of the group. Returning to the concept of *levels of culture* discussed previously in the chapter may be helpful in understanding individualism versus collectivism. Locus of decision making may be considered as a series of concentric circles (Figure 9-3). In the center is the smallest circle: the individual. At this level the individual considers mainly himself or herself when making a decision. The next circle represents a slightly larger group: usually the family. Many cultures expect the individual to consider what is best for the family when making a decision. The next circle represents a larger group: the community. This community could be an ethnic group, a religion, or even the individual's country. Some cultures expect people to consider the best interests of the entire, expansive group.

Examples of the ways that people use these different levels of consideration when making a decision are easy to find in OT practice. An individualistic elder is one who makes decisions about when and how he will be discharged home without consulting his or her spouse or family. These elders might believe that their spouse or family has a responsibility to care for them—a value that may not necessarily be shared. Another elder who considers his or her family when making a decision may refuse to be discharged home out of consideration to his or her grown children because they would have to adjust their lifestyles to accommodate the elder's needs. Another elder may decide to attempt to continue living independently to defy society's stereotype of dependence of elders.

Another way of thinking about individualism versus collectivism is to consider the degree of privacy a person seeks. Elders from cultures that highly value privacy may

be quite perplexed by the number of health care professionals who seem to know about their issues. Conversely, elders from other cultures who do not have rigid standards of privacy may feel isolated if they are not permitted to have constant contact with family or friends. The OT culture values independence, privacy, and individualism, but these values may be in conflict with an elder's needs if not carefully considered. One of the paradoxes of medical care in the United States is that, at the same time that we defend privacy rights in documentation, we assume that the individual will be completely comfortable undressing or toileting in our presence, and we do not give thought to the possibility that the elder may feel embarrassed by these experiences.

Sources of anxiety reduction

Every human being is subject to stress. How do individuals handle stress and reduce anxiety? Most people turn to four basic sources of security and stability: interpersonal relationships, religion, technology, and the law.[37,39-41] A person who must make a decision about an important health-related issue or adapt to a traumatic event is under stress. COTAs will find it helpful to know where or to whom elders turn for help and advice. If an elder is going to ask his or her spouse or family for advice, the COTA should include that spouse or family in therapy from the beginning of intervention so that they clearly understand the issues involved.

Elders who rely on religion as a source of anxiety reduction often need COTAs to help them obtain special considerations regarding religious practices. Understanding every nuance in the elder's religion is not as important as acknowledging the importance and appreciating the comfort that the elder finds in religious observances.

Reliance on technology as a source of anxiety reduction can be manifested when elders seek yet another medical test to confirm or refute a diagnosis. These clients may rely on medication as the solution to their problems or may collect a myriad of adaptive equipment or "gadgets." OT practitioners often have a bias toward relieving anxiety by prescribing the use of adaptive equipment without considering fully the extent to which the elder truly needs it.

Issues of equality/inequality

An important characteristic of all cultures is the division of power. Who controls the financial resources, and who controls decision making within the family? A sacred tenet in the United States is that "All men are created equal." Despite this tenet, prejudice against many groups still exists. All cultures have disadvantaged groups. Unequal status may be defined by economic situation, race, age, sex, or other factors. Members of socially and economically advantaged classes may project a sense of entitlement to health care services and may treat COTAs and other health care workers as servants. Conversely, members of a poverty-stricken underclass may eye COTAs with suspicion or defer to any recommendation out of fear of retaliation through withdrawal of needed services.

COTAs also should analyze issues of male and female equality. Female COTAs, in particular, may find it useful to know the way women are regarded in the elder's culture. In most cultures, men are more likely to be obeyed and trusted when they occupy positions of authority, but this is not always true for women.[42,43] COTAs must understand who will be best suited to act as a caregiver on the basis of the elder's cultural values regarding gender roles. A COTA who is of the opposite sex of the elder may decide to initiate OT intervention around issues less likely to bring up conflicts regarding privacy or authority until more rapport is built and the elder is able to appreciate the COTA's genuine concern for his or her welfare.

Another factor to be considered is status awarded people because of age. Ageism refers to the belief that one age group is superior to another. Often the younger generation is more valued. The physical appearance of age is frequently avoided through the use of cosmetics to conceal and surgery to reverse manifestations of age. Some people attempt to delay the natural developmental process through adopting healthier lifestyles of exercise, diet, rest, and so on. The avoidance of the appearance of age can contribute to the undervaluing of elders. Stereotypical descriptors such as "senile," "dependent," or "diseased" are used to describe the aging population as needy people. Because of these views of age, it can be easy for the COTA to assume a position of power over elders and place them in a position of inferiority and need of services to justify the existence of the profession.[44] McKnight[45] described how "ageism" has resulted in the view that age is a problem to be avoided. He argued that our assumptions and stereotypical myths surrounding the results of normal development contribute to ageism. These stereotypes of elders cast them as "less" in terms of sight, hearing, memory, mobility, health, learners, and even productive members of society. In contrast, McKnight described how his mother-in-law, whom he refers to as "Old Grandma," views "old":

> ... *finally knowing what is important ... when you are, rather than when you are becoming ... knowing about pain rather than fearing it ... being able to gain more pleasure from memory than prospect ... when doctors become impotent and powerless ... when satisfaction depends less and less on consumption ... using the strength that a good life has stored for you ... enjoying deference ... worrying about irrelevance.*[45] (p. 27)

COTAs must be prepared to overcome and critically reflect on their own bias related to growing old to provide culturally sensitive care to the elders they serve.

Use of time

Time is consciously and unconsciously formulated and used in each culture. Time is often treated as a language, a way of handling priorities, and a way of revealing how people feel about each other. Cultures can be divided into those who prefer a monochronic use of time and those who prefer a polychronic use of time.[46,47] Elders from monochronic cultures will probably prefer to organize their lives with a "one thing at a time" and "time is money" mentality. For these elders, adherence to schedules is highly important. They are likely to be offended if they are kept waiting for an appointment or if they perceive that the COTA is attending to too many issues at once. People from a monochronic culture prefer having the COTA's undivided attention and expect time to be used efficiently. These people are not necessarily unfriendly but prefer social "chit-chat" to be kept to a minimum if they are paying for a particular technical service. In contrast, elders from a polychronic culture organize their lives around social relationships. For them the time spent with someone is directly correlated to their personal value. Often these elders feel rushed by schedules. They may be late for an appointment because they encountered an acquaintance whom they did not want to offend by rushing off to a therapy appointment. With these elders, COTAs may find that sessions are most effective when a lot of conversation takes place. People from polychronic cultures may also wish to know many details about the COTA's life as a way of showing that they value the professional. When elders of a polychronic culture arrive late for an appointment, they may be offended if the COTA refuses to squeeze them into the schedule.

Communication Style

The meaning people give to the information they obtain through interaction with others largely depends on the way that information is transmitted. Cultures differ in the amount of information that is transmitted through verbal and nonverbal language. Cultures also differ in regard to the amount of information that is transmitted through the context of the situation.[48] Context includes the relationship to the individual with whom one is communicating. For example, after living together for more than 50 years, an elder couple does not always have to spell things out for each person to know the other's feelings. Each partner may know the other's feelings simply by the way that the other person moves and the tone of his or her voice. Their shared experiences over 50 years have given them high context; therefore, meaning is not lost when words are not spoken.

Hall[46] has noted that high-context cultures rely less on verbal communication than on understanding through shared experience and history. In high-context cultures, fewer words are spoken and more emphasis is placed on nonverbal cues and messages. High-context cultures tend to be formal, reliant on hierarchy, and rooted in the past; thus, they change more slowly and tend to provide more stability for their members.[49] When words are used in high-context cultures, communication is more indirect. People in these cultures usually express themselves through stories that imply their opinions.[48]

In contrast, persons from low-context cultures typically focus on precise, direct, and logical verbal communication.

These persons may not process the gestures, environmental clues, and unarticulated moods that are central to communication in high-context cultures. Low-context cultures may be more responsive to and comfortable with change but often lack a sense of continuity and connection with the past.[49]

Misunderstanding may easily arise when COTAs and elders, family members, or caregivers use a different level of context in their communication. Persons from high-context cultures may consider detailed verbal instructions insensitive and mechanistic; they may feel they are being "talked down to." Persons from low-context cultures may be uncomfortable with long pauses and may also feel impatient with indirect communication such as storytelling. It is the responsibility of the COTA to become aware of the style of communication of the elder, family member, or caregiver and adapt to that style. COTAs must note that nonverbal communication such as facial expressions, eye contact, and touching may have completely different meanings in different cultures. COTAs can learn these things by listening carefully, observing how the family interacts, and adapting OT practice style as new discoveries are made about the elder's culture.

CASE STUDY

Mrs. Pardo is a 70-year-old Filipino woman who was admitted to a skilled nursing facility after an infection developed in her right hip. She had a total hip replacement 3 weeks before being transferred to the skilled nursing facility. Because of the infection, Mrs. Pardo had received little therapy. A week ago, the OTR was finally able to complete an OT evaluation. Melissa, a newly hired COTA, is continuing the OT program. When discussing the case with Melissa, the OTR stated that, although Mrs. Pardo has been trained in getting from a supine position to a sitting position at the edge of the bed and in dressing, her family routinely provides this care. The OTR has not discussed with Mrs. Pardo or her family the need for these activities to be done independently. Part of Melissa's responsibility, according to the OTR, is to "convince them to not fuss over her so much."

Melissa reviewed Mrs. Pardo's medical record before meeting her. It appeared that Mrs. Pardo's condition was stable, and the infection was under control. Several professionals had documented that she was quite weak and deconditioned, presumably because of prolonged bed rest. Melissa reviewed the OT evaluation results and intervention goals, which seemed quite straightforward. The general objective was for Mrs. Pardo to become independent in ADL functions and transfers while observing specific hip precautions for at least 6 more weeks. These precautions included touch-toe weight bearing on the right leg, as well as avoiding right leg internal rotation and right hip flexion greater than 60 degrees. Melissa also noted that Mrs. Pardo was a widow who lived with one of her five adult daughters.

One of Mrs. Pardo's daughters and two of her adolescent grandchildren were present when Melissa met Mrs. Pardo. When Melissa introduced herself, Mrs. Pardo smiled and introduced her relatives. She also told Melissa she reminded her of someone she had met years ago while working as a sales representative for an American firm. Once Mrs. Pardo found out where Melissa was from she asked if Melissa knew the relatives of an acquaintance of hers, who was from Melissa's town. Finally, Melissa stated she was there to work on transfers and dressing. Because Melissa wanted to see how Mrs. Pardo performed these activities independently, she asked the relatives to leave the room for a few minutes. Once they left, Melissa sensed a change in Mrs. Pardo. Although she followed all of Melissa's directions quickly, she seemed to be avoiding eye contact. When Melissa asked her if everything was all right, Mrs. Pardo responded affirmatively. Melissa observed that Mrs. Pardo required minimal assistance to get out of the hospital bed, sit in a commode chair, and dress herself with a gown while observing all hip precautions. Noting that Mrs. Pardo appeared fatigued, Melissa said she would return at 3:00 p.m. to work on Mrs. Pardo's self-bathing ability. Melissa asked whether Mrs. Pardo was aware of any scheduling conflicts, to which Mrs. Pardo responded, "No." When Melissa left the room, she asked Mrs. Pardo's daughter if she would be available to observe the bath that afternoon. The daughter said she would be there without fail.

Later that afternoon Melissa entered Mrs. Pardo's room at the same moment that a different daughter was helping Mrs. Pardo get into bed. Alarmed that hip precautions were not being followed, Melissa immediately asked the daughter to let her take over and demonstrate the appropriate method of transferring to the bed. The daughter angrily stated that Mrs. Pardo was too tired for therapy and proceeded to complete the task without Melissa's assistance. Melissa was taken aback and told Mrs. Pardo she would return in the morning for the bath.

That evening Melissa could not stop thinking about the afternoon's events. She was aware that she had somehow offended Mrs. Pardo's daughter, and she wondered why Mrs. Pardo had gone back to bed knowing that Melissa would be coming to work with her at 3:00 p.m. Melissa decided to carefully analyze what had happened. She remembered how friendly and talkative Mrs. Pardo had been at the beginning of the session, which was perhaps a sign that she valued relationships highly and wanted Melissa to know she was appreciated. Then Melissa thought about the change in Mrs. Pardo when her family left and wondered if she felt alone without family to support her. Why had Mrs. Pardo said that everything was all right but then avoided eye contact? Was this her way of letting Melissa know that she did not want to do the task without directly opposing the plan for the session? Melissa thought about the tasks they had accomplished and wondered whether Mrs. Pardo had ever before been required to get out of a hospital bed, sit on a commode in front of another person, and dress in a hospital gown. Did these tasks have anything to do with her real life? Finally, Melissa remembered how she had entered the room while Mrs. Pardo's daughter was helping her get into bed. Melissa realized that she had blurted out orders without even introducing herself. Had she caused the daughter to feel embarrassed and incompetent? Was the daughter's anger a way of regaining control?

After evaluating the situation, Melissa concluded that Mrs. Pardo probably could not relate to the artificial ADL tasks presented to her. She also suspected that Mrs. Pardo relied on family members for support in making decisions and reducing anxiety. Mrs. Pardo also seemed to value the feelings of other people and avoided direct confrontation. The daughter might have been angry because Melissa confronted her directly. Melissa decided that the next day she would approach the intervention session with Mrs. Pardo differently. First, she would schedule the session when a family member could be present.

She also planned to spend some time simply conversing with Mrs. Pardo and her family members, and she planned to spend more time chit-chatting during the session. Melissa decided to take Mrs. Pardo to the simulated apartment in the rehabilitation department, where they could work in a more realistic home setting with a real bed and chair, and Mrs. Pardo could also work on dressing with her own clothes.

The next day, Melissa carried out her plan with great success. Melissa had realized that Mrs. Pardo was an associative thinker who needed new tasks to be associated with more familiar routines. Melissa had also realized that Mrs. Pardo valued family ties and social relationships greatly and consequently would not risk offending others with a direct refusal. In addition, Melissa realized that Mrs. Pardo relied on family as a source of anxiety reduction. Finally, Melissa had recognized that Mrs. Pardo was from a polychronic culture that valued a more social than prescriptive approach to rehabilitation.

CONCLUSION

Descriptions of particular cultural values or beliefs about aging have not been detailed in the chapter because such generalizations are inherently bound to foster assumptions and create stereotypes.[50] Even if stereotypes are positive, they may discourage practitioners from discovering the unique personality and aspirations of a client because they become shortcuts to communication. For example, sociologists have said that Hispanic families are a close-knit group and the most important social unit.[51] The term *familia* usually goes beyond the nuclear family and includes not only parents and children, but also extended family. Individuals within a family have a moral responsibility to aid other members of the family who experience financial problems, unemployment, poor health conditions, and other life issues. If the COTA assumes this to be true about an elderly Hispanic patient, she may jump to the conclusion that family training needs to begin immediately and not inquire whether the elder would prefer to be completely independent and live alone. The same value that may lead family members to take care of a grandparent may be leading the elder to avoid becoming a burden for others. Likewise, the assumption that a Japanese elder may prefer a highly structured and predictable daily routine, a Japanese cultural feature described by some scholars[52] may lead the COTA to not offer opportunities for spontaneous activities. Finally, the assumption that an elderly refugee from Sudan would prefer to let her husband make decisions about her care, as is customary in some Muslim cultures,[13] may lead the COTA to ignore that this couple customarily shared decision making and were mutually supportive. While it is advisable that the COTA be informed about the many features of cultures around the world, such knowledge should always be considered tentative and not a replacement for asking questions and letting the elder guide the selection of goals and interventions in the therapeutic process.

The chapter provides a framework that COTAs can use to approach elders from diverse backgrounds. Concepts

BOX 9-1

Attitude Self-Analysis

- Do I believe it is important to consider culture when treating elders?
- Am I willing to lower my defenses and take risks?
- Am I willing to practice behaviors that may feel unfamiliar and uncomfortable to benefit the elder with whom I am working?
- Am I willing to set aside some of my own cherished beliefs to make room for others whose values are unknown?
- Am I willing to change the ways I think and behave?
- Am I sufficiently familiar with my own heritage, including place of family origin, time of, and reasons for immigration, and language(s) spoken?
- What values, beliefs, and customs are identified with my own cultural heritage?
- In what ways do my beliefs, values, and customs interfere with my ability to understand those of others?
- Do I view elders as a resource in understanding their cultural beliefs, family dynamics, and views of health?
- Do I encourage elders to use resources from within their cultures that they see as important?

of culture and diversity have been discussed, with special attention given to the ways that these differences can contribute to the elder's ability to obtain meaning in therapy. Emphasis also was placed on the fact that both *culture* and *diversity* are very broad and complex terms. Consequently, a cultural model was presented to aid COTAs in designing individualized OT services for each elder. COTAs may use this information as a guide for culturally sensitive practice and remain open to new experiences that they encounter with each elder. Before attempting to treat elders from other backgrounds, COTAs must become aware of and analyze their own prejudices and biases about the dimensions of life that create diversity (Box 9-1). Such inner reflection should always accompany the exploration of the client's values, beliefs, and preferences (Box 9-2).

■ CHAPTER REVIEW QUESTIONS

1 Explain why it is difficult to define the term *culture*.
2 Give examples of ways in which you have learned and shared a particular value.
3 Give examples of values and beliefs that connect individuals with the various other levels of culture, including family, community, and country.
4 Explain how appreciating diversity can affect OT intervention with elders.
5 Describe your own cognitive style and explain how you base your actions on faith, fact, or feelings. Also,

BOX 9-2

Exploring the Elder's Values, Beliefs, and Preferences

Observation

- If possible, before beginning intervention with an elder, take some time to observe him or her from afar. How does the elder interact with others? How do family members and friends interact with the elder? To what degree is the communication direct? How frequent does eye contact appear to be? While the COTA should not simply mimic the elder's gestures, they should serve as cues to potentially preferred forms of interaction.
- Are there particular objects the elder has brought with him or her to the hospital? Are there any objects that seem to be prominently featured in the elder's home? Note any specific items and consider them of value, even though you may not at first understand why the elder chose them. Seek to integrate these items into therapy sessions.

Interaction

- Always approach the elder respectfully with a greeting. Ask the elder how he or she would prefer to be greeted and/or addressed. Note that even if an elder encourages you to use his or her first name that you do not immediately take other freedoms.
- Ask the elder how he or she understands the reasons for therapy. Ask questions to obtain the elder's explanatory health model:
  - What happened that you now were referred to therapy?
  - What do you think you/your body needs in order to heal?
  - What have you already tried to help yourself recover?
- Always ask the elder whether she or he would prefer to have someone present during therapy sessions. Note that an elder may not feel comfortable answering truthfully if relatives and/or friends are in the room, so ask the question when the elder's privacy can be protected.
- Always ask the elder whether a planned activity is acceptable before initiating it. Explain the goals and inquire whether there are preferred activities that are more meaningful/useful to the elder in his or her everyday life.
- Build trust slowly. Encourage the elder to tell you his or her life story in increments while working on a therapeutic activity. Follow the elder's lead; if he or she prefers to focus quietly on the task, do not insist on having a conversation.
- Share your personal story sparingly and only when or if the elder asks you to. Remember that the relationship should be centered on the elder, and your story should build trust not simply make idle conversation.
- Be careful with the frequency with which you ask questions. Permit the elder to answer fully, and pause before asking another question. Assess the level of comfort with answering questions and adjust accordingly.
- Express interest and openness about the ethnic and cultural heritage of the elder, and assess the level of comfort he or she has in speaking about it. Ask the elder to help you better understand his or her heritage. Be very careful that your gestures do not inadvertently communicate disgust. Remember that the elder is relaying information that for him or her is familiar and often a source of identity. Be culturally humble and communicate your desire to learn from the elder.
- Paraphrase what the elder tells you, particularly if related to decisions about his or her care. This will permit you to check your understanding and assure the elder that you care.

describe how you arrive at decisions about your own health behaviors and what you rely on to reduce anxiety in difficult times.

6 Describe at least three ways in which issues of equality and inequality may affect OT intervention with elders.

7 Explain ways in which you tend to behave on a monochronic and polychronic bases. Describe how this tendency may interfere with your ability to provide intervention to elders.

8 Describe at least three other strategies that Melissa could use with Mrs. Pardo that would take into consideration Mrs. Pardo's cultural context.

REFERENCES

1. American Occupational Therapy Association, 2008. Occupational therapy practice framework: Domain and process, 2nd ed. American Journal of Occupational Therapy 62 (6), 625-683.

2. Parvis, L., 2005. Understanding Cultural Diversity in Today's Complex World. Lulu Press, Morrisville, NC.

3. Rozak, T., 2009. The Making of an Elder Culture: Reflections on the Future of America's Most Audacious Generation. New Society, Gabriola Island, BC, Canada.

4. American Occupational Therapy Association, 2004. Definition of occupational therapy practice for the AOTA model practice act. Retrieved November 16, 2009, from http://www.aota.org/members/area4/docs/defotpractice.pdf.

5. Accreditation Council for Occupational Therapy Education, 2006. Accreditation standards for and educational program for the occupational therapy assistant. Retrieved November 16, 2009, from http://www.aota.org/Educate/Accredit/StandardsReview.aspx.

6. American Occupational Therapy Association, 2005. Occupational therapy code of ethics. American Journal of Occupational Therapy 59, 639-642.

7. Black, R., Wells, S., 2007. Culture and occupation: A model of empowerment in occupational therapy. AOTA Press, Bethesda, MD.

8. Bonder, B.R., Martin, L., Miracle, A.W., 2004. Culture emergent in occupation. American Journal of Occupational Therapy 58, 159-168.

9. Kielhofner, G., 2008. A Model of Human Occupation: Theory and Application, 4th ed. Lippincott Williams & Wilkins, Baltimore.
10. Peters-Golden, H., 2008. Culture Sketches: Case Studies in Anthropology. McGraw-Hill, New York.
11. Winkelman, M., 2009. Culture and Health: Applying Medical Anthropology. John Wiley & Sons, San Francisco.
12. Baumesiter, R., 2005. The Cultural Animal: Human Nature, Meaning, and Social Life. Oxford University Press, New York.
13. Gregg, G., 2008. Culture and Identity in a Muslim Culture. Oxford University Press, Oxford, England; Belmont, CA: Thompson Wadsworth.
14. Ross, H.C., 1993. The Art of Arabian Costume: A Saudi Arabian Profile. Players Press, San Francisco, CA.
15. Gardiner, H., Kosmitzki, C., 2008. Lives Across Cultures: Cross-Cultural Human Development. Pearson, Boston.
16. Haviland, W., Prims, H., Walrath, D., McBride, B., 2007. Cultural Anthropology: The Human Challenge, 12th ed. Wadsworth Publishing, Belmont, CA.
17. Kim, G., Chiriboga, D., Jang, Y., 2009. Cultural equivalence in depressive symptoms in older White, Black, and Mexican-American adults. Journal of the American Geriatrics Society 57 (5), 790-796.
18. Erez, M., Gati, E., 2004. A dynamic, multi-level model of culture: From the micro level of the individual to the macro level of a global culture. Applied Psychology: International Review 53 (4), 583-598.
19. Gatewood, J., 2001. Reflections on the nature of cultural distributions and the units of culture problem. Cross-Cultural Research: The Journal of Comparative Social Science 35 (2), 227-241.
20. Hasselkus, B., Rosa, S., 1997. Meaning and occupation. In: Christiansen, C., Baum, C. (Eds.), Enabling Function and Well-Being, 2nd ed. Slack, Thorofare, NJ.
21. Padilla, R., 2000. Considering culture in rehabilitation. In: Kumar, S. (Ed.), Multidisciplinary Approach to Rehabilitation. Butterworth/Heinemann, Oxford, England, pp. 123-154.
22. Anagnostou, Y., 2009. A critique of symbolic ethnicity: The ideology of choice? Ethnicities 9 (1), 94-122.
23. Bucher, R., 2009. Diversity Consciousness: Opening Our Minds to People, Cultures, and Opportunities, 3rd ed. Prentice Hall, Englewood Cliffs, NJ.
24. Kimbro, R., 2009. Acculturation in context: Gender, age at migration, neighborhood ethnicity, and health behaviors. Social Science Quarterly 90 (5),1145-1166.
25. Johnson, A., 2005. Privilege, Power, and Difference, 2nd ed. McGraw-Hill, New York.
26. United States Census Bureau, 2009. American community survey: 2008 data set. Retrieved November 16, 2009, from http://factfinder.census.gov/home/saff/main.html?_lang=en&_ts=.
27. Administration on Aging, 2008. A profile of older Americans: 2008. U.S. Department of Health and Human Services, Washington, DC.
28. Mosher, W., Chandra, A., Jones, J., 2005. Sexual behavior and selected health measures: Men and women 15-44 years of age, United States. Advanced Data No. 362. U.S. Department of Health and Human Services/Centers for Disease Control, Atlanta, GA.
29. Horowitz, J., Newcomb, M., 2001. A multidimensional approach to homosexual identity. Journal of Homosexuality 42 (2), 1-20.
30. Hostetler, A., 2009. Single by choice? Assessing and understanding voluntary singlehood among mature gay men. Journal of Homosexuality 56 (4), 499-531.
31. Starks, T., Gilbert, B., Fischer, A., Weston, R., DiLalla, D., 2009. Gendered sexuality: A new model and measure of attraction and intimacy. Journal of Homosexuality 56 (1), 14-30.
32. Pew Forum on Religion and Public Life, 2008. U.S. religious landscape survey: Religious affiliation: Diverse and dynamic. Pew Research Center, Washington, DC.
33. DeNavas-Walt, C., Proctor, B., Smith, J., 2009. Current population reports, P60-P236: Income, poverty, and health insurance coverage in the United States: 2008. U.S. Census Bureau, Washington, DC.
34. Gropper, R., 1996. Culture and the Clinical Encounter: An Intercultural Sensitizer for the Health Professions. Intercultural Press, Yarmouth, ME.
35. Allen, C., 1985. Occupational Therapy for Psychiatric Diseases: Measurement and Management of Cognitive Disabilities. Little, Brown, Boston.
36. Allen, C., Earhart, C., Blue, T., 1992. Occupational therapy goals for the physically and cognitively disabled. American Occupational Therapy Association, Rockville, MD.
37. Hofstede, G., Hofstede, G., 2005. Cultures and Organizations: Software of the Mind: Intercultural Cooperation and Its Importance for Survival. McGraw-Hill, New York.
38. Althen, G., 2002. American Ways. Intercultural Press, Yarmouth, ME.
39. Hall, E., 1981. Beyond Culture. Anchor, New York.
40. Harris, M., 1998. Theories of Culture in Postmodern Times. AltaMira Press, Pueblo, CO.
41. Morrison, T., Conaway, W., 2006. Kiss, Bow, or Shake Hands: How to Do Business in Sixty Countries, 2nd ed. Bob Adams, Holbrook, MA.
42. Bateson, M.C., 2001. Full Circles, Overlapping Lives: Culture and Generation in Transition. Ballantine, New York.
43. Johnson, N., 2007. Leadership through policy development: Collaboration, equity, empowerment, and multiculturalism. In: Chin, J., Lott, B., Rice, J., Sanchez-Hucles, J. (Eds.), Women and Leadership: Transforming Visions and Diverse Voices. Malden Blackwell, Boston, pp. 141-156.
44. Hasselkus, B.R., 2002. The Meaning of Everyday Occupation. Slack, Thorofare, NJ.
45. McKnight, J., 1995. The Careless Society: Community and Its Counterfeits. Basic, New York.
46. Hall, E., 1984. The Dance of Life: The Other Dimensions of Time. Anchor, New York.
47. Zimbardo, P., Boyd, J., 2008. Time Paradox: The New Psychology of Time. Simon & Schuster, New York.
48. Tseng, W., Streltzer, J., 2008. Cultural Competence in Healthcare: A Guide for Professionals. Springer, New York.
49. Luquis, R., 2008. Health education theoretical models and multicultural populations. In: Pérez, M., Luquis, R. (Eds.), Cultural Competence in Health Education and Health Promotion. Jossey-Bass, San Francisco, pp. 105-124.
50. Cruikshank, M., 2009. Learning to Be Old: Gender, Culture and Aging, 2nd ed. Rowan & Littlefield, Lanham, MD.
51. De Meante, B., 2009. Why Mexicans Think & Behave the Way They Do!: The Cultural Factors that Created the Character & Personality of the Mexican People. Phoenix, Blaine, WA.
52. Chou, R., Feagin, J., 2005. The Myth of the Model Minority: Asian Americans Facing Racism. Paradigm, Brookline, MA.

10

Ethical Aspects in the Work with Elders

LEA C. BRANDT

KEY TERMS

client autonomy, informed consent, ethical dilemma, ethical distress, distributive justice, least restrictive environment, benefits, burdens, ethics committee, confidentiality, empathetic relationships, whistle-blowing, American Occupational Therapy Association (AOTA) Ethics Commission (EC), National Board for Certification in Occupational Therapy (NBCOT), state regulatory boards

CHAPTER OBJECTIVES

1. Discuss steps for ethical consideration.
2. Become familiar with the language of ethics.

3. Refine and explain personal and professional ethical commitments.

Sheila, Maryann, and Chris are three friends who graduated from the same occupational therapy assistant (OTA) program a few years ago. They have gathered to discuss ethical conflicts they each have been experiencing where they work. Maryann works in a long-term care facility, Sheila works at a psychiatric hospital, and Chris is employed with a rehabilitation hospital. Recently, his employer expanded to home care, so Chris has begun seeing clients in their homes, as well as in the clinic.

In this chapter, the three certified occupational therapy assistants (COTAs) mentioned previously discuss a variety of ethical questions arising from the complexities of their job demands. These discussions include a series of steps for ethical consideration that students and clinicians can use in responding to ethical challenges in their practices. Some of the language of ethics is reflected in the Occupational Therapy Code of Ethics and Ethics Standards.[1] Other ethics commentaries that guide professional practice are introduced in the chapter. The author hopes that COTAs will take the opportunity to refine and explain the ethical commitments that shape their practice when working with elders and understand that being confronted with ethical conflict is inevitable in all areas of occupational therapy (OT) practice. Therefore, in addition to one's ongoing cultivation of clinical reasoning skills, it is equally important to develop skills related to ethical decision making.

AN OVERVIEW: ETHICS AND ELDER CARE

The health care environment is in the midst of great change. In recent years, OT practice has been especially influenced by the pressure to do more with less and through new medical technologies. In one way, these pressures have contributed positively to OT practice. For example, increased attention to the way health care dollars are spent has made OT practitioners focus more carefully on which interventions to use and the rationale for using them. While some technologies, such as improved joint replacement componentry, have enhanced clinical outcomes other technologies capable of sustaining life sometimes pose complex questions that clients, practitioners, and society are ill prepared to answer. The ethics of continuing to provide artificial nutrition and hydration to a person in a persistent vegetative state are one example. Other questions concern the ethics involved with equal access to the health care system for all persons.

Cost-control strategies also can create ethical challenges for practitioners. Traditionally, health care professionals have provided services based on the clinical needs of clients. Increasingly, however, financial constraints impede the practitioner's ability to uphold this commitment. For instance, cost controls on health care expenditures are sometimes linked to salary incentives in managed care organizations, which can tempt practitioners away from their professional responsibilities. Often third-party payers dictate the number of paid visits a patient may receive for a particular condition, and the number is not always indicative of clinical need. If a practitioner recommends more visits than allocated, clients may be required to pay some or all of the additional amount out of pocket, which may result in an insurmountable financial burden. Other ethically problematic cost-driven practices include "creative" documentation for reimbursement and accepting referrals for marginally necessary or needless interventions. Creative documentation refers to the practice of exaggerating a problem, altering a diagnosis, or implying a better prognosis so that more client visits can be approved. When actual fraud exists, such practices are also liable to legal inquiry and punishment.

Frequently, cost controls can translate into fewer staff for more clients. When these staffing changes contribute to inadequate supervision or require COTAs to use modalities for which they are not sufficiently trained, COTAs are placed in another ethically questionable position in terms of their professional standards of practice.

In addition to the clinical and financial environment of practice, special ethical concerns come up for COTAs who work with elders. Elders have a wide range of health care needs, and their occupational goals are diverse. Therefore, elders require personalized intervention plans, which may call for the practitioner to develop particular ethical sensitivities given the resources, practice environment restrictions, and client context.

Consider the example of ethical decision making in health care. Generally, in the United States, most people believe that adults should be the primary decision makers about their own health care because client autonomy is important. In the health care setting, autonomy refers to the idea that adults have the right to be involved in determining their plan of care and relevant intervention decisions. To ensure that clients have the information they need to make decisions consistent with good clinical outcomes, practitioners must communicate effectively regarding the benefits and burdens of potential interventions. While the value of client autonomy is expressed in many ways, informed consent serves as a cornerstone for an appropriately applied concept of autonomy. True informed consent hinges on respect for client autonomy and the practitioner's ability to effectively communicate potential outcomes.

To support a client's autonomous choice, health care providers must be careful to get informed consent from clients before doing a procedure, especially if the procedure has potential negative risks. The higher the risk, the more thorough the informed consent process should be. Before consenting, clients need to know the risks and benefits of the procedure, whether there are alternatives, and the way their health will be affected if intervention is refused. Once clients have this information, autonomy necessitates that they be allowed to accept or refuse the intervention. Further, respect for autonomy does not include offering interventions that are not clinically indicated. Instead, when clients demand interventions not supported by evidence-based practice, it is the practitioner's ethical responsibility to explain why the intervention cannot be provided and discuss how the burdens outweigh the benefits of intervention.

How is client autonomy translated into care for elders? Elders vary in their capacities for independent function

and thought, and thus their capacities for autonomous decision making. Some elders are no longer able to make decisions on their own behalf. Often the extent of this inability and its consequences for decision making are unclear. This state of fluctuating ability for decision making is often referred to as *diminished capacity*. Of course, a decline in physical independence is not always accompanied by mental dependency. COTAs must remember that clients who have lost most of their physical independence may still retain the ability to make independent decisions.

In addition, elders may retain the ability to make decisions in one situation and not in another. Decision-making capacity is situation-dependent and should therefore constantly be reassessed in practice. Caregivers need to appreciate that an elder's capacity for independent decision making may fluctuate because of his or her physical or mental conditions. For instance, patients with Alzheimer's disease, Parkinson's disease, or stroke may be more fully alert at certain times of the day than at other times.

Elders also vary in their capacities to respond to different kinds of decision-making tasks. In a nursing home, for example, a resident who is able to walk to a dining hall without assistance at the appropriate time may be unable to choose a balanced diet. Another resident may have the mental capacity to decide what to eat but is unable to keep reliable bank records. The task, the circumstance, and clients' mental and emotional state will determine their decision-making capacities.

Client decision making is only one area of ethical concern for COTAs. Through an exploration of the situations presented by the three COTAs, Chris, Sheila, and Maryann, the chapter presents a number of other issues. The chapter is organized around a four-step method for working through an ethical problem (Box 10-1). Each step is illustrated with specific cases experienced by the three friends.

AWARENESS: WHAT IS GOING ON?

The first step in approaching an ethical problem is to figure out what is going on. This may seem obvious at first, but actually the situation can be quite complicated, and, before COTAs take action, they must consider a number of factors.

BOX 10-1

Steps for Ethical Consideration
Awareness: What is going on?   *Reflection:* What do I think should happen?   *Support:* With whom do I need to talk?   *Action:* What will I do?

What Kind of Ethical Problem Is It?

COTAs may find it helpful to start by figuring out the kind of problem they are facing. Clinical ethicists often differentiate between two kinds of problems: an ethical dilemma and ethical distress.[2] An ethical dilemma refers to a situation in which there are two or more ethically correct options for action. However, with each choice, the COTA compromises something of value. Ethical distress refers to a situation in which the COTA knows which course of action to take but feels constrained to not carry it out. Often the constraint is imposed by someone who has more institutional authority than the COTA. Some situations may evoke both an ethical dilemma and ethical distress. Issues regarding distribution of scarce resources often result in both types of ethical problems. Distributive justice problems arise when there is not enough of something that is valued. The COTA must distribute the item or service in a fair way, or in the language of ethics, a "just" way (Box 10-2).

Who Is Involved?

The question of individuals involved must be considered when approaching an ethical problem. Usually the COTA is involved, and most likely the COTA's client is involved. But who else has a stake in the ethical problem that the COTA faces? It is not enough to know only who is involved; COTAs must also investigate their beliefs and values to anticipate areas of agreement and disagreement about the proposed course of action. The client's family often needs to be involved in medical decision making, but involvement may result in an ethical dilemma for the COTA.

For example, the family of one of Chris's home care clients asks him for help in pursuing long-term care placement for a client who has begun to wander from his home and has gotten lost several times. Chris knows that his client values his independence and will resist the move to a facility; however, Chris recognizes that the client might endanger himself. Chris must first question the client's decision-making capacity. Does the fact that the client wanders indicate that he lacks capacity? Does the client have the right to stay in his home even if Chris and the client's family believe it is a poor or unsafe choice? Respecting client choice is difficult when one does not agree with that choice or the decision could result in harm. However, often clients make decisions that we must respect even if we do not agree. Is this an instance when he should respect the wishes of the client? At what point should decision-making capacity be questioned? Does the client's family have the right to make decisions for their loved one? What other values, besides the client's autonomy, should Chris consider? In addition to Chris, the family, and the client, who else is likely to be involved?

Which Laws and Institutional Rules Apply?

There are distinct differences between the law and ethics. Ethical action stems from making morally good choices,

BOX 10-2

Examples of Ethical Problems

Ethical dilemma

Maryann works in a long-term care facility. A client who has had a stroke asks Maryann whether she will regain fine motor control of her hand. If Maryann tells her she probably will not regain all of her fine motor control, the client is likely to fall into a deep depression. If Maryann does not tell her the full extent of her prognosis, she probably will find out anyway, and then her trust in Maryann might diminish.

What are two of the actions Maryann could take?

What values are compromised if either action is taken?

Ethical distress

Sheila works at a psychiatric hospital. She has just learned that her client is to be discharged the following day. She knows he lives alone and will most likely not be able to regulate his medications appropriately. Sheila voices her concerns, but her supervisor tells her that the client's insurance coverage has run out, so they have no choice but to discharge him.

Is it ethically wrong to discharge this client? Why or why not?

What barrier(s) does Sheila confront when questioning the discharge plan?

Ethical dilemma and ethical distress: Distributive justice

Chris works at a rehabilitation clinic but has begun seeing clients in their homes as well. One of Chris's clients has been admitted to the rehabilitation program with clear payment guidelines from his insurance company: There will be no reimbursement for equipment of any type. The client needs a wrist support splint, but this item is considered equipment by the insurance company.

Should Chris ignore the need for a splint because of restricted payment guidelines?

Can you name at least three other scarcities in health care that are likely to raise issues of distributive justice for you as a COTA?

whereas the law usually deals with right and wrong as a principle of justice.[3] Ethics can be said to hold practitioners to a higher standard than the law. Certainly, throughout history there have been laws that are ethically problematic and ethical standards that are not recognized by the law. Sometimes laws and institutional rules both help clarify the role of COTAs in a given ethics problem. Some laws are federal, meaning that they apply in every state, but other laws apply only within a particular state's jurisdiction. Many institutions have legal counselors who can answer questions about specific legal issues. Supervisors also can help clarify the legal and institutional responsibilities of COTAs. Generally, institutions have established guidelines and rules that specify the expectations that they have for staff, clients, and administrators. COTAs are responsible for knowing which laws and policies apply to their practice and, according to the profession's Code of Ethics,[4] are responsible for complying with those regulations.

The influence of law in guiding ethical practice is illustrated in a case regarding the use of restraints that Sheila was asked to help resolve at the psychiatric hospital where she works. Sheila's client is a 68-year-old woman who was admitted to the acute care psychiatry department because of agitation and uncontrollable behavior. The client's charted diagnosis read, "Axis I schizoaffective bipolar type, axis III hypertension, degenerative joint disease, chronic obstructive pulmonary disease, chronic constipation, head trauma (grade 9; no further details)." Staff members have expressed that they do not particularly like this client; they often construe her behavior as violent. The client calls other residents and staff derogatory names; she also tells lies about them and accuses them of mistreating her. At times, she claims she is unable to walk and demands use of a wheelchair. She often stages a fall by throwing herself from the wheelchair onto the floor. The staff recommends that she be restrained in a chair for her own safety.

When Sheila brought this case to her friends for discussion, Maryann pointed out that given the client's age her case was most likely covered by Medicare. She goes on to state that she thinks this means that legally, like the staff in her nursing home, the staff in the psychiatric hospital should follow the guidelines for restraints defined by the Omnibus Budget Reconciliation Act (OBRA) of 1987. Maryann explained that this federal legislation requires health care providers to ensure client safety in the least restrictive environment. Sheila voiced her suspicion that maybe the restraints were being used as punishment, not client safety, but was not sure whether OBRA applied to psychiatric facilities. Chris then posed the following question, "Regardless of the legal implications shouldn't we strive for what is most ethical?" The others agreed that striving for the least restrictive environment is certainly ethically indicated, but it also would not hurt to understand how OBRA applies to psychiatric facilities. The three friends began thinking of ways that OT could help in designing the least restrictive environment for this client and whom to contact regarding OBRA guidelines. "After all," said Chris, "even unpleasant clients deserve the right to make choices and have some liberty, as long as they are not hurting others." While this case demonstrates how the law and ethics may support a single course of action, it also shows that there is a distinct difference between applying ethical standards and the law. When in doubt it is best to ethically reason through options in line with the standard of care set by the profession. OT practitioners should always strive to provide ethical care, which is often a higher standard than what is legally required. Chris, Sheila, and Maryann question whether there are situations when there would be a conflict between what is legally required and what is ethically indicated. How should a COTA respond if this type of conflict persists?

What Guidance Do the Occupational Therapy Ethics Standards Provide?

In her 1966 Eleanor Clarke Slagle lecture, Elizabeth Yerxa[5] asked, "What image do you see when you think of a professional? A person who always wears clean white shoes or someone who can spout off the origins and insertions of every muscle in the body or one who can discuss Freudian theory with a psychiatrist? No, professionalism is much more than appearance and intellectual accomplishments. It means being able to meet real needs. It means being unique. It means having and acting upon a philosophy."

The Occupational Therapy Ethics Standards provide a philosophical and practical translation of how to maintain professionalism in practice.[1] The Code of Ethics,[4] one of the documents in the Ethics Standards, outlines principles that are similar to a list of desired behaviors for OT practitioners. OT practitioners must demonstrate concern for the well-being of their clients and respect their clients' rights. OT practitioners must be competent, comply with laws and rules that apply to OT practitioners, and provide accurate information about services they provide. Finally, OT practitioners must be fair and discreet and demonstrate integrity with colleagues and other professionals.

Not only is the Occupational Therapy Code of Ethics a guide for behavior, it is also a regulatory code in that guidelines for conduct are stated and sanctions are provided for failure to comply with the code. These sanctions are stated in the Enforcement Procedures for the Code of Ethics.[6] Often the principles stated in the Code of Ethics are also found in local, state, and federal laws.

The Occupational Therapy Code of Ethics and related ethics standards provide ethical guidance in all areas of OT practice. However, it is recognized that these standards of practice are only one component of understanding and applying ethical reasoning. Practitioners need to go beyond following rules and regulations. They must attempt to demonstrate moral character and empathetic respect for clients. In fact, ethical practice, professional judgment, awareness of economic constraints, and evidence-based practice are all interrelated processes of OT practice.[7]

What Are My Options?

OT practitioners need to be aware of the range of ethical options available to them before deciding what action should be taken in a given case. As noted, sometimes the ethical options for a COTA are outlined by law. In some instances, practitioners may feel their ethical options are limited by their own personal religious prohibitions and beliefs. However, conflicts of conscience between personal and professional duties often result in a quandary where the ethical course of action is not clear. Some circumstances would ethically require practitioners to provide intervention even when it may conflict with their own moral sensitivities, while other situations would not. Some examples of conflicts of conscience in health care include a pharmacist refusing to distribute the morning-after pill, a fertility specialist refusing to artificially inseminate a gay woman, a nurse providing substandard care to a prisoner who is a known child molester, or a physician refusing to dialyze an intravenous drug user suffering from end-stage renal disease. What are some situations that may result in a conflict of conscience for OT providers?

When conflicts of conscience exist, clinical ethicists may suggest that health care providers, clients, and families try to estimate the consequences of a given option. These consequences can be weighed against the consequences of other options. The ethically preferable course of action will be that which carries the greatest probability of a good outcome (benefits) and the least amount of damage (burdens).

This calculation of consequences is illustrated with a case that Chris discussed with Maryann and Sheila. At the rehabilitation hospital where Chris works, the burn unit was considering the best way to treat a comatose 85-year-old man. The team was trying to decide whether to treat the client's severe burns or to provide him with palliative care until he died. To decide which course to take, the burn unit team was considering whether the burdens of intervention, including excruciating pain from grafts and range-of-motion exercises, were ethically warranted given his questionable survival. They also wondered about the quality of his life if he did survive. It was clear he would never return to his home and would need nursing facility care for the rest of his life. The client's family felt that this prospect of the future would be demoralizing for their relative because he had always cherished his independence. But some members of the staff argued that with rehabilitation the client might learn to adapt to and even enjoy a more social environment. Questions that arose for Chris out of this example include the following: What burdens are created by aggressive intervention in this case? What benefits are created by such intervention? What burdens are created by palliative care? What benefits are created by palliative care? Most importantly, how would the team determine how the patient would weigh benefits and burdens if he speaks for himself? Chris also understood that generally, unless there was a reason to believe that the family had a conflict of interest, they would be the presumed appropriate surrogate decision maker.

In accordance with professional values, COTAs should calculate these ratios of benefits and burdens in light of the client's well-being, not in terms of the staff's convenience or the client's estate. This kind of assurance is necessary for maintaining a bond of trust between health professionals and their clients, who expect professionals to work on behalf of their best interests.

Best interest with regard to elderly clients who have at some point held decision-making capacity would be to apply standards of substituted judgment. This is generally the case when working with elders who have recently lost decision-making capacity or appear to show diminished capacity. Based on the substituted judgment standard, Chris should support the rest of the health care team and family in making decisions based on what the client would presumably want if he were able to communicate his wishes. This analysis would include discussions with the family regarding conversations they may have had with the client before the incident, and/or reflecting on how the client lived his life to determine what he would want given the prognosis. Dialogue with the family would also give the health care team insight as to the family's motivations for recommending palliative care versus aggressive intervention.

Reflection: What Do I Think Should Happen?

After COTAs are aware of all of the facts and options in a given case, they must decide what they want to happen and must be able to explain their position. First, COTAs must determine what actions seem most wrong or right. This process may begin as a gut feeling that persists. Sensitivity to such feelings is an important component for reflective ethical practice. In addition, the legally defined roles of COTAs or their religious tenets may affect their ethical inclinations. Ethical reflection involves careful and critical examination of feelings and values, a rational estimate of benefits and burdens, and a sense of professional duty. This reflection is most effective when the COTA has engaged in dialogue with the client and/or family to factor in the client's wishes and motivations.

Often this stage of ethical consideration requires some emotional and even physical detachment as COTAs step back from the problem to reflect on their ethical commitments and reasoning. Sometimes the urgency of a situation requires rapid reflection; nonetheless, clinical ethicists recommend that a period of time be taken for serious consideration of preferences and motivations for choosing a given course of action. Each person should find personal methods of reflection that best fit his or her reasoning style.

Some health professionals find it useful to talk through a problem with a group of trusted advisors. In addition to colleagues from the other health professions, COTAs should include the registered occupational therapist (OTR) as a team partner in working through these difficult conflicts. Such a group can be informal, like the group of COTAs highlighted in the chapter, or more formal, such as an institutional ethics committee. Typically, ethics committees are composed of a multidisciplinary group of health care professionals, administrators, legal counsel, and a community representative. Just as with an informal group of peers, these committees may be helpful in considering the options for addressing a particular ethical dilemma or reviewing the ethics of decisions that have already been made. In most instances, these committees provide a recommendation for resolution, and it is up to the health care team to decide how they wish to move forward based on that recommendation.

When choosing to talk over an ethics problem with someone else, COTAs must respect the confidentiality of those involved. COTAs should make every effort to see that information about clients, colleagues, or institutions is shared in a way that does not reveal anyone's identity unless required to effectively provide intervention for that client. The client's name should not be used with persons not involved directly with the client's care. Similar discretion needs to be taken when the behavior of an institution or a peer is discussed.

Free writing is another method used for ethical reflection.[8] Free writing involves writing whatever comes to mind without worrying about language, spelling, and grammar. Usually the exercise is limited to 10 minutes, during which the writer does not stop writing. The key is to suspend the usual breaks in writing and let uncensored thoughts pour onto the page. The usefulness of this technique is in uncovering deep moral and ethical feelings. This technique may reveal previously unrealized opinions or persuasive reasons for a stance. The free writing technique requires only that COTAs trust themselves to be revealed.

Two weeks ago, Maryann was placed in a difficult position with one of her favorite clients, Mrs. Henry. Three months earlier, Mrs. Henry had come to the facility after experiencing a stroke. Despite Maryann's best efforts to help Mrs. Henry regain endurance and sitting balance, Maryann's supervising OTR concluded that Mrs. Henry was not likely to improve any further and recommended discontinuing her therapy. However, Mrs. Henry's family asked Maryann to continue the interventions. They could tell how much their mother enjoyed the attention. They were worried that Mrs. Henry would lose hope and her health would deteriorate further. Maryann explained that without demonstrable improvement, Medicare was not likely to reimburse the facility for this therapy. In response, the family appealed to Maryann's sense of loyalty to their mother, asking her to be creative about how she documented the effect of the therapy. Maryann faced an ethical dilemma between loyalty to someone she cared for and the obligation to truthfully document OT intervention. She decided to free write for 10 minutes to better determine a response (Box 10-3). To her surprise, she found her response was guided by her ethical preference.

Caring professionals are often confronted with the limits of their empathetic relationships with clients. Especially in long-term care environments, professionals may find that relating to their clients through the rigid shield of professional distance is unrealistic and uncomfortable. Conversely, clients must be protected from a caregiver's

BOX 10-3

Maryann's Free Writing

Let's see. It's 1:48, so that gives me until 1:58. I can't believe I'm writing this. This feels really stupid. OK. OK. The thing is, I don't know what to do for Mrs. H. She's such a sweet old lady. Even though she can't speak, she communicates with her eyes. They shine so gratefully when we are together. I can tell she appreciates my work. But it really bugs me that her family has pressured me to document progress when there isn't any. I am the one who brought up reimbursement, that probably wasn't the best decision. I wouldn't want other people to think of my family as a paycheck. Instead of inferring that I am withholding intervention strictly based on money, I should have spoke to the family about my professional obligations regarding provision of clinically beneficial care and why I can't ethically continue to see patients who were not making progress. I can see their point, and in fact I want to do anything at all to help her because I really care about her, but I think they would understand that my professional time needs to be spent seeing clients who can benefit from occupational therapy intervention. I do feel really close to Mrs. H., and want to help her but it would be a lie to say she is improving from the therapy. But I don't want to give up hope. This isn't any more clear than when I started writing. What time is it? Don't stop to look. Keep writing. OK. So. What am I supposed to do? The Code says #1, we are supposed to work for each patient's well-being but it also says I should provide proper individualized care ... ok that is confusing. The code is clear about telling the truth. So what help is that? I could get my OTR to fudge a bit on the chart, at least for a couple of weeks. But that is obviously a lie and fraud. What is the bottom line? Why is it that caring for Mrs. H. seems incompatible with telling the truth? Why not keep seeing Mrs. H., stopping by her room after hours to cheer her up. I wouldn't be doing therapy or compromising my responsibility to my employer, because it would be after work hours. I'd be there as her friend. I think that's what I'll do. I'll just have to tell the family that the therapy will end, but I won't desert their mother. And maybe I can help teach them how they can work with her so she feels like she is getting attention. Of course, if she shows improvement I can always work with the OTR to have her re-evaluated and put back on the caseload, which I can also tell the family. That gives me hope. I can't believe it, but I actually feel lighter. And in exactly 10 minutes to the second!

over-involvement, as in the extreme case of sexual liaisons, and also from a caregiver's subjective biases, as in the case of discrimination. Finding a balance between genuine caring for clients and realistic boundaries for professional involvement is a lifelong goal for all health care professionals that requires ongoing ethical introspection. Reflective ethical practice suggests that before responding to an ethical issue, when possible COTAs must step away from the urgency of the problem to gain perspective about their responsibilities.

Support: With Whom Do I Need to Talk?

Although ethical issues admittedly involve mindful reflection, they should not be considered in isolation from others. Ethical commitments are shaped by social influences, including upbringing, professional codes, and the circumstances of a given event. Likewise, the outcomes of most ethical decisions have social effects. Before acting according to moral convictions, COTAs should solicit the support of others who will be affected by the issue. In almost all instances of ethics in health care, this means communicating with the client, the client's family, and other staff members. Sometimes the organization's ethics committee can provide institutional support for a COTA's position. Others who are more directly involved in a given issue may have more influence than the COTA when voicing their ethical positions. In addition, others may justifiably have more decision-making authority given the particular circumstances under consideration. The usual practice in the United States is to prioritize the wishes of adult clients who have decision-making capacity above those of others, even when the adult's wishes run counter to expert opinion. Other professionals on the health care team, by virtue of status, training, and tradition, also may claim decision-making authority. This decision-making authority does not translate into moral authority, and COTAs should also recognize that they have a professional duty to facilitate dialogue and raise awareness of a potential ethical conflict.

When COTAs have limited influence, they must express their position and the reasons that support it so that others have the benefit of these insights. Also, by expressing their positions, COTAs can sometimes avoid the experience of ethical distress, when asked to participate in an intervention that conflicts with their ethical views. The more rational the COTAs' arguments in support of their position, the more persuasive COTAs will be in defending their objections, even if the course of events cannot be changed. In cases of ethical distress, communication has been identified as a primary strategy in reducing negative outcomes associated with this phenomenon. In addition to bringing important information to the table for discussion, COTAs may also acquire information that supports a decision to which they were initially opposed.

In cases in which COTAs are asked to do something that is ethically questionable, they have the responsibility to involve those with supervisory jurisdiction over them. COTAs should document such communications, especially if there are legal ramifications or if job security is at risk. Following is an example of this kind of dilemma.

In the last year, since his rehabilitation clinic changed to a managed care model, Chris has observed that he is increasingly asked to do interventions that OTRs previously did. Most of the time Chris appreciates the opportunity for more responsibility and feels comfortable doing what is asked of him. However, recently he was asked by the referring physician to work with a client who needed paraffin baths for her arthritic fingers. After he explained the situation, Chris and his friends discussed the issue.

"Absolutely not! You haven't had any training for this modality, and you might burn the client or something," said Sheila.

"It's not only unfair that they asked you to do this, isn't it illegal? I know you work across the state line in your facility, but I know in my state we have to be certified in physical agent modalities as does the supervising occupational therapist. You need to find out what your state practice act says! They are just trying to save money by asking you to do this instead of asking an OTR," added Maryann.

"That may well be," replied Chris, "but I still have to deal with it one way or another."

"So what are you going to do?" asked Maryann.

"Well, I like my job and I don't think this is worth quitting over, at least not without first communicating my distress and the legal implications to my supervisor. Like you, Maryann, I worry that I might hurt someone inadvertently, and this goes against my sense of professional duty to do no harm. Also in this case the legal liability is key, I could lose my license as could the supervising OT. I think that once I communicate this conflict to my supervisor and talk about how this could negatively impact staffing in the long run she will support me. After all, if the clinic loses both me and the supervising OT because we did not comply with our practice act or AOTA standards of practice the clinic will be in worse shape."

"We're behind you on this one, buddy. The other OT practitioners at the clinic will be, too. I bet if you e-mailed the AOTA Ethics Commission, their staff liaison would back you up," suggested Sheila.

"But whatever you do, I think you better carefully document everything that is said and done so there is a clear record of your reasons for refusing and your efforts to negotiate a change in your assignment," cautioned Maryann.

Action: What Will I Do?

Inevitably, even in the most complex ethics cases, COTAs need to take some action. In ethics, doing nothing can also be perceived as an action. If the previous steps have been considered in good conscience and the clinical benefits have been prioritized, COTAs usually have an ethical basis for action. COTAs may retain a sense of uncertainty, but at least they will have the comfort of knowing that they have given deep thought to their position to articulate the basis for their action. Generally speaking, COTAs will most likely not have to act alone because of the input received from others. In addition, COTAs must realize that because they are working under the supervision of an OTR, their action or inaction will impact both treating OT practitioners. Conversely, even though COTAs work closely with the OTR there is still a level of ethical accountability for one's personal action or inaction.

Take for example the following issue of reporting errors. It can be difficult to admit when one is wrong, but often the consequences of not reporting mistakes are much worse. Sheila decides to tell Chris and Maryann about a recent event that happened at the psychiatric hospital involving a colleague.

"Well, I wasn't going to bring this up today as I don't want you guys to think poorly about where I work, but we recently had a really terrible situation occur and I feel kind of conflicted about the outcome. I mean, I know I have probably made a similar mistake and yet, one of my friends was recently terminated by the hospital because she didn't follow policy and a patient died."

"What, you're kidding! Somebody died in an occupational therapy session?" Maryann exclaimed.

Sheila replied, "Well, not exactly during the session, but this colleague was working with a patient who was unsteady from all of the psychotropic medications she was taking and of course, elders often react differently to meds than younger patients. Anyway, the patient lost her balance while working on lower body dressing and bumped her head on the nightstand. The COTA was very apologetic, sat her down and ran to get the supervising OTR. She asked the OTR if they should go get a nurse or the doctor, but the patient seemed fine and her family was arriving for a visit. They decided that she was OK and just told her family to call the nurse if she started feeling sick to her stomach or dizzy. Unfortunately, the patient went to sleep, suffered an intracranial hemorrhage and subsequently died later that evening. Both the COTA and OTR lost their jobs for not following hospital policy, were involved in a civil lawsuit, were given a two-year probation by the state licensing board and received a public censure by the AOTA Ethics Commission."

"Wow, I don't even know what our policy is for reporting a fall in the home health setting. This is something I obviously need to find out," Chris stated with chagrin.

Sheila confided, "It is sad that this had to occur for me to understand how I can actually demonstrate unethical behavior in failing to act. I always assumed if you have good intentions, that is enough. It seems like a really harsh outcome for a seemingly small mistake. If only they had reported the fall to the nurse or doctor."

While frequent, errors in health care practice can be difficult to report because they often result in embarrassment and shame, which create a barrier for disclosure. As with other health care professions, what matters most is how OT practitioners take responsibility and learn from their mistakes. Disclosure is an important first step to foster learning from errors; and it often leads to positive outcomes for clients, OT providers, and future practice.[9]

While self-disclosure is difficult, arguably reporting the unethical behavior of a client's family, a professional colleague, or an institution is one of the most difficult actions to take. Nevertheless, if unethical conduct has been observed, COTAs have an ethical obligation to report this behavior to the authorities. In some states, this obligation is underscored by law. Thus, if COTAs know of a wrongdoing and do not report it, the law also considers them guilty.

This is the case with reporting elder abuse. In addition to the ethical obligation to limit harm to clients under their care, there are legal requirements obligating COTAs and other health care professionals to report elder abuse to the proper authorities. Almost all states have mandatory reporting laws that apply to OT practice. While laws have been enacted over the course of the last 40 years with the inception of the Older Americans Act of 1965, elder abuse is consistently underreported. Elder abuse can range from financial exploitation to violence and be inflicted by a family member, a care provider, or even an institution. It is a COTA's ethical responsibility to protect vulnerable populations, which includes reporting abusive situations involving elderly clients.

Reporting another's unethical behavior is sometimes referred to as *whistle-blowing*. Especially when the COTA's job may be threatened, it can take courage to follow through with such a report. If possible, COTAs should work with the support of others, especially those in a supervisory position. Obviously, this is difficult when a supervisor is the person being reported. Regardless of the circumstance, COTAs should make sure to document their actions so that their systematic efforts to address the problem are well established, especially if the COTA is in a less powerful position than the person being reported. Sometimes in a twist of logic, the whistle-blower becomes a scapegoat, or is blamed for another's unethical behavior. If COTAs have kept good records of their attempts to correct or resolve the situation, they will be more easily cleared of such an accusation.

Often, coworkers also will have observed unethical behavior and may feel similarly vulnerable. COTAs can sometimes increase the effectiveness of their responses if they work with others. When sharing information with others to gain support for their actions, COTAs must respect the confidentiality of persons and institutions by providing information fairly and appropriately. If warranted, the authorities will dispense an appropriate punishment for wrongdoing after an investigation.

Who are the relevant authorities? This may differ depending on the entity being reported. In the case of elder abuse, each state has a protective services agency and referral to agencies is available from the national Eldercare Locator, a public service of the U.S. Administration on Aging. Many states also have online directories that list local reporting numbers. It is important to work with managers and administrators when making reports to ensure that organizational policies are followed in the reporting process.

When reporting other health care professionals, the State Regulatory Board should be contacted. In many cases, state boards, created by state legislatures, have the power to intervene if they determine the public to be at risk because of a practitioner's incompetence, lack of qualifications, or unlawful behavior. State boards can publicly reprimand a practitioner or, if warranted, may even prohibit someone from practicing in that state.

With regard to OT practice, the AOTA Ethics Commission (EC) has prepared a detailed discussion of where to go to seek guidance about reporting unethical conduct. It names three major bodies with jurisdiction over professional behavior.[1] COTAs may call or write the AOTA EC. After discussing the possible violation of the Ethics Standards, COTAs can decide whether to file a formal complaint with the EC. The EC is responsible for writing the profession's Ethics Standards and for imposing sanctions on AOTA members who do not comply. Depending on the seriousness of the unethical behavior, the EC will suggest public censure, temporary suspension of membership, or revocation or permanent loss of membership.[6]

The National Board for Certification in Occupational Therapy (NBCOT) is responsible for certifying OTRs and COTAs. Depending on the significance of the unethical behavior that is reported, and after a thorough and confidential investigation, the NBCOT may also take action against the practitioner in question. The most severe punishment available through the NBCOT is permanent denial or revocation of certification. (The NBCOT maintains a Web page with up-to-date information at http://www.nbcot.org.)

Finally, COTAs should gather copies of their state's licensure laws, the AOTA Code of Ethics,[4] and other documents from the AOTA that can help clarify ethical issues. Documents such as the Standards of Practice for Occupational Therapy,[10] Guide for Supervision of Occupational Therapy Personnel in the Delivery of Occupational Therapy Services,[11] and Roles and Responsibilities of the Occupational Therapist and Occupational Therapy Assistant During the Delivery of Occupational Therapy Services[12] also can give COTAs a basis for their ethical arguments.

CONCLUSION

Working with elders carries special rewards and responsibilities. Clinical and ethical competency is necessary to maximize clients' functional capacities and contribute to the dignity and self-worth required for autonomous decision making. COTAs bring comfort to their clients through skillful intervention and by acting as the client's advocate in ensuring ethical care. A healing bond of trust is reinforced each time clients witness COTAs responding with a sense of ethical commitment in the fulfillment of their clients' needs.

BOX 10-4

Tips for Ethical Decision Making
■ Ensure that involved parties have their voices heard.
■ Ethical dilemmas cannot be collapsed into legal questions.
■ Clinical reasoning must accompany ethical analysis.
■ Expertise in the clinical health care arena should not be generalized to ethics.
■ Disclose and be aware of own moral values and bias.

The chapter reviewed ethical challenges in elder care settings and presented a step-by-step method for responding in a conscientious, informed manner. In addition to the steps involved in the ethical reasoning process, the chapter provided the reader with several tips to assist in ensuring thoughtful ethical reflection and application (Box 10-4). The COTA has an ethical duty to ensure that the client's voice is heard as well as the voice of those who may be speaking for the client. This is especially important in OT practice with elders who may at times present with diminished decision-making capacity but who have throughout their lives demonstrated a pattern of independent judgment, indicative of who they are as autonomous persons. While it is important to understand the legal parameters for ethical decision making, COTAs must ensure that ethical reasoning prevails in ensuring professionalism in practice. Ethical dilemmas cannot be collapsed into legal questions. So, too, is it important to understand the relationship between good ethical decisions and strong clinical practice. Many ethical dilemmas at the bedside are informed by clinical indicators. The COTA's ethical responsibility includes ensuring that intervention is consistent with what is clinically indicated. COTAs may often face situations impacted by power differentials within the health care team. Yet, COTAs must remember that authority in the clinical arena does not always translate to decision-making authority, and one should not generalize expertise in the clinical health care arena to ethics. Finally, it is imperative that COTAs recognize the influence that personal beliefs may have on practice. Therefore, disclosure of bias is ethically required. Health care professionals, including COTAs, need reminders that ethics is about how we should act in consideration of others, not necessarily how we feel or believe. The author hopes that readers will follow the strategies described when responding to events in their practices to ensure ethical outcomes for their clients.

CHAPTER REVIEW QUESTIONS

1 Recall the discussion that Sheila, Maryann, and Chris had about one of Sheila's clients at the psychiatric center who was being placed in restraints. At the end

of that conversation, Chris stated, "After all, even unpleasant clients deserve the right to make choices and have some liberty, as long as they are not hurting others." What ethical term did you learn earlier in the chapter that summarizes Chris's statement? Would this term apply to the following statement, "After all, even unpleasant clients deserve the right to make choices and have some liberty, as long as they are not hurting themselves"? Why or why not?

2 Reread the case of Chris, the COTA expected to use paraffin baths with a client.
  a Identify the benefits and burdens to the client if Chris were to administer the paraffin bath.
  b Based on your calculations, is it ethical for Chris to do the procedure?
  c Whom, if anyone, would you involve in supporting your decision if you were asked to use a modality for which you had not been trained?

3 Imagine that you are sitting with the three COTAs discussing the case that is described in the following. Suggest how you would guide their response to the ethical challenges facing Chris.

  Chris is concerned about recent changes in his supervision at the rehabilitation clinic, especially in the new home care work he is doing. He never sees his supervising OTR anymore. She does her evaluations in the evenings or on weekends, when he is not at work. She wants him to mail his notes for her to cosign, but he worries about client confidentiality, especially if the notes got lost in the mail. However, Chris is most concerned about some of the intervention being ordered for his older home care clients. He often feels pushed to provide three or four units (15 minutes) of intervention when his older clients seem able to tolerate only one or two units per session. He suspects that the extra interventions are motivated by financial reasons and not by the well-being of his clients.
  a Awareness
    1 What kind of ethical problem(s) is Chris facing?
    2 Who is involved?
    3 What laws and institutional rules apply?
    4 What guidance does the AOTA Code of Ethics give?
    5 What are Chris's options?
  b Reflection
    1 Suggest strategies that Chris can use for reflection.
    2 Provide reasons for your preferred response(s) to the problem(s) he faces.
  c Support
    1 Suggest strategies Chris might use for building support.
  d Action
    1 What should Chris do?

REFERENCES

1. American Occupational Therapy Association, 2008. Reference Guide to the Occupational Therapy Ethics Standards: 2008 Edition. AOTA Press, Bethesda, MD.
2. Purtilo, R., 2005. Ethical Dimensions in the Health Professions, 4th ed. WB Saunders, Philadelphia.
3. Slater, D.Y., 2004. Legal and ethical practice: A professional responsibility. OT Practice September 6, 13-16.
4. American Occupational Therapy Association, 2005. Occupational Therapy Code of Ethics. American Journal of Occupational Therapy 59, 639-642.
5. Yerxa, E., 1967. 1966 Eleanor Clarke Slagle Lecture: Authentic occupational therapy. American Journal of Occupational Therapy 21, 1-9.
6. American Occupational Therapy Association, 2007. Enforcement procedures for the Occupational Therapy Code of Ethics. American Journal of Occupational Therapy 61, 679-683.
7. Lopez, A., Vanner, E.A., Cowan, A.M., Samuel, A.P., Shepherd, D.L., 2008. Intervention planning facets—Four facets of occupational therapy intervention planning: Economics, ethics, professional judgment, and evidence-based practice. American Journal of Occupational Therapy 62, 87-96.
8. Goldberg, N., 2001. Thunder and Lightning: Cracking Open the Writer's Craft. Doubleday, New York.
9. Mu, K., Lohman, H., Scheirton, L., 2006. Occupational therapy practice errors in physical rehabilitation and geriatrics settings: A national survey study. American Journal of Occupational Therapy 60, 288-297.
10. American Occupational Therapy Association, 2005. Standards of practice for occupational therapy. American Journal of Occupational Therapy 59, 663-665.
11. American Occupational Therapy Association, 1999. Guide for supervision of occupational therapy personnel in the delivery of occupational therapy services. American Journal of Occupational Therapy 53, 592-594.
12. American Occupational Therapy Association, 2002. Roles and responsibilities of the occupational therapist and occupational therapy assistant during the delivery of occupational therapy services. OT Practice 7 (15), 9-10.

Working with Families and Caregivers of Elders

ADA BOONE HOERL, BARBARA JO RODRIGUES,
RENÉ PADILLA, AND SUE BYERS-CONNON

KEY TERMS

social support system, family, caregivers, education, role changes, stress, community,
resources, abuse, neglect

CHAPTER OBJECTIVES

1. Define the role of the certified occupational therapy assistant (COTA) in family and caregiver training.
2. Understand role changes within family systems at the onset of debilitating conditions in elders.
3. Discuss communication strategies that maximize comprehension during elder, family, and caregiver education.
4. Identify stressors that affect quality of care, ability to cope, and emotional responses in the elder-caregiver relationship.
5. Identify techniques to minimize caregiver stress.
6. Define and identify signs of elder abuse and neglect, and discuss reporting requirements.

Barbara woke up startled by the noise in the other room. She rose quickly, draped her robe over her shoulders and hurriedly walked out of the room, trying not to wake her husband. She had an anxious feeling that her mother may have fallen again. She had not had a full night's sleep for over 3 months since Dottie moved in with them. After having a stroke, Dottie had been at a nursing home for rehabilitation, and the therapists had concluded she could no longer live on her own. Dottie became very depressed, and each time Barbara visited she tearfully pleaded with her, "Please don't put me away at an old folks home, I couldn't bear it." Barbara felt quite distressed. As the mother of three children and a full-time grade-school teacher, she was already very busy but felt guilty about even contemplating an assisted living facility for her mother. She knew her mother could not afford to move to such a facility. Barbara spoke with her two brothers who lived out of state and both promised to help with the costs if Barbara took their mother in. Barbara consulted with her family and they all agreed to bring Dottie home to live with them. "We can set her up in the dining room. I can make some temporary walls," offered Mike, Barbara's husband. "Yes, that will let Grandma be close to the kitchen and family room," added Sandy, the youngest daughter, now a sophomore in high school and captain of the cheerleading squad. "I can drive her to therapy twice a week," volunteered Jimmy, a senior in high school and star quarterback of the football team. "I can come home

on the weekends if needed," added Patty, a freshman living in the college dorm in a town close by. A case manager helped Barbara get in contact with an agency that provided a caregiver for part of the day while Barbara was at work. Physical and occupational therapies were scheduled after a home evaluation. Barbara was relieved—it seemed everything was going to work out.

Early one morning about 2 weeks after Dottie moved in, the phone rang while Barbara was getting ready to leave for work. "I am sorry, I'm not going to be able to come today—my child is sick" said the attendant. The agency did not have a replacement. Barbara turned to her husband, who said, "I'll drop the kids off at school—you let your work know you can't come in today. I'll make arrangements to stay home tomorrow if necessary." Barbara called her school to ask that a substitute teacher be called in. She had a few paid vacation days left and although she was planning some special activities with her students, there would be no harm in waiting a day. "This will give me and mother an opportunity to sort through and organize all the old photos," said Barbara as the rest of the family left for the day.

After helping Dottie with her breakfast, bath, and getting dressed, Barbara pulled out the boxes of old pictures and spread them on the kitchen table. Dottie picked up one of a young woman at her wedding, and said, "This is when you got married—you looked beautiful." Barbara took the picture and responded, "That's not me,

Mom—that's you and Daddy!" After looking at several other photos, Barbara realized Dottie was quite confused about who the people in the photos were. "That's your son Peter, and this is your other son John," Barbara pointed out, adding, "Do you remember the names of their wives?" "Of course I do," responded Dottie. Barbara pushed, "What are their names?" Dottie looked blank for a little, and then responded, "Why are you asking me all these questions? You know their names." She stood up and walked to the family room and sat down on the sofa. Throughout the day, Barbara noticed other signs of confusion. By the end of the afternoon, Dottie seemed very tired and asked help to get to bed. By the time the rest of the family got home, Dottie was asleep in her converted room and remained there for the rest of the evening.

That night, as Barbara was getting ready to go to bed, she heard a crashing sound in the other room. She ran to the dining room and found Dottie sitting on the floor by the bed, Barbara called for Mike's help and together they were able to return Dottie to her bed. Although she did not seem to be in any pain, Dottie appeared dazed and did not seem to recognize Barbara, calling her by a different name. Mike and Barbara decided it would be wise to call Dottie's doctor, who recommended Dottie be taken to an emergency room right away so she could be evaluated.

At the hospital it was determined that there were no fractures, but that Dottie had experienced another small stroke. Once again, Dottie was transferred to a nursing home so she could receive intensive rehabilitation for a few days. Although the therapists noticed a little more confusion as compared to the previous rehabilitation course, they thought Dottie could return home with the same previous arrangements. Confusion was much more noticeable when Dottie returned home. She often could not find her way around the house and seemed unable to complete small tasks without constant verbal direction. She often would get up out of the chair and wander around the house without an apparent planned destination. The attendant reported that several times Dottie had attempted to leave the house during the day.

Barbara was very worried, but the doctor assured her there was not much else that could be done for Dottie except to structure her environment so that Dottie could have some routines and so her safety could be maximized. Another home evaluation was done and a registered occupational therapist (OTR)/COTA team worked with the family to remove tripping hazards and set up Dottie's room so she could find everything she needed in plain sight. Once Dottie returned, it was clear she could not be left alone in the house for any period of time, so the family sat down to work out a schedule so that someone was in the home at all times in the evening. Because of the heavy sports involvement of the children, it soon became apparent that they would not be able to watch Dottie very often. Therefore, it fell on Barbara and Mike to be home each

evening. This meant that only one parent could be present at the children's frequent events. Barbara felt it necessary to resign as president of the high school's booster club and later also to take a break from her book club and other regular activities so that she could stay at home with her mother.

As the weeks went by, Dottie fell twice more in the middle of the night as she tried to get up to use the restroom. It seemed to Barbara and Mike that Dottie was getting more and more confused as each day passed. In the middle of the night she would accept only Barbara's help, so Barbara began setting her alarm at 2:00 a.m. to help her mother to the bathroom and get her back to bed. Barbara would then try to sleep for a couple of hours before it was time to get up and get the family ready for the day. During some mornings Dottie would become anxious as Barbara said goodbye and the attendant reported it would take a couple of hours before Dottie could focus on her self-care and other daily routines. Barbara began wondering whether they would be able to leave Dottie in someone else's care so they could take their annual family vacation in a couple of weeks. She felt guilty that she wanted a break.

More than 50 million people provide care for a chronically ill, disabled, or aged family member or friend during any given year.[1] The term *caregiver* refers to anyone who provides assistance to someone else who is in some degree incapacitated and needs help. *Informal caregiver* and *family caregiver* are terms that refer to unpaid individuals such as family members, friends, and neighbors who provide care. These individuals can be primary or secondary caregivers, full-time or part-time, and can live with the person being cared for or live separately. Formal caregivers are volunteers or paid care providers associated with a service system.[2]

Families are the major provider of long-term care, but research has shown that caregiving exacts a heavy emotional, physical, and financial toll.[3] Many caregivers who work and provide care experience conflicts between these responsibilities. Twenty-two percent of caregivers are assisting two individuals, whereas 8% are caring for three or more.[2] Almost half of all caregivers are over age 50, making them more vulnerable to a decline in their own health, and one-third describe their own health as fair to poor.[1]

To provide optimal care, COTAs must consider the many factors that influence an elder's occupational performance. When planning intervention, the OTR/COTA team consider not only client factors and performance skills, but also the contexts and environments that may affect the elder's occupational performance potential.[4] Social support systems such as spouse and family can significantly affect the outcome of occupational therapy (OT) intervention.[5] COTAs must be able to interact with elders and their social support systems, especially the family, and treat elders and their families as units of care.

ROLES FOR CERTIFIED OCCUPATIONAL THERAPY ASSISTANTS

For COTAs to define their roles in facilitating family interaction, they must first understand the family caregiver's role. Family members are not necessarily inherently skilled at caregiving. Frequently this role is unfamiliar and possibly unwanted. Caregivers must do more than simply keep elders safe and clean and ensure that their daily physical needs are met. They must also help elders maintain socialization and a sense of dignity. These tasks can be overwhelming for a family member who has little or no experience with debilitating and chronic illness. Ensuring that caregivers and elders work together effectively is crucial.[6] COTAs should act as facilitators, educators, and resource personnel.

Development of elders' and caregivers' skills is achieved through selected activities with graded successes facilitated by COTAs. Activities that include family members and caregivers should be introduced as early as possible in the OT program to minimize dependence on COTAs. Facilitating interdependence between elders and their families and caregivers will ease the transition from one level of care to the next.

Effective elder, family, and caregiver education is a central component of care.[7] Knowledge is empowering and encourages elders, family members, and caregivers to be responsible. Activities selected during the early stages of intervention need not be complex. They may include directions on positioning, simple passive range-of-motion exercises, and communication strategies. As early as possible, it is important that the relationships between elders, family members, and caregivers not focus solely on the elder's functional limitations but on remaining skills, interests, and goals. Helping family members accept functional changes as part of a normal process rather than as a catastrophic decline can encourage preservation of relationships.[8,9] More training can follow as discharge planning progresses and the role of the caregiver becomes more clearly defined.[10]

Elder, family, and caregiver education is often required for all areas of occupation as described in the Occupational Therapy Practice Framework (see Chapter 7).[4] It is most effective to continually help elders, family members, and caregivers to consider OT intervention strategies focused on performance skills (such as sensory, motor, cognitive, or communication skills) in the context of meaningful occupations. Changes needed in the elders' or family routines and habits are more easily accomplished when they are consistent with their values, beliefs, and spirituality. Therefore, it is essential for the OTR/COTA team to have a good grasp of the elder's current preferences, past occupational participation, and future goals. COTAs may help elders, family members, and caregivers understand the physician's diagnosis and prognosis of the medical condition and its functional implications. Insight

regarding the specific physical, cognitive, and psychosocial impairments will aid caregivers in providing safe and appropriate assistance. Sometimes understanding the reasons for doing a certain task is more important than demonstrating proficiency in its performance.[11] For example, understanding principles of wrist protection that can be applied to every situation is more important for caregivers than correctly supervising the elder's use of radial wrist deviation to open a door each and every time. To maximize the effectiveness of the education, COTAs need to develop communication strategies (Box 11-1).

COTAs also act as resources for elders, family members, and caregivers. Depending on facility role delineation, COTAs may provide information about community and support services, as well as medical equipment vendors, paid caregivers, and respite programs. In collaboration with OTRs, COTAs may also serve as liaisons with other services. (Some resources are listed in the Appendix.)

COTAs can learn much about elders', family members', and caregivers' values, desires, and insights through frequent and close interaction. Elders may be unable to express themselves for many reasons. Some limitations

BOX 11-1

Considerations for Effective Communication

- Initially, make frequent, brief contacts to develop the relationship. This will familiarize the elder, family members, and caregivers with COTAs and their purpose.
- Manage the environment in which communication occurs. Minimize distractions and interruptions.
- Use responsive listening techniques. Maintain good eye contact, intermittently acknowledge statements made, and use body language that allows all parties to listen and respond. Be an active listener.
- Use common terminology that nonmedical individuals understand. If a common term is available, use it. For example, use *shoulder blade* for *scapula*. Otherwise, define and explain concepts in simple terms.
- Always respect client confidentiality. If able, secure permission from clients before discussing details with others.
- Use open-ended questions to encourage self-expression. Be comfortable with brief silences.
- Organize your ideas and avoid skipping between subjects. Focus on one topic at a time, and clarify what you do not understand.
- Provide education that will enable elders and their families to make informed choices. Do not offer advice or your personal opinion. Always acknowledge the right of choice.
- Communicate with respect and warmth. Be supportive. Respond to feedback when given.
- Do not promise if you cannot deliver.

may be premorbid, whereas others, such as aphasia, may result from illness. COTAs may act as advocates for elders, helping meet needs that might otherwise go unacknowledged. COTAs may also act as advocates for family members and caregivers.

Like elders, families and caregivers may have needs that become evident only after close and frequent interaction. Because each individual's ability to provide caregiving differs, the OTR/COTA team must consider everyone's abilities when planning for facility discharge and family training.

All members of the treatment team, including COTAs, must educate elders, family members, and caregivers about the team's treatment recommendations. Recommendations may include plans for discharge, supervision, follow-up treatment, and home/community programs, all of which must be clearly documented. When elders, families, and caregivers choose not to follow the team's recommendation, it is crucial to document all responses and actions to serve as a legal record if anyone is harmed. The more elders, family members, and caregivers are included in the formulation of plans, the more likely they are to comply with home programs and other discharge recommendations.[10]

ROLE CHANGES IN THE FAMILY

Greater therapeutic outcomes are achieved when intervention does not focus solely on elders but also includes families and caregivers.[12] This is especially important when family lifestyle changes are required because of elders' functional declines.[13]

Ideally, elders will consult family members when caregiving needs become evident. However, many variables affect a family system's abilities to meet the elder's needs. Some of these variables may include the treatment setting itself, cognitive deficits, psychological issues, the prior quality of family relationships, cultural and social influences, geographic distance, scheduling conflicts, financial resources, and advanced directives. COTAs must take all of these factors into consideration during collaborative planning.[10,14]

COTAs must consider role changes that occur for both elders and family during the course of an illness. OT should be designed around elders' and family members' skill levels. From that foundation, COTAs can facilitate adjustment to disability. With the onset of illness or disability, elders may feel a loss of independence, which can mean a major change in their sense of control and their role within the family.[15]

Role changes also occur within the family unit during an elder's illnesses.[16] Spouses may feel a deep sense of loss of a partner and may resent being solely responsible for previously shared tasks. In addition to a sense of loss, children must deal with the role reversal of being a parent to their own parent. Elders' disabilities and needs for caregiving may come at a time in children's lives when,

for the first time, they find themselves free of family responsibilities and are planning for their own retirement. Family members are usually unprepared for the sudden changes that may occur with acute illnesses.[17]

Roles within the family unit tend to be adjusted and adapted to gradually when elders have chronic or degenerative diseases.[18] However, as the functional impairments accumulate into a major disability with significant activity limitations, modifications in roles are required.[19] Not knowing the length of the illness is often a source of added frustration. In addition, chronic conditions may involve long-term adaptations that demand a greater degree of self-care and responsibility on the part of elders and caregivers.[20]

Caregiver Stresses

An entire generation is moving into the caregiving role for their aging parents.[1,7] These caregivers are changing their lives to assist their parents through the illness process. In addition to grieving for their parent, these caregivers may also be experiencing a loss of their own independence, privacy, financial security, safety, and comfort within their own homes. These losses may leave caregivers ultimately feeling guilty about their inadequacies or angry toward the debilitated elder.[8]

Life changes for caregivers and their families. This changing process may be gradual, beginning with the elder experiencing mild confusion and only requiring assistance with bills. The change also may be sudden and immediate, with the elder surviving a stroke and needing total physical care. The care required may be temporary or permanent with no hope for rehabilitation. No matter what the situation, this change of life is stressful for everyone involved.[13]

Advice from physicians, nurses, and therapists and attempts at self-education about an unfamiliar illness also can add stress. The need to learn the language of health care workers can be stressful, especially for caregivers for whom English is a second language or caregivers who are functionally illiterate.

Stress also may be increased by family members who offer suggestions for caring for elders. When decisions are made by several relatives but one family member or caregiver is responsible for following through with the group's decisions, the caregiver can easily become overwhelmed and feel resentful.

Elders who need caregiving may require various levels of assistance, and their conditions may change frequently. At times little assistance may be needed, but there may be long periods when much more assistance is required (Figure 11-1). Other family members may not understand the fluctuating assistance levels, and their perceptions of the work required to maintain the elder at home may not be accurate.[12,21]

Family members may not understand their own emotions or those of the primary caregiver. Family members

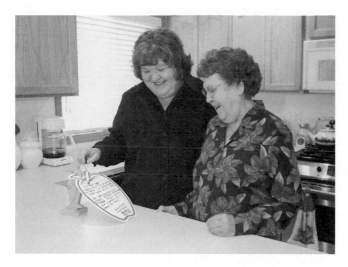

FIGURE 11-1 Caregiving may require various levels of assistance. This 90-year-old elder needs only a reminder to function in her environment while her daughter is at work.

may deny feelings of guilt, frustration, anger, or grief. They also may be in denial about the level of care required and may not be ready to assist. Family members who are unable to understand their own emotions or the illness and needs of the elder may become angry with the caregiver for not allowing the elder more independence.[16] They may be resentful and suspicious of the caregiver's motives or intentions, which can devastate caregivers and reduce the level of care they are willing to provide.

The demands and constraints of caregiving can become overwhelming. Caregivers may feel isolated and believe that they must be the sole providers of care. They may think they have no time for friends or support systems. Responsibilities can quickly become burdens, and caregivers may feel that they are not providing the needed assistance and are failing in their responsibilities to the elder.[22] Caregivers may refuse assistance from others because they feel the home is not clean enough for others to visit, or they believe they are the only ones who can properly care for the elder. Caregivers may forget that the level of care they now provide is the result of months of practice and learning through trial and error. COTAs must become adept at identifying signs of caregiver stress to ensure that the elder's needs are being met (Box 11-2).

Family Resources

COTAs should continually assess the family's needs and resources and offer the best referrals possible, keeping in mind that family members may feel isolated and disconnected or may be reluctant to ask for assistance. It may first be necessary to assist family members in identifying their needs and willingness to accept assistance. The suggestion that they read a book about caregivers or attend a caregiver support group may be met with resistance. However, COTAs must provide support and guidance

BOX 11-2

Signs of Caregiver Stress

- Too much stress can be damaging to both the caregiver and the elder. The following stress indicators experienced frequently or simultaneously can lead to more serious health problems.
- The caregiver may deny the disease and its effect on the person who has been diagnosed: "I know Mom's going to get better."
- The caregiver may express anger that no effective treatments or cures currently exist for chronic conditions such as Alzheimer's disease* and that people do not understand what's going on: "If he asks me that question one more time, I'll scream."
- The caregiver may withdraw socially from friends and activities that once brought pleasure: "I don't care about getting together with the neighbors anymore."
- The caregiver may express anxiety about facing another day and what the future holds: "What happens when he needs more care than I can provide?"
- The caregiver may experience depression, which eventually breaks the spirit and affects coping ability: "I don't care anymore."
- The caregiver may be exhausted, which makes it nearly impossible to complete necessary tasks: "I'm too tired for this."
- The caregiver may experience sleeplessness caused by worrying: "What if she wanders out of the house or falls and hurts herself?"
- The caregiver may express irritability, which may lead to moodiness and trigger negative responses and reactions: "Leave me alone!"
- Lack of concentration on the part of the caregiver makes it difficult to perform familiar tasks: "I was so busy, I forgot we had an appointment."
- The caregiver experiences mental and physical health problems: "I can't remember the last time I felt good."

Adapted from the Alzheimer's Association. (1995). Ten signs of caregiver stress. Chicago: Alzheimer's Association.
*For more information on Alzheimer's disease and services provided by the Alzheimer's Association, call 1-800-272-3900.

while family members go through the process of realizing their own needs. When family members are ready to ask for assistance, COTAs must be ready with reliable resources and referrals. Successful experiences encourage families to use available community resources. COTAs must help family members and caregivers understand that caring for themselves and accepting help will ultimately help them care for the elder. Caring for themselves and accepting help may also make it possible to offer care at home for a longer period (Box 11-3; Figure 11-2).

Many community and national resources are available for families and caregivers. Support groups, publications,

BOX 11-3

Ways to Reduce Caregiver Stress

- Get a diagnosis as early as possible.
- Symptoms may appear gradually, and if a person seems physically healthy, it is easy to ignore unusual behavior or attribute it to something else. See a physician when warning signs are present. Some dementia symptoms are treatable. Once you know what you are dealing with, you will be able to better manage the present and plan for the future.
- Know what resources are available.
- For your own well-being and that of the person for whom you are caring, become familiar with care resources available in your community. Adult day care, in-home assistance, visiting nurses, and Meals on Wheels are just some of the community services that can help.
- Become an educated caregiver.
- As the disease progresses, different caregiving skills and capabilities are necessary. Care techniques and suggestions can help you better understand and cope with many of the challenging behavior and personality changes.
- Get help.
- Trying to do everything by yourself will leave you exhausted. The support of family, friends, and community resources can be an enormous help. If assistance is not offered, ask for it. If you have difficulty asking for assistance, have someone close to you advocate for you. If stress becomes overwhelming, do not be afraid to seek professional help. Support group meetings and help lines are also good sources of comfort and reassurance.
- Take care of yourself.
- Caregivers frequently devote themselves totally to those they care for and, in the process, neglect their own needs. Pay attention to yourself. Watch your diet, exercise, and get plenty of rest. Use respite services to take time off for shopping, a movie, or an uninterrupted visit with a friend. Those close to you, including the one for whom you are caring, want you to take care of yourself.
- Manage your level of stress.
- Stress can cause physical problems (blurred vision, stomach irritation, high blood pressure) and changes in behavior (irritability, lack of concentration, loss of appetite). Note your symptoms. Use relaxation techniques that work for you, and consult a physician.
- Accept changes as they occur.
- Elders change and so do their needs. They often require care beyond what you can provide at home. A thorough investigation of available care options should make transitions easier, as will support and assistance from those who care about you and your loved one.
- Do legal and financial planning.
- Consult an attorney and discuss issues related to durable power of attorney, living wills and trusts, future medical care, housing, and other key considerations. Planning now will alleviate stress later. If possible and appropriate, involve the elder and other family members in planning activities and decisions.
- Be realistic.
- The care you provide does make a difference. Neither you nor the elder can control many of the circumstances and behaviors that will occur. Give yourself permission to grieve for the losses you experience, but also focus on the positive moments as they occur and enjoy your good memories.
- Give yourself credit, not guilt.
- You are only human. Occasionally, you may lose patience and at times be unable to provide all of the care the way you would like. Remember, you are doing the best you can, so give yourself credit. Being a devoted caregiver is not something to feel guilty about. Your loved one needs you, and you are there. That is something to be proud of.

Adapted from the Alzheimer's Association. (1995). Ten signs of caregiver stress. Chicago: Alzheimer's Association.
For more information on Alzheimer's disease and services provided by the Alzheimer's Association, call 1-800-272-3900.

videos, and resources can be found in virtually every large community. In rural areas, organizations may be contacted by phone, in writing, or through computer technology. (An extensive resource and referral list is included in the Appendix.)

RECOGNIZING SIGNS AND REPORTING ELDER ABUSE OR NEGLECT

Unfortunately, abuse and neglect of elders do occur.[23] Between 1 and 2 million Americans age 65 and older have been injured, exploited, or otherwise mistreated by someone on whom they depended for care or protection.[24] Estimates of the frequency of elder abuse range from 2% to 10%.[25] All professionals working with elders must be informed of their responsibilities and prepare themselves to act on the elder's behalf if suspicion of abuse or neglect arises. Federal definitions of elder abuse have been included in the Older Americans Act since 1987. Each state also has its own definition of elder abuse through legislation on adult protective services. COTAs should contact their state's ombudsman or Adult Protective Services Office for more detailed and specific guidelines. Only general definitions and guidelines are presented in this chapter. Elders have a right to direct their own care, refuse care, and receive protection from being taken advantage of or hurt by others.

The National Center on Elder Abuse (NCEA) of the U.S. Administration on Aging has identified and defined

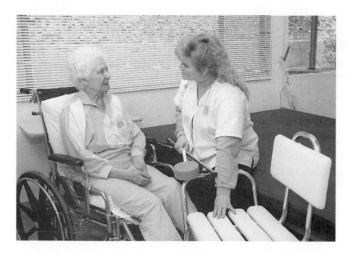

FIGURE 11-2 Careful discharge planning can help elders and caregivers feel less overwhelmed with changes.

seven types of elder abuse.[26] *Physical abuse* is nonaccidental use of physical force that results in bodily injury, pain, or impairment. This may include acts of violence such as striking, shoving, shaking, slapping, kicking, pinching, and burning. Inappropriate use of drugs and physical restraints, force-feeding, and physical punishment of any kind also are considered physical abuse. *Sexual abuse* is nonconsensual sexual contact of any kind with an elder. It includes unwanted touching, all types of sexual assault or battery, coerced nudity, and sexually explicit photographing. *Emotional* or *psychological abuse* is willful infliction of mental or emotional anguish by threat, humiliation, or other verbal or nonverbal abusive conduct. This may include things such as verbal assaults, insults, threats, intimidation, humiliation, and harassment. The NCEA also includes treatment of elders like infants and isolating them from family and friends or from their regular activities as emotional/psychological abuse. *Neglect* is the willful or nonwillful failure by caregivers to fulfill their obligations or duties as caretakers. *Abandonment* is the desertion of elders by the people who have assumed responsibility for providing care for them. *Financial* or *material exploitation* is an unauthorized use of an elder's funds, property, or resources. This may include such things as cashing an elder's checks without permission, forging an elder's signature, misusing or stealing an older person's money or possessions, coercing or deceiving an elder into signing any document and the improper use of conservatorship, guardianship, or power of attorney. Finally, *self-abuse* and *neglect* are behaviors of elders directed at themselves that threaten their own health or safety, such as refusing to eat or drink, or provide oneself with adequate clothing, shelter, personal hygiene, or medications.

Abuse may occur in the home or community setting, as well as in residential care, skilled nursing facilities (SNFs), or day health programs. In an effort to protect elders, every health care provider must be aware of signs and indicators of abuse. Indicators of abuse have been outlined in many documents available through agencies on aging (Table 11-1).[27]

Many states have enacted mandatory reporting laws that require professionals who regularly work with elders, including health workers such as COTAs, law enforcement personnel, and human service personnel, to report suspected abuse. State and local agencies designated to receive and investigate reports and provide referral services to victims, families, and elders at risk for abuse include the Adult Protective Services Agency, long-term care ombudsman programs, law enforcement or local social service agencies, area agencies on aging, aging service providers, and aging advocacy groups. If elder abuse is suspected, these agencies can assist COTAs.

COTAs must report physical abuse if they witness an incident that reasonably appears to be physical abuse; find a physical injury of a suspicious nature, location, or repetition; or listen to an incident related by an elder or dependent adult. An immediate telephone call followed by a written report is often required. This report should include identifying information about the person filing the report, the victim, and the caregiver. In addition, the incident and condition of the victim and any other information leading the reporter to suspect abuse must be included. Although many facilities have designated personnel to carry out reporting, it is each individual's duty to report suspected abuse. Failure to report is a legally punishable misdemeanor in states with mandatory reporting laws. Further, COTAs have an ethical responsibility to demonstrate a concern for the safety and well-being of the recipients of their services,[28] and failure to do so may result in disciplinary action by a professional organization of which the COTA is a member.[29]

The COTA's responsibility does not end with this report. Connecting the elder and/or the family with community resources to help cope with trauma, address conflicts, and so on. Referral should be done in a way that is acceptable to the elder. Many churches, community centers, and organizations such as the Area Agency on Aging can assist in locating resources to support elders to continue living safely in their communities. The Appendix of this text contains a listing of organizations that provide such resources.

CASE STUDY

After the last fall, Barbara called Dottie's physician and got a referral for home-based occupational therapy services. Paul, the OTR, called Barbara to set up the initial visit. "I am sorry; I can't miss another day of work. Can't you come on Saturday?" asked Barbara. After Paul explained that the agency provided services on weekdays only, Barbara responded, "OK, I give up. I am too tired to argue. But it will have to be first thing in the morning—I can't miss a whole day of work." Paul made arrangements for Diana, a recently hired COTA, to join him during the home visit because she would be picking up the case if they determined services were indeed needed.

TABLE 11-1

Signs and Symptoms of Abuse	
Type of abuse	**Signs and symptoms**
Physical	bruises, welts, lacerations bone fractures open wounds, cuts, punctures, untreated injuries in various stages of healing sprains, dislocations, and internal injuries/bleeding broken eyeglasses laboratory findings of medication overdose or underutilization of prescribed drugs elder's report of being hit or mistreated elder's sudden change in behavior caregiver's refusal to allow visitors to see an elder alone
Sexual	bruises around the breasts or genital area unexplained venereal disease or genital infections unexplained vaginal or anal bleeding torn, stained, or bloody underclothing elder's report of being sexually assaulted or raped
Emotional/ psychological	being emotionally upset or agitated being extremely withdrawn and non-communicative or non-responsive unusual behavior usually attributed to dementia (e.g., sucking, biting, rocking) elder's report of being verbally or emotionally mistreated
Neglect	dehydration, malnutrition, untreated bed sores, and poor personal hygiene unattended or untreated health problems hazardous or unsafe living condition/arrangements (e.g., improper wiring, no heat, or no running water) unsanitary and unclean living conditions (e.g., dirt, fleas, lice on person, soiled bedding, fecal/urine smell, inadequate clothing) elder's report of being mistreated
Abandonment	desertion of an elder at a hospital, a nursing facility, or other similar institution desertion of an elder at a shopping center or other public location elder's own report of being abandoned
Financial/ material exploitation	sudden changes in bank account or banking practice; unexplained withdrawal of large sums of money by a person accompanying the elder inclusion of additional names on an elder's bank signature card unauthorized withdrawal of the elder's funds using the elder's ATM card abrupt changes in a will or other financial documents unexplained disappearance of funds or valuable possessions substandard care being provided or bills unpaid despite the availability of adequate financial resources discovery of an elder's signature being forged for financial transactions or for the titles of his or her possessions sudden appearance of previously uninvolved relatives claiming their rights to an elder's affairs and possessions unexplained sudden transfer of assets to a family member or someone outside of the family provision of services that are not necessary elder's report of financial exploitation
Self-neglect	dehydration, malnutrition, untreated or improperly attended medical conditions, and poor personal hygiene hazardous or unsafe living conditions/arrangements (e.g., improper wiring, no indoor plumbing, no heat, no running water) unsanitary or unclean living quarters (e.g., animal/insect infestation, no functioning toilet, fecal/urine smell) inappropriate and/or inadequate clothing, lack of necessary medical aids (e.g., eyeglasses, hearing aids, dentures) grossly inadequate housing or homelessness

Adapted from National Center on Elder Abuse. (2007). Major types of elder abuse. Washington, DC: U.S. Administration on Aging.

On the designated date, Paul and Diana arrived at the home, and Dottie's attendant opened the door. "I am sorry, I wasn't told anyone would be coming today," said the attendant. "I will have to call Miss Barbara." Within an hour, Barbara arrived at the house and apologized for her delay. "I am very sorry, I completely forgot about this appointment."

While they waited for Barbara, Paul and Diana sat in the living room with Dottie and began the initial interview. "Dottie, please tell us how it came about that a call for occupational therapy services was made? What has been going on?" asked Paul. Dottie responded, "I do not know. I have been doing fine—I can handle everything I need to do." Clarice, the attendant, reminded Dottie, "Don't forget you fell a few times, Dottie. Tell them about that." Dottie at first seemed confused, but then offered, "Oh, yes, I fell getting out of bed because someone had left things on the floor and I tripped. But that was just an accident. It's not going to happen again." Paul asked Dottie to describe her typical day, which she did in large strokes. "I get up and try to help with breakfast before the kids leave. Then I take a shower and get dressed and then watch my morning TV shows. Sometimes I go to visit friends. Then I cook lunch and start with cleaning the house. My daughter is too busy, you know, and she brought me to live here so I could help her. They are all so busy all the time." Paul and Diana noticed that Clarice, who was sitting behind Dottie, shook her head several times as Dottie described her routines. Diana asked, "Have you needed any help to shower and get dressed?" Dottie shook her head and answered, "Well, I don't really need help, but my daughter has Clarice stay with me to keep me company, so I let her help me sometimes."

By the time Barbara arrived, Dottie had told Paul and Diana about her life before her first stroke. Up to that point she had been living alone and was very active in her church. She never missed one of her grandchildren's games. She drove a car up to about a month before the stroke. She gave up driving because she felt her eyesight was becoming problematic. She enjoyed cooking, sewing, and gardening. Since the stroke, she had not been outside of the house except for medical appointments, and just recently she attempted to do some sewing once her work was brought from her own home.

When Barbara arrived, Paul asked if they could talk as Dottie demonstrated how she got dressed, accessed the bathroom, and prepared a simple snack. Barbara responded, "That is why Clarice is here. Mom doesn't need to do most of that. We just need her to walk better so she doesn't fall. That is what worries me the most. She can't be alone because she will fall." Paul and Diana asked Dottie to show them where she slept, and once there asked her to demonstrate how she got in and out of bed. Dottie agreed to do so, but when she began sitting up from the bed, Barbara jumped in and provided assistance. Paul encouraged Barbara to let Dottie demonstrate her abilities and, with some struggling, finally she was able to get herself to sitting on the edge of the bed. A similar pattern of Paul asking Dottie to demonstrate a skill and Barbara jumping in to assist her was evident when Dottie dressed and accessed the bathroom.

When the group was on the way to the kitchen, Barbara again noted, "We don't let mother do much cooking. She gets confused and it ends up being more work for me in the end." When Barbara was distracted, Paul took Diana aside and asked her to observe Dottie make a peanut butter and jelly sandwich while he took Barbara to the living room to talk to her. In the living room, Paul asked Barbara how she was dealing with Dottie's functional changes. Barbara tearfully confessed, "I am

exhausted. I am so worried she will hurt herself; she just can't be left alone. We can't afford to pay for an attendant all the time, and I keep missing work. I don't sleep because she needs to get up at night to go to the bathroom, and she is so hard headed—she just will not use the commode by the bed. She only lets me or Clarice help her with dressing or her bath. I don't want to put her in a skilled nursing facility, but I don't know if I can keep her either!"

In the kitchen, Diana observed Dottie walk to the refrigerator, open the door, and stare into space. Diana asked what steps she needed to follow to make the sandwich and Dottie seemed confused. "Get what you need for a peanut butter and jelly sandwich," Diana encouraged. Still, Dottie appeared confused, so Diana instructed her to find each of the needed materials one by one. Once everything was assembled on the counter in front of her, Dottie was able to assemble a sandwich without any other problems. Diana asked her what she usually cooked, and Dottie answered, "Nothing anymore, Barbie doesn't let me do anything anymore."

■■ CASE STUDY QUESTIONS

1 What are the major issues going on with Dottie and her family?
2 What communication strategies could the treatment team use to integrate the different viewpoints of Dottie and her family?
3 What intervention strategies should the team implement to meet Dottie's needs as well as those of the family?

■■ CHAPTER REVIEW QUESTIONS

1 While working at a skilled nursing facility you approach a new elder who says, "My husband just left me here all alone. Oh, please help me, I want to go home." How should you respond?
2 You work in a rehabilitation unit. You recommend a tub transfer bench for an elder with hemiplegia. Medicare will not cover the expense of this bench. The family says, "We'll just rig something up when we get home." How should you respond?
3 You are working on an Alzheimer's disease special unit. An elder comes up to you, grabs your arm and says, "Momma, where have you been? I've been so afraid." As the elder continues to cling to your arm, you notice the elder's family members are watching. The elder's behavior escalates whenever a family member approaches. How should you respond?
4 The grown daughter of an elder approaches you and states, "My father has been an alcoholic all my life. He has been so mean to my mother. His being in the hospital is the first peace she's had in years. Please don't let my father come home." How should you respond?
5 You have worked closely with an elder for 2 weeks. After a week-long vacation you return to learn that the elder has refused treatment most of the week you were absent. The elder had stated: (Refer to item #6.)

6 "I don't want anyone new! My family doesn't know how to help me." What steps should you have taken to minimize the elder's dependence on you?

7 On admission of their 87-year-old widowed father to an acute-care hospital, three adult children state that it is their desire to take him home and share the caregiving responsibilities when he is ready for discharge. During the 3-week hospitalization, staff members have seen the children visit only once. They also have not returned repeated phone calls by the social worker. What input should the COTA give to the treatment team in preparation for discharge?

REFERENCES

1. Hammer, L., Neal, M., 2008. Working sandwiched-generation caregivers: Prevalence, characteristics, and outcomes. Psychologist-Manager Journal 11 (1), 93-112.

2. National Alliance for Caregiving & American Association of Retired Persons, 2008. Caregiving in the U.S. Retrieved December 12, 2009, from http://www.caregiving.org/data/04finalreport.pdf.

3. Robison, J., Fortinsky, R., Kleppinger, A., Shugrue, N., Porter, M., 2009. A broader view of family caregiving: Effects of caregiving and caregiver conditions on depressive symptoms, health, work, and social isolation. Journals of Gerontology 64 (6), 788-798.

4. American Occupational Therapy Association, 2008. Occupational therapy practice framework: Domain and process, 2nd ed. American Journal of Occupational Therapy 62, 625-683.

5. American Occupational Therapy Association, 2007. AOTA's statement on family caregivers. American Journal of Occupational Therapy 61, 710.

6. Christie, J., Smith, G., Williamson, G., Lance, C., Shovali, T., Silva, L., et al., 2009. Quality of informal care is multidimensional. Rehabilitation Psychology 54, 173-181.

7. Bookman, A., Harrington, M., 2007. Family caregivers: A shadow workforce in the geriatric health care system? Journal of Health Politics, Policy and Law 32, 1005-1041.

8. Eloranta, S., Routasalo, P., Ave, S., 2008. Personal resources supporting living at home as described by older home care clients. International Journal of Nursing Practice 14, 308-314.

9. Stewart, M., Barnfather, A., Neufeld, A., Warren, S., Letourneau, N., Liu, L., et al., 2006. Accessible support for family caregivers of seniors with chronic conditions: From isolation to inclusion. Canadian Journal on Aging 25, 179-192.

10. Bauer, M., Fitzgerald, L., Haesler, E., Manfrin, M., 2009. Hospital discharge planning for frail older people and their family. Are we delivering best practice? A review of the evidence. Journal of Clinical Nursing 18 (18), 2539-2546.

11. Wilkins, V., Bruce, M., Sirey, J., 2009. Caregiving tasks and training interest of family caregivers of medically ill homebound older adults. Journal of Aging and Health 21 (3), 528-542.

12. Brown, J., Sintzel, J., Arnault, D., George, N., 2009. Confidence to foster across cultures: Caregiver perspectives. Journal of Child & Family Studies 18 (6), 633-642.

13. Evercare and National Alliance for Caregiving, 2006. Study of caregivers in decline: Findings from a national survey. Retrieved December 12, 2009, from http://www.caregiving.org/data/Caregivers%20in%20Decline%20Study-FINAL-lowres.pdf.

14. Dedhia, P., Kravet, S., Bulger, J., Hinson, T., Sridharan, A., Kolodner, K., et al., 2009. A quality improvement intervention to facilitate the transition of older adults from three hospitals back to their homes. Journal of the American Geriatrics Society 57 (9), 1540-1546.

15. Kuba, C., 2006. Navigating the Journey of Aging Parents: What Care Receivers Want. Routledge, New York.

16. Koerner, S., Kenyon, D., Shirai, Y., 2009. Caregiving for elder relatives: Which caregivers experience personal benefits/gains? Archives of Gerontology and Geriatrics 48, 238-245.

17. Stephens, M., Franks, M., 2009. All in the family: Providing care to chronically ill and disabled older adults. In: Qualls, S., Zarit, S. (Eds.), Aging Families and Caregiving. John Wiley & Sons, Hoboken, NJ, pp. 61-84.

18. Giunta, N., Scharlach, A., 2009. Caregiver services: Resources, trends, and best practices. In: Qualls, S., Zarit, S. (Eds.), Aging Families and Caregiving. John Wiley & Sons, Hoboken, NJ, pp. 241-268.

19. McCabe, M., Firth, L., O'Connor, E., 2009. A comparison of mood and quality of life among people with progressive neurological illnesses and their caregivers. Journal of Clinical Psychology in Medical Settings 16 (4), 355-362.

20. Cohen-Mansfield, J., Wirtz, P., 2009. The reasons for nursing home entry in an adult day care population: Caregiver reports versus regression results. Journal of Geriatric Psychiatry and Neurology 22 (4), 274-281.

21. Gitlin, L., Corcoran, M., 2005. Occupational therapy and dementia care: The home environmental skills-building program for individuals and families. AOTA Press, Bethesda, MD.

22. Jacinto, G., 2010. The self-forgiveness process of caregivers after the death of care-receivers diagnosed with Alzheimer's disease. Journal of Social Service Research 36 (1), 24-36.

23. Abbey, L., 2009. Elder abuse and neglect: When home is not safe. Clinics in Geriatric Medicine 25 (1), 47-60.

24. Cooper, C., Selwood, A., Livingston, G., 2008. The prevalence of elder abuse and neglect: A systematic review. Age and Ageing 37 (2), 151-160.

25. Lachs, M., Pillemer, K., 2004. Elder abuse. Lancet 364, 1192-1263.

26. National Center on Elder Abuse, 2007. Major types of elder abuse. Retrieved December 12, 2009, from http://www.ncea.aoa.gov/NCEAroot/Main_Site/FAQ/Basics/Types_Of_Abuse.aspx.

27. Ploeg, J., Fear, J., Hutchison, B., MacMillan, H., Bolan, G., 2008. A systematic review of interventions for elder abuse. Journal of Elder Abuse & Neglect 21 (3), 187-210.

28. American Occupational Therapy Association, 2005. Occupational Therapy Code of Ethics. American Journal of Occupational Therapy 59, 639-642.

29. American Occupational Therapy Association, 2007b. Enforcement procedures for the Occupational Therapy Code of Ethics. American Journal of Occupational Therapy 61, 679-685.

12

Addressing Sexual Activity of Elders

HELENE L. LOHMAN AND DAVID PLUTSCHACK

KEY TERMS

sexuality, values, myths, homosexuality, sexually transmitted diseases,
physiological changes, nursing facilities, permission, limited information,
specific suggestions, intensive therapy model

CHAPTER OBJECTIVES

1. Discuss the ways that values can influence attitudes about elder sexuality.
2. Identify primary myths about elder sexuality.
3. Discuss how elder homosexuals have been ignored by society.
4. Describe normal, age-related, sexual, physiological changes.
5. Describe sexually transmitted diseases and the elder population.
6. Discuss the treatment team members' roles in addressing elders' sexual concerns.
7. Discuss the ways elders' sexuality is commonly dealt with in nursing facilities.

8. List the components of the permission, limited information, specific suggestions, and intensive therapy model (PLISSIT), and discuss ways that the certified occupational therapy assistant (COTA) can apply this model.
9. Identify strategies for elder sexual education.
10. List intervention and safety sides for addressing sexual concerns of elders who experience strokes, heart disease, and arthritis.
11. Increase personal comfort to discuss elder sexual concerns.

Heather is a COTA employed at an acute care hospital. A large part of her caseload is elders who have sustained total hip replacements. Intervention approaches are routine, and transfers, home situation, and safety precautions are typically addressed with people who have total hip repairs. One day a circumstance happened that resulted in Heather changing her intervention approach. Heather was working with Sam, an elder who had sustained a right total hip replacement. After Heather went through the protocol for total hip replacements, she asked him if he had any questions. "Yes," he responded, "my wife and I want to know when we can have intimate relations." Heather felt a surge of emotions. She felt perplexed because she did not know how to respond. She recalled blushing with embarrassment, stammering through a sentence stating that she would get back with Sam and abruptly leaving the room. Afterward Heather reflected about the situation. She wondered why she felt so embarrassed and what she could have done differently. She questioned whether she harbored feelings that elders should not be sexually active. After further reflection, Heather took the initiative to learn more about sexuality and elders and to incorporate this knowledge into intervention.

COTAs that provide thorough intervention first get to know elders as human beings and develop an understanding of the person's daily life routines. Part of the daily life routines of many elders may involve sexual functioning. Sexual activity is categorized as an activities of daily living (ADL) function, according to the second edition of the Occupational Therapy Practice Framework: Domain and Process[1] and is defined as "engaging in activities that result in sexual satisfaction."[1] Sexual expression can be an important part of a person's life at any age and is related to a person's self-concept, self-esteem, and body image (Figure 12-1).[2] However, despite sexuality being so integral to human sexual expression, it may be ignored in clinical intervention for many reasons, including discomfort with one's own sexuality or with an elder or disabled person remaining sexually active. Other reasons may include a lack of understanding of normal sexual changes with aging and a lack of knowledge about sexual function with regard to age and disability. Dealing with the elder's concerns about sexual function should be part of intervention. This chapter helps the COTA learn about this important but often ignored area of ADL intervention. Furthermore, the chapter helps clarify myths and misconceptions.

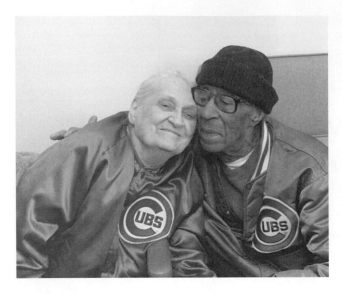

FIGURE 12-1 Sexuality involves touch, hugs, and other forms of expression.

VALUES ABOUT SEXUALITY

Each generation has certain values reflective of society, although such values are not necessarily uniformly held by all members of that generation. All individuals also have their own value systems.[1] The Traditionalists (born between 1922 and 1945) are from a generation that was generally not well educated on sexuality and often did not discuss sexuality freely.[3,4] For some members of this generation, sex was considered only a necessity for procreation and not a source of enjoyment. These are deeply held values that can influence the elder's comfort level when discussing sexual feelings during clinical intervention. In addition, COTAs may feel uncomfortable discussing sexual concerns with elders because sexuality may not have been an open topic for some members of their generation either. But generational values change, and it is predicted that the Baby Boomer generation, especially the women from that generation, may embrace more openness about sexuality.[5] Exercises 12-1 and 12-2 should be completed before further reading to explore values regarding elders and sexuality.

MYTHS ABOUT ELDERS AND SEXUAL FUNCTIONING

The media have provided people with misinformation and myths about elder sexual functioning. Television, magazines, and Internet advertisements encourage people to ignore or to cover up the aging process. Greeting cards make fun of aging and suggest that lying about age is acceptable. Some media sources encourage myths about sexuality such as "the dirty old man syndrome." In addition, myths can be perpetuated by family members, peers, or elders themselves. With this inundation of misinformation, many people believe myths instead of truths about

the sexual functioning of elders. Exercise 12-3 helps determine personal myths about elders and sexuality.

Discussion of Myths

Findings from a recently updated survey study in 2005 by the American Association of Retired Persons (AARP) (n = 1682)[6] provide perspective about some of these myths about geriatric sexuality. A key finding was that 56% of persons age 45 and older of both sexes considered sexual relationships as contributing to their quality of life.[6] However, a greater percentage of elder men and younger male respondents than women valued sexual activity as contributing to their quality of life.[6] Nevertheless, sexuality was perceived as an integral part of these elders' lives, not something they avoided. Furthermore, many elder men and women found their partner to be attractive; men 70 years of age or older reported this 53% of the time, whereas women of the same age reported this 49% of the time.[6] In addition, women older than 70 years were more likely to describe their partners as romantic as compared with their younger counterparts (41% older than 70 years compared with 34% 45-49 years and 38% 50-59 years).[6] Thus, these findings contradict the societal myths that equate age with unattractiveness and lack of romance. Health decline and lack of partners were major contributing factors to decreased sexual activity.[6]

The AARP study[6] together with other literature[7,8] suggest that for women sexual activity often stops because of lack of a partner. Kinsella and colleagues[9] found in 2006 that only 40% of women age 65 and older were married compared to 72% of men in the same age group. When examining elders age 75 and older the gap between women and men grows even larger, with 28% of women and 68% of men reporting being married.[9] In addition, some elder women believe the myth that they are unattractive and therefore should remain abstinent from sexual relationships. Previous research by AARP[10] found that the current elder generation's values are strongly against women being sexually active without a husband, but more current research conducted by AARP[6] shows this trend is changing among the elder population. The results of the 2005 AARP study found a 7% decrease from the 1999 study in the viewpoint of opposition for sexual relations outside of marriage in individuals age 45 years and older.[6,10]

Both older men and older women may experience pressure from their children to remain abstinent. Some adult children may find it difficult to think of their parents as having normal sexual desires, especially if the parent is in a nursing facility.[4,11]

Most men experience occasional impotence or erectile dysfunction by the time they are elder[12,13] because of fatigue, stress, illness, or alcohol.[14] However, erectile dysfunction is not considered to be a normal part of aging.[8] In the AARP study, 15% of men age 45 years and older admitted to being diagnosed with erectile dysfunction.[6] Men can continue to have normal sexual activity

■ Exercise 12-1: Generational Sexual Attitudes/Values Inventory

Answer the following questions while considering your generation, the Baby Boomer generation (born between 1946 and 1964), and the Traditionalist generation (born between 1922 and 1945). Fill in "yes" or "no" for each question, then discuss or contemplate your findings. (For more information on generational cohorts, please refer to Chapter 1.)

1. It is appropriate to openly discuss sexual needs and concerns.	Your generation Yes (Acceptable) ___ No (Unacceptable) ___	Current elder generation Yes (Acceptable) ___ No (Unacceptable) ___
2. Sexual activity is acceptable in a non-marriage situation.	Your generation Yes (Acceptable) ___ No (Unacceptable) ___	Current elder generation Yes (Acceptable) ___ No (Unacceptable) ___
3. Sexual activity is appropriate if the purpose is physical pleasure.	Your generation Yes (Acceptable) ___ No (Unacceptable) ___	Current elder generation Yes (Acceptable) ___ No (Unacceptable) ___
4. Sexual activity is for procreation only.	Your generation Yes (Acceptable) ___ No (Unacceptable) ___	Current elder generation Yes (Acceptable) ___ No (Unacceptable) ___
5. The naked body is very private. Nudity is unacceptable.	Your generation Yes (Acceptable) ___ No (Unacceptable) ___	Current elder generation Yes (Acceptable) ___ No (Unacceptable) ___
6. Women should discuss their sexual needs with their partners.	Your generation Yes (Acceptable) ___ No (Unacceptable) ___	Current elder generation Yes (Acceptable) ___ No (Unacceptable) ___
7. It is appropriate for women to initiate sex.	Your generation Yes (Acceptable) ___ No (Unacceptable) ___	Current elder generation Yes (Acceptable) ___ No (Unacceptable) ___
8. Masturbation is a normal sexual act.	Your generation Yes (Acceptable) ___ No (Unacceptable) ___	Current elder generation Yes (Acceptable) ___ No (Unacceptable) ___
9. Sexual activity between people of the same sex is acceptable.	Your generation Yes (Acceptable) ___ No (Unacceptable) ___	Current elder generation Yes (Acceptable) ___ No (Unacceptable) ___
10. Sexual activity between adults of different generations is unacceptable.	Your generation Yes (Acceptable) ___ No (Unacceptable) ___	Current elder generation Yes (Acceptable) ___ No (Unacceptable) ___

These questions are adapted from a module by Goldstein, H., & Runyon, C. (1993). An occupational therapy module to increase sensitivity about geriatric sexuality. *Physical and Occupational Therapy in Geriatrics*, 11(2), 57-75.

■ Exercise 12-2: Personal Values Assessment

This exercise helps identify personal values and attitudes. Answer the following questions. On completion of this exercise, any uncomfortable feelings may be handled by using this chapter as an educational tool to help dispel myths and misconceptions and to clarify normal physiological changes resulting from aging. After reading the chapter, the COTA can retake this personal value assessment to determine whether uncomfortable feelings have decreased.

	Agree	Disagree
1. Elders in nursing facilities should not be sexually active.	Agree	Disagree
2. My grandparents (or parents) should not be sexually active.	Agree	Disagree
3. It is acceptable for elder men to remain sexually active.	Agree	Disagree
4. It is acceptable for elder women to remain sexually active.	Agree	Disagree
5. It is immoral for elders to engage in recreational sex.	Agree	Disagree
6. Sexual education is not necessary for elders.	Agree	Disagree
7. Sexual education is not necessary for nursing facility staff.	Agree	Disagree
8. Nursing facilities should provide large enough beds for couples to sleep together.	Agree	Disagree
9. Nursing facilities should provide privacy for residents who desire sexual activity.	Agree	Disagree

These questions are adapted from a scale developed by White, C. B. (1982). The aging sexuality knowledge and attitudes scale (ASKAS): A scale for the assessment of attitudes and knowledge regarding sexuality in the aged. *Archives of Sexual Behavior*, 11(6), 491-502.

■ **Exercise 12-3: Myths about Geriatric Sexuality**

For each question below, answer *T* if the statement reflects a myth or *F* if the statement does not reflect a myth.

Question	True	False
1. Elders are no longer interested in sexuality.	True	False
2. Elders no longer engage in sexual activity.	True	False
3. Elders engage in a wide variety of sexual activity, including intercourse, cuddling, caressing, mutual stimulation, and oral sex.	True	False
4. Elders in nursing facilities should be segregated according to sex; sexual functioning should be prohibited.	True	False
5. Elder women are unattractive.	True	False
6. More elder men remain sexually active than elder women.	True	False
7. Elders are too frail to engage in sexual activity.	True	False
8. Inability to maintain an erection (erectile dysfunction) is not a natural consequence of aging.	True	False
9. All elders are heterosexual.	True	False

Data from Comfort, A., & Dial, L. (1991). Sexuality and aging: An overview. *Clinics in Geriatric Medicine*, 7(1), 1-7; Goodwin, A. J., & Scott, L. (1987). Sexuality in the second half of life. In P. B. Doress & D. L. Siegal (Eds.). *The Midlife and Older Women Book Project: Ourselves Growing Older*. New York: Touchstone; Hammond, D. (1989). Love, sex, and marriage in later years. In E. S. Deichman & R. Kociechki R. (Eds.). *Working with the Elderly: An Introduction*. Buffalo, NY: Prometheus; Morrison-Beedy, D., & Robbins, L. (1989). Sexual assessment and the aging female. *Nurse Practitioner*, 14(36); and Pfeiffer, E., Verwoerdt, A., & Wang, H. S. (1968). Sexual behavior in aged men and women. *Archives in General Psychiatry*, 19, 753-758.
Answers to Exercise 12-3 questions: 1. T; 2. T; 3. F; 4. T; 5. T; 6. F; 7. T; 8. F; 9. F.

throughout their lives. Minor physiological changes may have some effect on sexual functioning. For example, a benefit from physiological aging can be delayed ejaculation, which can increase sexual pleasure for the partner.[15,16]

For elder men who have erectile dysfunction, medications can help, such as Viagra (Pfizer U.S. Pharmaceuticals Group, New York), which increases the vascular flow to the genitals. However, caution must be taken in prescribing Viagra or any other medication because erectile dysfunction is complex, involving physical and psychological factors. In addition, Viagra, like any medication, has side effects and interactions with other medications.[12,13] The elder should discuss with a physician the benefits as well as the risks involved in taking Viagra or other medication for erectile dysfunction. Media coverage using promotions by celebrities about taking Viagra has had a positive impact on opening discussions about erectile dysfunction.[15]

Most elders, especially the young old (that is, those 65 to 75 years of age), have active lives in which sexuality can remain an important component. Most likely, if a couple has always been sexually active, they will continue to be so as they grow older. As with any age group, communication is important for a positive sexual relationship. Frailty and disability do not automatically necessitate cause for an elder to be abstinent, although as findings from the AARP study suggest, having a disability or health problem does contribute to decreased sexual activity.[6]

ELDER HOMOSEXUALS

Society has often ignored homosexuality in elders. Overall, society has embraced a "heteronormativity" viewpoint, or "a general perspective which sees heterosexual experiences as the only, or central view of the world."[17] Obviously, the elder cohort is diverse in terms of income, race, health status, and sexual orientation. Within this cohort

the elder homosexual population also has a diverse background.[18] The invisibility of the homosexual population is reflected in the paucity of research about homosexual elders.[19,20] In occupational therapy literature, only a few articles have considered the homosexual experience,[21-24] and even fewer have considered elder homosexuals.[17] Progress in occupational therapy research and literature in these areas has been minimal, considering the growing number of elders identifying themselves as homosexual.

Many elder homosexuals may be uncomfortable sharing about their sexuality, having grown up in a time when overt prejudice was expressed toward homosexuals.[12,19] Homosexuality was defined as a mental illness by the American Psychiatric Association until 1973.[12] Discrimination continues to exist with examples of lesbian couples who want to live together in long-term care facilities being denied rooms.[19] Social Security does not recognize a lifelong companion for benefits, and many medical and other legal decisions are made by family members rather than a person's partner.[18]

COTAs can help dispel myths by simple actions such as the use of more inclusive language. As Harrison[17] suggests, asking who are the significant others in a person's life rather than who is a person's spouse can help create a more open conversation. Times are changing and there are now organizations that advocate for elder homosexuals, such as the National Association of Lesbian and Gay Gerontology, Lesbian and Aging Issues Network, and a Lesbian and Gay Aging Network with the American Society on Aging.[17,18]

NORMAL AGE-RELATED PHYSIOLOGICAL CHANGES IN MEN AND WOMEN

With normal aging, physiological changes might affect sexual functioning. Knowledge of these changes may help

BOX 12-1

Age-Related Physiological Changes and Sexual Responses

Women

1. Decrease in rate and amount of vaginal lubrication may possibly lead to painful intercourse.[8,15,25]
2. Orgasmic phase decrease may occur in elder women, resulting in a decrease in orgasm intensity.[15,16]
3. Structural changes or atrophy may occur in the labia or uterus, in addition to a reduction in the expansion of the vagina width and length.[8,16,25,26]
4. Thinning of the lining of the vagina can result in irritation and painful intercourse.[8]
5. Sexual stimulation from the nipples, clitoris, and vulva may decrease with age due to a decrease in sensation.[15]

Men

1. Erection is slower, less full, and disappears quickly after orgasm. Erection has a longer refractory period. A man in his eighties may need to wait several days as compared with a man in his twenties, in whom refractory period is a few minutes.[27,28]
2. Elder men may experience a decrease in penile rigidity.[27,28]
3. A decreased volume of sperm occurs; although fertility level is decreased, men do not become sterile.[16,29]
4. Decreased penile sensitivity results in increased need for direct penile stimulation over other forms of stimulation such as visual, psychological, or manual.[28,30]
5. Ejaculatory control enhanced, and ejaculation may occur every third episode of sexual activity as a result of less concern about orgasm.[16]
6. Ejaculation and orgasm is less strong.[8,16]
7. Decrease in ejaculatory testosterone occurs, although most elder men have the minimal level for sexual functioning.[8]
8. Reduced size of testicles and increased size of prostate gland.[28,30]

Adapted from Goldstein, H., & Runyon, C. (1993). An occupational therapy module to increase sensitivity about geriatric sexuality. *Physical and Occupational Therapy in Geriatrics*, 11(2), 57-75.

the COTA counsel the elder (Box 12-1). Not all of these changes happen to every elder, and the degree varies among individuals.[31] Lindau and colleagues[7] surveyed 3,005 adults ranging from ages 57 to 85 years and found that 39% of women reported issues with vaginal lubrication and 34% of women were unable to reach an orgasm; erectile dysfunction (37%) ranked the highest among men.[7] In addition, COTAs should be aware of the concept "use it or lose it." Elders who remain sexually active may not experience some of these physiological changes or not to the same degree as elders who do not remain sexually

active. Furthermore, these physiological changes are just one aspect of sexuality. Sexuality, including sexual functioning, is complex and involves psychological, spiritual, social, and cultural dimensions of a human being.[2,32] The ways a person reacts to and perceives these physiological changes ultimately affect sexual functioning. COTAs can apply this knowledge to educate elders. For example, a commercially available lubricant can supplement decreased vaginal secretion and can help reduce abrasion from thinning of the vaginal lining. Lubrication may also prevent dyspareunia, or painful intercourse.[26] Kegel exercises (pelvic floor exercises) help preserve vaginal tone in women, can aid in the intervention of erectile dysfunction in men, and can reduce symptoms of incontinence in both genders.[33-35] COTAS can instruct the elder to do these exercises several times daily, such as three times daily for 10 increments with tightening the muscles for 3 to 4 seconds. Instruct the elder to think about holding back urine to do the exercise correctly.[36]

SEXUALLY TRANSMITTED DISEASES AMONG THE ELDER POPULATION

An often overlooked aspect of sexual activity in the elder population is the prevalence and prevention of sexually transmitted diseases (STDs). The AARP study[6] shows increasing numbers of elders are sexually active without being married, which puts them at a risk for STDs. A Centers for Disease Control and Prevention (CDC) study[37] estimated 15% of new diagnoses of HIV/AIDS in 2005 were among individuals age 50 or older.[6] A lack of information among the elder population about sexual activity poses a risk for transmitting STDs. Without the risk of pregnancy, many older adults forgo using safe sex techniques such as condoms.[38]

Prevention and education with elders should be incorporated with intervention. Promoting the use of condoms and other safe sex techniques is important in discussions of sexuality with elders. COTAs working in long-term care facilities can educate elders on the importance of safe sex techniques as well as the proper use of condoms. COTAs can also collaborate with other health care professionals to facilitate education on safe sex among the elder population.

ROLE OF INTERVENTION IN SEXUAL EDUCATION

COTAs, registered occupational therapists (OTRs), and elders should collaborate to address concerns about sexuality. In addition, COTAs should be aware of other team members' areas of expertise. Sexual dysfunction such as erectile problems, ejaculatory disturbances, anorgasmia (lack of orgasm), and pain during intercourse may be caused by side effects of medication and other physiological reasons.[39] The physician and pharmacist must be notified about these concerns. Sexual dysfunction has a psychological component.[40] Therefore, the client should

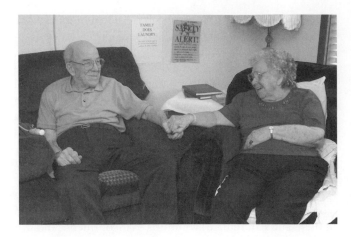

FIGURE 12-2 Sharing a room in a long-term care facility, these elders are able to enjoy the companionship of their lifelong spouse.

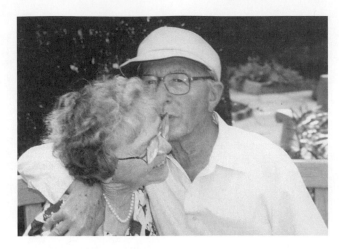

FIGURE 12-3 Sexual expression is an important part of a person's life at any age.

be referred for counseling with a social worker or psychologist who has expertise with elders who have disabilities and sexual dysfunction. In addition to the OTR/COTA team, some physical therapists and nurses may educate the client about sexual positioning. Speech therapists may assist elders who have difficulties with communication.[41,42]

ADDRESSING ELDER SEXUALITY IN A NURSING FACILITY

Trends in public policy and in professional literature suggest a more accepting attitude of sexual activity in nursing facilities (Figure 12-2). Federal laws regulate privacy for institutionalized patients, namely the Omnibus Budget Reconciliation Act[43] passed in 1987.[44] Professional literature since the 1990s has generally encouraged a more accepting attitude of sexuality in nursing home settings.[11] However, despite these positive trends, challenges still exist in nursing home facilities. These challenges include availability of privacy,[11] dealing with sexual behavior of residents who have cognitive impairments,[44-46] and addressing sexual concerns of residents with chronic conditions.[47] In addition, negative attitudes and viewpoints against sexual activity of elders are expressed by some staff,[4,44,45] spouses, and residents.[11] Staff may express their disapproval in many ways. One subtle way is by joking about sexual activity, which may serve as a means to make elders conform to the expectation of asexuality in some nursing facilities.

In some institutional settings, envisioning elders being interested in sex is difficult, and the elders themselves may be intolerant of peer engagement in sexual behavior.[11,15] Generational beliefs or societal expectations may influence these attitudes.[47] Mulligan and Palguta[48] found that male elders in nursing home facilities displayed continued interest in sex and were sexually active if a partner was available.

Sexuality does not only include sexual intercourse. It also involves kissing, touching, hugging, masturbation, and expressing oneself as a sexual being.[49,50] COTAs participating in program planning can suggest dances and other social events that encourage romance and human touch. They can encourage elders to be well dressed and well groomed. In addition, COTAs should always be aware of respecting client privacy. Shutting a curtain between beds or going to another room for intervention with personal ADL functions helps preserve privacy rights.

Elders should reside in a supportive environment that encourages sexual expression and involvement in sexual activity.[47] Residents should have a say in nursing home standards, especially setting standards for sexual behavior within the community[11,51] because most nursing home residents and staff support sexual rights.[47]

Finally, education can help dispel myths and misconceptions about sexuality and elders.[52] COTAs who have positive attitudes and are educated about sexuality and elders can help dispel the ageist attitudes sometimes held by nursing home staff, family members, or the elders themselves (Figure 12-3).

EDUCATING AND COUNSELING THE ELDER CLIENT

The Permission, Limited Information, Specific Suggestions, and Intensive Therapy Model

Intervention models may help provide sexual education to elders. The permission, limited information, specific suggestions, and intensive therapy (PLISSIT) model developed by Annon[53,54] is a useful format for presenting sexual education information (Box 12-2).

COTAs can use the first, second, and third stages of this model during intervention. The elder must be assured

BOX 12-2

The PLISSIT Model

- P = Permission.
- This stage involves listening in a nonjudgmental, knowledgeable, and relaxed manner as the client discusses sexual concerns. General questions can be asked in an intake or screening evaluation (for example, "Do you have any concerns about the effects of your disease on sexual function?").
- LI = Limited information.
- At this level, elders can be educated about normal physiological changes with aging, myths and stereotypes about the elder population, and sexuality and psychosocial factors that may inhibit or stress the elder.
- SS = Specific suggestions.
- At this level, COTAs may make appropriate suggestions for improved sexual functioning. Elders also may need to be referred to specialists such as social workers, psychologists, and physical or occupational therapists.
- IT = Intensive therapy.
- This level of counseling involves the expertise of a skilled social worker, psychologist, or psychiatrist.

Data from Annon, J. S. (1974). The behavioral treatment of sexual problems: Brief therapy [brochure]. Honolulu, HI: Kapiolani Health Services; Annon, J. S. (1976). *The Behavioral Treatment of Sexual Problems: Brief Therapy.* New York: Harper & Row; and Lohman, H., & Runyon, C. (1995). *Counseling the Geriatric Client about Sexuality Issues in Counseling and Therapy: Lesson 5.* New York: Hatherleigh.

of confidentiality throughout the educational process. In the first stage of the PLISSIT model, permission, the COTA applies therapeutic listening skills. The verbal and nonverbal body language of the COTA must show comfort with the topic. COTAs can ask questions using clear and direct language in a nonthreatening manner to encourage communication about sexual functioning during the ADL assessment.[4] In addition, the COTA can convey that sexuality is a normal part of every human's needs throughout a lifetime.[55] Elders who are interested in discussing sexuality may have general questions about normal sexual changes with aging or common myths. The spouse or partner should be encouraged to join the discussion.

In the second stage of the model, the COTA can apply limited information by relating knowledge of sexuality gleaned from this chapter and other relevant sources. The COTA can provide specific suggestions in the third stage. Many suggestions to help elders who have disabling conditions and their partners maintain sexual function are discussed in the chapter. The COTA should refer the elder who needs psychological support at any point of the education process to the appropriate counselor. The fourth stage of the model, intensive therapy, involves the

skills of a trained counselor and is especially important for those elders experiencing sexual dysfunction.

Role of the Certified Occupational Therapy Assistant in Sexual Education

To provide elders with adequate sex education, COTAs must have a general knowledge about medical conditions, awareness of psychological issues, and an understanding of the importance of good communication. Understanding the effects of a disease or disabling condition on sexual performance is necessary. COTAs must remember that the manifestations of a disease or condition differs with each person, and often sexual functioning has to do with how a person adapts to life changes.[14] The following are some general education suggestions:

1. Encourage elders to maintain good communication with their partners in all aspects of their lives, not just about sexuality.[16]
2. Encourage elders to experiment with different sexual positions for comfort.[16]
3. Provide instruction on energy conservation techniques. Suggest resting before sexual activity.[56]
4. Encourage elders with decreased energy to explore other forms of sexual expression such as caressing, masturbation, and oral sex.[16]
5. Reassure elders that once they are medically stable and their physician has assessed them, they can reassume sexual activity.[33]
6. Talk with elders about any fears that they may have about resuming sexual functioning.[38]

The specific sexual concerns of elders who have experienced cerebrovascular accidents (CVAs), heart disease, and arthritis are discussed in the following sections.

Safety Considerations with Sexual Activity

- Medications, drugs, alcohol, and smoking can be a cause of sexual dysfunction. COTAs should encourage elders to consult with their physicians or pharmacists to discuss sexual dysfunction related to these areas.
- Elders who sustained strokes may have motor, sensory, and psychological dysfunctions. Sensory and motor dysfunctions should be considered with suggestions for positioning with sexual activity.
- With a cardiac condition, encourage elders to consult with physicians before returning to sexual activity. COTAs should educate elders on the precautions for sexual activity after a cardiac condition: chest pain, shortness of breath, excessive fatigue, and continuous increase in blood pressure after sex or heart palpitations lasting longer than 15 minutes after sex.[33,57,58] If elders experience these symptoms, they should seek immediate medical assistance.
- Arthritis can cause pain, fatigue, and joint inflammation during sexual activity. Elders should

BOX 12-3

Intervention Gems and Elder Sexual Activity

- Sexuality activity is an ADL listed in the Occupational Therapy Practice Framework II.[1] It is a normal part of aging and should be incorporated into intervention if elders desire. Generational values as well as individual values influence attitudes and beliefs about sexuality.
- The current generation of elders, the Traditionalists, grew up in a time when sexuality was not openly discussed. With some members of the Baby Boomer generation, sexuality may be more openly discussed in intervention sessions.
- Discussing sexuality and sexual activity is a sensitive subject and may cause some health care professionals to become uncomfortable. COTAs must be comfortable discussing sexuality with intervention, including sexual positioning, sexual orientation, and psychological aspects of sexuality.
- Develop a rapport with elders before discussing sexual activity, and address sexuality based on the PLISSIT Model.
- Elders may not have an adequate amount of knowledge about sexual activity after sustaining a condition, and therefore education is an important aspect of intervention. Education about positioning, energy conservation, sexually transmitted diseases, and safe sex techniques can be incorporated into an elder's intervention.
- COTAs can also collaborate with the treatment team as well as educate staff of the importance of incorporating sexuality within the elder's intervention plan.

- The effects of a stroke can have motor, sensory, and psychological manifestations that may affect an elder's ability to participate in sexual activity. Common compensatory techniques for sexual intercourse include lying on the affected side so the unaffected arm is free, using pillows under the affected side, the use of touch for individuals with aphasia, and a non-distracting environment for individuals with cognitive impairments.
- Elders with cardiac condition may have fear of sustaining a recurrent heart attack during sexual activity. Elders with cardiac conditions should consult a physician before beginning sexual activity. If cleared to resume sexual activity, COTAs can instruct elders on the use of relaxation techniques and energy conservation during sexual activity.
- Pain, fatigue, joint inflammation, and anxiety can all hinder sexual activity with elders who have arthritis. COTAs can instruct elders with arthritis to use energy conservation techniques and rest to decrease pain during sexual activity. Heat pads or warm baths can be effective preparatory methods to decrease pain during sexual activity.
- Elders with hip replacements should be instructed to abide by hip precautions during sexual activity.
- Elders with knee replacements often prefer a side-lying position for comfort. Pillows can also be used with elders with knee replacements to maintain comfort and for safety.

be instructed on sexual positions that reduce the risk of these debilitating factors.

- Safety concerns with sexual activity and other activities are necessary for elders to follow after total hip replacements. Review with elders that with any sexual or life activity they should not flex the affected hip more than 90 degrees[59,60] and that the affected hip should not be adducted or externally rotated.[59,61]
- COTAs need to recognize when to refer elders with sexual concerns that would benefit from additional services to appropriate professionals (Box 12-3).

EFFECTS OF HEALTH CONDITIONS ON ELDER SEXUALITY

Cerebrovascular Accident

COTAs commonly work with elders who have sustained CVAs or strokes. Dealing with sexual concerns after a stroke is often ignored.[41,62,63] Addressing sexuality should be one of many aspects of a thorough evaluation. Just as

the outcomes after a stroke are complex and different for each person, so are the impacts of a stroke on sexuality. It is not unusual for someone after a stroke to experience a decreased desire for sexual activity and decreased satisfaction with sexual activity.[12,64,65] A study of 109 men who had a stroke found a decrease in erectile function, sexual desire, and ejaculatory function after stroke, but a lack of sexual desire was the main cause of limitations in sexual intercourse.[66] Changes after a CVA have been linked to a person's attitude about sexual activity and to fears about having erectile dysfunction, experiencing rejection, or having another stroke.[41,65-67] Changes in one's body image and one's coping skills can be psychological manifestations.[41,67,68] Being aphasic, having functional changes, displaying difficulties in arousal, and taking certain medications that have side effects on sexual performance also can influence sexual activity.[69] Many of these changes may indicate a need for intervention about sexuality, and COTAs can play a strong role because of their background in working with people who have had CVAs. However, in considering any intervention, COTAs should keep in mind the concept that sexual dysfunctions after a

CVA will likely result from multiple causes[67]; therefore, use of clinical reasoning skills[70] and a team-based approach[41] will be important.

COTAs should observe for motor abnormalities and other symptoms that can affect sexual function, including hemiplegia; perceptual, cognitive, and visual spatial disturbances; speech problems; emotional manifestations; and sensory deficits. For example, if elders are depressed, they may have no interest in sex. Anxiety may cause sexual performance problems such as male impotence and decreased female lubrication leading to painful intercourse. If elders have unilateral neglect, they may ignore one side of the body during sexual performance. Expressive aphasia may result in difficulty stating sexual needs. Sensory deficits such as esthesia or hyperesthesia on the affected side may affect sexual pleasure.[41,71] Motor disturbances such as muscle weakness or hypertonia can make sexual performance awkward.[41,71] (See Chapter 19 for a detailed discussion about CVA.)

After identifying the symptoms that affect sexual performance, the OTR and the COTA should collaborate with the elder to develop specific intervention suggestions. For example, clients with hemiplegia are sometimes advised to lie on the affected side so that the unaffected arm is free to caress the partner,[41,72] or to just find a comfortable position.[16] Simple adaptations such as using pillows under the affected side, use of a vibrator, raising the headboard, and adding a bed trapeze can help with motor manifestations of the CVA.[41,71] Touch and other forms of nonverbal communication are useful with elders who have expressive aphasia.[16] The partners of elders with visual field deficits should be encouraged to approach from the impaired side and use touch on both sides. Minimizing environmental distractions during sexual activity may help elders with cognitive deficits involving concentration.[73]

Beyond the physical effects of a CVA, some elders may experience low self-esteem and depression. These symptoms can affect sexual desire and performance.[41,67,74] Elders who are in some way dependent on a partner may feel ambivalent about resuming a sexual relationship because of role changes.[41,75] In addition, elders may worry about sustaining another CVA.[67,76] Results of a study of 103 individuals who had a stroke for the first time found 65% of the individuals had a fear of experiencing another stroke while engaging in sexual activity.[76] Elders with these psychological manifestations may require counseling.

Heart Disease

Heart disease is one of the most common chronic ailments affecting the elder population.[77] Elders can have acute cardiac conditions, such as myocardial infarctions (MI), or chronic cardiac conditions, such as hypertension. With either type of cardiac condition the possible impact on sexuality should not be ignored. Elders should consult their physician for recommendations about sexual activity

and cardiac conditions.[30] DeBusk and colleagues[78] developed a classification system to use as a guideline for physician's recommendations to manage sexual activity in patients with cardiac disease. With this classification system, patients are divided into low, medium, or high cardiac risk. Patients with low risk, such as having controlled hypertension or mild stable angina, are recommended to safely resume sex. Patients with moderate risk, such as sustaining a recent MI or displaying moderate angina, require further cardiac evaluation. Patients in the high-risk category, such as having unstable angina or hypertension, are recommended to be stabilized before reassuming sexual activity.

Once stabilized, some elders with cardiac conditions may be instructed to resume sexual activity in a gradual manner.[58] For elders who gradually reassume sexual activity, alternative forms of sexuality other than intercourse can be suggested. However, before reassuming sexual activity, elders should be instructed by the medical team about precautions and when to notify their physician.

Examples of precautions for sexual activity are chest pain, shortness of breath, excessive fatigue, and continuous increase in blood pressure after sex or heart palpitations lasting longer than 15 minutes after sex.[33,58,62] The medical team also should be aware of negative side effects of common cardiac medications, herbal supplements, or illicit drugs that can influence libido or result in sexual dysfunction.[33,58,79]

Sustaining a cardiac condition can impact a person psychologically, resulting in fears about resuming sexuality. The resumption of sexual activity after a heart attack is believed by some people to cause future cardiac incidents and even death.[58,80] Findings from a study (n = 1774) published in the *Journal of the American Medical Association* helps clarify anecdotal information.[81] Sexual activity was found to contribute to MIs in a small number of the subjects (0.9%), and regular exercise was related to a decreased risk.[81] Elders need to be educated that the physical demands of sexual activity are equal to mild to moderate exercise ("heart rate rarely increases to greater than 130 beats per minute and systolic blood pressure is rarely greater than 170 mm Hg"[78]).

Relaxation is important because fears and anxieties are common after cardiac incidents, especially about resuming sexual relationships.[82] In addition, it is not uncommon to be depressed.[83] Sexual dysfunctions can develop because of these anxieties.[16,79] Sexual dysfunctions such as erectile problems also can result from physical reasons such as arteriosclerosis (hardening of the arteries).[27,63] Furthermore, one must consider the sexual activity of the person before the cardiac incident.[14] Using positions that require less energy expenditure and encouraging relaxation with sexual activity are helpful suggestions.[83] COTAs can teach elders stress reduction techniques. Energy conservation techniques also may be helpful for those who are gradually building up their endurance. It is also beneficial to wait 1 to 3 hours after meals to allow the heart to pump blood to assist with the digestive process.[58,83] Per the PLISSIT model,[53,54] COTAs may need to refer the elder to an expert to address any sexual dysfunction. (See Chapter 23 for a more detailed discussion about cardiac concerns and the elderly.)

Arthritis

Arthritis is another common chronic condition among elders. All types of arthritis, including osteoarthritis and rheumatoid arthritis, can influence sexual function with physical and psychological effects. Physical concerns can be pain, functional limitations, fatigue, medication side effects, and genital lesions with some types of arthritis. Psychological problems include but are not limited to depression, anxiety, and loss of self-esteem.[84-86] In addition, less opportunity to meet potential partners because of isolation and physical separation from one's partner because of repeated hospitalizations is another psychological concern.[84,85]

Elders with joint inflammation and pain may be particularly prone to sexual performance problems. A common intervention goal for people with rheumatoid arthritis is to maintain or increase functional abilities in all areas of life,[86,87] including sexual function. COTAs can make specific suggestions to help elders reduce joint pain and discomfort and preserve energy. Exercises to increase and maintain muscle strength affect the motor aspect of sexual performance. Elders should be encouraged to use a heating pad or tub bath before sexual activity to help decrease joint pain and inflammation. Elders and their partners also may experiment with various sexual positions that decrease joint pressure. Rest and energy conservation techniques may help make sexual performance less fatiguing. Finding the best time of day for sexual activity when the elder is less fatigued helps sexual performance.[60,86]

Joint Replacements

Elders with a history of arthritis commonly sustain joint replacements. Elders after total hip replacements are counseled to follow certain precautions in all areas of their lives, including sexuality. For an elder who has had a total hip replacement (posterolateral approach), it is important to review that with any sexual activity, or life activity, the elder should not flex the affected hip more than 90 degrees[59,60] and that the affected hip should not be adducted or externally rotated.[59,61] After the customary healing period of approximately 6 weeks and with physician approval, these elders can resume sexual activity as long as they follow precautions.

For intercourse, it is preferable with either sex that the elder with the total hip replacement be positioned supine (on back) with hips abducted (apart), knees in extension (straight), and legs in neutral (toes pointed up), and not in external rotation (toes pointed out).[60] Intercourse in a side-lying position for the involved elder woman is accomplished by lying on her unaffected side with a minimum of two pillows between her legs to keep them abducted. The involved man using a side-lying position should also lie on his unaffected side and should "use his partner's legs to support his affected leg." Thus, the man's affected leg is on top of his partner's leg during sexual intercourse. The elder man's partner should have a minimum of two pillows between her legs for support and to help her partner follow precautions.[60] Other suggestions are pillows between the knees to help maintain the hip joints in abduction,[88] and pillows under the knees while in a supine position can prevent extreme external rotation.[61]

After a total knee replacement, elders should be instructed to find the most comfortable position for intercourse. When the involved person is in a supine position, pillows can be placed under the knee, and the person can bend the knee within a comfortable range.[60] A side-lying position is often most comfortable after surgery, and pillow support under the knee is beneficial.[60]. Exercise 12-4 is a role play exercise to overview many of the concepts discussed in in the chapter. Its purpose is to help increase comfort level in addressing sexual concerns of clients in practice.

■ Exercise 12-4: Role Play

Addressing sexual concerns in intervention will become more comfortable with practice for COTAs. The purpose of this role-play exercise is to increase comfort levels when discussing sexual issues. It also serves as a review of chapter material. To begin the exercise, choose four people to be part of a radio talk show panel made up of knowledgeable professionals who are experts on the sexuality of elders. Then choose people who will read the scenarios listed in the following. Members of the radio talk show panel are allowed to consult notes and have a commercial break if they want to discuss a situation before responding.

Another method is to role play doing a live show on the Internet site Skype found at http://www.skype.com. Role play a synchronous session in which elders (played by students) from several community facilities call in their questions about sexuality, either using a webcam or a microphone.

Situations for Role Play:

■ I am 78 years of age and have rheumatoid arthritis. Over the years, I have developed increasingly painful joints, particularly in my hips. I am currently a widow but will soon marry a wonderful man. I would like to enjoy my new sexual relationship. Do you have any suggestions?

■ I am a 65-year-old man who had a heart attack 8 weeks ago. My doctor says that it is safe to begin sex again. Still, I have tremendous fears. Are these fears normal, and what can I do about them?

■ I am a nurse's aide who works in a nursing facility. I have recently noticed male and female patients taking an interest in each other. They are constantly holding hands and have been observed kissing. The other aides make fun of them and have told them to stop, but they continue openly expressing their affection. I feel that they have a right to express their romantic side. Who is right?

■ I am an 82-year-old man. My wife and I continue to have a satisfying sexual relationship. However, I have noticed in recent years that my first erection is slower and it takes me even longer to achieve an erection the second time. I am afraid to ask my physician about this. Am I normal?

■ I am a 64-year-old man who had a heart attack 2 years ago. I have been impotent since getting out of the hospital. What should I do?

■ I have a two-part question. I am 65 years old and have recently had a minor stroke. I am uncomfortable asking my physician about this. I have noticed over the years that sexual activity with my lover has become painful because of less vaginal lubrication. Is this normal, and is there anything I can do about it? Concerning the stroke, my left side is impaired and weakened. Do you have any suggestions for sexual positioning?

■ I am an 87-year-old lesbian. I can now more openly state that fact because times are changing. However, in most of my lifetime I have had to hide my sexuality. Because of having arthritis and high blood pressure, I have found it more difficult to get around and am now looking into relocating to an assisted living facility with my partner. With interviews at the facilities we have been open about our sexual relationship. Although none of the directors has directly stated that they do not want us to move into their facility, it has been obvious from their body language that we are less than welcome. We realize that we will likely experience some prejudice from other residents wherever we move. Do you have any suggestions on how to approach finding a place? Also, as long as you are consulting, do you have suggestions about my arthritis and maintaining sexual relations with my partner?

■ CHAPTER REVIEW QUESTIONS

1 Discuss common myths related to elder sexuality.
2 Discuss the viewpoint held by society about elder homosexuals.
3 Discuss issues related to STDs and the elder population.
4 Identify some of the normal age-related physiological changes for women and some simple intervention suggestions for them.

5 Identify some of the normal age-related physiological changes for men.
6 List the members of the treatment team and discuss ways the team can work together to address elders' sexual concerns.
7 Discuss the ways that attitudes of health care workers in nursing home facilities affect elder sexuality.
8 Describe ways COTAs help facilitate elder sexual expression in a nursing home setting.
9 List and describe the parts of the PLISSIT model.
10 Describe ways COTAs may apply the PLISSIT model in intervention.

REFERENCES

1. American Occupational Therapy Association, 2008. Occupational therapy practice framework: Domain and process, second ed. American Journal of Occupational Therapy 62, 625-683.
2. Pangman, V.C., Sequire, M., 2000. Sexuality and the chronically ill older adult: A social justice issue. Sexuality and Disability 18 (1), 49-50.
3. Goodwin, A.J., Scott, L., 1987. Sexuality in the second half of life. In: Doress, P.B., Siegal, D.L. (Eds.), The Midlife and Older Women Book Project: Ourselves Growing Older. Touchstone, New York, pp. 79-99.
4. Langer, N., 2009. Late life love and intimacy. Educational Gerontology 35 (8), 752-764.
5. Jacoby, S., 2005, July/August. Sex in America. *AARP the Magazine 1-2*. Retrieved from http://www.aarpmagazine.org/lifestyle/relationships/sex_in_america.html/page=1.
6. American Association of Retired Persons (AARP), 2005. Sexuality at midlife and beyond: 2004 update of attitudes and behaviors [WWW page]. URL http://assets.aarp.org/rgcenter/general/2004_sexuality.pdf.
7. Lindau, S., Schumm, P., Laumann, E., Levinson, W., O'Muircheartaigh, C., Waite, L., 2007, August. A study of sexuality and health among older adults in the United States. New England Journal of Medicine 357 (8), 762-774.
8. Meston, C.M., 1997. Successful aging: Aging and sexuality. Western Journal of Medicine 167 (4), 285-290.
9. Kinsella, K., Wan H., U.S. Census Bureau, 2009. An aging world: 2008 (Report No. P95/09-1). U.S. Government Printing Office, Washington, DC.
10. American Association of Retired Persons (AARP), 1999. AARP modern maturity sexuality survey—summary of findings [WWW page]. URL http://www.research.aarp.org/health/mmsexsurvey_l.html.
11. Gibson, M.C., Bol, N., Woodbury, M.G., Beaton, C., Janke, C., 1999. Comparison of caregivers', residents' and community-dwelling spouses' opinions about expressing sexuality in an institutional setting. Journal of Gerontological Nursing 25 (4), 30-39.
12. Allen, W., 2008. Sexuality. In: Ferrini, A.F., Ferrini, R.L. (Eds.), Health in the Later Years. 4th ed. McGraw-Hill, New York.
13. Starr, B.D., 2002. Sexuality. In: Schulz, R. (Ed.), The Encyclopedia of Aging: A Comprehensive Source in Gerontology and Geriatrics, forth ed. Vol. 2. Springer, New York.
14. Lerner, S., 2000. Sexuality and myths: A study of aging factors. Focus on Geriatric Care and Rehabilitation 13 (10), 3-12.
15. Agronin, M.E., 2004. Sexual disorders. In: Blazer, D.G., Steffens, D.C., Busse, E.W. (Eds.), The American Psychiatric Publishing Textbook of Geriatric Psychiatry, third ed. American Psychiatric, Washington, DC, pp. 303-317.

16. Laflin, M., 2002. Sexuality and the elderly individuals. In Lewis, C.B. (Ed.). Aging: The Health-Care Challenge, fourth ed. FA Davis, Philadelphia.

17. Harrison, J., 2001. "It's none of my business": Gay and lesbian invisibility in aged care. Australian Occupational Therapy Journal 48, 142-145.

18. Kimmel, D.C., 2006. Homosexuality. In: Schulz, R. (Ed.), The Encyclopedia of Aging: A Comprehensive Resource in Gerontology and Geriatrics, vol. 1, fourth ed. Springer, New York.

19. Wojciechowski, C., 1998. Issues in caring for older lesbians. Journal of Gerontological Nursing 24, 28-33.

20. Wright, S., Canetto, S., 2009. Stereotypes of older lesbians and gay men. Educational Gerontology 35 (5), 424-452.

21. Birkholtz, M., Blair, S., 1999. "Coming out" and its impact on women's occupational behavior—a discussion paper. Journal of Occupational Science 62, 68-74.

22. Jackson, J., 1995. Sexual orientation: Its relevance to occupational science and the practice of occupational therapy. American Journal of Occupational Therapy, 54, 26-35.

23. Jackson, J., 2000. Understanding the experience of non-inclusive occupational therapy clinics: Lesbians' perspectives. American Journal of Occupational Therapy 54, 26-35.

24. Walsh, A., Crepeau, E., 1998. "My secret life": The emergence of one gay man's authentic identity. American Journal of Occupational Therapy 52:563-569.

25. Zeiss, A.M., Kasl-Godley, J., 2001. Sexuality in older adults' relationships. Generations 25, 18-25.

26. Johnson, L.E., Alline, K.M., 2007. Sexual health. In: Ham, R.J., Sloane, P.D., Warshaw, G.A., Bernard, M.A., Flaherty, E. (Eds.), Primary Care Geriatrics: A Case-Based Approach, fifth ed. Mosby Elsevier, Philadelphia, pp. 401-407.

27. Tenover, J.L., 2009. Sexuality, sexual function, androgen therapy, and the aging male. In: Hazzard, W.R., Halter, J.B. (Eds.), Hazzard's geriatric medicine and gerontology, sixth ed. McGraw-Hill Medical Pub. Division. New York. pp. 1634. Retrieved from http://www.accessmedicine.com.cuhsl.creighton.edu/content.aspx?aID=5118079

28. Schiavi, R.C., Rehman, J., 1995. Sexuality and aging. Urologic Clinics of North America 22 (4), 711-726.

29. LeVay, S., Valente, S.M., 2006. Human Sexuality, second ed. Sinauer Associates, Sunderland, MA.

30. Miracle, A., Miracle, T.S., 2009. Sexuality in late adulthood. In: Bonder, B.R., Bello-Haas, V.D. (Eds.), Functional Performance in Older Adults, third ed. FA Davis, Philadelphia.

31. Glass, C., Dalton, A., 1988. Sexuality in older adults: A continuing education concern. Journal of Continuing Education in Nursing 19, 61-64.

32. DeLamater, J., Karraker, A., 2009, February. Sexual functioning in older adults. Current Psychiatry Reports 11 (1), 6-11. doi:10.1007/s11920-009-0002-4.

33. Mueller, L.W., 1997. Common questions about sex and sexuality in elders. American Journal of Nursing 97 (7), 61-64.

34. Sivalingam, S., Hashim, H., Schwaibold, H., 2006. An overview of the diagnosis and treatment of erectile dysfunction. Drugs 66 (18), 2339-2355.

35. Weiss, B.D., 2005. Selecting medications for the treatment of urinary incontinence. American Family Physician 71 (2), 315-322.

36. Mayo Clinic, n.d.. Kegel exercises: How to strengthen pelvic floor muscles. Retrieved February 5, 2010, from http://www.mayoclinic.com/health/Kegel-exercises/WO00119.

37. Centers for Disease Control and Prevention (CDC), 2008. HIV/AIDS among persons aged 50 and older [WWW page]. URL http://www.cdc.gov/hiv/topics/over50/resources/factsheets/over50.htm.

38. Atkinson, P.J., 2006. Intimacy and sexuality. In: Meiner, S.E., Lueckenotte, A.G. (Eds.), Gerontologic Nursing, third ed. Mosby Elsevier, St. Louis, MO, pp. 268-280.

39. Camacho, M.E., Reyes-Ortiz, C.A., 2005. Sexual dysfunction in the elderly: Age or disease? International Journal of Impotence Research 17, S52-S56.

40. Laumann, E.O., Nicolosi, A., Glasser, D.B., Paik, A., Gingell, C., Moreira, E., Wang, T., 2005. Sexual problems among women and men aged 40-80 y: Prevalence and correlates identified in the global study of sexual attitudes and behaviors. International Journal of Impotence Research 17 (1), 39-57.

41. Farman, J., Friedman, J.D., 2004. Sexual function and intimacy. In: Stroke Rehabilitation: A Function-Based Approach. 2nd ed. Mosby, St. Louis, MO, pp. 533-549.

42. Lohman, H., Runyon, C., 1995. Counseling the Geriatric Client about Sexuality Issues in Counseling and Therapy: Lesson 5. Hatherleigh, New York.

43. Omnibus Budget Reconciliation Act (OBRA), 1987. Health Care Financing Administration. Health Care Administration, Baltimore.

44. Reingold, D., Burros, N., 2004. Sexuality in the nursing home. Journal of Gerontological Social Work 43 (2/3), 175-186. doi:10.1300/J083v43n02_12.

45. Doyle, D., Bisson, D., Janes, N., Lynch, H., Martin, C. 1999. Human sexuality in long-term care. The Canadian Nurse 95 (1), 26-29.

46. Tzeng, Y., Lin, L., Shyr, Y.L., Wen, J., 2009. Sexual behaviour of institutionalised residents with dementia–a qualitative study. Journal of Clinical Nursing 18 (7), 991-1001.

47. Ghusn, H., 1995. Sexuality in institutionalized patients. Physical medicine and rehabilitation: State of the art reviews, 9, 2. Hanley & Belfus, Philadelphia.

48. Mulligan, T., Palguta, R.F., 1991. Sexual interest, activity, and satisfaction among male nursing home residents. Archives of Sexual Behavior 20 (2), 199-204.

49. Ginsberg, T.B., Pomerantz, S.C., Kramer-Feeley, V., 2005, September. Sexuality in older adults: Behaviours and preferences. Age and Ageing 34 (5), 475-480.

50. Lyder, C.H., 1991. Examining sexuality in long-term care. Journal of Practical Nursing 41 (4), 25-27.

51. Roach, S., 2004. Sexual behaviour of nursing home residents: Staff perceptions and responses. Journal of Advanced Nursing 48 (4), 371-379. doi:10.1111/j.1365-2648.2004.03206.x.

52. Lohman, H., Aitken, M., 1995. Influence of education on knowledge and attitude toward older adult sexuality. Physical and Occupational Therapy in Geriatrics 13, 51.

53. Annon, J.S., 1974. The behavioral treatment of sexual problems: Brief therapy [brochure]. Kapiolani Health Services, Honolulu, HI.

54. Annon, J.S., 1976. The Behavioral Treatment of Sexual Problems: Brief Therapy. Harper & Row, New York.

55. Kessel, B., 2001. Sexuality in the older person. Age and Ageing 30, 121-124.

56. Hordern, A., Currow, D., 2003. A patient-centered approach to sexuality in the face of life-limiting illness. Medical Journal of Australia, 179 (Suppl. 6), S8-S11.

57. Miller, C.A., 2009. Nursing for Wellness in Older Adults. 5th ed. Lippincott Williams & Wilkins, Philadelphia.

58. Steinke, E.E., 2000. Sexual counseling after myocardial infarction. American Journal of Nursing 100 (12), 38-44.

59. Pratt, E., Gray, P.A., 2007. Total hip arthroplasty. In: Maxey, L., Magnusson, J. (Eds.), Rehabilitation for the Postsurgical Orthopedic Patient, second ed. Mosby, St. Louis, MO.

60. Whittington, C., Mansour, S., Sloan, S.L., 2001. Sex After Total Joint Replacement: A Guide for You and Your Partner. Media Partners, Atlanta, GA.

61. Coleman, S., 2002. Hip fractures and lower extremity joint replacement. In: Pedretti, L.W., Early, M.B. (Eds.), Occupational Therapy: Practice Skills for Physical Dysfunction, fifth ed. Mosby, St. Louis, MO.

62. Miller, L., 2008, February 4. Let's talk about sex. OT Practice 13 (2), 7-8.

63. Miracle, A., Miracle, T.S., 2001. Sexuality in late adulthood. In: Bonder, B.R., Wagner, M.B. (Eds.), Functional Performance in Older Adults. 2nd ed. FA Davis, Philadelphia.

64. Edmans, J., 1998. An investigation of stroke patients resuming sexual activity. British Journal of Occupational Therapy 61 (1), 36-38.

65. Korpelainen, J.T., Nieminen, P., Myllyla, V.V., 1999. Sexual functioning among stroke patients and their spouses. Stroke 30, 715-719.

66. Jung, J.H., Kam, S.C., Choi, S.M., Jae, S.U., Lee, S.H., Hyun, J.S., 2008. Sexual dysfunction in male stroke patients: Correlation between brain lesions and sexual function. Urology 71 (1), 99-103.

67. Monga, T.N., Ostermann, H.J., 1995. Sexuality and sexual adjustment in stroke patients. Physical Medicine and Rehabilitation State of the Art Reviews 9 (2), 345-359.

68. Wilz, G., 2007. Predictors of subjective impairment after stroke: Influence of depression, gender, and severity of stroke. Brain Injury 21 (1), 39-45.

69. Cheung, R.T., 2008. Sexual dysfunction after stroke: A need for more study. European Journal of Neurology 15 (7), 641.

70. Mattingly, C., Fleming, M.H., 1994. Clinical Reasoning: Forms of Inquiry in a Therapeutic Practice. FA Davis, Philadelphia.

71. Zukas, R., Ross-Robinson, L., 1991. Sexuality and the disabled woman. Occupational Therapy Practice 2 (4), 1-12.

72. Burgener, S., Logan, G., 1989. Sexuality concerns of the post-style patient. Rehabilitation Nursing 14 (4), 178-195.

73. Neistadt, M.E., Freda, M., 1987. Choices: A Guide to Sexual Counseling with Physically Disabled Adults. Robert E. Krieger, Malabar, FL.

74. Somers, K.J., Philbrick, K.L., 2007, June. Sexual dysfunction in the medically ill. Current Psychiatry Reports 9 (3), 247-254.

75. Mooradian, A.D., 1991. Geriatric sexuality and chronic diseases. Clinics in Geriatric Medicine 7 (1), 113-131.

76. Tamam, Y., Tamam, L., Akil, E., Yasan, A., Tamam, B., 2008. Post-stroke sexual functioning in first stroke patients. European Journal of Neurology: The Official Journal of the European Federation of Neurological Societies 15 (7), 660-666. Retrieved from MEDLINE database.

77. U.S. Department of Health and Human Services (DHHS), 2008. A profile of older Americans: 2008. Author, Washington, DC.

78. DeBusk, R., Drory, Y., Goldstein, I., Jackson, G., Kaul, S., Kimmel, S., et al. 2000. Management of sexual dysfunction in patients with cardiovascular disease: recommendations of The Princeton Consensus Panel. The American Journal of Cardiology 86 (2), 175-181. Retrieved from MEDLINE database.

79. Steinke, E.E., Jaarsma, T., 2008. Impact of cardiovascular disease on sexuality. In: Moser, D.K., Riegel, B. (Eds.), Cardiac Nursing: A Companion to Braunwald's Heart Disease. WB Saunders, St. Louis, MO.

80. Mandras, S.A., Uber, P.A., Mehra, M.R., 2007, October. Sexual activity and chronic heart failure. Mayo Clinic Proceedings 82 (10), 1203-1210.

81. Muller, J., Mittleman, M., Maclure, M., Sherwood, J., Tofler, G., 1996. Triggering myocardial infarction by sexual activity. Low absolute risk and prevention by regular physical exertion. Determinants of Myocardial Infarction Onset Study Investigators. JAMA: The Journal of the American Medical Association 275 (18), 1405-1409.

82. Westlake, C., Dracup, K., Walden, J., Fonarow, G. 1999. Sexuality of patients with advanced heart failure and their spouses or partners. The Journal of Heart and Lung Transplantation: The Official Publication of the International Society for Heart Transplantation 18 (11), 1133-1138. Retrieved from MEDLINE database.

83. American Heart Association, 2009. Sexual activity and heart disease or stroke [WWW page]. URL http://www.americanheart.org/presenter.jhtml?identifier=4714.

84. Isik, A., Koca, S.S., Ozturk, A., Mermi, O., 2007, June. Anxiety and depression in patients with rheumatoid arthritis. Clinical Rheumatology 26 (6), 872-878.

85. Lim, P.A.C., 1995. Sexuality in patients with musculoskeletal diseases. Physical Medicine and Rehabilitation: State of the Art Review 9 (2), 401-415.

86. Helewa, A., 2004. Management of persons with rheumatoid arthritis and other inflammatory conditions. In: Walker, J.M., Helewa, A. (Eds.), Physical Rehabilitation in Arthritis, second ed. WB Saunders, St. Louis, MO, pp. 191-212.

87. Yasuda, Y.L., 2002. Rheumatoid arthritis and osteoarthritis. In: Trombly, C.A. (Ed.), Occupational Therapy for Physical Dysfunction, fifth ed. Lippincott Williams & Wilkins, Baltimore.

88. Lawson, S., 2006. Hip fractures and lower extremity joint replacement. In: Pendleton, H. McHugh, Schultz-Krohn, W. (Eds.). Pedretti's Occupational Therapy: Practice Skills for Physical Dysfunction, sixth ed. Mosby, Philadelphia, pp. 1020-1035.

13

Use of Medications by Elders

BRENDA M. COPPARD, KELLI COOVER, AND MICHELE FAULKNER

KEY TERMS

self-medication, over-the-counter, polypharmacy, adverse drug reactions,
side effects, drug interactions

CHAPTER OBJECTIVES

1. Identify factors that predispose elders to adverse drug events, and discuss strategies to detect medication problems.
2. Define *polypharmacy* and identify recommended interventions to diminish drug-related problems of polypharmacy in elders.
3. Identify classes of medications commonly associated with adverse drug reactions in elders.
4. Identify and describe skills needed for safe self-medication.
5. Apply the OT Practice Framework: Domain and Process, second edition, to analyze self-medication for individuals with various conditions.
6. Explain the ways that adaptive devices compensate for skills needed for safe self-medication.
7. Describe elder and caregiver education needs regarding self-medication.

Ashley is a certified occupational therapy assistant (COTA) working in a skilled nursing facility 3 days a week. Her time for seeing the residents is dependent upon the needs of the facility. One of the residents she follows is Anna, a 79-year-old woman with a history of a recent stroke, high blood pressure, depression, and insomnia. Ashley has noticed changes in Anna's alertness and behavior, based on the time of day that she is seen for intervention. When Ashley follows Anna in the morning, she seems very tired, unfocused, and often complains of dizziness. Ashley has found such morning therapy sessions to be less productive toward meeting Anna's intervention goals. When she sees Anna in the afternoon, she seems to be almost a completely different person, exhibiting much more energy and enthusiasm to do intervention tasks. Ashley began to question the inconsistency of Anna's behaviors. Could Anna be experiencing poor sleep, resulting in the morning fatigue? But why the dizziness? Is Anna more depressed? If that is the case, why does she seem to be in a much better mood in the afternoon? Ashley also questions whether the behavioral differences could be related to the medications that Anna is taking. Ashley decides to consult with the treatment team about Anna's inconsistent behavior and her dizziness.

The other health care practitioners on the treatment team are a physical therapist, a nurse, a speech therapist, and a pharmacist. There is much discussion about Anna because other members of the treatment team have noticed her inconsistent behavior, too. Some members

suggest asking for lab work to review lab level values. The pharmacist, Roger, looks at Anna's medications and points out a possible correlation between the timing and the dosages of the medications with the behaviors that Anna is exhibiting. He questions whether Anna is experiencing some common side effects from the medications that she is taking and informs the team that he plans to consult about Anna's medication with her physician. The following week when Ashley follows Anna for the morning intervention sessions, she is much better focused. Ashley learns that as a result of the team meeting, Anna's medications were readjusted.

COTAs often work with elders on a daily basis in a variety of treatment settings. Because COTAs spend a considerable amount of time with the elder population, they are a valuable asset in addressing medication routines. COTAs also may convey vital information regarding medications and side effects to the health care team. When specific medication information is required, advice should be sought from a pharmacist or other medication expert. Common medications and medication-related problems encountered by elders are discussed in the chapter. Skills for self-medication and intervention programs for elders and caregivers are also discussed.

FACTORS AFFECTING MEDICATION RISK IN ELDERS

Elders consume the majority of prescription and over-the-counter (OTC) medications in the United States. Because of the aging population and individuals are living longer, often with chronic diseases that require medication therapy, it is no surprise that over 40% of elders in the community take at least five prescription medications.[1] When OTCs are included, the number of medications consumed per day often exceeds 10 or more. It is important to note that natural products (such as health foods, supplements, and vitamins) may also be consumed by this population. Yet because they are erroneously not considered medications by some, they may not be reported when an elder is questioned about medication use.

POLYPHARMACY

Several components contribute to the incidence of polypharmacy (use of multiple medications in a single individual). Sometimes the use of many medications is the right thing for patients to control their diseases and ensure a better quality of life. However, there are risks associated with polypharmacy. Drug interactions happen with increased frequency the more drugs that a person consumes. These interactions may include the increase or decrease in effectiveness of one drug caused by another or a more pronounced manifestation of an adverse event due to the elder taking two drugs that have a similar side-effect profile. In addition, sometimes new medications are introduced for the specific reason of offsetting a troublesome effect caused by another. Providing new medications may be appropriate, but this scenario often occurs because the problem is not recognized as drug-induced. Risk factors that contribute to polypharmacy include the use of multiple physicians with different specialties who may prescribe similar medications, the use of multiple pharmacies, inappropriate medication reconciliation upon discharge from the hospital, and the fact that elders often have multiple conditions requiring medication therapy.

PHYSIOLOGY AND THE AGING PROCESS

Many factors are involved in the increased incidence of medication-related adverse events in elders. With aging, kidney and liver functions decline. Many medications are excreted by the kidney and metabolized, or degraded, by the liver. Therefore, changes in organ function may frequently lead to drug accumulation in the body. This accumulation may result in toxic levels of drugs. To avoid drug accumulation, it is imperative that consideration be given to modifying doses for older individuals.

Although not all of the reasons are well understood, older persons tend to be more sensitive to the effects of certain medications. Body composition (lean tissue to fat ratio) changes as we age. Changes in body composition may result in alterations in how the body distributes a medication, making more or less of the drug available to have an effect. This is true for both the desired effects and for unwanted side effects. The adage "start low, go slow" should generally be used when initiating a new medication therapy in an older person.

ELDER MEDICATION USE AND IMPLICATIONS FOR THE COTA

When medical records are available, COTAs should always check the medication section to determine which medications are being used. This information helps COTAs be aware of possible side effects and drug interactions that might be observed with clinical intervention. COTAs should contact the elders' physicians and pharmacies with any medication-related concerns or questions. (Common drug-related abbreviations and definitions are listed in Table 13-1. Medications commonly used by elders are listed in Table 13-2. Note that this is not an all-inclusive listing of medications used by elders or those that may contribute to side effects. Only generic names are listed, and they should be cross-referenced with trade names when necessary.)

Cardiovascular diseases (high blood pressure, congestive heart failure, irregular heart rhythm, chest pain, heart attack, and stroke) are common in the older population. Medications used to treat these diseases may alter a patient's blood pressure and/or heart rate, resulting in dizziness and the potential for falls. One class of medication, the diuretics, may cause excessive urination. As such it is recommended that nighttime dosing be avoided because of the risk of falls and interruption in rest. COTAs may notice that the client needs frequent breaks during therapy to use the restroom, and that the timing of the medication dose may need to be altered to avoid this. Persons taking one or more of the medication types mentioned previously should be closely monitored during therapy for the emergence of side effects, and consideration should be given to routine monitoring of blood pressure by the COTA. In addition, many of these same clients will be using medications to treat high cholesterol.

TABLE 13-1

Common Drug-Related Terminology	
Abbreviations	**Definitions**
PO	By mouth
IM	Intramuscular
IV	Intravenous
SC or SQ	Subcutaneous
PR	Rectally
SL	Sublingually (under the tongue)
QD or Q Day	Once a day
BID	Twice daily
TID	Three times daily
QID	Four times daily
QOD	Every other day
PRN	As needed
AC	Before meals
PC	After meals

TABLE 13-2

Disease States, Medications, and Common Side Effects

Disease States	Medications	Common Side Effects
Cardiovascular (high blood pressure, congestive heart failure, high cholesterol, irregular heart rhythm, chest pain, heart attack, stroke)	ACE inhibitors (e.g., lisinopril, enalapril, captopril, benazepril, ramipril, fosinopril) Angiotensin receptor blockers (ARBs): (e.g., losartan, valsartan, irbesartan, candesartan, olmesartan) Beta blockers (e.g., metoprolol, carvedilol, atenolol, propranolol) Calcium channel blockers (e.g., amlodipine, felodipine, nifedipine, diltiazem, verapamil) Cholesterol medications (e.g., atorvastatin, simvastatin, lovastatin, rosuvastatin, pravastatin, gemfibrozil, fenofibrate, niacin, ezetimibe) Diuretics (e.g., hydrochlorothiazide, triamterene, furosemide, bumetanide, chlorthalidone, torsemide) Miscellaneous (e.g., clonidine, doxazosin, prazosin, terazosin, minoxidil)	Low blood pressure, dizziness, muscle pain, low heart rate, irregular heart rate, drowsiness, urinary frequency or incontinence, increased fall risk, fluid in the extremities/swelling, cough
Blood thinning agents	Warfarin, clopidogrel, aspirin, ticlopidine, prasugrel, enoxaparin, heparin, dalteparin	Bleeding, bruising
Pain medications	Nonsteroidal drugs (e.g., aspirin, ibuprofen, naproxen, celecoxib, meloxicam, diclofenac, ketorolac) Narcotics (e.g., codeine, hydrocodone, oxycodone, morphine, fentanyl, methadone) Miscellaneous (e.g., acetaminophen, tramadol)	Bleeding, bruising, gastrointestinal pain, swelling of the extremities, dizziness, drowsiness, increased fall risk, confusion, nausea, constipation, hallucinations
Psychiatric medications	Antidepressants (e.g., sertraline, fluoxetine, venlafaxine, mirtazapine, bupropion, citalopram, escitalopram, amitriptyline, trazodone) Antipsychotics (e.g., quetiapine, risperidone, haloperidol, olanzapine, aripiprazole) Anti-anxiety agents (e.g., diazepam, alprazolam, lorazepam, buspirone) Drugs for cognitive impairment (e.g., donepezil, rivastigmine, galantamine, memantine)	Drowsiness, dizziness, confusion, seizures, extrapyramidal side effects, nausea, diarrhea, weight loss
Sleep disorders	Diazepam, alprazolam, temazepam, lorazepam, trazodone, zolpidem, eszopiclone, zaleplon, diphenhydramine	Drowsiness, dizziness, increased fall risk, amnesia, hallucinations
Diabetes	Metformin, glipizide, glyburide, pioglitazone, rosiglitazone, insulin, exenatide, sitagliptin	Low blood sugar, dizziness, tremor, sweating, headache, confusion, nausea
Urge incontinence	Tolterodine, oxybutynin, dicyclomine, solifenacin, darifenacin, trospium	Dry mouth, dry eyes, urinary retention, constipation, elevated heart rate, inability to perspire

Some of these drugs may cause diffuse muscle pain when they are started, with a dose increase, or with the addition of another medication, which may increase blood levels of the former. The COTA can help identify this type of drug-induced musculoskeletal pain and see to it that it is addressed by the appropriate individual because, in some cases, the consequences of this side effect can be severe and even life threatening.

Drugs that affect the blood's ability to clot are also frequently used in persons with cardiovascular diseases. The COTA must be aware that the client is using one of these agents as the risk of a serious bleed is increased and therapy may have to be adjusted. One sign associated with the use of these medications is easy bruising. This is not necessarily unexpected, but if the COTA believes that the amount of bruising is excessive, he or she may wish to refer the patient to have the medication therapy evaluated.

Another common complaint of elders is pain, which can be either chronic (such as arthritis pain) or short-term because of an acute injury. The use of OTC pain medications is common when elders choose to self-treat. These medications include acetaminophen, aspirin, ibuprofen, and naproxen. Commonly observed side effects associated with these agents include gastrointestinal distress (which may be a symptom of a more serious condition such as a stomach ulcer) and increases in blood pressure because some of these medications can cause fluid retention. With more severe pain, prescription medications are used. Most prescription pain medications (primarily narcotics such as codeine, hydrocodone, oxycodone, and morphine) exert their action in the central nervous system and therefore may cause dizziness, drowsiness, and confusion. These symptoms add to the risk of falls and may make successful therapeutic intervention by the COTA a challenge if the client is unable to fully participate because of cognitive impairment.

Many older persons experience a variety of psychosocial, psychiatric, and cognitive disorders. Drugs that may be used to treat such diagnoses include antipsychotics, antidepressants, anti-anxiety agents, and medications used to slow the progression of cognitive impairment, such as those used in the treatment of Alzheimer's dementia. These medications are all active in the central nervous system and therefore have the potential to affect sensorium, alertness, and balance. Additionally, some of them may have effects on other body systems causing disturbances in sleep and bodily functions (dry eyes, dry mouth, urinary retention, constipation, elevated heart rate, and the inability to perspire). Some of the agents used to treat psychosis also cause extrapyramidal symptoms that may manifest as abnormal movements of the limbs, head, neck, and the tongue. Sometimes these symptoms can be controlled with another medication or by discontinuing the offending agent. However, other times the benefit of continuing the medication may outweigh the risk associated with developing these symptoms, and the client and COTA may need to find a way to work around them. Furthermore, use of these medications is likely to aid the COTA in working with a client when symptoms of these types of disorders are controlled.

Sleep disturbances are frequently encountered by the older person. Such disturbances include the inability to fall asleep, early morning awakening, and daytime drowsiness. Sleep-inducing medications are often used to help older persons sleep. However, it is important to note that as people age, they need fewer hours of sleep, and education of elders is necessary to help them differentiate between insomnia and the normal aging process as it pertains to sleep. Some sleep agents may cause clients to be drowsy during the morning hours, which may interfere with the therapy process. Proper sleep hygiene (going to bed and getting up at the same time each day, minimizing daytime napping, using the bed for sleep and sex only, and avoidance of caffeine and exercise late in the day) can make a large difference in the client's ability to fully participate in therapy. If daytime drowsiness is a concern, the COTA may wish to inquire about the use of sleep agents

(both prescription and OTC) to determine whether a change needs to be made.

As persons age, the diagnosis of diabetes becomes more common. Drugs used for the treatment of elevated blood glucose are associated with several side effects that may be observed by the COTA. The most common of these is hypoglycemia, or low-blood glucose. Symptoms associated with hypoglycemia include sweating, dizziness, weakness, tremor, elevated heart rate, and confusion. These symptoms may be more common if the client has not had a normal amount of food before therapy. Additionally, diabetes can cause impaired sensation in the extremities, also known as neuropathy. This can result in numbness or extreme pain and may present a substantial challenge for the COTA. It is important that therapy be tailored for elders with impaired sensation to ensure that they remain safe during therapy and in their living environment. Medications are available to help with the pain of neuropathy, and the COTA may wish to refer patients if the pain interferes with quality of life.

Although not a normal part of aging, urinary incontinence may be frequently encountered in the elderly population. Incontinence presents its own challenges such as those associated with frequent toileting and skin breakdown as a result of excessive exposure to moisture. Medications used to treat one type of incontinence, overactive bladder or "urge" incontinence, can cause a multitude of side effects similar to those mentioned as associated with the psychoactive medications (dry eyes, dry mouth, urinary retention, constipation, elevated heart rate, and the inability to perspire).

STRATEGIES FOR MINIMIZING MEDICATION PROBLEMS IN ELDERS

There are multiple reasons why older adults may be at higher risk for medication problems than younger persons. It is imperative that health care providers ensure that clients can safely manage their medications. Psychiatric diagnoses, such as dementia and depression, are common in this population and may affect the client's ability to manage drug therapy without assistance. Often the first indication that there may be a problem in this area is the inability to manage other daily tasks such as keeping good finances or managing basic household responsibilities.

The older generation is often apprehensive when it comes to questioning health care providers, and this may lead to a lack of active participation in their own care. In many cases, a medication regimen can be simplified, but if the health care provider is not asked to do this, it is unlikely to occur. Additionally, if information about medications or their side effects is not readily offered, an older person might not directly ask about such things, and this may lead to underrecognition of side effects. It is also important that clients understand why they are taking each medication and its intended purpose so that they may self-monitor for problems.

There are many reasons that clients may not adhere to a medication regimen as prescribed. Over-adherence may occur, either by mistake because clients cannot remember whether a medication has already been taken, or because they may believe that "if a little is good, more must be better." On the other hand, under-adherence also occurs for various reasons. Avoidance of side effects may lead a client to skip doses. Additionally, if money is a concern, clients may choose to alter their regimen by deliberately taking a medication less often than recommended. Cutting pills in half and taking partial doses is another common occurrence when saving money is an issue.

Self-treatment of symptoms or side effects with OTC medications may also result in problems. Although OTC medications are available without a prescription, it is incorrect to believe that they are without risks. Drug interactions may occur with medications that have previously been prescribed. It is also incorrect to believe that "natural" products are inherently safe because they, too, may interact with other drugs and cause side effects that may be more difficult to recognize because of a lack of regulation and standardization.

APPLICATION OF THE OCCUPATIONAL THERAPY PROCESS TO SELF-MEDICATION

Medication routines of clients are often not addressed by OT.[2] This is evident in the lack of literature on self-medication programs and OT interventions with medication routines. Medication routines are instrumental activities of daily living (IADL). According to the Occupational Therapy Practice Framework: Domain and Process (second edition), medication routines are classified as a health management and maintenance IADL.[3] Thus, assessment of routines and instruction in proper use of medication should be dealt with as part of activities of daily living (ADL) routines.[4] Participation in one's medication routine includes obtaining medication, opening and closing containers, following prescribed schedules, taking correct quantities, reporting problems and adverse effects, and administering correct quantities by using prescribed methods.

CLIENT FACTORS

Values, beliefs, spirituality, body functions, and body structures that reside within the client and may affect performance in medication routines should be analyzed by the registered occupational therapist (OTR) and COTA. This section overviews how each of these client factors can potentially impact one's medication routine.

Values, Beliefs, and Spirituality

A variety of factors related to adherence to medication routines has been researched, including people's values and beliefs. The self-regulations theory[5,6] is a patient-centered understanding to such factors that affect adherence. The theory suggests that people attempt to understand their illness by developing a representation of their illness, its causes, its effects, the duration of the illness, and whether the illness can be cured or controlled. In this view, it is thought that people are motivated to reduce their health-related risks and will work on eliminating health threats in ways that are congruent with their perceptions.

In addition to forming representations of illness, it is hypothesized that clients also form representations of their treatments.[7] Researchers have demonstrated the link between values and behaviors.[8-10] Decisions about taking medication are likely to be affected by the beliefs about the medicines, the illness, and the treatment providers.[11] Values are often the underpinnings of behaviors. People typically decide what is important for them and then act on such decisions. Although a paucity of literature exists on the influence of spirituality on medication routines, persons diagnosed with terminal illnesses have reported a high level of spirituality (and they have been correlated highly with psychological adaptation and positive health outcomes).[12-14]

Bodily Functions

Bodily functions are "physiological functions of body systems (including psychological functions)" (p. 635).[3] Bodily functions affect one's ability to perform and participate in an occupation. Medication routines require extensive performance from multiple bodily functions, including the following:
- Mental functions
- Sensory functions and pain
- Neuromusculoskeletal and movement-related functions
- Cardiovascular, hematological, immunological, and respiratory system function
- Voice and speech function
- Digestive, metabolic, and endocrine system function
- Genitourinary and reproductive functions
- Skin and related structure functions

Mental Functions

Both long-term and a working memory[15] are required for independent self-medication. Elders need long-term memory to understand which condition is being treated and the purpose for the medication(s) they take. Understanding and remembering the nature of the regimen also is required for self-medication. Elders use long-term memory to remember where the medication is stored. Working memory, which includes simultaneous storing and processing of information, is needed to avoid under medication or overmedication. This frequently occurs when elders do not remember whether they took a medication. Various items such as programmable alarms or auditory devices that exclaim, "time to take your pill," and pill storage boxes can aid self-medication. Home health aides and pharmacists may assist in filling self-medication boxes.

A fee may be charged for this service. One advantage of involving home health aid or a pharmacist is that they can make sure the elder is actually taking the medicine, as prescribed, when it is time to refill the storage container.

A great deal of problem solving is needed to properly self-medicate. Elders must decide whether to contact the physician when changes in a condition occur. For example, Ken goes to his physician because he wonders whether his frequent headaches indicate that his blood pressure medication is not working or whether he needs a new prescription for his glasses. Problem solving also is needed to determine when refills need to be obtained and how to safely store medication. Even more complex is the problem solving that is needed to determine Medicare prescription plan options.[16] Some pharmacies and health care agencies will provide individualized consults for elders who need assistance in understanding and choosing such plans.

Elders must be motivated to comply with their medication regimen. Depression, uncertainty, misunderstanding, financial worries, lack of confidence, side effects, and social or cultural taboos are all factors that may contribute to a lack of motivation. For example, Hazel, a 74-year-old woman with a history of heart failure and high blood pressure, sometimes takes her captopril tablets once a day instead of three times a day. Hazel does this when she feels "better" to save money. In addition, some elders are embarrassed by the diagnosis of depression, or other emotional disorders, and are reluctant to take prescribed antidepressants or other medicines used to treat psychological problems.

Sensory Functions and Pain

Visual perception skills may be required by elders who take multiple medications. Visual perception skills include color discrimination, depth perception, and figure-ground perception. Visual acuity and perception are required to distinguish between different containers of medication and to read instruction labels. If needed, glasses should be worn when elders self-medicate. Adaptations may be used to assist elders who have visual impairments (Figure 13-1). Magnifying lenses and large type or contrasting print may be helpful. For severe visual impairments, different size, different shape, or multicolor containers can be used for medication storage. Instructions for administration can be tape recorded to relay information that cannot be read. Depth perception skills are needed to obtain pills in a multipartition container. Figure-ground perception also is needed to see white pills in a white pill box. COTAs should suggest that elders use colored pill containers for white pills.

According to the Deafness Research Foundation, there is a relationship between age and hearing loss. For example, 30% of adults who are ages 65 to 74 years and 47% of adults age 75 years and older have a hearing impairment.[17] COTAs should remember this when educating elders, family members, and caregivers. The ability

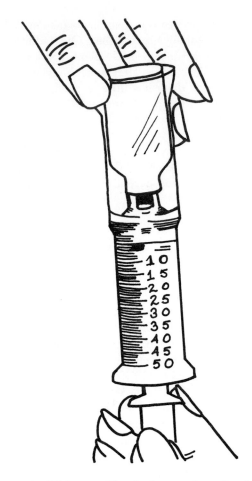

FIGURE 13-1 This magnifier device consists of a plastic cylinder in which the medication and syringe fit at each end and permits elders with visual impairments to view amounts easily.

to hear is important for elders to understand patient education, medication dosages, and changes. COTAs should provide both verbal and written instructions when educating elders. For example, Kathy, a COTA, meets with Vladimir, who has difficulty hearing, to review his discharge program. She first checks to make sure Vladimir is wearing his hearing aid and then reviews the information in his client education packet. Kathy speaks slowly and clearly and is sitting directly at eye level with Vladimir. She also frequently asks Vladimir whether he has any questions and encourages him to repeat back to her what he understands (see Chapter 16).

Neuromusculoskeletal and Movement-Related Functions

Usually a great deal of fine motor coordination, finger dexterity, and some degree of strength are needed to open and close medication containers and use syringes. Fine grasp patterns are required when picking up pills or tablets. Therefore, elders with conditions such as rheumatoid arthritis or Parkinson's disease may have difficulty opening childproof containers. Non-childproof tops can be provided by the pharmacist, if requested. If nonsafety caps are dispensed by the pharmacist, it is essential that elders store their medication out of the reach of children.

Manipulating medication containers requires strength. Occasionally, a medication routine involves crushing pills or splitting them in half. Such assists as pill crushers and pill splitters can help an elder who has poor hand strength. Elders should never use a razor blade to cut tablets. Many medications are released over time (known as *extended* or *sustained release*) and should not be crushed. A pharmacist is an invaluable resource person to find out whether a tablet can be crushed. Furthermore, sometimes a liquid form of the medication (if available) may be a better choice for an elder who needs to crush several medicines.

Elders taking medications need to have a way of getting prescriptions filled on a regular basis. Elders who do not drive or are wheelchair-bound may need to seek out community resources to obtain rides to medical appointments and the pharmacy. Some pharmacies will deliver medications for a fee. In addition, some communities have volunteer programs that provide this transportation service at no cost. For example, Antonio is unable to drive because of his poor vision, but he is able to renew prescriptions by using a free transportation service provided by his church. Automated systems are available at many pharmacies, which allow people to renew their prescriptions over the phone. Some pharmacies also provide automatic refill service for maintenance prescription medications.

It is estimated that 35% to 68% of persons over age 65 have some degree of swallowing dysfunction.[18] Patients and caregivers (N = 477) were surveyed about swallowing medicine. Results of the survey included 68% of persons reported opening a capsule or crushing a tablet, whereas 64% reported not taking their medication because of difficulty swallowing. Health professionals must facilitate medication routines of patients who cannot properly swallow medications by reviewing regimens, omitting medications that are unnecessary, and determining alternative forms of medications when needed.

Cardiovascular, Hematological, Immunological, and Respiratory System Function

Some medications, including nebulizers and inhalers, require the ability to inhale medication through the mouth or nostrils. Inhalers are used to deliver medication directly to the lungs. A nebulizer is a type of inhaler that is used to spray a fine mist of medication through the use of a mask. A mouthpiece is often connected to a machine and plastic tubing to deliver the medication to the person. Inspiration must be satisfactory to receive the medication.

Voice and Speech Functions

Elders must be able to communicate their medication regimen with health care providers and caregivers. Health care providers must reciprocate communication in an effective manner. Demonstration, web-based, verbal, and written formats can be used for communication. Elders may find it helpful to keep names, phone numbers, and addresses of health care providers and agencies in a regular place so they are available for emergencies. Posting this information on the refrigerator may also be helpful. For example, Greta has been deaf since birth but is able to communicate by using a notebook that contains information regarding her past and present medical condition. She stores this notebook in a drawer in the nightstand by her bed. She also has notified family members where the notebook is located in case of an emergency.

Skin and Related Structure Functions

Some topical medications must not be applied to open wounds. Thus, the skin must be free from wounds, abrasions, and cuts.

ACTIVITY DEMANDS

Medication routines involve activity demands. According to the Occupational Therapy Practice Framework, activity demands are "aspects of an activity, which include the objects and their properties, space, social demands, sequencing or timing, required actions and skills, and required underlying body functions and body structure needed to carry out the activity" (p. 638).[3] Aspects of activity demands include the following:

- Objects and their properties
- Space demands
- Social demands
- Sequence and timing
- Required actions and performance skills
- Required body functions
- Required body structures

Table 13-3 offers examples of activity demands typically involved in medication routines.

Performance Skills

Performance skills include the abilities demonstrated while performing the actions.[3] Skills include motor and praxis, sensory perceptual, emotional regulation, cognitive, and communication and social skills. Examples of performance skills required during medication routines are presented in Table 13-4.

OCCUPATIONAL THERAPY PROCESS

According to the Occupational Therapy Practice Framework,[3] evaluation, intervention, and outcomes comprise the process of occupational therapy. Evaluation includes the occupational profile and analysis of occupational performance. Intervention constitutes the plan, implementation, and review. Finally, the outcomes are the determination of success of the desired outcomes. The following outlines the process as applied to medication routines.

The occupational profile is "the initial step in the evaluation process that provides an understanding of the

TABLE 13-3

Activity Demands and Examples Related to Medication Routines

Activity demand aspect	Examples related to medication routine
Objects and their properties	Common objects used in medication routines include pill bottles, pill storage boxes, syringes, inhalers, tubes, gloves, etc.
Space demands	Space to complete a medication routine commonly requires appropriate lighting to see what one is doing, ample room to manipulate any equipment or objects used, and proper space for medication storage. Occasionally, medication must be stored in special environments—for example, environments that adhere to recommended temperature ranges and restricted exposure to sunlight.
Social demands	Medication routines require communicating when one may need medication to refill prescriptions or report outcomes or concerns to one's physician(s).
Sequence and timing	Medication routines often require timing of medication. Occasionally, medications must be taken properly throughout the day. For example, sequencing the medication routine involves selecting the container, opening the container, securing the medication tablet, and swallowing the medication.
Required actions and performance skills	Skills used to perform medication routines include opening and closing containers, manipulating any objects needed in medication routines, etc.
Required body functions	Body functions needed in medication routine often include mental, neuromusculoskeletal, and speech functions.
Required body structures	Body structures often needed to perform medication routines include use of hands, eyes, etc.

TABLE 13-4

Examples of Skills Needed for Medication Routines

Skill	Example
Motor and praxis skills	Planning and executing movements to successfully open and close medication containers; maintaining balance while taking medication; adjusting posture, for example, to extend neck when applying eye drops.
Sensory perceptual skills	Sensing that a pill is on your tongue and ready to be swallowed; feeling relief after an anti-itch cream has been applied to an itchy and irritated area; seeing the volume marks on a syringe.
Cognitive skills	Ability to recognize when one needs a prescription refill; ability to remember taking medication, judging whether the symptoms being addressed are getting better, worse, or staying the same.
Communication and social skills	Ability to communicate with family, caretakers, pharmacists, and physicians about one's medication routine; ability to answer questions posed by health care providers and caretakers about medication routine.

client's occupational history and experiences, patterns of daily living, interests, values, and needs. The client's problems and concerns about performing occupations and daily life activities are identified, and the client's priorities are determined" (p. 646).[3] COTAs often assist in gathering information from the client during the profile. Questions and items to be used as part of the occupational profile related to medication routines include the following:

■ Tell me about any medications you take. Don't forget to include prescriptions, OTC medications, supplements, and natural products.
■ Tell me about any vitamins or nutritional supplements you use.
■ Describe your routine of taking medications.

■ Describe any concerns you might have about your medication routine.

Depending on the issues that arise from the occupational profile, the therapist may determine to analyze the person's performance related to the medication routine. Analysis of occupational performance is "the step in the evaluation process during which the client's assets, problems, or potential problems are more specifically identified. Actual performance is often observed in context to identify what supports performance and what hinders performance. Performance skills, performance patterns, context or contexts, activity demands, and client factors are all considered, but only selected aspects may be specifically assessed. Targeted outcomes are identified" (p. 646).[3] For example, a therapist may suspect that the elder's grip strength is insufficient to open a medication container and thus test grip strength using a dynamometer or asking the person to open his or her medication container(s). Based on the analysis of occupational performance, the therapist is able to plan intervention.

The intervention plan consists of "a plan that will guide actions taken and that is developed in collaboration with the client. It is based on selected theories, frames of reference, and evidence. Outcomes to be targeted are confirmed" (p. 646).[3] For example, the therapist may use a rehabilitative frame of reference and focus on the person's abilities and compensate for disability. Thus, the therapist may decide that the person's grip strength is not sufficient to open childproof medication containers and has the client practice opening a container that is not childproof. The therapist may provide information on how to request such containers for future prescriptions. This action is the intervention implementation, or the "ongoing actions taken to influence and support improved client performance. Interventions are directed at identified outcomes. Client's response is monitored and documented" (p. 646).[3] The therapist will then review "the implementation plan and process as well as its progress toward targeted outcomes" (p. 646).[3] The following section addresses ideas for medication intervention with elders.

ASSISTIVE AIDS FOR SELF-MEDICATION

Many commercial or homemade aids can assist individuals with self-medication.[19] Each aid has advantages and disadvantages.

Commercial Aids

Calendars

Calendars are helpful for tracking medication schedules. A pocket calendar or a calendar hung near the place where medication is taken can be used to mark each time medication is taken. At the end of the day, marks are counted to make sure that the medication schedule was followed. The advantage of using calendars is that the medications are stored in their original containers and remain properly labeled. Calendars are also inexpensive and readily available. The disadvantage of using a calendar is that it requires some basic reading, comprehension, and memory skills to mark the calendar each time medications are taken.[19]

Pill storage boxes/storage boxes

For people who take medications on a regular basis, a pill box or pill reminder is a useful item. Pill storage boxes are containers with compartments in which to put medications (Figure 13-2). Pill boxes are easy to use and can be useful to adhere to one's medication schedule regardless of whether one is at home or traveling. Pill boxes are organized daily, weekly, or monthly. Some have the capacity to organize medications throughout the day (e.g., breakfast, lunch, and dinner). Added features such as locks or timers and alarms can be ideal when safety is a concern

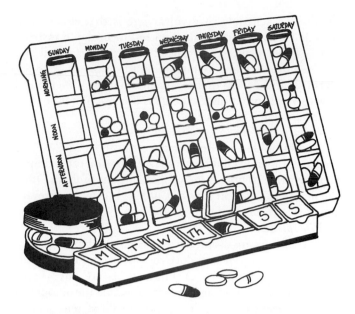

FIGURE 13-2 Various pill boxes are available with compartments for single or multiple daily and weekly doses.

or when a cognitive reminder is needed. Some boxes are made to look like jewelry. There is certainly one likely to be available to suit one's needs and style.

Pill boxes require manual dexterity skills to open and close and to manipulate pills. Visual discrimination also is required to identify desired pills. Pill boxes usually do not provide tight storage for medications that require tight containers, such as nitroglycerin. In addition, the pills are no longer in labeled, childproof containers.

There are advantages and disadvantages for using daily and 7-day pill boxes.[19] An advantage of a daily pill box is a better chance of taking all daily doses. Any errors made in setting up this pill box would be experienced for one day only. A disadvantage of a daily pill box is that each compartment could contain several unlabeled pills. The elder would have to identify the medication(s) by physical appearance. This is a serious safety concern if pills are similar in size, shape, or color, especially if the elder has impaired vision or is easily confused.

Weekly pill boxes store medication for 7 days. The design of some pill boxes allows the separation of multiple daily doses. These boxes often consist of four rows and seven columns. The four rows are marked with times of the day (morning, noon, evening, and bedtime), and the seven columns are marked with the day of the week. The advantage of using a 7-day pill box is that setup is required once a week only. The disadvantage is that setup requires more accuracy.[19] If there is a mistake, it may occur seven times.

A pill box with an alarm is an option for elders who must take their medication at specific times. The advantage of this type of pill box is that it alerts elders of the medication schedule. A disadvantage is that elders must be able to read, understand, and follow in-depth instructions. These devices often need to be programmed and may require very fine manipulation to set the clock or the alarm. If the device breaks, repairs may be difficult and expensive. Another disadvantage is the risk of not hearing the alarm when it sounds.

Insulin holders

Insulin holders are intended for one-handed use. The device holds an insulin bottle so that a person can manipulate a syringe to obtain the proper amount of fluid. Often the device has suction cups or a nonskid surface to prevent the device from sliding on a table top.

Pill splitters

Pill splitters are useful devices when a pill must be split for proper dosage or to reduce the pill size for easier swallowing (when appropriate). Pill splitters are often lightweight and use a leverage design to reduce the amount of strength needed to use it. As previously stated, a razor blade should never be used to cut a tablet.

Pill crushers

A pill crusher is a device used to pulverize tablets into a fine powder. Similar to the design of pill splitters, pill crushers use a leverage system so that an abundance of strength is not required. Pill crushers can be beneficial when individuals have difficulty swallowing whole tablets. (Remember that not all tablets can be crushed or split.)

Talking and shaking alarms, watches, and prescription bottles

For elders who experience difficulty remembering to take their medications or what their medication routine is, several devices such as talking or shaking alarms and talking prescription bottles may be beneficial. Talking alarms are devices that are programmed to send a "beep," voice message, or visual cue when it is time to take a medication. Shaking alarms can be clipped to the bedding to wake elders when it is time to take their medication. The device can be put in one's pocket when in public and it will provide a quiet vibration to indicate the medication time. A talking prescription bottle is a device attached to a prescription bottle. A pharmacist or physician records the prescription information into the device. To operate, one pushes a button on the device to play a recorded message about the contents; how many pills to take, when, and what for; and any warnings. The talking prescription bottle is intended for those who have low vision or hearing impairments. It is also beneficial for elders for whom English is a second language or for elders who have difficulty reading.

Homemade Aids

Medication diary

A medication diary is another aid for tracking medication use (Table 13-5).

TABLE 13-5

Contents of a Medication Diary	
Section	**Information**
1: Demographics	Name Date Address Phone number Date of birth Medication allergies: date of occurrence and type of reaction Vaccinations (year, date) Flu shots (year, date)
2: Health care providers	List names and phone numbers of all health care providers (tape their business cards here).
3: Past medications	List all medical conditions that required treatment with medication over the years. List all medical conditions that currently require treatment with medication.
4: Special equipment	List all adaptive or special equipment required (such as a nebulizer, ostomy products, and incontinence products). Include the brand, size, and model, and the supplier's name and phone number.
5: Recent medications	Enter the name of new medications used, the date, the reason the medication is being used, the strength of the medication, and how often the medication is taken each day. Keep track of any dosage changes, discontinuation, the date, and the reason for the change or discontinuation.
6: Over-the-counter medications	List any over-the-counter medications used for the eyes, ears, skin, and other organs and tissues. Enter how often the medications are used.
7: Questions for health care providers	List any questions to ask the doctor or pharmacist.

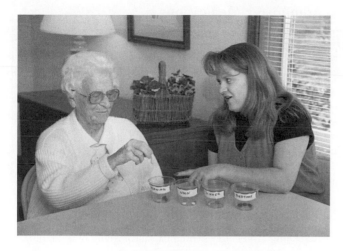

FIGURE 13-3 Storage pill cups can be made at home by simply using small plastic or paper cups.

COTAs may assist elders in making a diary, which can be kept in a notebook. This information can then be shared with other health care professionals, as needed.

Storage cups

Storage cups can be made at home by using small plastic or paper cups that are stacked and ordered according to the number of times the medication must be taken throughout the day. The cups should be marked in relation to when medications are taken (for example, morning, noon, dinner, and bedtime) (Figure 13-3). After the morning medication is taken, the "morning" cup is moved to the bottom of the stack. This allows the next medication dose to be on the top. This system requires that elders have good manual dexterity, visual-perceptual, and memory skills. A similar system can be made using egg cartons. For liquid or powder medications, a system can be set up using small, labeled, airtight containers. Using a homemade system is simple and inexpensive. However, using a homemade system may cause medication to be exposed to improper storage conditions.[19] Also, pills in open view may tempt small children who live in or visit the elder's home. This risk can be reduced by storing the medication out of view and reach.

SELF-MEDICATION PROGRAM

A formal self-medication program may prevent problems with polypharmacy.[2] The program is designed to (1) use an interdisciplinary team approach, (2) educate elders about their medications, (3) develop elders' motor skills for proper administration, (4) offer practice opportunities to elders, (5) assess elders for any adaptive devices that may be useful, and (6) evaluate elders' skills in medication administration before discharge.

The elders' intervention plan should include interventions to maximize independence with self-medication. Depending on elders' limitations and deficits, COTAs should engage them in simulated medication tasks. An example of such a task is using small, colored candy pieces to practice color discrimination and fine prehensile patterns. Reading and comprehending general labels can aid in reading medication labels. Opening and closing medication containers should be practiced. In addition, elders should master any adaptive aids before being discharged from OT.

Relatives, friends, and home care personnel who assist in the delivery of medications often have not been included in discussions of medications.[20] Family and caregivers should be able to name the elder's medications, describe the purpose of each medication, and describe any precautions associated with each medication. COTAs can refer to Box 13-1 to help educate family and other caregivers. Box 13-2 addresses safety issues for COTAs' consideration.

CASE STUDY

Pat is an 83-year-old woman living at home with her 85-year-old husband. Pat is currently under the care of two physicians: her primary medical physician and a psychiatrist. Pat has a recent history of falls and has significant bruising on her forehead. One of her falls occurred in the middle of the night while she was attempting to walk to the bathroom. Additionally, she complains of dizziness and pain in her knees, which affects her ability to participate in events outside of her home.

Two weeks ago Pat fell and fractured her hip. Her mental status fluctuates. Her husband is in charge of administering medications. Her problems and medications are listed as follows:

Disease state	Medication	Dosage
Congestive heart failure	Furosemide (diuretic or water pill)	40 mg po bid
	Metoprolol XL (beta blocker)	100 mg po once daily
	Lisinopril (ace inhibitor)	10 mg po once daily
Anxiety	Lorazepam (anti-anxiety)	0.5 mg po tid
Osteoarthritis	Naproxen (pain reliever)	500 mg po bid
Depression	Sertraline (antidepressant)	50 mg po once daily
Insomnia	Diphenhydramine (nonprescription sleep aid)	25 mg po hs prn
Prevention of blood clots after surgery	Warfarin (blood thinner)	2.5 mg po once daily

■ CASE STUDY QUESTIONS

1 Which medication-related problems might be of concern to COTAs?
2 Could any of Pat's current medical problems be caused by her medications? If so, which medications cause which side effects? (Refer to Table 13-2.)
3 What other factors may place Pat at risk for polypharmacy and medication-related problems?
4 The COTA is concerned about the frequency of Pat's falls and the risk for another hip fracture but is unsure whether any medications are contributing to the falls. What is a

BOX 13-1

Guidelines for Caregivers Who Administer Medications

Elders most at risk to experience problems with medications are those who are:

- Seeing more than one physician
- Taking many medications
- Using more than one pharmacy

Keep track of the following information on the elder(s) you are caring for:

- All of the prescription drugs the elder is taking
- All of the nonprescription (OTC) drugs the elder is taking
- All other medicinal items the elder uses from a health food store or supermarket
- When and how much medicine to give
- What results to expect from the medicine
- Any physical or mental change in the elder (report to physician)
- What to do if a dose is missed

Prescriptions

The need for the medications should be reevaluated at least every 3 to 6 months.

Do not save unused medication for future use without the physician's approval. Take the entire course of any antibiotic that is prescribed.

Do not share medications with anyone. Closely check expiration dates and dispose of expired medicine.

If you are not clear about what the directions you are given mean, clarify them with your pharmacist or the prescriber. For instance, look at the following directions:

- Take as directed.
- Take before meals.
- Take as needed.
- Take four times a day.
- What does four times a day really mean?
- Does it mean every 6 hours? Does it mean with meals and at bedtime?
- Does before meals mean before each meal or on an empty stomach?
- How often is it safe to take a medication prescribed on an "as needed" basis?

These are the types of questions that a patient or caregiver should ask.

Written directions should always be given, and "take as directed" should not be considered adequate direction.

To reduce the risk for aspiration and swallowing problems, never give tablets or capsules while the elder is lying down. Always give medications with plenty of fluids to reduce stomach upset unless directed otherwise.

Medication storage

Store medications properly. Keep them in a cool, dry place, away from the sunlight and away from children. Keep the label on the medication container until all medicine is used or destroyed. If traveling, take the original medicine container with you in case of an emergency.

Medication disposal

Do not flush medications down the toilet unless the label or instructions specifically tell you to do so. Find out whether there is a drug take-back program in your community by calling your city or county. If such a program is not available, discard medications as follows:

Take the drugs out of their original containers. Mix them with an undesirable substance (kitty litter, used coffee grounds). Seal the mixture in a disposable container and place in the trash. Make sure that personal information and prescription numbers are made illegible, and discard the original medication containers.

Take precautions with the following:

- Chewable tablets: Elders often do not like chewable tablets because they can interfere with dentures. One option is to have the elder suck on the tablet to dissolve it. Chewable tablets should not be swallowed whole.
- Crushing tablets or opening capsules: Many pills should not be crushed because they are designed to be long-acting. Other pills should not be crushed because the contents may cause stomach upset or inflammation.

Always check with the pharmacist. Occasionally, a liquid substitute is available.

- Liquid medications: Because liquid medications are difficult to measure accurately, ask the pharmacist for a measuring device to ensure the correct dose.
- Applying ointments: Because medications applied to the elder's skin will have an effect on your skin, wash hands after each application. Use gauze or gloves to apply.
- Applying patches: Always remove old patches. Know how often and where to apply the patch on the body. Remove old patches gently because elders have delicate skin. Notify the pharmacist if the skin becomes irritated or the patch does not stick.
- Giving injections: Practice administration techniques with a nurse or pharmacist.
- Tube feedings: Tube feedings with medication require special instructions. Liquid medications, if available, work best when medicine needs to be given down a feeding tube. Some medications may actually directly interact with the enterable supplement. Contact the pharmacist for instructions on exactly how to give the medication.

Discharge plans from the hospital or nursing home

This can be a very confusing time! Medications often change while the elder is in the hospital. Everyone must know which medications to take and which not to take.

- Know about any generic drugs. Tablets or capsules may look different and have a different name, but the medications contain the same ingredient in the same amount. Keep an accurate list or bring all of the medications when visiting every doctor. Shop at one pharmacy to avoid medication duplication. If moving to another area, ask the pharmacist to forward your prescription records to your new pharmacist.
- Monitor the elder's nutrition, diet, and fluids. Pay attention to the elder's appetite, and notify the physician if there are any concerns such as weight gain or loss. Know whether the elder requires a special diet, including foods/liquids to avoid and to encourage. Administer medication by offering plenty of liquids, unless otherwise instructed.

BOX 13-2

Safety Gems for COTAs to Consider with Medication Provision and Elders

- Critically consider and bring forward concerns about possible common medication side effects for symptoms that the elder may be exhibiting.
- Be aware of possible medication side effects that may cause symptoms that could lead to safety issues such as falls or cognitive impairment. (Refer to Table 13-2.)
- Share results of assessments (particularly cognitive, communication skills, neuromuscular and movement, and sensory assessment findings) with members of the treatment team to help inform others about the elder's ability to safely manage and self-administer medications.
- Communicate any medication issues, such as the alteration of medications to save money or difficulty with a particular dosage form (for instance, those that need to be swallowed), with appropriate team members.
- Make appropriate adaptations so that elders can safely take medications.

reasonable course of action to address this plausible medication-related concern?

5 What skills for safe self-medication are affected in Pat's case?
6 What assistive devices may help with her medication routine and why?
7 Who should be involved in a self-medication program to help Pat with her medications?

CHAPTER REVIEW QUESTIONS

1 Considering the information in the chapter, explain why the COTA is an important player in the health care team to address medication issues with elders.
2 What are some reasons for polypharmacy among elders?
3 What is one side effect of each of the following: diuretics, OTC and prescription pain relievers, antidepressants/antipsychotics, and insulin? (Refer to Table 13-2.)
4 What resources and personnel are available to address the concerns or questions of COTAs regarding medications?
5 Explain skills needed for safe self-medication.
6 What aids are available to elders with poor vision, memory, or hearing, or lack of transportation?
7 What should be included in a medication diary?
8 What are some essential components to a self-medication program?
9 What information should COTAs provide to educate caregivers?

REFERENCES

1. Wilson, I.B., Schoen, C., Neuman, P., Strollo, M.K., Rogers, W.H., Chang, H., et al., 2007. Physician-patient communication about prescription medication nonadherence: A 50-state study of America's seniors. Journal of General Internal Medicine 22, 6-12.
2. Potts, J.M., 1994. Developing a patient self-medication program for the rehabilitation setting. Rehabilitation Nursing 19, 344.
3. American Occupational Therapy Association, 2008. Occupational therapy practice framework: Domain and process, 2nd ed. American Journal of Occupational Therapy 62, 625-683.
4. Lewis, S.C., 1989. Elder Care in Occupational Therapy. Slack, Thorofare, NJ.
5. Diefenbach, M.A., Leventhal, H., 1996. The common-sense model of illness representation: Theoretical and practical considerations. Journal of Social Distress and the Homeless 5, 11-38.
6. Leventhal, H., Benyamini, Y., Brownlee, S., Diefenbach, M., Leventhal, E.A., Patrick-Miller, L., et al., 1997. Illness representations: Theoretical foundations. In: Petrie, K.J., Weinman, J.A. (Eds.), Perceptions of Health and Illness: Current Research and Applications. Harwood Academic, Singapore, pp. 19-45.
7. Gauchet, A., Tarquinio, C., Fischer, G., 2007. Psychosocial predictors of medication adherence among persons living with HIV. International Journal of Behavioral Medicine 14 (3), 141-150.
8. Church, R.M., 1987. Pharmacy practice in the Indian Health Service. American Journal of Hospital Pharmacy 44 (4), 771-775.
9. Lefley, H.P., 1990. Culture and chronic mental illness. Hospital and Community Psychiatry 41 (3), 277-286.
10. Whetstone, W.R., Reid, J.C., 1991. Health promotion of older adults: Perceived barriers. Journal of Advanced Nursing 16 (11), 1343-1349.
11. Horne, R., 1997. Representations of medication and treatment: Advances in theory and measurement. In: Petrie, K.J., Weinman, J. (Eds.), Perceptions of Health and Illness: Current Research and Applications. Harwood Academic, London, pp. 155-187.
12. Margolin, A., Schuman-Olivier, Z., Beitel, M., Arnold, R.M., Fulwiler, C.E., et al., 2007. A preliminary study of spiritual self-schema (3-S[+]) therapy for reducing impulsivity of HIV-positive drug users. Journal of Clinical Psychology 63 (10), 979-999.
13. Ironson, G., Stuetzle, R., Fletcher, M.A., 2006. An increase in religiousness/spirituality occurs after HIV diagnosis and predicts slower disease progression over 4 years in people with HIV. Journal of General Internal Medicine 21 (Suppl 5), S62-S68.
14. Leach, C.R., Schoenberg, N.E., 2008. Striving for control: Cognitive, self-care, and faith strategies employed by vulnerable black and white older adults with multiple chronic conditions. Journal of Cross-Cultural Gerontology 23 (4), 377-399.
15. Andiel, C., Liu, L., 1995. Working memory and older adults: Implications for occupational therapy. American Journal of Occupational Therapy 49, 681-686.
16. Tseng, C.W., Dudley, R.A., Brook, R.H., Keeler, E., Hixon, A.L., Manlucu, L.R., Mangione, C.M., 2009. Elderly patients' knowledge of drug benefit caps and communication with providers about exceeding caps. Journal of the American Geriatric Society 57, 848-854.
17. Deafness Research Foundation, 2008. Statistics. Retrieved January 27, 2010, from http://www.drf.org/Statistics.
18. Kelly, J., D'Cruz, G., Wright, D., 2009. A qualitative study of the problems surrounding medication administration to patients with dysphagia. Dysphagia 24, 49-56.
19. Meyer, M.E., 1993. Coping with medications. Singular, San Diego, CA.
20. Wieder, A.J., Wolf-Klein, G.P., 1994. When medications change, tell the caregiver, too. Geriatrics 49, 48.

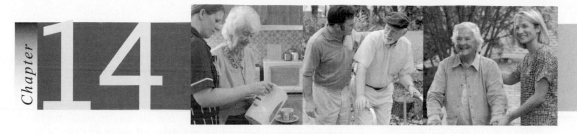

Considerations of Mobility

TRACY MILIUS, CANDICE MULLENDORE, IVELISSE LAZZARINI, CYNTHIA GOODMAN, LOU JENSEN, SANDRA HATTORI OKADA, PENNI JEAN LAVOOT, MICHELE LUTHER-KRUG, AND MARY ELLEN KEITH

KEY TERMS

restraints, restraint reduction, environmental adaptations, psychosocial approaches, activity alternatives, fall prevention, aging in place, environmental hazards, mobility, transit, driving, pedestrian, paratransit, wheelchair assessment, wheelchair selection, bariatric wheelchair assessment

CHAPTER OBJECTIVES

1. Discuss the Omnibus Budget Reconciliation Act regulations pertaining to the use of physical restraints.
2. Describe the steps in the establishment of a restraint reduction program.
3. Describe the role of the certified occupational therapy assistant in restraint reduction.
4. Outline the basic steps in evaluating the fit of a wheelchair.
5. Describe the major precautions to consider when elders should use wheelchairs.
6. Describe essential considerations when evaluating and fitting a bariatric person with a wheelchair.
7. Identify three reasons that elder adults are at a greater risk for falls than the general population.

8. Identify environmental, biological, psychosocial, and functional causes of falls.
9. Describe key considerations during the evaluation process for elder adults at risk for falls.
10. Describe recommended and evidence-based interventions to prevent falls.
11. Discuss potential desired outcomes of fall prevention interventions.
12. Discuss ways elders may gain access to public transportation.
13. Describe ways elders may become safer pedestrians.
14. Describe a driving evaluation, and identify criteria for this assessment.
15. Describe visual and physical changes in elders that may affect their ability to drive.

TRACY MILLIUS, CANDICE MULLENDORE, AND IVELISSE LAZZARINI

PART 1 Restraint Reduction

The use of physical restraints in health care practice has been common for many years.[1] The American health care system has used physical restraints throughout the continuum of care ranging from hospital emergency rooms, psychiatric units and med-surgical units, to nursing homes and other institutions. However, there continues to be mounting evidence of patient safety risks related to the use of physical restraints.[2]

In 1987, the Omnibus Budget Reconciliation Act of 1987[3] (OBRA) was implemented, and it forbid the use of physical restraints for the purposes of discipline or staff convenience in nursing homes. However, the use of physical restraints continues in nursing homes in the United States, but it is declining. In 2006 the Centers for Medicare & Medicaid Services (CMS) tightened the regulations regarding the use of restraints by requiring health

BOX 14-1

Negative Effects of Restraints

Psychosocial	Physical
Depression	Hazards of immobility
Lethargy	Incontinence
Withdrawal	Constipation
Anxiety	Disturbed spell pattern
Distress	Loss of balance
Fear	Falls
Panic	Pressure ulcers
Anger	Bone demineralization
Agitation	Loss of muscle tone and mass
Increased aggression	Respiratory difficulties
Reduced opportunity	Pneumonia
for social contact	Infection
Threat to identity	Thrombophlebitis
Embarrassment	Dehydration
Humiliation	Impaired circulation
Demoralization	Respiratory problems
Decreased feelings of	Orthostatic hypotension
dignity	Decreased appetite
Decreased sense of	Decreased ability to care for
self-esteem	self
Decreased autonomy	Abrasions
Helplessness	Cuts
Dependence	Bruises
Regression	Decreased functional status
Increased confusion	Loss of freedom
Increased disorientation	Death caused by suffocation
Increased disorganized	or strangulation
behavior	Broken human spirit

care workers to undergo more extensive training about the appropriate use of restraints to help ensure patient safety.[4] CMS also launched a 2-year campaign to reduce the use of restraints in nursing homes because of the high risks of harm associated with restraint usage.[5] According to the U.S. Department of Health and Human Services Agency for Healthcare Research and Quality, the amount of long-stay nursing home residents who have physical restraints has decreased from 10.4% in 2000 to 5% in 2007 (Box 14-1).[6]

OMNIBUS BUDGET RECONCILIATION ACT REGULATIONS

OBRA was drafted to protect elders from abuse and to promote choice and dignity. The ultimate goal of OBRA is that each person reaches his or her highest practical level of well-being. A reduction in the use of restraints is only a small part of this intent. OBRA requires caregivers to develop an individualized plan of care that supports each elder in the least restrictive environment

possible.[4,7,8] Certified occupational therapy assistants (COTAs) should become familiar with OBRA guidelines regarding restraints.

OBRA defines two types of restraints: chemical and physical. "Physical restraint can be any manual method, such as any physical or mechanical device, that restricts the patient's freedom of movement."[4] Some examples of physical restraints with the elderly may include restrictive chairs with full lap trays and small wheels that limit mobility, vests used to secure patients to their chairs or beds, wrist or ankle restraints, or bedrails. "Chemical restraints are described as a drug or medication when it is used as a restriction to manage the patient's behavior or restrict the patient's freedom of movement and is not a standard treatment or dosage for the patient's condition."[9]

Restraints are permitted only when they enable greater functional independence, restrict the elder from interfering with the provision of life-saving treatment, or are necessary because less restrictive devices have failed. A documented medical need and physician's order for restraints must exist. Clients must be released at least every 2 hours, and the restraints can be used as a temporary intervention only.[4]

Despite these guidelines, the improper use of restraints continues in the United States. COTAs have an ethical and legal obligation to report elder abuse, which includes using restraints as punishment for clients or as a convenience to staff. COTAs should also participate in educating others about restraints and may wish to initiate a restraint reduction program in their own facility and offer restraint alternatives.

ESTABLISHING A RESTRAINT REDUCTION PROGRAM

Reducing restraints is a complex matter. COTAs must evaluate and appropriately address ethical considerations, regulatory and professional standards, legal liability concerns, and health care team members' education regarding restraint use. It is also important to identify areas for, and participate in, research concerning physical restraints to assist staff nurses and other members of the health care team with making informed decisions regarding patient care.[10]

Philosophy

The philosophical premises of an educational program aimed at restraint reduction include beliefs about quality of care, commitment to understanding the meaning of behavior, and desire to shift practice from control of behavior to individualized approaches to care. If a change is to occur, an educational program aimed at restraint reduction must recognize the potential contributions of all staff members, use an interactive teaching style, and promote discussion and problem solving. Results of testing a restraint education program suggested that altering staff beliefs and increasing knowledge produced a change in restraint practices, at least in the short-term.[11]

A fundamental philosophical concept in the care of elders is the empowerment of both elders and staff. This empowerment is expressed in collaborative solutions to problems. The ability to contribute to solutions allows elders their dignity and adds meaning and quality to their lives.[12] Making choices, including the choice to take a risk, is an essential part of life and contributes to maintaining self-respect.

In addition, it is also paramount to teach family members about the potentially harmful effects of restraint use and the regulatory restrictions and oversight on using restraints. While family members may incorrectly believe that a restraint prevents injury, COTAs or other health care provider plays an important role in educating family members on the aspects of patient autonomy and freedom of movement.

Policy

Health care providers' written policies and procedures should be consistent with each of the requirements listed in the regulations. Yearly mandatory training for staff should be provided, and all training and education programs should be documented. Documentation of events of restraint use should meet required regulations.[10]

When a facility makes a philosophical decision to reduce restraint use, education must be incorporated to help change the organizational culture and to provide strategies for the successful removal of restraints.[13]

Education

Practitioners must teach these concepts not only because they have been mandated by federal regulation, but also because, as Brungardt[14] indicates, elders' function cannot improve "if they are tied down or drugged up." Physical restraints are generally harmful to residents because of the negative effects on multiple body systems and interference with normal functioning, including a resident's capacity to walk, get food, get fluids, change position, toilet, and socialize. Specific physical consequences of restraint use are numerous as well and may include death, injuries, falls, physical deconditioning, incontinence, malnutrition, dehydration, and bone demineralization. Muscle atrophy, skin tears, pressure ulcers, contractures, cardiac rhythm disturbances, and infection can be other consequences of being restrained.[15]

An effective education program includes an experiential component, such as applying a variety of restraints to participants. Few individuals can imagine choosing restraints as an appropriate intervention for themselves. Feeling the helplessness and degradation of being restrained sensitizes staff to the use of restraints on elders. Education should use and affirm participants' life

experiences. Including board members, volunteers, and all facility employees (kitchen workers, bookkeepers, administration, chaplains, and maintenance workers) in this educational program has been identified as a factor leading to the decreased reliance on restraints.[16,17] The CMS Federal Register[18] indicates that staff must be trained regarding restraint use and regulations, and all training must be documented.

Steps for Success

The key to eliminating the use of restraints is individualized care, which depends on staff knowing the resident as a person. One strategy for fostering staff-resident relationships is the consistent assignment of staff to residents, which may help promote individualized care. Staff members responsible for care planning should try and document various options to avoid the use of restraints (Box 14-2).[15]

BOX 14-2

Suggestions to Facilitate a Successful Restraint-Free Environment

- Develop a restraint committee involving all disciplines and departments in the facility.
- Determine the goal for the restraint reduction program. Is it to minimize restraints or completely ban restraints?
- Develop a strategic plan including protocols for specific restraint cases.
- Recruit specialists (gerontological nurse specialist, occupational therapy personnel, etc.) for consultation.
- Determine a protocol for how restraints are ordered by physicians.
- Limit restraint usage to a 24-hour trial. If the restraint usage exceeds that time period, consult with the physician.
- Provide documentation of both alternatives and reasons for restraint usage when requesting physician's orders.
- Implement a gradual process of change when starting the restraint reduction program.
- Start with the easiest cases first and move on to more difficult cases once initial success is achieved.
- Complete ongoing resident assessments. Provide restraint alternatives and interventions based on an individualized resident-specific approach. Include family participation. Learn from others who have successful restraint reduction programs.

From Joanna Briggs Institute. (2002). Physical Restraint—Part 2: Minimization in Acute and Residential Care Facilities, *Best Practice*, 6(4). Asia, Australia: Blackwell.

All members of the team, including families, staff from each shift, consultants, contract personnel, ombudsmen, state surveyors, physicians, and elders themselves, should be included in all stages of the program. Dialogue between these participants from the beginning makes the transition to restraint-free care much smoother. All team members play an important role. Family members can, for example, describe the elder's previous routines and preferences. Kari and Michels[12] assert that certified nursing assistants (CNAs) have essential knowledge of elders and that their usual lack of influence in decision making negatively affects the quality of care.

CNAs may be the team members who first notice behavioral changes and the need for removal of restraints in elders.[16] Strumpf and colleagues[11] indicate that respect for the dignity of the CNA's work is vital for any significant reduction in the use of restraints. An interdisciplinary team assessment of the need for restraint is helpful in reducing reliance on restraints.[17,19]

The most successful restraint-free programs have adopted permanent staffing.[20] This model assigns daily a "primary" CNA (and registered nurse, housekeeper, therapist, among others) to each elder. When these staff members are not working, they should have regular replacements. Permanence in staffing fosters relationships between elders, families, and staff who contribute to feelings of safety and connectedness. Permanent staff are particularly important to elders with cognitive impairment. Initial success will help staff members feel confident about continuing restraint reduction. Family involvement that ranges from simply being notified of the restraint reduction to formal family educational programs has proven effective in a reduction program.[13]

Rader[21] has found that the biggest obstacles to eliminating restraints are fears, biases, and unwillingness to change. She proposes that caregivers, clients, advocates, and regulators work together to create new interventions on the basis of the elder's perspectives and wishes. Reducing restraints should be only the beginning of providing safe care in a dignified and less restrictive environment that promotes the elder's abilities.[22,23]

ROLE OF THE CERTIFIED OCCUPATIONAL THERAPY ASSISTANT

In collaboration with a registered occupational therapist (OTR), COTAs may assess the need for restraints, consult with staff about alternatives to restraint, and provide intervention to eliminate restraint use. The type or technique of restraint used must be the least restrictive intervention that will be effective to protect the patient, staff member, or others from harm.[4]

Assessment

Once the need for intervention is documented and an occupational therapy (OT) order has been received, the OTR/COTA team performs an evaluation. Specific assessments of posture, alignment, balance, strength, and visual acuity are necessary. Assessments of head control, trunk stability, upper extremity support, and the ability to self-propel are added to evaluate seating needs.[24,25] Perceptual and cognitive assessments should be included only as appropriate. Practitioners should not embarrass or agitate cognitively impaired elders by assessing areas already documented as deficient.

Consultation

The assessment may reveal minimal intervention needs, perhaps consultation only. Patterson and colleagues[26] include the roles of advocate, observer, teacher, information specialist, team problem solver, and identifier of resources and alternatives in their definition of consultant. They also report that the combination of consultation with formal restraint reduction training significantly reduces the use of restraints. COTAs are uniquely qualified to function as consultants in developing alternatives to restraints, especially if they are familiar with restraint reduction principles, OBRA regulations, and the basic principles of positioning. For example, an elbow air splint may be all that is necessary for an elder who continually scratches at sutures on a healing incision. Although an air splint is certainly restrictive, it allows more movement than wrist restraints, thereby meeting the criterion for "least restrictive environment." Because wound healing is temporary, the air splint is a temporary measure. A protocol for use of the air splint should be provided. The care plan should document the reason that the splint is being used, the way it will be used, and the way it will be reassessed by the nursing staff.

COTAs may recommend other environmental, psychosocial, and activity-related alternatives (Table 14-1). The alternatives outlined are not a complete list. Options are limitless, depending on the COTA's creativity. Each measure considered should provide as much free choice and control as possible for elders. Eigsti and Vrooman[27] claim that the basic ingredient in reducing restraint use is teaching the staff to understand and believe that alternatives exist.

ENVIRONMENTAL ADAPTATIONS

There are several strategies that can be used to modify the environment to move toward making it restraint free. For example, using chairs that are at the right height, depth, and level of backing for each resident to have comfortable and safe seating can reduce the risk and need for restraints. Furthermore, individualizing the chairs each resident uses in the dining room or other public areas can help provide a match with the residents' needs.[15]

An inexpensive and less restrictive alternative for the confused elder who rises unsafely from a chair might be a personal alarm. Several such alarms are on the market. They do not prevent the elder from rising, but they do alert staff. An elder's attempt to rise usually occurs for

TABLE 14-1

		Alternatives to Restraints
Environmental alternatives	*Chairs*	Deep seats Tilted Recliners Rockers Gliders Bean bag Adirondack type Customized
	Beds	Water or concave-type mattress Create bed boundaries with swim noodles under sheets or body pillows Positioning cushions Individual height mattresses, including floor mattresses Trapeze for bed mobility
	Monitoring Systems	Television monitoring Enclosed courtyards Alarms Exit alarms Door buzzers Nursery intercom Personal alarms for bed or chair Wandering alarms at doorways and exits Pressure-sensitive pads Positional alarms Limb bracelet alarms
	Signs	Directional Stop or Keep Out Identifying (elder's name)
	Safety Adaptations	Nonskid surfaces Low bed Mattress or sleep mat on floor ¾ to ½ length bed rails (instead of full length) Lowered or no bed rail Accessible call lights Move furniture and other obstacles from walkways Accessible light switches Safe walking routes Encouraged use of handrail Bedside commode or urinal Items within reach Shoes or nonskid socks worn in bed
	Personalized Room	Familiar furniture Familiar objects to hold Meaningful pictures and photographs
	Other Adaptations	Lighting (easy to turn on switches and access) Locked exit doors Cloth barrier doorways attached with Velcro Activity area at end of corridors Bean bags (different sizes) Pillows Foam Nonslip mats Firm wheelchair seats Air-splints "Wrap-around" walkers with seats

Continued

TABLE 14-1

Alternatives to Restraints—cont'd		
Psychosocial alternatives	*Behavioral Strategies*	Remotivation Reality orientation (if helpful) Frequent reminders Active listening Responding to agenda behavior
	Decrease or Increase	Interactions Visiting Sensory stimulation (especially noise such as that from overhead paging, television, radio, among others) Identification of antecedent to the unwanted behavior and appropriate measures to address
	Activities	Companionship Encourage resident/staff interactions Consistent staff for familiarity Decreased sensory stimulation Decreased noise Structured daily routines Self-care Permit or encourage wandering and pacing Exercise Bowling Nature walks Wheelchair aerobics, dances, ball games Ambulation programs Toileting every 2 hours Nighttime activities Volunteer and family assistance Buddy system Activity kits Diversional opportunities Relaxation techniques Massage Therapeutic touch Warm bath Music specific to elder tastes

a reason and warrants attention from the caregiver. However, a personal alarm may frighten or agitate the elder or surrounding residents. Therefore, the use of the alarm should be with caution and take into account the environment, elder, and other residents.

Many facilities have discovered that nursery intercoms are an inexpensive and effective way to monitor safe ambulators who wander. Directional signs may help these elders locate their rooms and deter them from entering someone else's room. An alternative to direction signs are signs with familiar pictures instead of words.

Providing cues to help orient residents who wander may also be helpful. Cues can include memory boxes by a resident's door, personal furnishings that residents will recognize, or large visual signs or pictures for bathrooms and other frequently sought areas.[15] Simple velcro signs can be placed across doorways that wandering residents should not enter (i.e., exit doors). These signs are generally red or yellow and may read "Stop" (Figure 14-1). These visual cues help the wandering resident return to another area of the building.

There are many new types of beds on the market that will allow a facility to reduce bed rail use and decrease incidence of falls. For residents at a higher risk for falls, the new beds can be adjusted from standard height to 7 inches off the floor, so that when falls do occur, they will not cause serious injury. Safety alarms, special mattresses and pillows, and thick rubber bedside mats can also be installed. Placing squeak toys between the sheets and mattress pads reminds residents when they are getting too close to the edge of the bed. When side rails must be used, staff can set foam "swim noodles" between the mattress

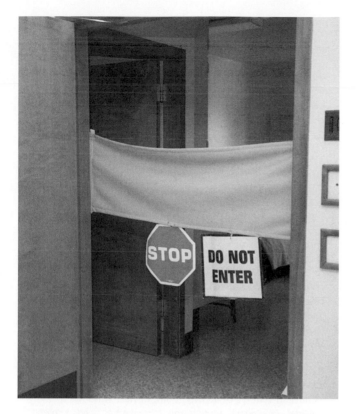

FIGURE 14-1 Environmental adaptations should help restrict elders with Alzheimer's disease from wandering into other people's rooms without restricting access to corridors.

and side rail to reduce the risk of a resident getting trapped against the rail.[29]

PSYCHOSOCIAL APPROACHES

Qualitative studies[1] and other literature[15] indicate negative experiences of people who have been restrained, including emotional distress, loss of dignity and independence, dehumanization, increased agitation, and depression. Residents may experience emotions ranging from frustration and anxiety to anger and terror when restrained. Therefore, psychosocial approaches to reduce restraint use are important.

Wandering or attempts to get up from a chair may be part of an elder's agenda behavior and may lead to agitation if the elder is restrained. Evans and colleagues[30] indicate that the keys to responding successfully to agenda behavior are to allow elders to act on their plans, identify a point at which they may accept a suggestion or guidance, and allow them to keep their dignity throughout an incident. The important difference in the result of this approach compared with others is that allowing the elder to play out the behavior provides a sense of identity and promotes feelings of belonging, safety, and connectedness. This diminishes the elder's need to seek those feelings elsewhere. Further incidences of wandering are

subsequently decreased or eliminated.[31] Brungardt[14] adds that this method works well if the elder's welfare is considered before the needs or routines of the facility.

ACTIVITY ALTERNATIVES

Activity zones with recreational activities, such as multisensory theme boxes, and offering substitute physical activities that interest residents such as dance, exercise, or rocking, may be ways to engage residents in something of interest and reduce the occurrence of wandering. Providing cues to help orient residents who wander may also be helpful. Cues can include memory boxes by a resident's door, personal furnishings that residents will recognize, or large visual signs or pictures for bathrooms and various frequently sought areas.[15]

Providing meaningful activity alternatives can decrease behavior such as restlessness that has traditionally led to the use of restraints. An activity kit, perhaps in the form of a sewing basket, briefcase, fanny pack, or tackle box, may be helpful. The kit may be assembled by family members who are familiar with the elder's interests.[21,32] The idea is to provide something familiar, comfortable, and safe that engages the elder's attention.

INTERVENTION

Although not all referrals require intervention beyond consultation, the assessment may identify a need for ongoing intervention. Examples of intervention to eliminate the need for restraints include the development of self-care techniques, upper body positioning, and seating adaptations.

Because restraint use is associated with the inability to perform self-care, elders and their caregivers should be taught strategies for accomplishing this goal. Determining the routines the elder followed in the past to maintain a sense of continuity and predictability is particularly important. Because part of the objective is to reduce anxiety and agitation, self-care must be done according to the elder's agenda and routine rather than those of the COTA or facility.

Elders with hemiplegia are often provided with half-tray style lapboards to assist with upper body positioning. Because these elders need the best support possible for their upper extremities, this is one of the few cases in which it may be advantageous to begin with the most restrictive device, a full lapboard, and adapt if necessary. If a full lapboard causes agitation or seems too restrictive (perhaps the elder is unable to use a urinal independently), a swing-away half lap tray may be used. Another solution is a foam wedge or cylindrical bean bag, which can extend the width of the armrest for safe positioning without a lapboard. As with any restrictive device, however, less than perfect positioning may be necessary to accommodate the elder's choice.

Another specific OT intervention aimed at reducing the need for restraints is a positioning assessment for elders who are wheelchair-bound. Ill-fitting wheelchairs contribute to restraint use, which can lead to an abnormal sitting posture and the eventual loss of function.[33] For example, wheelchairs usually found in nursing homes were not designed for independent mobility or long-term sitting. Necessary adaptations for comfort and function include dropping the seat so that elders can reach the floor with their feet, replacing the sling seat with a firm seat and cushion, and replacing the sling back with a firm back. A narrower chair may help elders propel themselves more comfortably.[34] Knowledge of the principles of positioning is essential. (Basic alignment principles applicable to any elder are outlined in Chapter 19.) Once adaptations have been designed and implemented, the elder's verbal, behavioral, and postural response must be observed. The system should be reassessed and adapted as necessary until the positioning goals have been met. Documentation should accompany every step of this process, especially if the elder declines the intervention. With very difficult cases, consultation with a seating expert may be helpful. However, even the nonexpert can make many "low-tech" foam supports. More detailed information on wheelchair positioning is included in Part 4 of the chapter.

Relatively inexpensive foam is available in large sizes at the local building or craft store and can easily be cut and shaped with an electric knife. This type of foam works well for the addition of width to an armrest, the fabrication of forearm wedges to elevate edematous upper extremities, or the provision of lightweight lateral trunk support. Egg crate foam is another inexpensive material suitable for limited purposes. Neither of these low-density foams is adequate to support entire body weight while sitting or during episodes of spasticity. For long-term positioning, manufactured cushions of mixed density foam, gel, or air cushions are more durable and are recommended for both comfort and maintained skin integrity. The therapeutic role of orthotic devices in achieving proper body position, balance, and alignment and improving overall functional capacity without the potential negative effects of restraint use is recognized by the Health Care Financing Administration (HCFA).[7,8] This recognition does not provide the license to use wedges, reclining chairs, or seat belts as restraints, even for cognitively intact elders. However, it does allow the legitimate use of positioning devices to increase function, given a demonstrated necessity. Any adaptation should maintain the dignity of elders and augment their quality of life.

CASE STUDY

Mary, a 79-year-old woman with the diagnosis of dementia resides in a long-term care facility. Other medical history includes multiple transient ischemic attacks (TIAs) and skin breakdown on the buttocks area. Mary requires total assist

transfers from the bed to the wheel chair. Her current wheel chair positioning includes a pressure relief cushion and a self-release pelvic belt to prevent sliding forward in the wheel chair. Mary is able to self-release the pelvic positioning belt; therefore, the belt is not considered to be a restraint. However, when she releases it because of agitation or trying to take herself to the bathroom, she tends to slide forward in her chair and is at risk for falls. To prevent this from happening, the nursing staff have requested that the pelvic belt be replaced with one that Mary is not able to release herself. The new pelvic belt then becomes a restraint. The nursing staff order the OTR/COTA team of Marc and Diana to address this case.

Because Marc and Diana are aware of restraint reduction guidelines, they provide interventions to promote optimal positioning using the least restrictive methods. They install a manual tilt pack on the wheel chair to reduce sliding forward and remove the pelvic positioning belt. They also install a drop seat to allow Mary's feet to touch the ground and self-propel throughout the facility. They provide a wedge cushion for optimal positioning. To involve the other members of the health care team, they educate nursing on proper positioning devices and techniques.

Finally, they focus on the resident and encourage Mary to self-propel her wheel chair for increased independence. They talk with staff about engaging Mary in various activities throughout the day and evening and suggest moving her to various interesting areas during the day (high traffic areas, such as nursing stations or activity room, or near windows to see outside). As a result, Mary is able to make her needs known when placed near the nursing station and enjoys increased independence with mobility. The pelvic belt is replaced by a recliner back, drop seat, and wedge cushion. These interventions collectively position Mary correctly and reduce her incidences of sliding forward and fall risk. Most importantly, Mary does not have a restraint.

QUESTIONS ABOUT CASE STUDY

1 How is addressing Mary's wheelchair positioning in this study related to restraint reduction?
2 How did Marc and Diana help maintain Mary's dignity and quality of life?
3 How did the OTR/COTA team work as part of the interdisciplinary team to eliminate Mary's restraint and improve her functional abilities?

CONCLUSION

COTAs have a responsibility to clearly state their professional opinion and recommendations regarding restraint reduction. Clients must choose whether to act on that advice. True restraint reduction requires an examination of attitudes about the rights of elders, especially those with cognitive impairment, to make choices and take risks. COTAs must be willing to become advocates for elders. An understanding of OBRA regulations and positioning principles and the ability to be flexible and creative within a team framework permit COTAs to contribute effectively to restraint elimination programs. If COTAs have honestly attempted to increase function and honor the dignity of the elders they serve, they will have followed not only the letter of the law, but also the intent and spirit.

CYNTHIA GOODMAN

PART 2 **Wheelchair Seating and Positioning: Considerations for Elders**

In 1997, approximately 19% of individuals age 65 years and older relied on a wheelchair for their mobility within the household and community.[35] As the population in this age range continues to grow, this percentage is expected to increase rapidly. More recent data indicate that 2.2 million community dwelling people use wheelchairs, of which 58% use manual wheelchairs.[36] Persons age 65 years or older and living in nursing homes or facilities are reported to be greater than 50% of the total population.[37] The highest rates of manual wheelchair use is in the elderly. People greater than age 65 years (57.8%) use manual wheelchairs. Of note, more than two-thirds of power chair users are not the elderly.[38] The use of assistive devices, such as wheelchairs for mobility, has increased with the population growth, technological advances, and initiatives in public policies.[35] Public policies such as the Technology Related Assistance for Individuals with Disabilities Act (1998) and the Rehabilitation Act Amendments of 1986 have contributed to the increased access to wheelchairs by elders. The use of a wheelchair for mobility in the home or community, or both, is important in improving individuals' level of independence and their ability to participate in chosen occupations.

Health professionals frequently have a "one size fits all" approach to wheelchair seating and positioning. This is often true with elders because Medicare has strict guidelines regarding wheelchair rental and purchase. However, elders have numerous conditions associated with aging that increase the likelihood of complications from improper wheelchair seating and positioning. Such conditions include joint replacements, osteoarthritis, osteoporosis, musculoskeletal changes, including kyphosis and scoliosis, cerebrovascular accident, Alzheimer's disease, amyotrophic lateral sclerosis, Parkinson's disease, dementia, chronic obstructive pulmonary disease, diabetes, congestive heart failure, and hypertension.[39]

A wheelchair should be selected with the unique needs of the individual person in mind. The overall outcomes for a person in a proper position in his or her wheelchair include increased independence, prevention of skin breakdown, decreased need for caregiver(s), and a general overall improvement in quality of life.[40] The result of an elder seated improperly in his or her wheelchair can be fixed or flexible deformities, as well as a decrease in overall function.[41]

A proper wheelchair seating and positioning assessment should be conducted by an OTR. The COTA may collaborate in this process. Areas considered in such an assessment include diagnosis, prognosis, age, cognition, perception, level of independence with activities of daily living (ADL) and occupations, functional mobility, body weight distribution, posture, sensory status, presence of edema, skin integrity, and time spent in the wheelchair. It is important that the elder be involved in the decision about a wheelchair.

Until recently, there were not much data on outcome satisfaction of wheelchair use. It has been found that the utilization of wheeled mobility devices depends on a number of factors such as the user's demographics, health factors, wheelchair characteristics and environmental factors, and the quality of service and delivery.[42-44] The involvement of the user in the selection process and the satisfaction related to the mobility device play a significant role in the use or the abandonment of the device.[45,46]

Proper assessment and selection of a wheelchair are paramount for the satisfaction and utilization of the device. There are a number of key components to a proper assessment.[36,47] They are pre-mat assessment and interview, mat physical assessment, objectives and goals, determine the parameters of options (clinical reasoning), possible options, trial of equipment, prescription and letter of necessity, delivery and fitting, and follow-up.[47] The interview with the elder and caregiver and the gathering of background information help get a complete picture of the clinical situation and the elder's goals for the use of the wheelchair along with the concern of whether the elder already has a wheelchair.[36] There are future considerations when positioning a person of any age and size. They include tilt versus recline, is the elder agitated or cognitively impaired, clinical indicators/medical necessity, and bariatric client considerations.[47]

Key issues to address when assessing and selecting a wheelchair for a bariatric elder are center of gravity, additional assessment measurements, and specific issues of the bariatric elder, such as stability and mobility, overall width, adjustability for changing shapes, and transportability.[47] The one-size-fits-all approach will not work with bariatric elders because of the varying weight distribution. Dr. Kevin Huffman, a bariatric consultant and board certified bariatric physician, indicates that generally bariatric women carry weight below the waist, whereas men carry weight above.[48]

The center of gravity of bariatric individuals tends to be more forward than that of a non-bariatric person.[48]

The axle is often of the rear wheel on a number of wheelchairs. When working with a bariatric elder, it is important to have an axle that moves to allow for the center of gravity to move forward to accommodate the elder's center of gravity.[47]

Seat depth is also important because of the posterior redundant tissue that often makes it difficult for bariatric elders to sit all the way back in their chair. They often appear to be tilted as they are leaning back to touch the back of their chair. There are specific measurements needed to accommodate the posterior redundant tissue and posterior shelf of the client.[49] The OT practitioner needs to look at the back support and determine how to accommodate the shape and space of the buttock.[49] It is also important to ask how and where the wheelchair will be used. A significant issue is environmental access.[49] The OT practitioner will need to access the environment so as to ascertain the accessibility of the wheelchair in the elder's environment.

Wheelchair abandonment is more likely to occur when the individual's needs are not addressed.[50,51] Once a proper wheelchair has been determined, the COTA must help monitor the patient in all of the areas previously assessed.

Certain aspects of wheelchair seating and positioning are of particular importance to elders. Because of musculoskeletal changes, the elder's posture needs to be monitored continuously. In addition, elders are more at risk for skin breakdown. Therefore, the COTA should help monitor this and educate the elder about the need for pressure relief on a regular schedule. The COTA may also be responsible for making sure the components of a wheelchair are working properly. If a needed repair is identified, the COTA can help facilitate a follow-up visit with the wheelchair vendor.

Skin breakdown can occur quickly with elders. There are several types of skin breakdown related to improper seating, including abrasion, pressure, and shearing. Abrasion occurs when the skin rubs against a surface and causes damage to the tissue.[41] An example of this may be when an overweight individual sits in a standard-size wheelchair, and his or her hips rub against the armrest. In addition, rubbing against any sharp areas can cause an abrasion. Elders generally have fragile skin, and an abrasion can occur with very little rubbing.[41] A COTA should be aware of this risk and evaluate if any abrasions occur.

Pressure occurs when the forces of two surfaces act against each other. In an optimal wheelchair seating system, pressure will be equally distributed between the person and the seating system. Unfortunately, this equal distribution can be difficult to achieve and maintain, and therefore pressure sores may develop. A pressure sore occurs when the blood circulation to an area is decreased. Subsequently, oxygen does not flow to those cells and death of the cells may occur. After death of the cells occurs, necrosis takes place, and a pressure sore results. Pressure sores develop from the inside out, generally in areas with bony prominences. The ischial tuberosities and sacrum are areas in which pressure sores commonly occur because of improper seating. A COTA should be aware of this risk and continually monitor whether an elder is at risk for pressure sores. Elders who are particularly slender may be at more risk for a pressure sore. All elders should be seated on some type of wheelchair cushion after a proper OT evaluation.

Shearing is another cause of skin breakdown. Shearing also occurs when two surfaces rub against each other. It is not uncommon for shearing to happen with elders seated improperly in sling wheelchairs. The sling does not adequately support the pelvis, and elders may slump in their chair, causing shearing at the ischial tuberosities and sacral areas. In addition, the risk for shearing in those same areas and in the spinous processes increases with a chair that reclines.[41]

The COTA can help elders learn how to monitor their skin for potential breakdown. Any areas of redness, particularly over bony prominences, can quickly turn into an abrasion or pressure ulcer. The COTA can advise the elders and their caregivers about how to complete a skin inspection. The COTA also can help adapt or modify mirrors to help elders view their skin.

The COTA should also be mindful that a bariatric client has redundant tissue that may get pinched or stuck in crevices, and hence the COTA will need to check for potential areas and consult with the OTR on how to accommodate this. Oftentimes the bariatric client has skin integrity issues in regards to the legs. A padded articulating calf support that is adjustable will help.[48] The COTA needs to make sure to protect the client from all sharp objects and parts with the addition of padding in strategic locations on the chair.

It is important for the COTA to be aware of the optimal seating position. The most important element of proper seating is the position of the pelvis. The pelvis is the base of support when one is sitting. The pelvis should be in a neutral position with weight equally distributed between the left and right ischial tuberosities. The trunk should have slight lordosis in the lumbar area, slight kyphosis in the thoracic region, and a small amount of cervical extension.[41]

The elder's femurs should be in neutral position, with a slight abduction of the hips and 90 degrees of flexion at the hip, knee, and ankle. The arms should be supported by the armrests with the elbows slightly forward of the shoulders.[41] The armrests should be an adequate height to support the arms but not to elevate the shoulders (Figure 14-2).

Improved posture in a wheelchair can help physiological functions such as breathing, swallowing, and digestion.[40] In addition, adjusting posture can improve socialization by simply changing the elder's eye gaze to allow for more interactions in the environment. Comfort is often improved with proper seating, which may also

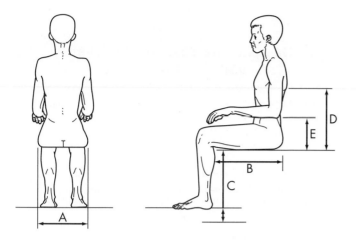

FIGURE 14-2 General guidelines for wheelchair measurement. A, Seat width. B, Seat depth. C, Seat height. D, Backrest height. E, Armrest height. *(Adapted from Wilson, A. B. Jr. (1992). Wheelchairs: A Prescription Guide. New York: Demos.)*

impact elders' tolerance and endurance to sit in their wheelchair for longer periods.

The COTA can observe the posture of elders in their wheelchair and make note of any abnormalities such as posterior tilt of the pelvis, sliding forward in the wheelchair, leaning to one side, inadequate arm support, and the inability to self-propel in the wheelchair. If a COTA identified problems in an elder's current wheelchair system, a referral to an OTR would be indicated for the reevaluation of the seating system. The negative impact of poor seating on frail elders is summarized in Table 14-2.[40]

Because of insurance restrictions, elders often find themselves in rental wheelchairs with sling upholstery. Sling-upholstered wheelchairs were not designed to be primary or long-term seating systems; they were designed to transport people through short distances.[40] People seated for long periods in sling-upholstered wheelchairs often develop poor posture, including posterior pelvic tilt

TABLE 14-2

Negative Impact of Poor Seating on Frail Elders		
Seating problem	**Result on body**	**Potential negative impact**
Wheelchair too tall	Feet do not touch the floor Inability to move self Migration of pelvis out of chair	Agitation Circulatory problems Edema in legs Decreased activity Poor sitting posture Increased restraint use Pain
Poor back support	Compression of trunk, chest, abdomen Sliding out of chair Increased posterior pelvic tilt	Skin breakdown on back and sacrum Impaired digestion, elimination, chewing, swallowing, breathing, and coughing
Wheelchair too heavy	Inability to move chair Requires more energy to move chair	Decreased activity, socialization Fatigue
Wheelchair too wide	Shifting pelvis from side to side Leaning out of chair Inability to access hand rims	Sheering of skin Poor posture, circulation Increased restraint use Pain Agitation
Hammocking effect	Pelvic obliquity Scoliosis Sliding out of chair Requires more energy to stay in chair	Poor posture and circulation of sling seat Increased restraint use Decreased wheelchair tolerance Pain Sheering of skin Fatigue Agitation
Foot rests too high	Lack of femoral support Unequal pressure distribution Increased ischial tuberosity pressure	Poor posture Pain Skin breakdown

From Rader, J., Jones, D., & Miller, L. (2000). The importance of individualized wheelchair seating for frail older adults. *Journal of Gerontological Nursing, 26*, 24-32.

and kyphosis, in the thoracic and lumbar regions. This type of posture increases the possibility of skin breakdown and limits elders' ability to engage in their occupations. Simple remedies, such as inserting a solid seat or back, or both, can significantly improve the situation for elders. COTAs can help identify problems associated with poor wheelchair seating and positioning and help recommend changes to improve independence.

Pain and agitation also have been associated with improper positioning of elders in wheelchairs.[52] As a result, elders with these symptoms may find themselves with restraints in their wheelchairs. Unfortunately, this usage of restraints can cause further agitation and can decrease the elder's level of alertness and ability to participate in occupations. Other elders may find themselves sliding or leaning in the wheelchair. Caregivers often use seating restraint to help with posture.[40] The use of a restraint to correct posture does not address the cause for the misalignment, which is poor seating and positioning. Therefore, the COTA should be careful when monitoring the elder's posture in a wheelchair. See Part 1 of the chapter for a review of the proper usage of restraints, and see Box 14-3 for common seating observations.[40]

COTAs can also help determine elders' functional levels in their current seating system. Because of insurance restrictions from Medicare noted earlier, elders often are set up with heavy, standard-sized wheelchairs that can impede their ability to participate in activities. A study of nursing home residents by Simmons and colleagues[53] indicated a positive correlation between hand-grip strength and wheelchair endurance. This study revealed that simple modifications, such as extending brake handles, modifying seat-to-floor height, and prescribing lightweight wheelchairs when appropriate, would increase the elder's participation within the nursing home.

If a COTA notices a decrease in an elder's functional activity, it would be important to determine whether the seating system is impairing the elder's ability to participate

BOX 14-3

Observations That Should Trigger a Seating Assessment

Leaning or sliding in chair
- Use of a tie-on restraint
- Use of geri-chair or recliner as restraint
- Crying and yelling behaviors in wheelchair-bound elders
- Agitation and restlessness in wheelchair-bound elders
- Seatbelts that go over or above the abdomen
- Tray tables, lap pillows, wedges, or bolsters used for positioning

From Rader, Jones, & Miller. (2000). The importance of individualized wheelchair seating for frail older adults. *Journal of Gerontological Nursing*, 26, 24-32.

in certain activities. Of particular importance would be to determine whether the elder's strength has decreased. A decrease in any level of strength may also mean a decrease in the elder's ability to transfer to and from a wheelchair and/or self-propel to activities. The COTA can discuss with elders what factors are impeding their participation in activities. It may be that a simple solution, such as extending the hand brakes or oiling the flip-up footplates, can facilitate increased participation in an activity.

CONCLUSION

A good wheelchair seating system can support improvements in posture, comfort, independence, and endurance, while preventing skin breakdown. Furthermore, a good system can help elders increase their tolerance for being in the wheelchair, increase socialization, and decrease the burden on caregivers.[40] The COTA should work closely with elders, caregivers, the OTR, and the interdisciplinary team to ensure an optimal wheelchair seating system for each elder, no matter their size or shape.

LOU JENSEN AND SANDRA HATTORI OKADA

PART 3   **Fall Prevention**

Elsa is a 74-year-old woman who was recently widowed. Elsa is independent in most of her basic ADL but had required her husband to assist her in getting into and out of her bathtub. Since his death, Elsa has attempted this task by herself but has had several near falls. She was accustomed to relying on her husband Robert for many instrumental activities of daily living (IADL) such as housework, yard maintenance, shopping, and driving.

Elsa has the reputation among her friends as being a wonderful cook, but, in recent years, she was finding herself relying on her husband to be her "eyes in the kitchen" as Elsa's macular degeneration was progressing, making it increasingly difficult to read the dial on the stove and to see while she prepared meals. After her husband's death, Elsa has had increasing difficulty keeping up with her home maintenance. Additionally, she does not want to burden her friends and neighbors for transportation, so she has drastically decreased time spent in activities outside of her home such as medical appointments, church activities, and other social events. This decrease in physical activity coupled with situational depression has left Elsa feeling isolated, weak, and fearful of the future.

Recently, Elsa was visiting on the phone with her daughter who lives out of state and admitted that she has fallen inside her home twice in the last week. Elsa's daughter is quite concerned and encouraged her mother to visit with her physician. Elsa is hesitant, stating, "The next thing you know, I'll have to move into a nursing home, and I can't bear to leave my house. If I leave here, I'm afraid my memories of Robert will quickly fade away."

Falls among the elderly are a complex and significant health problem that can lead to participation restrictions, activity limitations, altered living situations (e.g., premature nursing home admissions), injury, and even death. A fall is "an unexpected event in which the participant comes to rest on the ground, floor, or lower level."[54] Roughly one out of every three adults age 65 and older experience at least one fall per year.[55,56] This ratio increases to one half of elders age 80 and older.[57] Accidental falls are the leading cause of nonfatal injuries treated in hospital emergency departments in all adult age groups and account for 40% of hospital admissions for older adults.[58] Of those elders hospitalized for injuries related to a fall, about half are discharged to nursing homes.[59] Elders who sustain a hip fracture as a result of a fall have a 34% mortality rate within 1 year of the fracture.[60] Falls are the leading cause of death from injury in those age 65 and older.[58] Falls that do not cause physical injury often cause a fear of falling that results in a decrease in occupational participation and independence,[61] and impairments in client factors such as strength and balance because of a decrease in overall activity level.[62]

The effect of a fall on the life of an elder alone emphasizes the importance of including fall prevention into the care plan of any elder. However, the financial impact of falls on the health care system and society adds additional justification for addressing this important health problem. The estimated total direct cost annually of all fall injuries for people age 65 and older exceeds $19 billion.[63]

On an individual level, costs associated with a fall-produced fracture are $58,120 for the first year and $86,967 for a lifetime.[64] As the elder population increases in the next 30 years, so will the incidence of falls and the costs associated with them. Therefore, it is important for COTAs to be knowledgeable about the risk factors and causes associated with falls, as well as how the OT process can be used to effectively reduce falls in the elderly.

RISK FACTORS AND CAUSES OF FALLS

Falls are multifactorial in nature and can have a variety of precipitating causes (Box 14-4). Elders are particularly vulnerable to falls because of the increased prevalence of

BOX 14-4

Causes of and Risk Factors for Falls in Elderly Persons

Cause	Risk Factor
Accident and environment-related	Lower extremity weakness
	History of falls
Gait and balance disorders or weakness	Gait deficit
	Balance deficit
Dizziness and vertigo	Use of assistive device
Drop attack	Visual deficit
Confusion	Arthritis
Postural hypotension	Impaired ADL
Visual disorder	Depression
Syncope	Cognitive impairment
	Age >80 years

Data from Rubenstein and Josephson. (2006).

intrinsic risk factors such as comorbid clinical conditions, multiple medication regiments, and age-related physiological changes (e.g., decreased vision and decreased muscle strength). More important, a delicate balance exists between intrinsic factors and common environmental hazards; even a small disruption in this dynamic system can lead to a devastating fall. For example, a so-called accidental trip over a new throw rug may cause a fall that could be attributed to the throw rug (i.e., the environment). However, the fall could have been more likely because the elder had impaired vision, lower extremity weakness, and balance deficits (i.e., intrinsic risk factors). Falls in the elderly population can occur in a variety of environments, including the home, community, hospital, or nursing home, although numbers are higher for those in institutional settings.[65]

Environmental Causes

Accidents related to the environment are the primary cause of falls among elders, comprising 31% of falls.[65] Over one-third (39%) of falls occur in the home.[66] Disease processes associated with aging are often strong determinants for falls, but environmental factors in the home may be a more common cause.[67] About 30% of older adults are aging in place (growing old at home), a 32% increase from previous decades.[68] A poorly kept home or yard may be an environmental sign of age-related changes. As people age, they may lose the endurance, strength, and cognitive ability to structure tasks and deal with their environment. Common environmental hazards in the home include poor lighting or glare, uneven stairs, lack of handrails by stairs, and uneven or unsafe surfaces (frayed rug edges, slippery floors in the shower and tub, polished floors, cracks in cement, high doorsteps, and so on). Other hazards may involve old, unstable, or low furniture (chairs, beds, or toilets); pets; young children; clutter or electric

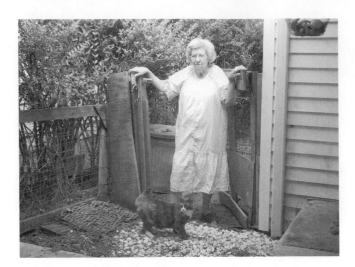

FIGURE 14-3 Common potential hazards that may cause falls include rugs and pets that may get under foot.

cords in walkways; inaccessible items; and limited space for ADL functions (Figure 14-3). New, used, or improperly installed equipment and unfamiliar environments may also be hazardous.

According to Carpenter and colleagues,[66] approximately 55% of falls in the elderly population occur outside of the home. Common areas in the community where falls occur include public buildings, streets, sidewalks, transferring to or from transportation, or another person's home. In addition, the greatest proportion of persons with repeated falls occur in the community, specifically on the street or sidewalk. The most common activities that elderly persons engage in when they fall include walking on uneven ground, tripping (over curbs, rugs, or objects), and slipping on wet surfaces. Other examples of activities associated with falls include lifting heavy objects, reaching, balancing on items of unstable support (overturned box), or turning quickly. Therefore, the COTA should take into consideration the context and environment, as well as the activity engaged in during a fall when determining a fall prevention plan.[66]

Biological Causes

Sensory

Visual changes associated with aging that may influence falls include decreases in depth perception, peripheral vision, color discrimination, acuity, and accommodation. Approximately 30% of persons age 65 and older have visual impairments.[69,70] As the elderly population grows, so will the number of persons with visual impairments. A visual impairment can affect a person's ability to participate in functional mobility in the home and in the community.

Stairs may become more difficult to maneuver. Knowing the location of the next step and judging its depth can become a big challenge. That 75% of all stair accidents occur while descending the stairs, most in the second half of the flight, is also noteworthy.[25,71] New bifocals or trifocals may require adjustment time, and looking down stairs requires constant head and eye adjustments.

Medical conditions affecting vision include macular degeneration, cataracts, diabetic retinopathy, glaucoma, and stroke.[69] These conditions may manifest as scotomas (blind spots), which impair safety in mobility. Objects on the floor, such as pencils and telephone cords, may not be apparent. Elders with visual impairments may also run into furniture. Decreased visual input caused by disease processes may result in a decrease in postural stability.[72] In turn, this affects an elder's balance and may contribute to the greater incidence of falls among this population.

A disorder involving spatial organization or figure ground may cause an elder to perceive a change in rug color or flooring as a stair and glare on the linoleum as spilled liquid. A dark stairway may be perceived as a ramp. Misinterpreting this information may cause a misjudged step and a fall. (Chapter 15 provides more detailed information on age-related changes in vision and recommended adaptations.)

Vestibular disorders that cause dizziness and vertigo may also contribute to falls in the elderly. Benign paroxysmal positional vertigo (BPPV) is a mechanical vestibular problem caused by displaced otoconia in the inner ear as a result of trauma or age.[73] BPPV can cause severe dizziness and vertigo, especially with changes in position or head movements. An elder, particularly one who has a history of falls, may be susceptible to this disorder. Indeed, BPPV is the most common cause of vertigo in persons over age 65 years.[73]

Neurological/Musculoskeletal

Conditions that affect posture and body alignment cause changes in center of gravity, gait, stride, strength, and joint stability, all of which increase the risk for falls. Age-related changes in postural control include decreased proprioception, slower righting reflexes, decreased muscle tone, and increased postural sway.[72] Changes in gait include decreased height of stepping. Men tend to have a more flexed posture and wide-based, short-stepped gait, whereas women tend to have a more narrow-based, waddling gait.[74] Medical conditions that affect instability include degenerative joint disease, deconditioning, malnutrition, dehydration, and neurological disorders such as neuropathy, stroke, Parkinson's disease, and dementia.[25,71,74] Elderly women are more susceptible to brittle bones, with a greater incidence of osteoporosis after menopause. In the case of brittle bones, it may be a fractured bone that causes the fall rather than vice versa. However, falls in the elderly cause 90% of the incidence of hip fractures.[75] Musculoskeletal conditions that contribute to falls in the elderly include osteoarthritis, spondylosis, and a general decrease in joint range of motion.[74]

To compensate for changes in gait and decreased balance, elders may "furniture glide" by holding on to

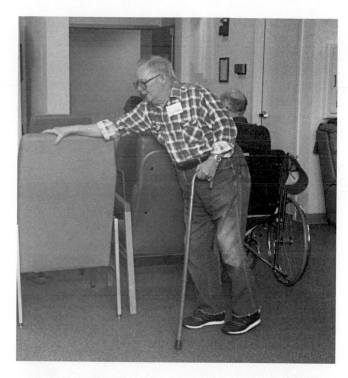

FIGURE 14-4 Elders often "furniture glide" by holding on to furniture to compensate for changes in gait and decreased balance.

furniture for support while they walk (Figure 14-4). They may also drag a foot or lose their balance toward their weaker side (stroke), have a shuffling gait (Alzheimer's disease), or fall forward (Parkinson's disease) during ADL training. Older adults may hold onto faucets or towel racks to get into the tub or shower or lean against the shower wall for stability while bathing.

Cardiovascular

Age-related changes include orthostatic hypotension, which affects approximately 30% of the elder population.[71] Other medical conditions that cause blood pressure changes include hypertension, neuropathy, and diabetes. In addition, these changes can occur as side effects of certain medications. Arrhythmias may cause up to 50% of syncopal episodes in elders.[71] Elders may experience a greater incidence of dizziness or light-headedness, with lower cardiac output, autonomic dysfunction, impaired venous return, and prolonged bed rest. Underlying cardiac disease is the most common cause of syncope that may result in a fall.[57] Together with extrinsic or environmental factors, these biological or intrinsic factors are the primary causes of falls among elders.[25,65,76]

Cognitive/Psychosocial Causes

Psychosocial and cognitive risk factors that may influence falls include poor judgment, insight, and problem-solving skills; confusion; and inattention resulting from fatigue, depression, and dementia. Other factors may include reactions to psychotropic medications, fear of falling,

unfamiliarity with a new environment or caregiver, and a strong drive for independence. Elders and their families may not comply with recommended safety modifications because of cultural or personal preferences, aesthetic values, and limited financial or social resources. Consequently, both the caregiver and the client are at greater risk for having a fall.

Depression and psychotropic medications have both been associated with an increased fall risk. Depression increases the risk of falling twofold,[65] presumably because of an inattention to the environment and a disregard for safety. A systematic review and meta-analysis of drugs and falls revealed an increased risk of falls when associated with psychotropic drug use in elders.[77] A later meta-analysis concluded similarly, noting that not enough has been done in the past decade to address this fall risk factor.[78]

Functional Causes

Performing ADL functions becomes increasingly challenging for elders. About 18% of the elder population report difficulties with ADL, and 26% report difficulties with IADL.[79] Functional mobility problems that may lead to falls include difficulty with performing transfers (to or from a lounge chair, bed, toilet, tub or shower, wheelchair, and car), dressing and bathing (especially the lower body), reaching, sitting, standing, and walking unsupported. Other factors may include the lack of assistive aids for ambulation or an inability to use them. Elders with dementia may forget where they left a cane or walk carrying their walker rather than using it for support. Old, lost, borrowed, or smudged glasses may impair vision. Poorly fitting shoes, loose pants with dragging hems, and flimsy sandals with nylons can affect balance. Falls most commonly occur in places where elders perform most self-care activities: by the bed and in the bathroom.[25,76]

Knowledge of the most common risk factors and causes of falls in the elderly can significantly inform the OT process, as described in the second edition of the Occupational Therapy Practice Framework: Domain and Process.[80] COTAs are important team members in all parts of the process and therefore must understand components of a comprehensive fall risk assessment, fall prevention and reduction interventions, and meaningful ways to measure the outcomes of interventions designed to reduce falls in the elderly.

EVALUATION

Because falls in the elderly typically result from a combination of several intrinsic and extrinsic risk factors, multiple precipitating causes, and in a variety of environments, fall prevention is an issue for the entire health care team. Team members, including the COTA, can collaborate to perform an accurate evaluation of the client and to obtain a detailed fall history before designing a fall prevention program. Shumway-Cook and colleagues[81] found that only half of older adults who fell claimed to have discussed the fall with their health care provider. In this same study, only three-fourths of elders who did discuss their fall with their health care provider were questioned about the cause of the fall, and less than two-thirds received information on fall prevention. Reasons for this communication breakdown may be varied. Elders may be ashamed to admit that they have fallen, or may fear they will be forced to leave their home or lose their independence if they disclose a fall. Conversely, elders may not consider it important or relevant to report a fall in which no injury was sustained. However, open and honest communication is important to successfully address fall prevention. The OTR/COTA team can collaborate to obtain a complete occupational profile that includes fall-related history and must make the establishment of therapeutic rapport a priority to ensure that the information is complete and accurate.

COTAs, in collaboration with OTRs, are well-equipped to assess elders' fall risk, educate on fall prevention strategies, and provide other resources. In addition to assessing client risk factors related to body structures and functions and performance skills, an interview to obtain an accurate history of falls is necessary. Clients should be asked to describe the frequency, timing, and location of their fall(s), the activities they were involved in during their fall(s) and any devices or equipment used, their medical history and symptoms, and medications taken and their side effects.[25,82] If the elder reports no history of falling, care should still be taken to identify risk factors. When asking about functional status, COTAs should not only ask whether the elder is able to perform ADL functions but also observe the way these are done. In other words, the OT evaluation process includes obtaining a detailed occupational profile and analyzing occupational performance.[80] For example, when the COTA asked Elsa whether she could get off the toilet by herself, she responded that she was independent with toileting. When the COTA asked her to demonstrate this transfer, Elsa hooked her cane on a towel rack to pull herself off of the toilet. The COTA was able to determine a high risk for falling only because the transfer was observed. If the COTA had simply accepted Elsa's report of independence, she would not have been able to recommend a raised toilet seat and toilet rails or replacement of the towel racks with sturdy grab bars.

The extensiveness of the evaluation process and team members involved depends on the planned fall prevention strategy. A team approach may be the most beneficial method to address fall prevention. For example, OT practitioners are well-suited to address safe performance of daily occupations. A referral to physical therapy may be indicated to address weakness, balance and coordination deficits, and overall endurance. A nutritionist or dietitian may be included to determine the adequacy of a client's diet and whether modifications that would improve overall health and strength need to be made. Pharmacists can review medications and potential side effects that may lead to an increased risk of falling. Referrals to any number of medical specialists could be indicated if a client has an underlying medical condition that affects their fall risk. Once the necessary referrals are made and the team has established goals with the client, intervention can begin.

FALL PREVENTION INTERVENTIONS

Rubenstein and Josephson[65] have classified current fall prevention interventions for the elderly into five broad categories: multidimensional fall risk assessment and risk reduction; exercise-based intervention; environmental assessment and modification; institutional approaches; and multifactorial approaches, including medical management of the elder. COTAs can be involved, in varying degrees, in each of these interventions.

Review of the Evidence

Several Cochrane systematic reviews of the available evidence for preventing falls in older people have been conducted in recent years. In a review of 111 trials involving 55,3030 community-dwelling participants, exercise-based interventions (group or individual) that targeted two or more performance skills (e.g., strength, balance, flexibility, or endurance) reduced the rate of falls and risk of falling in the elderly.[56] Multifactorial interventions also reduced the rate of falls in older community-dwelling adults. Interventions designed to improve safety in the home were found to be effective in reducing falls in high-risk elder populations only, such as persons with visual impairment.

A separate review, using 41 trials (25,422 participants), was conducted by Cameron and colleagues[83] for older people in institutions. For elders in nursing homes, exercise-based and multifactorial interventions produced variable results on reducing falls. These interventions were most successful when implemented by a coordinated health care team. The evidence did suggest that the prescription of vitamin D and a medication review by a pharmacist reduced falls. For elders in hospitals, interventions that targeted multiple risk factors and supervised exercise were effective in reducing falls.

Multidimensional Fall Risk Assessment and Risk Reduction

The goal of the multidimensional approach for fall prevention in the elder population is to target the multiple risk factors associated with falls to reduce fall risk. This approach can be used for both individuals and populations. For example, a multidimensional fall prevention program can be offered to a population of community-dwelling well elders to educate them on ways to prevent falls and to screen elders to determine their fall risk. Health fairs and community educational programs are two examples of a population-based multidimensional approach for fall prevention. Conversely, an individualized multidimensional fall prevention program may be instituted for an elder who has a history of falls or is at high risk for falling. In either case, fall risk assessment precedes intervention and consists of a fall history, general medical and medication history, and an assessment of client factors and performance skills.

Exercise-Based Intervention

As mentioned previously, exercise-based interventions have been found to effectively reduce falls in elders.[56,84] General strengthening programs incorporated in the elder's daily routine can help decrease deconditioning, especially that caused by a sedentary lifestyle. In addition to OT-led exercise programs, COTAs may also refer elders to physical therapy for general lower extremity strengthening and balance exercises.[72] Community exercise programs, such as dancing, water aerobics, swimming, and walking clubs, are also appropriate recommendations.

Activities that target balance can be incorporated into the OT treatment plan. A careful balance of activities designed to remediate balance with those that allow compensation needs to be considered. Tai Chi is a form of exercise that has been shown to be effective in reducing falls and improving balance.[56,85,86]

Gradual increases in activity are recommended for people with conditions that affect endurance (such as cardiac conditions and deconditioning). Strategically located sturdy chairs may be useful for elders who require rest periods when going from one room to another. Sitting while bathing and avoiding long hot baths are also recommended. A commode chair by the bed may save energy. Activities that involve straining and holding one's breath (such as during toileting, strenuous transfers, or exercise) can cause light-headedness and should be monitored.

Environmental Assessment and Modifications

OT practitioners, with their focus on the importance of the environment on occupation, are well-equipped to perform home assessments and make modification to improve safety and reduce fall risks in elder populations. Home safety checklists can be provided as a preventive measure for well elders. Often, however, home safety assessments are more beneficial in detecting potential environmental hazards and making individualized recommendations to clients to improve safety.

Bathroom modifications may include a tub or shower bench with armrests and back, a handheld shower hose, grab bars, or a raised toilet seat. Throw rugs should be removed, or nonskid backing should be applied under them. Nonskid stripping or rubber mats can be placed on tub or shower floors. Sliding glass doors should be removed to allow for wider access into the tub. A shower curtain may be hung from a pressure mounted bar to provide privacy if the glass doors are removed. Heat-sensitive safety valves also can be installed to prevent scalding. If the elder uses a wheelchair and the door to the bathroom is too narrow, a rolling shower bench or commode chair with wheels may help. Placing a commode chair by the bed may eliminate unsafe night transfers to the bathroom toilet. A three-in-one commode chair is an inexpensive solution. This type of commode is light and can be used at bedside, over the toilet, or in the tub or shower. Caregivers should remember, however, that emptying the commode bucket and lifting and relocating the commode can be difficult for elders. They should be discouraged from using soap dispensers, towel racks, and toilet paper holders for support. Hygiene items should be placed within reach. Mirrors may be tilted or lowered for better viewing during ADL functions. Doors under the sink should be removed to give the elder more leg room while sitting in front of the sink.

Similar precautions should be taken in the kitchen. Step stools should be avoided, and frequently used utensils and dishes should be rearranged so they are within safe reach. Use of energy conservation techniques during meal preparation may decrease the risk for falling because of fatigue or orthostatic hypotension. Simple meal preparation packages are widely available in grocery stores. Use of a microwave can help decrease the amount of time an elder spends standing at a stove to prepare a meal.

About 30% of all falls in the elderly occur in the home.[66] Of those elders who fell during ADL, 22% had falls that occurred when they tried to get out of bed or up from a chair. The height of seats (beds, sofas, chairs) can be increased with firm cushions. Worn mattresses or cushions should be rotated. Chairs with armrests are recommended to facilitate rising from the chair. Chairs with wheels should be avoided, and the brakes of wheelchairs and commodes must be secured before transfers are attempted. Elders should lean forward in the wheelchair only when both feet are flat on the floor (not on the footrests). Electronic lift chairs are typically available in furniture stores.

Caregivers must ensure that stairs are well lit, with no glare, and equipped with railings running along the entire length of the stairwell on both sides. Stripping of various colors can be used at the edge of each step to distinguish them from each other. Safety grip strips may be placed on each step as well. Light switches should be within reach at both the top and bottom of the stairway. COTAs should discuss with elders safe ways to change a light bulb. User-friendly, touch-sensitive, and motion-sensor light switches are also available. Transition areas such as doorways, garages, and patios are common sites for falls. COTAs should look at the outdoor environment, transition areas, and the indoor environment to help prevent falls.

Interventions to compensate for visual loss include increased lighting with limited glare, improved contrast for steps and furniture, decreased clutter in walkways, and well maintained flooring. COTAs should anticipate elders' performance at different times of the day, with varied natural lighting and indoor lighting. Referrals to vision specialists may be appropriate to ensure that elders are wearing the appropriate eyewear.

Environmental modifications can also include modifications of the objects commonly used during ADL by the elder. COTAs should encourage elders to wear sturdy, comfortable, rubber-soled footwear (e.g., tennis shoes) to help obtain a more secure footing. Some elders may wear slip-on shoes because tying or fastening shoes is difficult. Assistive devices such as elastic laces or Velcro closures may help address this difficulty and provide the elder with more stable footwear to help prevent falls. When dressing, elders should pull pant legs above their ankles before standing. Pants should be pulled down after transferring from the wheelchair to the toilet to avoid tripping.

Elders with a reach of less than 6 to 7 inches are also limited in their mobility skills and are the most restricted in ADL functions.[74] Older adults who have difficulty reaching and carrying objects may require reachers, extended handles on bath brushes or shoe horns, carts, walker trays or bags, and sock aids. COTAs play an important role in educating elders in the proper use of these assistive devices so that the devices themselves do not become fall hazards. COTAs can also help the elder problem-solve unique situations. For example, they can determine the best way to attach the reacher to the walker or rearrange items around the living space so they are within reach. Higher electrical outlets also could be recommended to limit the need to reach and bend. Redesigning or rearranging an elder's environment is often an inexpensive and effective fall prevention technique. However, it is important to consider that rearranging furniture may disorient an elder, which could increase the possibility of a fall. Environment redesign should occur only with the consent of the elder, and follow-up visits are recommended to assess the transition.

Difficulty with transfers and mobility during ADL functions may require safety training with the cane, walker, or wheelchair. This is particularly important because many falls occur in transit during transfers. Elders with nocturia, a normal age change involving increased frequency of urination at night, have a particular need for night lights and a clear passage to the toilet. Before rearranging furniture to provide wider walkways, COTAs must first make sure elders do not need the furniture for stability when ambulating. A consultation with a physical therapist may help clarify the most appropriate and safe assistive device for ambulation.

Institutional Interventions

Institution interventions are fall prevention strategies implemented in institutions such as hospitals, nursing homes, and assisted living facilities. Hospitals often have screening procedures for all patients, which include assessing patients for their fall risk. Often, these screens include an evaluation of cognition and balance by a physician and/or OTR. For those patients found to be at high risk for

falls, bed or chair alarms, increased supervision (e.g., a sitter in the room or room placement close to the nursing station), low hospital beds, and the judicious use of restraints (e.g., bed rails, wrist restraints, and restraint vests) are all viable options for keeping the patient safe from falls. Additionally, early mobilization and participation in familiar ADL are recommended to address fall risk.

Nursing homes and assisted living facilities can also implement programs in addition to those mentioned previously to reduce fall risks. Examples include dedicated fall-reduction staff who can provide more supervision and multifaceted fall reduction interventions,[87-89] walking and other exercise-based programs to improve client factors, staff education and policies related to fall reduction and reporting, and so on. Previously discussed in the chapter were methods of restraint reduction and proper seating and positioning. Addressing these issues can also reduce falls among elders in institutional settings.

Multifactorial Interventions

Multifactorial interventions are those that incorporate several strategies into a coordinated fall prevention program. This is a useful approach for COTAs who want to ensure they are using a holistic, client-centered approach. Included in the OT plan of care should be referrals to other health professionals who are educated on managing the often complex medical issues of elders. Elders who report dizziness with a change in position may be experiencing a decrease in blood pressure that could result in a fall with or without syncope. A referral to the elder's physician would facilitate medical management of this problem. Meanwhile, the COTA should monitor the elder's blood pressure, and elders should be allowed to make slow transitions from supine to sitting or sitting to standing positions. A few minutes may be necessary to allow the blood pressure to accommodate to the change in head position. By teaching elders different techniques for dressing and bathing and instructing them in the use of long-handle devices, COTAs can help elders limit and modify their bending. A typical recommendation is that the elder get dressed while seated to help accommodate for orthostatic hypotension. The rest of the health care team should be informed of reports of dizziness and unstable changes in blood pressure.

COTAs, elders, family members, and caregivers should work together to identify activities important to elders that can be modified to prevent falls. Family members should be included because elders may depend on them to help with preparation and assistance. Elders may prefer to perform toileting activities independently but may not mind assistance with feeding. COTAs should identify personal and shared spaces in the elder's living environment. If family members do not want to modify the only bathroom in the home with a raised toilet seat and grab bars, a commode chair by the elder's bed may be appropriate. COTAs should help elders and their family members

BOX 14-5

Safety Tips
■ Consider referrals to others on the health care team. Periodic medication reviews by a pharmacist and medical check-ups by a physician are important safeguards against falls. ■ Exercise has been shown to reduce falls in the elderly. Be sure to proceed with exercise programs that take into account individual elder's comorbidities and functional status. ■ Consider issuing and educating on adaptive equipment (e.g., grab bars, tub benches or shower chairs, and bedside commodes) when full remediation is not possible. ■ Home safety assessments are beneficial to address occupations in context and to reduce environmental hazards such as poor lighting, excessive clutter, and unsafe walking surfaces.

Address safety measures and recommend that a cellular or cordless phone always be within reach of an elder at risk for falls (e.g., in a walker bag, fanny pack).

address safety concerns and practice giving assistance in a safe environment.

Additional areas to consider are the frequency and occurrence of falls. If elders experience repeated falls, their confidence levels may decrease, which could result in a decrease in participation in ADL and IADL.[67] The time of day that a fall occurs is also important information to obtain. About 64% of elders in a study reported falls in the afternoon to late afternoon period.[67] The afternoon is generally a time of increased activity for elders, and the assessment of ADL and IADL should address the time factor.

COTAs should make sure that strategies exist for emergency situations. Typical questions include the following: If a curtain is not drawn, will the neighbor know that this may be an indication of trouble? If an elder falls, will he or she know the proper way to get up from the floor if no injuries are apparent? Is a telephone within reach? Is a list of emergency phone numbers placed by the phone? If the elder is at home alone, are there emergency alert systems available to signal for help? Is a telephone reassurance program available in which a volunteer calls daily? Is it safer to soil clothes than risk an unassisted transfer to the toilet? All of these questions should be addressed to ensure the elder's safety before discharge from OT. See Box 14-5 for additional safety tips.

OUTCOMES

Identifying outcomes that are important to the client and that can be measured to demonstrate the effectiveness of OT intervention is an important step in the occupational therapy process. Ideally, outcomes are selected collaboratively by the client and OT practitioner(s) early in the therapy process. COTAs, with guidance from OTRs, can contribute to outcomes identification and use. The Framework[80] describes nine broad outcomes for any OT intervention, any of which may be appropriate, depending on which fall prevention strategy is used.

Prevention is an obvious outcome to select in fall prevention programs. The number of falls experienced by the client can be counted during a specified time frame and compared to the number of falls experienced by the client before intervention. These data can provide evidence of the effectiveness of the fall prevention intervention. However, not all clients have experienced falls before OT intervention but may have risk factors for falls. Therefore, this outcome alone may not be an adequate measure of success.

Adaptation, health, and wellness can be measurable outcomes in fall prevention programs. Secondary effects of such interventions may be a positive change, or adaptation, in body functions and performance skills such as strength, balance, visual acuity, or endurance. If deficits in these functions and skills were intrinsic risk factors for falls, an improvement may help decrease fall risk. For example, if a client had poor muscle strength and balance, and strengthening and balance activities were included in the intervention plan, appropriate outcome measures would be manual muscle testing or a balance or fall-risk assessment. Many valid and reliable balance assessments are available and can be easily administered.

Occupational performance and role competence are commonly used outcomes in OT practice and may be the client's desired outcomes for fall prevention interventions. For example, if safety with bathing or showering is addressed through environmental modifications, a client's occupational performance may improve from needing assistance with tub transfers to being independent with tub transfers as long as a tub transfer bench is used.

Self-advocacy may be a selected outcome. If a client discovers, through guidance from an OT practitioner, that he or she is no longer safe to ambulate in the community because of high fall risk, the ability to self-advocate for community transportation services may be an appropriate outcome.

Participation and quality of life should always be overarching outcomes for any intervention, including fall prevention. Simply helping a client improve endurance and balance does not ensure that he or she can safely and comfortably participate in desired life events and believe that he or she has an improved quality of life. COTAs must be sure to carry out interventions in their natural contexts and ensure that clients are able to participate in these contexts. Many standardized measures of participation and quality of life exist, as well.

Finally, occupational justice is defined as "access to and participation in the full range of meaningful and enriching occupations afforded to others."[80] Care must be taken to design fall prevention interventions such that clients have a reasonable balance between freedom from falls and participation in meaningful occupations. Fall prevention may be extremely challenging if a client has irreversible risk factors such as dementia or blindness. However, if the only answer to fall prevention appears to be a drastic reduction in physical activities so that falls are minimized, the client may potentially sacrifice or be denied access to meaningful living.

CASE STUDY

Let us revisit the case of Elsa. Elsa's daughter finally convinced her to visit with her physician about her recent falls. The physician ordered home health occupational and physical therapy services for Elsa. Based on what you know about effective fall prevention, answer the questions below.

1 What risk factors does Elsa have that contribute to her falling?
2 What further information would you want to have before designing a fall prevention intervention plan? Specifically, what further questions would you want to ask Elsa, and what assessments and/or functional observations would you want to observe?
3 Which fall prevention approach(es) would be most appropriate for Elsa? Describe two intervention activities for each approach.
4 Finally, consider what outcomes would be most appropriate for Elsa. What specific measures would you, along with the OTR and client, choose?

PENNI JEAN LAVOOT, MICHELE LUTHER-KRUG, AND MARY ELLEN KEITH

PART 4   Community Mobility

Most elders prefer the freedom of traveling by automobile (Figure 14-5). Driving is an important factor in their independence and mental health.[90] By the year 2030, one in five American drivers will be age 65 years or older.[91] In 2008, elders represented 15% of all licensed drivers in the United States and accounted for 15% of all traffic fatalities.[92] Most of these fatalities involving older drivers occur during the daytime (80%), on weekdays (72%), and involve other vehicles (69%).[92] Elders are becoming increasingly more reliant on automotive transportation. The reason could be that the majority of elders live in rural or suburban communities. Often in these communities there are limited or no resources available for transportation options for seniors. COTAs can help elders assess the resources within the elders' local communities.[93]

Elders may experience age-related changes that can negatively affect their ability to drive, including decreased visual acuity, color discrimination, depth perception, figure ground and peripheral vision, and increased sensitivity to glare.[94] Other factors that may influence driving and mobility include unrecognized disease processes, physical changes, psychosocial issues, medications, cognitive changes, reduction in hearing ability, and environmental issues such as small print on signs. Physical changes contributing to driving abilities of elders also include changes in sensation, range of motion, decrease in reaction time, and decrease in decision-making abilities.[95]

Age-related changes affect the mobility of elders, whether they are pedestrians, drivers, or users of public transportation. For example, pedestrians may have difficulty stepping up or down from curbs or crossing streets within the time allotted by crossing signals (Figure 14-6). Drivers may have difficulties merging, yielding the right of way, negotiating intersections, backing up, handling quick maneuvers, reading traffic signs, and making left turns.[96] Physical barriers may make public transportation inaccessible. All of these challenges may rob elders of the freedom and independence they may have enjoyed throughout their lives.

A common goal of OT is to assist elders in being as independent as possible in their homes and communities.[97] As with most adults, an elder regularly goes to the doctor's office, grocery store, places of worship, bank,

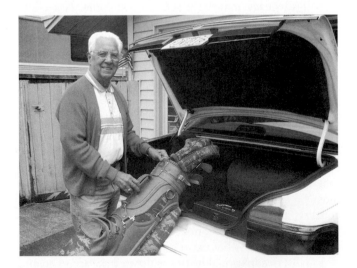

FIGURE 14-5 Most elders prefer to travel by automobile.

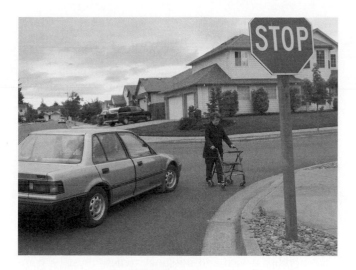

FIGURE 14-6 Elder Pedestrians may need more time to cross streets than other people.

Information-Gathering Questions
1. What method of transportation do you typically use to get around in the community?
2. Have you driven before, and do you currently drive?
3. Do you own and drive a car? What kind?
4. Have you noticed any difficulties operating a car?
5. When was the last time you were tested at the Department of Motor Vehicles?
6. When was the last time you had your vision tested?
7. Do you have any conditions that might affect your ability to operate a motor vehicle?
8. Are you familiar with your community?
9. Do you have difficulties driving at night or with glare?
10. How many miles do you drive a year?
11. In the past 5 years have you had any accidents? Moving violations? Please describe.
12. Have you ever used public transportation?
13. Would you be willing to use public transportation? If not, why?
14. Do you need any assistance to get in and out of a car or public transportation?
15. Do you know how to read a bus schedule?
16. Are you familiar with any community resources for transportation?

salon/barber, and pharmacy. These places may be around the corner or many miles from the elder's home. The role of the COTA in helping identify realistic goals and treatment plans for elders often includes increasing their ability to move in the community. To do this effectively, COTAs must explore as many options as possible for community mobility (Box 14-6). Community transportation options vary greatly among rural areas and cities.

PEDESTRIAN SAFETY

Walking safely is an important factor in community mobility. Elders account for 18.3% of all pedestrian fatalities.[92] COTAs should evaluate the ability of elders to walk outdoors. Box 14-7 lists precautions for safe walking in an elder's community.

Elders who use wheelchairs, walkers, and scooters usually have more difficulty and require more time conquering crosswalks, curbs, and uneven sidewalks. These elders need training to negotiate cutout curbs because electric scooters or wheelchairs may overturn when descending. Electric scooters with three wheels tend to tip more often than those with four wheels. A mobility expert should conduct an evaluation to determine the type of equipment needed. This evaluation should take into consideration the elder's cognition, physical impairments, home environment, seating and positioning needs, and the progression of disease. Whenever possible, COTAs should provide safety training with the exact type of mobility equipment that elders will be using in the community. COTAs also can help elders advocate for curb cuts or longer crossing times at various intersections to ensure independence and safety in the community. To this end, the city's Traffic Commission or the Architectural and Transportation Barriers Compliance Board can be of assistance.

Pedestrian Safety Tips
1. Always use a crosswalk.
2. Use the pedestrian push button and wait for the WALK sign to appear.
3. Before stepping into the roadway, search for turning vehicles, look left-right-left, and keep looking while crossing.
4. Wear bright (fluorescent) colors during daylight and wear reflective material and carry a flashlight if walking at night.

Adapted from the American Automobile Association. (1993). Walking through the years. Heathrow, FL: Traffic Safety and Engineering Department.

Elders who fatigue easily or are unable to walk long distances may consider using an electric scooter or wheelchair (Figure 14-7). Golf carts can be especially helpful for elders who live in a planned retirement community and stay within the closed community area. An obstacle course can be set up to determine the elder's ability to maneuver before this expensive device is purchased. An evaluation in wheelchair and scooter prescriptions by a specialist is also recommended before purchase.

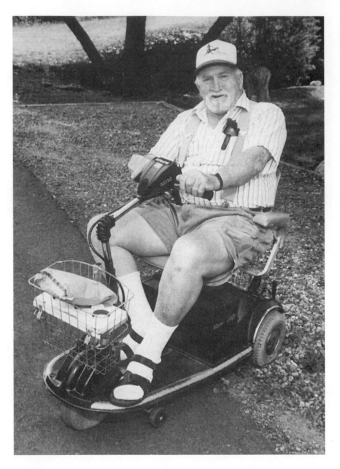

FIGURE 14-7 Elders may use electric scooters to move around freely in the community.

If elders need to transport a wheelchair or scooter in their personal vehicles, community mobility becomes much more complicated. Wheeled power mobility devices should be transported only in a van fitted with an electric lift or ramp of the appropriate size and weight. A driver rehabilitation professional should evaluate each case before a van or lift is purchased to prevent expensive mistakes such as incompatible equipment. A driver rehabilitation professional takes into account many factors, including the type of wheelchair or scooter that must be transported, whether the person needing the equipment will be a driver or passenger, and the length of time that the equipment will be needed. They can also determine the ability of the elder to operate the prescribed equipment. The diagnosis of the elder is also important. An elder with a progressive illness has different needs than an elder without a progressive illness. A driver rehabilitation professional can be found by contacting the Association of Driver Rehabilitation Specialists (ADED) (http:// driver-ed.org) or the AOTA Older Driver Initiative.

The driver rehabilitation professional can also provide resources for vendors who install adaptive equipment for vehicles in a particular geographic area. The National Mobility Equipment Dealers Association is a resource for locating these qualified vehicle modifiers/dealers. Before an electric lift, ramp, or scooter carrier is purchased, the prospective user should demonstrate an ability to perform the entire loading process using the recommended equipment. COTAs can assist elders by providing information on driver rehabilitation specialists in the area.

In contrast to power wheelchairs, power scooters can be transported in a variety of ways. They can be stored in the trunk of some cars or on the back of the vehicle. The COTA can refer the elder or caregiver to a driver rehabilitation professional to assist with assessing the safest loading devices, based on the balance and function of the elder client. The elder and caregivers must practice every step of this process before the equipment is purchased. The mobility device and personal vehicle must be compatible for safety reasons. Checking with the manufacturer of the vehicle to see whether it can handle the extra weight of a scooter carrier is necessary.

COTAs can assist the elder driver in applying for a disabled parking placard, usually issued by the Department of Motor Vehicles (DMV) of each state. This entitles the driver of the car to park close to buildings and may also include assistance at the gas station. Some elder drivers do not apply for this placard because they do not understand the application procedure. Other elders may not apply because of a perceived social stigma. It is important for the COTA to help the elder determine the requirements for a disabled parking placard. In many states, the form must be filled out and signed by a licensed physician.

ALTERNATIVE TRANSPORTATION

When planning OT intervention, COTAs must take into consideration the individual's lifestyle and needs.[97] This is especially true for elders who have never driven, are now unable to drive because of impairments, voluntarily decide not to drive, or want the option of using community transportation in addition to their personal vehicles. Elders who relied on others for transportation may need to learn to drive, especially if those people are no longer available. COTAs should help the elder investigate community transportation resources available where the elder currently resides or is planning to live. Information on alternative transportation can be obtained by calling city hall, a local senior citizens' center, the local DMV, local transportation agencies, the area's Office on Aging, and the local American Association of Retired Persons (AARP) offices. Independent living centers in the community may also be good sources of information. When calling these agencies, COTAs should help the elder obtain information about application procedures, cost, distance traveled, eligibility requirements, and the type of additional equipment available on the vehicles.

Title II of the Americans with Disabilities Act (ADA) addresses many needs of elders with disabilities. This act states that no qualified individual with a disability shall, by reason of that disability, be excluded from participating in or be denied the benefits of the services, programs, or activities of a public entity. According to the ADA, a qualified individual is defined as a person with a disability who meets the essential eligibility requirements for receiving services or participating in programs or activities provided by a public entity. The individual may meet these qualifications with or without reasonable modifications to rules, policies, or practices. They may also qualify with or without the removal of architectural barriers or the provision of auxiliary aids and services. Public entity refers to any state or local government or instrumentality of a state or local government. The paratransit and other special transportation services provided by public entities are designed to be usable by individuals with disabilities, be they physical or mental, who need the assistance of another individual to board, ride, or disembark from any vehicle on the system. Individuals for whom no fixed and accessible route transit (usually a public bus) is available are also eligible for paratransit and special transportation services. However, a fixed, accessible route transit should be used if available (Figure 14-8).[98]

Elders who have impairments that prevent them from traveling to or from a boarding location for fixed transportation may also be eligible for special services. Under the law, any individual accompanying the person with the disability may be eligible for paratransit services, provided that space is available and other people with disabilities are not displaced (Figure 14-9).[99] This means that if elders with a disability cannot use the available bus system, another transportation system that can pick them up directly from their home must be provided. COTAs working with elders who have a disability must know the ADA as it relates to transportation and accessibility. COTAs also should become knowledgeable about the paratransit services in the local community.

As good as paratransit services may be, they almost never help elders in leaving their homes. Regardless of whether elders are using a bus, paratransit service, or personal vehicle, their ability to safely exit their homes is of critical importance and must be evaluated to determine whether available services should be used. Information regarding this issue can be found in Part 2 of the chapter. The elder may be unable to climb stairs or even unlock or lock the door. COTAs should consider these factors and include them when training in the use of transportation services.

Some elders find the process of applying for special transportation services overcomplicated and confusing. COTAs should have applications available and know the eligibility requirements for these services. If possible, COTAs should schedule an outing with elders to use particular services and help them resolve any difficulties that arise. Elders may need encouragement to be assertive when they require assistance. If the outing is successful, elders are more likely to use the service independently or with a friend or family member.

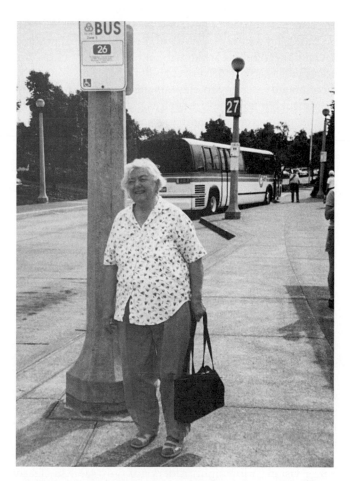

FIGURE 14-8 Elders may need to learn to use community transportation in addition to their personal vehicle.

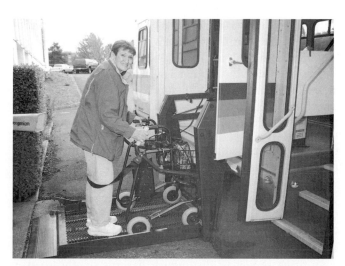

FIGURE 14-9 Public transportation may be a viable option for elders who may no longer be able to drive.

SAFE DRIVING

Aging is a highly complex process that varies tremendously among individuals. Chronologic age alone is not a good predictor of driving performance. The physical effects of aging in combination with a disability make driving safety an important issue. Although driving may seem simple because so many people do it, it is an extremely complex occupation that requires constant attention and concentration.[100] Driving involves a number of abilities. The abilities of sensing, deciding, and acting are critical in operating a vehicle. Drivers must perform a series of coordinated activities with their hands and feet while using input from their eyes and ears. Drivers must make many decisions on the basis of what they see and hear in relation to other vehicles on the road, other drivers, traffic signs, signals, and road conditions. These decisions result in the actions of braking, steering, and accelerating, or a combination of all three to maintain or adjust the position of the vehicle in traffic. Because fluctuations in traffic occur quickly, the coordination between decisions and actions must be smooth. Drivers make about 20 decisions for each mile traveled, demonstrating that the occupation of driving is complex and fast paced.[96,100] Age- or disability-related decreases in sensorimotor skills may compromise driving safety by reducing the speed with which an elder can sense, decide, and act in traffic.

The sense dimension of driving includes visual acuity, visual accommodation, field of vision, dark adaptation, color vision, visual searching, and hearing. Glare and illumination, as well as certain diseases of the eye, may also affect the way the driver senses environmental changes. Integrity of muscles and joints and reaction time are also intimately related to driving. Elders may not perceive, interpret, and react to sensory stimulation as acutely or quickly as younger people. Approximately 60% of all persons age 65 years and older have a visual impairment.[101] As the size of our elder population increases, the number of people with visual impairments will increase significantly. Visual impairments are a primary consideration in safe driving and should be assessed accordingly.

Vision is usually defined as visual acuity or the ability to see fine details. Static acuity (such as looking at an eye chart) is tested in driver licensing examinations. Dynamic acuity (subject or target moving) is more closely related to traffic accidents but is seldom tested. Up to age 40 or 50 years, little change occurs in visual acuity, but visual acuity declines markedly in individuals older than age 50.[102] By age 70 years, most elders have poor acuity without correction. The implications of this decline for driving are that drivers find distinguishing between objects increasingly difficult and need to be closer to objects to clearly perceive them.[103] To compensate for this, elders may drive slowly to distinguish hazards on the road in time to avoid them. Some diseases of the eye, such as macular degeneration or diabetic retinopathy, can be improved with devices such as a bioptic telescope system. Bioptic systems combine prescription eyewear with a small telescopic system. The eyewear lens portion is deemed the carrier that provides general vision, whereas the telescope aids in quick spotting of detail for the visually impaired patient. The telescope can be fabricated for one or both eyes.[104] COTAs should be aware that not all states approve bioptic driving and therefore should be aware of their state's visual standards.

Accommodation is defined as the ability to focus the eyes on nearby objects. With aging, changes in the lenses of the eyes and in the muscles that adjust them decrease their capacity for accommodation. For this reason, many elders need bifocal or trifocal eyewear, which affects driving because more time is required to change focus from near to distant objects, such as when looking from the instrument panel to the road and vice versa. A younger person can change focus in about 2 seconds, whereas adults older than age 40 years take 3 seconds or more. This delay is potentially hazardous. The retina of the normal eye receives about one half as much light at age 50 as at age 20 years and about one third as much at age 60 as at age 20 years.[105] This change is primarily because of a decrease in the size of the pupil. Elders who complain of night blindness have good reason not to drive at night because less light is available. Choosing well-lighted highways and instrument panels and keeping headlights, windows, and eyeglasses clean are helpful measures. A driver rehabilitation professional may recommend changes in the enhancement of the instrument panel to improve use such as marking various speeds on the odometer or modifying the speedometer with a magnifier.

Field of vision decreases with age, and this decrease can contribute to the possibility of collisions. For example, people who can see only directly ahead confront a greater risk for accidents at intersections because they cannot see vehicles approaching from the sides. Compensations for a decreased field of vision can include the use of special panoramic mirrors and the habit of turning the head more often to check for traffic. Many elders may also not be aware of their blind spot on the side of the vehicle. Reminders to look over the shoulder before all lane changes may be necessary.

Glare occurs when too much light or light from the wrong direction or source is present. If excessive light shines on a highway sign, the elder may not see it. Quick recovery from oncoming headlights is necessary for safe driving. In the elder driver, eye recovery is slower and sensitivity to glare increases. The windshields of a vehicle produce glare, and one way to reduce dashboard glare is to place a black cloth over the dash.

Dark adaptation is the process whereby eyes adjust for better vision in low light. Elders not only see less clearly in darkness but also require more time to accommodate to it.[106] This can be a particular problem when driving in and out of tunnels. Many elders decide on their own not to drive at night for this reason.

Elders may not identify the color of traffic signs or signals as well as younger people, especially when the light is dim or glare is present. This can be a problem because elders require additional time to read road signs, which diverts their attention from the road and traffic.[102]

Uncontrolled glare may mask oncoming traffic and limit the ability to see traffic lights, signs, and brake lights. Not controlling glare can make the driver less safe on the road. Some conditions can require more stringent control of light and glare. The color and properties of the filter are important, and the low vision specialist and the driver rehabilitation specialist can help determine the degree of glare problems and appropriate treatments, including sun filters, hats, adaptive visors, and other adaptive steps. A driver rehabilitation specialist may advise some patients to avoid driving just after sunrise and just before sunset, where low-lying sun might cause significant glare problems.

According to the AARP,[107] elders may be able to compensate for some visual limitations. They should have their vision checked at least yearly and avoid eyeglass frames that obstruct peripheral vision. Learning the general meaning of traffic signs by their shapes and colors and avoiding driving at night whenever possible are useful precautions. Various lens tints may be used to improve color recognition or the detection of objects, signs, and road users in low contrast areas.

Approximately 37% of people older than age 65 years experience some hearing loss.[108] This loss can cause problems during driving because horns, sirens, and train whistles may be difficult to hear. It may also prevent elders from realizing that the turn signal indicator is on when no turns are being made. Elders should have their hearing tested by a qualified professional. When adjusting to any hearing assistive device, elders should keep the volume of the car radio as low as possible, leave the air conditioning or heating units on the lowest possible setting, and visually check turn signals. Alerting systems and mirrors may also be used to improve awareness. (Resources for drivers with hearing difficulties are listed in the Appendix.)

The aging process also affects muscles and joints in ways that may affect driving. Elders may experience back pain, making it difficult to sit for long periods. Special cushions may be helpful. Arthritis may cause stiffness in the neck, which makes it painful when turning to check for traffic. Fatigue and discomfort are also problems that may distract elders and lessen their awareness of traffic conditions. Power steering and power brakes can help tremendously. A wide variety of mirrors is available to compensate for stiffness in the neck. Using tilt steering and arm rests may also help. A driver rehabilitation specialist can help determine whether modifications to their vehicle will help the elder who is experiencing a decrease in strength or in range of motion. Reaction time is

extremely important in safe driving. Reaction time is the time required by the eyes to see and the brain to process, decide what to do, and transmit the information to the proper body parts. For example, after seeing that the traffic ahead has stopped, a driver extends the right leg and pushes on the brake pedal. The ability to respond quickly may decrease with age, but specific safety measures can be used to compensate for the loss. One strategy is to maintain a safe distance from the car ahead. When stopping, the driver should be able to see the tires of the car in front. Other strategies are to avoid rush hour traffic and to take someone else along, especially when traveling to a new destination. If elders are upset or ill, they will probably have a slower reaction time. Education on compensatory techniques can help elders change unsafe habits. The AARP and the AAA offer various programs and courses for elder drivers (Figure 14-10). The driver safety course offered by the AARP covers many issues, including decreased reaction time, visual and hearing losses, the effects of certain medications, and hazardous situations.[107] The fee for these courses is nominal, and many insurance companies will offer a rebate on automobile insurance after successful completion of a driver safety course. However, these classes do not include behind-the-wheel testing. COTAs should discuss any concerns about the elder's ability to drive safely with the supervising OTR and physician whenever possible.

A behind-the-wheel evaluation is the best method for determining driver safety. A driving evaluation program that specializes in working with persons with disabilities can determine safety and equipment needs. The AOTA Older Driver Initiative and the ADED assist COTAs in locating driver evaluation programs. These programs can also instruct COTAs in the proper procedures for reporting unsafe or questionable drivers to the DMV of each state. COTAs should clearly document all

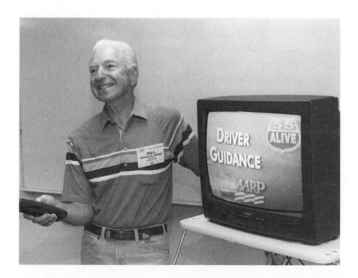

FIGURE 14-10 There are various programs and courses in the community to assist elder drivers.

recommendations to elders. For example, if the COTA recommends that an elder's driving ability be evaluated after a stroke, this recommendation must be clearly stated in the medical chart. To demonstrate thorough care, COTAs are advised to document the names of at least three resources given to the client.

A wide variety of equipment is available to help elders continue driving. This equipment is available from a variety of sources, including equipment catalogs, vendors, and automobile manufacturers (Table 14-3). (Refer to the Appendix for addresses of organizations to contact for additional resources.)

CASE STUDY

Mr. Thomas is 62 years old. One year ago he had a right cerebrovascular accident and has a nonfunctional left upper extremity. For long distances, he uses a manual wheelchair, which he pushes with his right lower extremity. For short distances, he slowly ambulates using a quad cane. Other medical conditions include a seizure disorder controlled by medication and a left hip joint replacement that causes pain and discomfort with prolonged sitting. A former physical education teacher, Mr. Thomas enjoys working with students at the high school level and is anxious to return to work in some capacity. His wife works full-time, and he receives occasional assistance in transportation from friends. Mr. Thomas believes he is ready to drive, but his wife is very concerned for his safety.

TABLE 14-3

Adaptive Equipment Ideas		
Difficulty	**Effect on driving**	**Resources to assist elder drivers**
Decreased neck ROM or pain when turning head	Limited scope of view of traffic around car	Install panoramic mirrors (Brookstone) or convex mirrors (can be installed by vendors); refer to driving program for evaluation; instruct client in use of head support
Decreased shoulder ROM or pain in shoulders	Difficulty steering, reaching for seat belt, and adjusting rearview mirror	Use arm supports already in vehicle; automobile upholsterer can build up existing arm supports to support elbows, which usually decreases client's shoulder pain; client may need effort of steering reduced, which can be determined by driving evaluation (driving program can refer to appropriate vendor for this modification); instruct elder in use of stick to adjust rearview mirror and tilt steering wheel
Decreased ROM or pain in fingers and hands	Difficulty turning key, opening door, adjusting radio, air conditioning, and so on; possible difficulty holding onto steering wheel safely	A wide variety of key holders and door openers is available from medical supply catalogs; knob extensions can be made by car vendors; refer client for driving evaluation to determine need for steering device or built-up steering wheel
Back pain	Decreased concentration caused by pain; difficulty turning to check traffic	A wide variety of cushions and lumbar supports is available from medical supply companies and vendors; these should be tried before purchase; driving programs can also evaluate and provide resources
Impairment or loss of both lower extremities	Inability to operate gas and brake pedals	Refer to driving program for evaluation of ability to use hand controls
Impairment or loss of right lower extremity	Difficulty using gas and brake pedals	Refer to driving program for evaluation of ability to use left foot accelerator
Impairment or loss of left upper extremity	Difficulty using turn signal and turning	Refer to driving program for evaluation of ability to use right crossover directional and spinner knob
Impairment or loss of right upper extremity	Difficulty steering, shifting gears in automatic or manual cars	Refer to driving program for evaluation of ability to use spinner knob
Hearing impairment	Inability to hear emergency sirens; failure to turn off turn signal	Elder drivers can purchase equipment to amplify sound of blinker; hearing aids can help clients better hear sirens
Cognitive impairment	Decreased judgment and decision making; slow reaction time; unsafe driving	Refer to driving program for detailed evaluation; discuss concerns with occupational therapist; document recommendations clearly
Visual impairment	Compromised ability to read signs; overly slow driving; generally unsafe driving skills	Refer to optometrist for vision checkup; if elder has low vision, refer to ophthalmologist or neuro-optometrist that specializes in low vision. Neuro-Optometric Rehabilitation Association (NORA) is a good resource for locating this area of specialty.

Adapted from Lillie, S. (1993). Evaluation for driving. In T. T. Yoshikawa & E. Lipton (Eds.). *Ambulatory Geriatric Care*. St. Louis, MO: Mosby.
ROM, range of motion.

Mr. Thomas received a driving evaluation, during which he exhibited difficulties such as weaving out of the lane and forgetting to turn off his turn signal. After driving for 20 minutes, he drifted across two lanes and lost his concentration. The driving instructor had to take over the steering wheel to pull the car over to the side of the road. Mr. Thomas stated that his "leg hurt."

After the evaluation, the deficits observed during driving were discussed. Mr. Thomas demonstrated insight into his difficulties and expressed the desire to begin training to improve his driving skills. Equipment needs included a spinner knob to allow him to steer with one hand and a right crossover directional device that enabled him to use his right hand for directional use. Training strategies included asking Mr. Thomas to tell the driving instructor when he was starting to have pain in his leg and to pull over when it was safe. He was reminded to turn off his directional signal after use and to look ahead while driving. After three training sessions, Mr. Thomas was able to demonstrate safe driving skills. He received a driving test from the DMV and passed. He is now able to return to part-time work and independent living.

■ CASE STUDY QUESTIONS

1 Considering the case of Mr. Thomas, identify some relevant recommendations for driving if he had experienced a spinal cord injury rather than a cerebrovascular accident.
2 Identify alternatives for transportation appropriate for Mr. Thomas if he had failed the driving evaluation.
3 Identify possible funding resources such as Vocational Rehabilitation Services for adaptive driving equipment and driver rehabilitation sessions.

■ CHAPTER REVIEW QUESTIONS

1 Explain the reason that Omnibus Budget Reconciliation Act regulations involving the use of restraints were drafted, and discuss related requirements for health providers.
2 Explain the steps to be taken in establishing a restraint reduction program.
3 Explain the role of the COTA in consultations regarding the use of restraints.
4 Describe at least three environmental adaptations that may help reduce the use of restraints.
5 Identify psychosocial approaches to reducing the use of restraints with an elder who wanders.
6 Explain the ways that activity aids in the reduction of restraints.
7 Describe the ideal position in which an elder should sit in a wheelchair.
8 Describe at least three additional considerations when monitoring the appropriate fitting wheelchair for a bariatric client.
9 List five precautions to consider when monitoring the appropriate fit of a wheelchair for an elder.
10 Identify three reasons that many falls go unreported.
11 Explain the reason that some elders and their family members are reluctant to change the environment

when personal safety and prevention of falls are a concern.
12 Explain the need for assessment of an elder's nighttime toileting skills.
13 Describe ways the home can be modified to prevent falls if elders have vision impairments and poor standing balance.
14 Identify three emergency strategies for an elder who lives alone and has a history of falls.
15 List the issues that must be considered when recommending community transportation.
16 Describe strategies to alleviate the elder's fear of using transportation.
17 Describe the actions of the COTA when the client's ability to be a safe driver is in question.

REFERENCES

1. Joanna Briggs Institute (JBI), 2002. Physical restraint—part 1: Use in acute and residential care facilities. Best Practice 6 (3), 1-6.
2. Mott, S., Poole, J., Kenrick, M., 2005. Physical and chemical restraints in acute care: Their potential impact on the rehabilitation of older people. International Journal of Nursing Practice 11 (3), 95-101.
3. OBRA Omnibus Budget Reconciliation Act, Pub. L. No. 100-20, 101 Stat. 1330 (1987).
4. Centers for Medicare & Medicaid Services, 2006. CMS publishes final patients rights rule on use of restraints and seclusion: Better, more extensive training of staff required. Retrieved March 18, 2010, from http://www.cms.hhs.gov/apps/media/press/release.asp?Counter=2057.
5. U.S. Department of Health & Human Services, Centers for Medicare & Medicaid Services, 2008. Release of report: Freedom from unnecessary restraints: Two decades of national progress in nursing home care (Ref: S&C-09-11). Retrieved from http://www.cms.gov/SurveyCertificationGenInfo/downloads/SCLetter09-11.pdf.
6. U.S. Department of Health and Human Services, Agency for Healthcare Research and Quality, 2009. National Healthcare Quality Report. (AHRQ Publication No. 10-0003). Retrieved from http://www.ahrq.gov/qual/nhqr09/nhqr09.pdf.
7. Health Care Financing Administration, 1995. Interpretive guidelines Rev. 250: Part II guidance to surveyors for long-term care facilities tag #s f221-241. U.S. Department of Health and Human Services, Washington, DC, pp. 44-53.
8. Health Care Financing Administration, 2001. 42 Code of Federal Regulations, Part 483 Subpart B, Requirements for long-term care facilities. U.S. Department of Health and Human Services, Washington, DC.
9. Morris, K., 2007. Issues and answers: Restraint use. Ohio Nurses Review 82 (4), 14-15.
10. Kleen, K., 2004. Restraint regulation: The tie that binds: Break free of potential litigation by recognizing patient rights related to physical restraints. Nursing Management 35 (11), 36-38.
11. Strumpf, N.E., Evans, L.K., Wagner, J., Patterson, J., 1992. Reducing physical restraint: Developing an educational program. Journal of Gerontological Nursing 18 (11), 21.
12. Kari, N., Michels, P., 1991. The Lazarus project: The politics of empowerment. American Journal of Occupational Therapy 45 (8), 719.
13. Joanna Briggs Institute (JBI), 2002b. Physical restraint—part 2: Minimization in acute and residential care facilities. Best Practice 6 (4), 1-6.

14. Brungardt, G., 1994. Patient restraints: New guidelines for a less restrictive approach. Geriatrics 49 (6), 43.
15. Reed, P., Tilly, J., 2008. Dementia care practice recommendations for nursing homes and assisted living, phase 2: Falls, wandering, and physical restraints. Alzheimer's Care Today 9 (1), 51-59.
16. Janelli, L.M., Kanski, G.W., Neary, M.A., 1994. Physical restraints: Has OBRA made a difference? Journal of Gerontological Nursing 20 (6), 17.
17. Strumpf, N., Evans, L., Bourbonniere, M., 2001. Restraints. In: Mezey, M. (Ed.), The Encyclopedia of Elder Care. Springer, New York, pp. 567-569.
18. Medicare and Medicaid Programs; Hospital Conditions of Participation: Patient Rights; Final Rule. 71 Fed. Reg. 71294 (2006) (to be codified at 42 C.F.R. pt. 483.13).
19. Mion, L.C., Mercurio, A., 1992. Methods to reduce restraints: Process, outcomes, and future directions. Journal of Gerontological Nursing 18 (11), 5.
20. J. Rader, personal communication, 1996.
21. Rader, J., 1995. In: Tornquist, E. (Ed.), Individualized Dementia Care: Creative, Compassionate Approaches. Springer, New York.
22. Werner, P., Koroknay, V., Braun, J., Cohen-Mansfield, J., 1994. Individualized care alternatives used in the process of removing restraints in the nursing home. Journal of the American Geriatrics Society 42 (3), 321.
23. Neufeld, R.R., Libow, L.S., Foley, W.J., Dunbar, J.M., Cohen, C., Breuer, B., 1999. Restraint reduction reduces serious injuries among nursing home residents. Journal of the American Geriatrics Society 47 (10), 1202-1207.
24. Ericson, L.L., 1991. Restraints in the nursing home environment. Occupational Therapy Forum 6 (4), 1.
25. Tideiksaar, R., 2001. Falls. In: Bonder, B., Wagner, M. (Eds.), Functional Performance in Older Adults. second ed. FA Davis, Philadelphia.
26. Patterson, J.E., Strumpf, N.E., Evans, L.K., 1995. Nursing consultation to reduce restraints in a nursing home. Clinical Nurse Specialist 9 (4), 231.
27. Eigsti, D.G., Vrooman, N., 1992. Releasing restraints in the nursing home: It can be done. Journal of Gerontological Nursing 18 (1), 21.
28. Reference deleted in chapter.
29. Maine care center reduces use of bed rails. 2004. Health Progress 85 (6), 32.
30. Evans, L.K., Forceia, M.A., Yurkow, J., et al., 1999. The geriatric day hospital. In: Katz, P., Mezey, M., Kane, R. (Eds.), Emerging Systems in Long-Term Care. Springer, New York.
31. Gallo, J.J., Busby-Whitehead, J., Rabins, P.V., et al., 1999. Reichel's Care of the Elderly: Clinical Aspects of Aging. fifth ed. Lippincott Williams & Wilkins, Philadelphia.
32. Plautz, R., Camp, C., 2001. Activities as agents for intervention and rehabilitation in long-term care. In: Bonder, B., Wagner, M., (Eds.), Functional Performance in Older Adults. second ed. FA Davis, Philadelphia.
33. Greenberg, D., 1996. Geriatric seating and positioning: Definitely a therapy task. Gerontology Special Interest Section Newsletter 19 (3), 1.
34. Jones, D.A., 1995. Seating problems in long-term care. In: Tornquist, E.M. (Ed.), Individualized Dementia Care: Creative Compassionate Approaches. Springer, New York.
35. Russell, J.N., Hendershot, G.E., LeClere, F., Howie, L.J., Adler, M., 1997. Trends and differential use of assistive technology devices: United States, 1994. Advance Data 292, 1-10.
36. Sabol, T.P., Haley, E.S., 2006. Wheelchair evaluation for the older adult. Clinics in Geriatric Medicine 22, 355-375.
37. Brechtelsbauer, D.A., Louie, A., 1999. Wheelchair use among long-term care residents. Annals of Long Term Care 1999 (7), 213-220.
38. Kaye, H.S., Kang, T., LaPlante, M.P., 2000. Mobility Device Use in the United States. Disability Statistics Report 14. U.S. Department of Education, National Institute on Disability and Rehabilitation Research, Washington, DC.
39. Krasilovsky, G., 1993. Seating assessment and management in a nursing home population. Physical and Occupational Therapy in Geriatrics 11, 25-38.
40. Rader, J., Jones, D., Miller, L., 2000. The importance of individualized wheelchair seating for frail older adults. Journal of Gerontological Nursing 26, 24-32.
41. Perr, A., 1998. Elements of seating and wheeled mobility intervention. Occupational Therapy Practice 3 (9), 16-24.
42. Hoenig, H., Landerman, L.R., Shipp, K.M., George, L., 2003. Activity restriction among wheelchair users. American Journal of Geriatrics Society 2003 (51), 1244-1251.
43. Hoenig, H., Landerman, L.R., Shipp, K.M., Pieper, C., Pieper C., Richardson, M., et al., 2005. Clinical Trial of a Rehabilitation Expert Clinician Versus Usual Care for Providing Manual Wheelchairs. Journal of American Geriatrics Society 53, 1712-1720.
44. Hoenig, H., Pieper, C., Zolkewitz, M., Schenkman, M., Branch, L.G., 2002. Wheelchair users are not necessarily wheelchair bound. Journal of Geriatrics Society 50, 645-654.
45. Scherer, M.J., Sax, C., Vanbiervliet, A., Cushman, L.A., Scherer, J.V., 2005. Predictors of assistive technology use: The importance of personal and psychological factors. Disability Rehabilitation 27, 1321-1331.
46. Phillips, B., Zhao, H., 1993. Predictors of assistive technology abandonment. Assistive Technology 5, 36-45.
47. Fontein, J., Mundy, P., 2008. Wheelchair positioning for all ages and sizes. PowerPoint presentation at Care Medical Care Fair, November 2008, www.pdgmobility.com.
48. Brackens, L., 2008. All bariatric patients were not created equal: Mobility Management Newsletter (10/01/2008), www.mobilitymgmt.com.
49. Fontein, J., Tanguay, S., 2009. Measurement, positioning and mobility considerations for bariatric customers. PowerPoint presentation at Care Medical Care Fair, November 2009, www.pdgmobility.com and www.mobilitymgmt.com.
50. Kittel, A., Di Marco, A. & Stewart, H. (2002). Factors influencing the decision to abandon manual wheelchairs for three individuals with a spinal cord injury. Disability & Rehabilitation, 24 (1-3), 106-114.
51. Batavia, M., Batavia, A. & Friedman, R. (2001). Changing chairs: anticipating problems in prescribing wheelchairs. Disability & Rehabilitation, 23 (12), 539-548.
52. Feldt, K.S., Warne, M.A., Ryden, M.B., 1998. Examining pain and agitation in aggressive cognitively impaired older adults. Journal of Gerontological Nursing 24 (11), 14-22.
53. Simmons, S., Schnelle, J., MacRae, P., Ouslander, J., 1995. Wheelchairs as mobility restraints: Predictors of wheelchair activity in non-ambulatory nursing home residents. Journal of American Geriatrics Society 43, 384-388.
54. Lamb, S.E., Jorstad-Stein, E.C., Hauer, K., Becker, C., 2005. Prevention of Falls Network Europe and Outcomes Consensus Group. Development of a common outcome data set for fall injury prevention trials: The Prevention of Falls Network of Europe Consensus. Journal of the American Geriatrics Society 53, 1618-1622.
55. Centers for Disease Control and Prevention, 2008. Self-reported falls and fall-related injuries among persons aged > or =65 years—United States, 2006. Morbidity and Mortality Weekly Report 57, 225-229.
56. Gillespie, L.D., Robertson, M.C., Gillespie, W.J., Lamb, S.E., Gates, S., Cumming, R.G., et al., 2009. Interventions for preventing falls in older people living in the community. Cochrane Database of Systematic Reviews, 2. Art. No.: CD007146.

57. Rubenstein, L.Z., Josephson, K.R., 2002. The epidemiology of falls and syncope. Clinics in Geriatric Medicine 18, 141-158.

58. Centers for Disease Control and Prevention, 2006. Fatalities and injuries from falls among older adults—United States, 1993-2003 and 2001-2005. Morbidity and Mortality Weekly Report 55, 1222-1224.

59. Rubenstein, L.Z., Solomon, D.H., Roth, C.P., Young, R.T., Shekelle, P.G., Chang, J.T., et al., 2009. Detection and management of falls and instability in vulnerable elders by community physicians. Journal of the American Geriatrics Society 57 (9), 1527-1531.

60. Min, L., Yoon, W., Mariano, J., Wenger, N., Elliott, M., Kamberg, C., Saliba, D., et al., 2009. The vulnerable elders—13 survey predicts 5-year functional decline and mortality outcomes in older ambulatory care patients. Journal of the American Geriatrics Society 57 (11), 2070-2076.

61. Jung, D., Lee, J., Lee, S., 2009. A meta-analysis of fear of falling treatment programs for the elderly. Western Journal of Nursing Research 31 (1), 6-16.

62. Laird, R.D., Studenski, S., Perera, S., Wallace, D., 2001. Fall history is an independent predictor of adverse health outcomes and utilization in the elderly. American Journal of Managed Care 7 (12), 1133-1138.

63. Stevens, J.A., Corso, P.S., Finkelstein, E.A., Miller, T.R., 2006. The costs of fatal and nonfatal falls among older adults. Injury Prevention 12, 290-295.

64. Frick, K.D., Kung, J.Y., Parrish, J.M., Narrett, M.J., 2010. Evaluation the cost-effectiveness of fall prevention programs that reduce fall-related hip fractures in older adults. Journal of the American Geriatrics Society 58, 136-141.

65. Rubenstein, L.Z., Josephson, K.R., 2006. Falls and their prevention in elderly people: What does the evidence show? Medical Clinics of North America 90, 807-824.

66. Carpenter, C., Scheatzle, M., D'Antonio, J., Ricci, P., Coben, J., 2009. Identification of fall risk factors in older adult emergency department patients. Academic Emergency Medicine 16 (3), 211-219.

67. Chang, J., Ganz, D., 2007. Quality indicators for falls and mobility problems in vulnerable elders. Journal of the American Geriatrics Society 55 (S2), S327-S334.

68. Administration on Aging, 2003. A profile of older Americans: 2002. U.S. Department of Health and Human Services, Washington, DC.

69. Desai, M., Pratt, L.A., Lentzner, H., Robinson, K.N., 2001. Trends in vision and hearing among older Americans. Aging Trends 2, 1-8.

70. Good, G., LaGrow, S., Alpass, F., 2008. An age-cohort study of older adults with and without visual impairments: Activity, independence, and life satisfaction. Journal of Visual Impairment & Blindness 102 (9), 517-527.

71. Light, K., Thigpen, M., 2010. Geriatric Rehabilitation: Evidence and Clinical Application. McGraw-Hill, New York.

72. Naqvi, F., Lee, S., Fields, L., 2009. Appraising a guideline for preventing acute care falls. Geriatrics 64 (3), 10-33.

73. Nolte, J., 2009. The Human Brain: An Introduction to its Functional Anatomy, 6th ed. Mosby Elsevier, Philadelphia.

74. Costarella, M., Monteleone, L., Steindler, R., Zuccaro, S., 2010. Decline of physical and cognitive conditions in the elderly measured through the functional reach test and the Mini-Mental State Examination. Archives of Gerontology and Geriatrics 50 (3), 332-337.

75. Carter, N.D., Kannus, P., Khan, K.M., 2001. Exercise in the prevention of falls in older people: A systematic literature review examining the rationale and the evidence. Sports Medicine 31, 427-438.

76. Tideiksaar, R., 1987. Fall prevention in the home. Topics in Geriatric Rehabilitation 3, 1.

77. Leipzig, R.M., Cumming, R.G., Tinetti, M.E., 1999. Drugs and falls in older people: A systematic review and meta-analysis: I. Psychotropic drugs. Journal of American Geriatrics Society 47, 30-39.

78. Woolcott, J., Richardson, K., Wiens, M., Marin, J., Khan, K., Marra, C., 2009. Meta-analysis of the impact of 9 medication classes on falls in elderly persons. Archives of Internal Medicine 169 (21), 1952-1960.

79. Fuller-Thomson, E., Yu, B., Nuru-Jeter, A., Guralnik, J., Minkler, M., 2009. Basic ADL disability and functional limitation rates among older Americans from 2000-2005: The end of the decline? Journals of Gerontology; Series A, Biological Sciences and Medical Sciences 64 (12), 1333-1336.

80. American Occupational Therapy Association, 2008. Occupational Therapy Practice Framework: Domain and Process. second ed. American Journal of Occupational Therapy 62, 625-683.

81. Shumway-Cook, A., Ciol, M.A., Hoffman, J., Yorkston, K., Chan, L., 2009. Falls in the Medicare population: Incidence, associated factors, and impact on health care. Physical Therapy 89, 324-332.

82. Tideiksaar, R., 1989. Geriatric falls: Assessing the cause, preventing recurrence. Geriatrics 44 (7), 57.

83. Cameron, I.D., Murray, G.R., Gillespie, L.D., Robertson, M.C., Hill, K.D., Cumming, R.G., et al., 2010. Interventions for preventing falls in older people in nursing care facilities and hospitals. Cochrane Database of Systematic Reviews, 1, Art. No.: CD005465.

84. Sherrington, C., Whitney, J.C., Lord, S.R., Herbert, R.D., Cumming, R.G., Close, J.C., 2008. Effective exercise for the prevention of falls: A systematic review and meta-analysis. Journal of the American Geriatrics Society 56, 2234-2243.

85. Kim, H., Han, J., Cho, Y., 2009. The effectiveness of community-based tai chi training on balance control during stair descent by older adults. Journal of Physical Therapy Science 21, 317-323.

86. Mihay, L.M., Boggs, K.M., Breck, A.J., Dokken, E.L., NaThalang, G.C., 2006. The effect of tai chi inspired exercise compared to strength training: A pilot study of elderly retired community dwellers. Physical and Occupational Therapy in Geriatrics 24 (3), 13-26.

87. Bouwen, A., De Lepeleire, J., Buntinx, F., 2008. Rate of accidental falls in institutionalized older people with and without cognitive impairment halved as a result of a staff-orientated intervention. Age and Ageing 37, 306-310.

88. Detweiler, M.B., Kim, K.Y., Taylor, B.Y., 2005. Focused supervision of high-risk fall dementia patients: A simple method to reduce fall incidence and severity. American Journal of Alzheimer's Disease and Other Dementias 20, 97-104.

89. Shimada, H., Tiedeman, A., Lord, S., Suzuki, T., 2009. The effect of enhanced supervision on fall rates in residential aged care. American Journal of Physical Medicine and Rehabilitation 88, 823-828.

90. Bartley, M., O'Neill, D., 2010. Transportation and driving in longitudinal studies on ageing. Age & Ageing 39, 631-636.

91. Savoye, C., 2001. States to try to help elderly stay behind the wheel. Christian Science Monitor, 93, 3.

92. National Highway Traffic Safety Administration, n.d. Traffic safety facts 2008 data: Older population (DOT HS 811 161). Author, Washington, DC. Retrieved October 25, 2010, from http://www-nrd.nhtsa.dot.gov/Pubs/811161.PDF.

93. American Occupational Therapy Association, 2005. Statement: Driving and community mobility. American Journal of Occupational Therapy 59, 666-670.

94. National Institutes on Aging, 2010. Age page. Retrieved October 25, 2010, from http://www.nia.nih.gov/HealthInformation/Publications/drivers.htm.

95. Borowsky, A., Shinar, D., Oron-Gilad, T., 2010. Age, skill, and hazard perception in driving. Accident Analysis & Prevention 42, 1240-1249.

96. Hunt, L.A., Arbesman, M., 2008. Evidence-based and occupational perspective of effective interventions for older clients that remediate or support improved driving performance. American Journal of Occupational Therapy 62, 136-148.

97. American Occupational Therapy Association, 2008. Occupational therapy practice framework: Domain and process. second ed. American Journal of Occupational Therapy 62, 625-683.

98. Hendrickson, C., 2005. Changes over time in community mobility of elders with disabilities. Physical and Occupational Therapy in Geriatrics 23 (2-3), 75-89.

99. Chia, D., 2008. Policies and practices for effectively and efficiently meeting ADA paratransit demand: A synthesis of transit practice. Transit Cooperative Research Board/ Transportation Research Board, Washington, DC.

100. Hoggarth, P.A., Innes, C.R., Dalrymple-Alford, J.C., Severinsen, J., Jones, R., 2010. Comparison of a linear and a non-linear model for using sensory-motor, cognitive, personality, and demographic data to predict driving ability in healthy older adults. Accident, Analysis and Prevention 42, 1759-1768.

101. Vitale, S., Cotch, M., Sperduto, R., 2006. Prevalence of visual impairment in the United States. Journal of the American Medical Association 295 (18), 2158-2163.

102. Ilett, G., 2010. Functional vision assessment. Optician 240 (6260), 24, 25.

103. Swamy, B., 2009. Vision screening for frail older people: A randomized trial. British Journal of Ophthalmology 93, 736-741.

104. BiopticDrivingUSA.com, 2010. An introduction: Driving with bioptic glasses. Retrieved November 9, 2010, from http://www.biopticdrivingusa.com/.

105. Cui, Q., O'Neill, W., Paige, G., 2010. Advancing age alters the influence of eye position on sound localization. Experimental Brain Research 206, 371-379.

106. Morrison, J., McGrath, C., 2008. Assessment of the optical contributions to the age-related deterioration in vision. Quarterly Journal of Experimental Physiology 93, 249-269.

107. American Association of Retired Persons, 2010. Vision changes and driving: Knowing what to expect and when to get eye exams help mature drivers continue to drive safely. Retrieved October 25, 2010, from http://www.aarp.org/home-garden/transportation/info-05-2010/dsp_article_vision_changes_driving.html.

108. Huang, Q., Tang, J., 2010. Age-related hearing loss or presbycusis. European Archives of Oto-Rhino-Laryngology 267, 1179-1791.

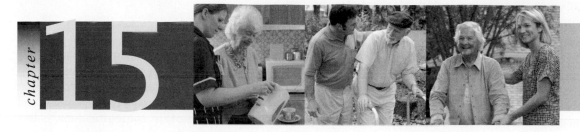

Working with Elders Who Have Vision Impairments

EVELYN Z. KATZ AND REBECCA BOTHWELL

KEY TERMS

cataracts, glaucoma, retina, lens, macular degeneration, diabetic retinopathy, visual acuity, contrast sensitivity, visual cognition, visual memory, pattern recognition, scanning, visual attention, oculomotor control, visual fields, eccentric viewing, scotoma, hemi-inattention, diplopia, strabismus

CHAPTER OBJECTIVES

1. Describe typical physiological changes affecting vision that occur with aging.
2. Name and describe the major ocular diseases affecting vision in elders.
3. Describe common vision deficits resulting from neurological insults in elders.
4. Describe psychosocial implications of vision impairments in elders, possible effects on rehabilitation, and on functional outcomes.
5. Describe the use of the Occupational Therapy Practice Framework's[1] dynamic, interactive process of evaluation, intervention, and outcomes to address functional deficits in elder clients resulting from visual impairments.
6. Identify general principles to enhance vision.
7. Identify environmental or contextual considerations and interventions to increase independence and safety in elders with low vision.
8. Identify general principles in intervention of visual dysfunction after brain insult.
9. Identify team members and community resources that registered occupational therapists (OTRs) and certified occupational therapy assistants (COTAs) may collaborate with to improve functional outcomes in elders with low vision.

CASE STUDY

Mrs. N. is an 82-year-old widow who lived alone in the two-story home that she shared with her husband for more than 50 years. At a visit to her ophthalmologist, she was told that her complaints of blurry vision with reading the mail and newspaper were due to dry macular degeneration, and that new glasses would not help her. The ophthalmologist informed her that there was nothing he could do to correct her condition.

Mrs. N. is now at a subacute rehabilitation facility following a recent knee replacement surgery, and the OTR/COTA team has been ordered to follow her. She tells them that she is a little afraid to be at home alone. She is having trouble seeing her appliance controls and the phone dial. Between her new knee replacement and her vision loss, she does not know whether she can navigate the steps in her home. She is nervous about going outdoors because she is having trouble seeing curbs and changes in walking surfaces, especially at dusk or on hazy days. She feels isolated and lonely. Her children are wondering whether she will be able to return home.

■ CASE STUDY QUESTIONS

Before reading the chapter, consider your own preconceptions about vision loss.

1. Do you think someone with partial sight, like Mrs. N., can function independently?
2. What would you do if you, like Mrs. N, could not read regular print, street signs, or the controls on your appliances?
3. If you were suddenly unable to do the things mentioned previously, list three specific activities with which you might experience difficulty.
4. Now, choose one of the activities you listed and try to complete it in a darkened room or with your vision partially obscured. Have someone time you while you do it. Afterward answer the following questions:
5. What feelings did you experience as you tried to complete the activity? Frustration? Irritation? Embarrassment?
6. Did it take you longer to complete the activity than it would without partially obscuring your vision?
7. Did you have to use other senses or make adaptations to complete the activity?

Visual impairments are common in the elderly population. One in six adults age 65 and older has a visual impairment, and this number is expected to double by the year 2030.[2] The odds of developing visual impairment worsen with age, as one in four adults age 75 years or older experiences either a moderate or severe visual impairment.[3] In addition to vision loss from ocular disease, many adults are affected by visual impairments resulting from head trauma, stroke, or neurological insult. Between 40% and 75% of individuals with head trauma or stroke are estimated to experience visual impairments requiring rehabilitation.[4] According to the Occupational Therapy Practice Framework: Domain and Process (2nd Ed.), seeing and related functions are addressed in the clients factors table as a body function under the sensory functions and pain category, and visual is listed in the Performance Skills table as a sensory perceptual skill.[1] These statistics along with the inclusion of vision in the Occupational Therapy Practice Framework[1] demonstrate the need for COTAs to possess a thorough understanding of the causes of vision loss and appropriate intervention techniques. Regardless of the particular setting, any COTA working with elders is likely to encounter many clients with visual impairments.

This chapter will provide information on the psychosocial effects of vision loss, effects of normal aging on vision, common conditions causing vision loss in elders, and visual dysfunction after neurological insult. The chapter also addresses the process for assessing elder clients' occupational performance and outcomes as well as general principles used in planning interventions to help elder clients achieve their functional goals. OTRs and COTAs function as part of a team that includes physicians, other health care providers, family/caregivers, and the elder client. The chapter addresses the roles of these team members and community resources.

PSYCHOSOCIAL EFFECTS OF VISION IMPAIRMENT

Almost 25% of adults with visual impairment report symptoms of depression compared with 10% of those without visual impairment.[5] The thought of losing one's vision is one of the most devastating disabilities imaginable. Without vision, the ability to perform many of the daily activities normally taken for granted is lost. Without vision, a means of social connectedness is lost because it is no longer possible to make eye contact or to read subtle facial expressions. The thought of vision loss conjures up a terrifying world of blackness. However, although most people think of vision loss as total blindness, most individuals with visual impairments are not totally blind. In fact, in one report, 80% of those who reported being legally blind had some degree of usable vision.[6] It is often difficult for family members, friends, and the general public to understand the limitations and capabilities of those with partial sight.[7] It is not uncommon for partially sighted individuals to be labeled as "fakes" when others observe that they are capable of one task that requires some degree of vision but are incapable of another task.[7] This confusion about the abilities of those with partial sight may produce more psychological distress than does total blindness.[7]

In addition to the ambiguity associated with being partially sighted, individuals often find it difficult to adjust to their vision loss because of the uncertainty of their condition. For many, it is difficult to know whether their vision will improve, stay the same, or get worse. There is often an internal struggle with a desire to be independent and the desire to be taken care of. In some situations, elders may want assistance but feel unable to ask for it. Elders struggling with vision loss may experience mood swings. Friedman[7] describes the stages of coping that individuals with vision loss experience as closely paralleling those that Kubler-Ross[8] describes in her study on death and dying. These stages include initial shock and denial, then guilt, bargaining, anger, depression, and, finally, adaptation.

Perski[9] describes a similar response of adaptation when he writes about the five-stage process of being a successful low vision patient. Perski[9] notes "there are definite psychological stages that many persons go through before they become a successful user of visual aids. Probably the first harsh reality that a low vision person must face is that a single pair of glasses will not help his or her vision. The reality that the person must hold a magnifying glass or use separate reading glasses and hold materials very close to his or her eye is often too much to bear."

EFFECTS OF THE NORMAL AGING PROCESS ON VISION

Although elders are more likely to experience visual impairments because of some specific ocular and neurological pathologies, they also experience many age-related changes that affect visual functioning. These normal changes must be taken into consideration when working with this population.

The retina is a multilayered lining of neural tissue on the innermost part of the eye (Figure 15-1). It receives visual messages and transmits them through the optic nerve to the brain.[10] The central area of the retina, or

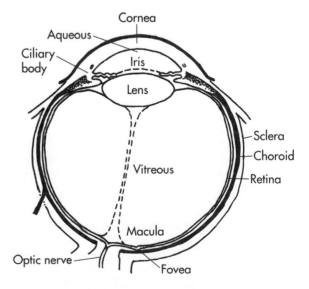

FIGURE 15-1   Anatomy of the eye.

TABLE 15-1

	Changes in Visual System Associated with Age	
Structural component	**Age-related change**	**Functional implications**
Cornea	Decreased fluid bathing cornea	Dryness, irritation
	Accumulation of lipids	Increased astigmatism with increased blurring of vision
Iris	Decreased permeability	May contribute to glaucoma
Ciliary muscles	Atrophy of muscles	Decreased mobility of lens causing decreased muscle effectiveness
Pupil	Decreased pupil size	Decreased light reaching retina; difficulty seeing dark objects or objects in dim light
	Decreased papillary reflex	Decreased dark adaptation and recovery from glare
Lens	Lens growth	Decreased accommodative ability
	Decreased refractive index of lenses	Uneven refracture properties can result in double vision in one eye
	Yellowing	Reduced amount of light reaching retina, changes in light composition alters color vision
Vitreous	Contracts	Increased chance of separation from retina or retinal detachment

Adapted from Zoltan, B. (2006). *Vision, Perception, and Cognition: A Manual for the Evaluation and Treatment of the Adult with Acquired Brain Injury,* 4th ed. Thorofare, NJ: Slack.

macula, has a concentration of cone cells that enable color vision and fine-detail discrimination. Rod cells are extremely sensitive to light and provide peripheral vision and night vision.[10] As the retina ages, it gradually loses neurons. Central or peripheral vision may be affected, depending on which retinal neurons die. The rate of retinal deterioration and the resultant visual field loss vary among individuals, but, generally, elders experience shrinkage of the peripheral field, experience difficulty with light and dark adaptation, and require increased time to switch from viewing near objects to far objects (accommodation) and to recover from glare. Because pupil size and function decrease with age, elders require more illumination for fine-detail tasks.[11] Many elders require three times more light than a person requires in his or her twenties or thirties.[12]

Changes may also occur in the lens of the eye with age (see Figure 15-1). The lens is responsible for properly focusing the image on the retina. It does this by changing shape according to the distance of the object being viewed.[13] As the lens ages, it loses some of its elasticity, making shape change or accommodation more difficult. This condition, called *presbyopia*, affects focal ability at near distances, making it difficult to read print or perform close-vision tasks.[14] The greatest change usually occurs between ages 40 and 45 years.[14] Reading glasses or bifocals are often prescribed at this time. In addition to this loss of elasticity, the lens also becomes yellower with age. This deeper yellow can affect the ability to differentiate between colors and discriminate objects with low contrast.[15]

SPECIFIC OCULAR PATHOLOGIES

In addition to the natural aging process, specific pathological eye conditions have a more profound effect on functional visual abilities. Four major conditions that

affect an elder's vision are cataracts, age-related macular degeneration (wet or dry), glaucoma, and diabetic retinopathy. Each of these conditions can cause visual impairment when they occur in isolation, but they commonly co-occur in elders, increasing the challenge to remain functionally independent (Table 15-1). More about general intervention ideas for any ocular condition will be presented later in the chapter.

Cataracts

A cataract is a clouding of the lens, the clear part of the eye that helps focus light, or an image on the retina. This clouding is related to aging and changes in the protein that, along with water, make up the lens. Protein clumps up in the lens, forming cataracts, which make vision blurry and dull by preventing adequate amounts of light from reaching the retina.[16] Cataracts can be treated successfully with surgery and are no longer considered to be a major cause of permanent visual impairment in developed countries. The most common procedure is the removal of the opacified lens followed by the insertion of an intraocular lens implant.[17]

If an elder is struggling with cataracts before surgery or if the elder is not a surgical candidate, interventions that control glare, increase lighting, and low levels of magnification can be helpful.

Macular Degeneration or Age-Related Macular Degeneration (ARMD)

Macular degeneration is the leading cause of vision loss in older Americans.[18] The macula is the central portion of the retina where the clearest vision is found. There are two types of macular degeneration: the "dry" (non-exudative or atrophic) type and the "wet" (exudative or hemorrhagic type). Dry age-related macular degeneration

(ARMD) is the result of yellowish deposits, or drusen, forming under the macula. This causes the macula to thin and dry out. As cells on the macula become non-functioning, elders experience a blurry, dark, or blank spot in the center of their visual field. The wet form of ARMD is caused by the rapid growth of small blood vessels beneath the macula. These blood vessels leak and cause scarring on the macula, resulting in vision loss.[18] The wet form of ARMD can sometimes be treated with photoco-agulation, laser surgery, or, more recently and effectively, by intraocular injection with Macugen, Lucentis, or Avastin (drugs that dry up the leaking blood vessels and slow their regrowth). Results of the Age-Related Eye Disease Studies (AREDS) suggest that progression of dry ARMD can be slowed by the intake of anti-oxidant sup-plements.[19] Current interventions can slow the rate of vision loss; however, there is no known intervention that prevents macular degeneration or that can reverse the loss of vision.[19] Because peripheral visual fields are usually spared, ARMD does not result in total blindness.[18]

Common problems experienced by elders with ARMD include difficulty distinguishing faces, reading signs, or seeing traffic signals (distance tasks), or reading regular print, writing, and doing needlework (near tasks). Elders with wet ARMD often experience distortion of the central visual field that may make straight lines appear wavy (metamorphopsia). This distortion can lead to balance and mobility problems. Visual hallucinations as a result of Charles Bonnet syndrome are sometimes experienced by elders with ARMD. The hallmark of these hallucinations is that they occur and disappear spontaneously with no known external cause, and they are recognized as unreal by the elder and are nonthreatening. Some elders have described seeing "fields of flowers in my living room," animals, or even people across the room.[20] Elders experi-encing Charles Bonnet syndrome may be reluctant to discuss their visual symptoms, fearing a label of mental instability or decreased cognitive function. They need to be reassured that this is not the case. Charles Bonnet syndrome has been found to affect elders with ARMD with severe loss of contrast sensitivity in both eyes.[21] COTAs working with elders who have macular degenera-tion should be aware of specific interventions for this diagnosis (Box 15-1).

Glaucoma

Glaucoma is a group of serious ocular conditions that involve excessively high pressure inside the eyeball. This increased pressure results from a buildup of excess fluid in the eye.[10] Increased intraocular pressure can eventually cause damage to the optic nerve or the blood vessels that supply the optic nerve.[10] One of the first effects of this optic nerve damage is usually a loss of vision in the periph-eral field (Figure 15-2). This loss of peripheral vision is often not noticed by the individual initially, and the disease frequently progresses substantially before it is noticed.[22]

BOX 15-1

Intervention Gems for Individuals with Macular Degeneration

Elders with macular degeneration usually experience problems with loss of detail, central vision early in their vision loss. Peripheral vision is usually spared, even in more advanced stages.

- Lighting—provide training with different types of task lighting: full spectrum incandescent, fluorescent, halogen, and LED as well as positioning of lighting source so that the elder can identify which one is preferred for an activity.
- Reduce glare in the elder's environment by eliminating bare or exposed light bulbs and highly polished or reflective surfaces; use light diffusing shades, blinds or curtains, and careful placement of furniture.
- Use color and contrast in the elder's environment to define objects and surfaces—a contrasting colored towel, draped on a chair can make it easier to see.
- Increase object size—large numbered phones, kitchen timers, medicine organizers, large print checks make ADL easier to complete with decreased central or detail vision.
- Decrease clutter, including visual clutter—clear paths from room to room and in front of furniture, counters, and appliances. Limit the number of items on countertops and tables. Limit use of bold patterns, which create visual clutter.
- Magnification—when possible, elders will need referral to a low-vision ophthalmologist or optometrist to prescribe the appropriate magnification devices for near, intermediate, and distance activities. However, magnifying lamps, nail clippers with attached low powered magnifiers, and inexpensive low powered magnifiers for craft and sewing may allow the elder to complete activities with decreased vision.
- Transportation options—train elders in use of alternative transportation. Many communities have paratransit systems for individuals who cannot drive or use conventional public transportation safely. Some communities offer reduced fare taxi programs for the visually impaired.

If left undetected and untreated, this loss can lead to total blindness. Elders should be encouraged to have routine ophthalmologic visits so that glaucoma may be diagnosed at an early stage. When the diagnosis is early, individuals respond well to medication and, if necessary, surgery to improve the balance of fluid in the eye.[10]

There are many types of glaucoma, but open-angle is the most common.[10] Other types include closed-angle or narrow angle, traumatic, and low-tension glaucoma.[10] Open-angle glaucoma involves an eye with normal

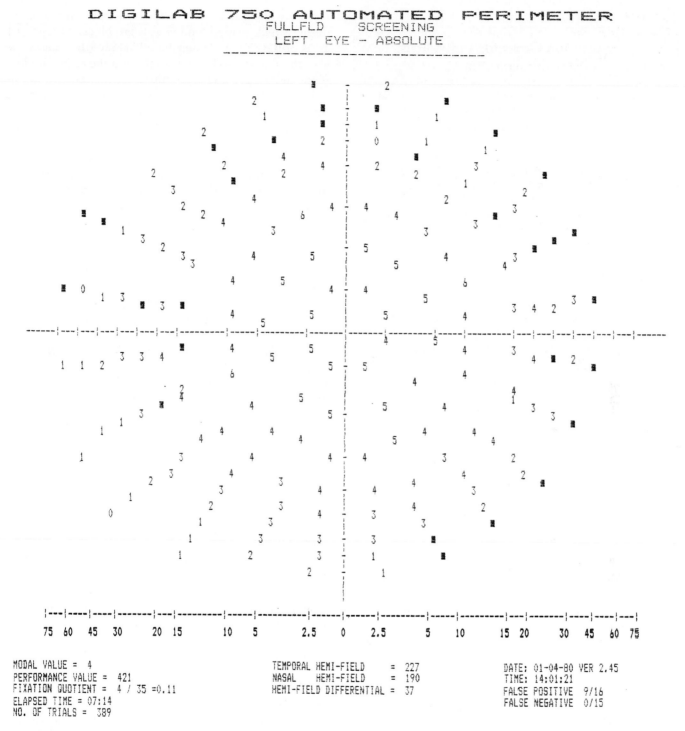

FIGURE 15-2 This printout from an automated perimeter test indicates visual loss in points marked with black squares. Note the peripheral distribution.

anatomy that, for unknown reasons, is not able to drain the fluid as efficiently as it produces it. This leads to a slow, gradual buildup of intraocular pressure over time.[10]

Closed, or narrow-angle, glaucoma is less common. This type of glaucoma progresses rapidly, and symptoms are immediately apparent. Nausea, headaches, severe redness of the eye, and pain may be symptoms of an acute

attack of narrow-angle glaucoma.[23] Emergency surgery is often required to reduce the intraocular pressure.

The functional implications of glaucoma vary greatly, depending on the severity of the disease. When diagnosis is early, glaucoma can be treated and many people may have little need to adjust their lifestyles. If the disease is allowed to progress, individuals may experience decreased

BOX 15-2

Intervention Gems for Individuals with Glaucoma

Most individuals with glaucoma do not experience problems with their vision until their disease is relatively advanced.

- Medication management is vital—train client in nonvisual techniques, labeling, organization, talking labels, and talking reminders or alarms for self-administering oral medicines and eye drops.
- Mobility problems (due to reduced peripheral vision)—address by use of contrast, reduce clutter/tripping hazards, train awareness of boundaries, and edges in environment; refer to orientation and mobility specialist for long cane (white cane) and nonsighted techniques for community mobility.
- Contrast and glare—Use of yellow, amber, or light plum glasses to increase contrast, decrease glare. Reduce reflective surfaces (glass tabletops, mirrors, highly polished floors, or counters), cover exposed light bulbs, windows, and angle task light sources to decrease glare.
- Low-power magnifiers—may help for small print or poor contrast materials.
- Increase object size for ease of identification.
- Bright colored objects will stand out if client has decreased contrast sensitivity.
- Organized scanning patterns—train client to scan in horizontal left to right, zig-zag, and circular patterns to locate obstacles, edges, and objects in their reduced visual field.

peripheral vision, difficulty adjusting to changing light, fluctuating and blurred vision, shadow-like halos around lights, and an increased sensitivity to glare.[24,25] If glaucoma goes undiagnosed, a person may lose all of his or her vision beginning with the peripheral field and eventually extending into the central visual field. Mobility and safety can be severely compromised in elders with advanced glaucoma. Referral to an orientation and mobility teacher may be appropriate for an elder experiencing decreased mobility because of vision loss at this stage. COTAs working with elders who have glaucoma should be aware of specific interventions for this diagnosis (Box 15-2).

Diabetic Retinopathy

Diabetic retinopathy, one of the complications of diabetes mellitus, is another leading cause of visual impairment in elders. Diabetic retinopathy has four stages: (1) mild nonproliferative retinopathy, the earliest stage in which microaneurysms occur as a small ballooning in the tiny vessels of the retina[19]; (2) moderate nonproliferative retinopathy, during which some blood vessels that nourish the retina are blocked; (3) severe nonproliferative retinopathy, during which many blood vessels are blocked, depriving areas of the retina of their blood supply (this causes the growth of new blood vessels to nourish the retina, leading to the next stage); and (4) proliferative retinopathy. In this most advanced stage, new blood vessels grow along the retina and along the surface of the vitreous gel that fills the inside of the eye. The new blood vessels are abnormal, with fragile walls that may leak and cause more severe changes in visual acuity. The new network of vessels and its accompanying fibrous tissue contract, and the vitreous may pull away from the retina causing further hemorrhage into the vitreous. This can also cause a retinal detachment, a serious condition requiring immediate attention and surgery to prevent vision loss.[19] If fluid leaks into the center of the macula, swelling and blurred vision can occur. This condition, known as macular edema, can happen at any stage of diabetic retinopathy, causing a significant distortion and loss of vision.[19]

Diabetic retinopathy may be treated either by photocoagulation, injection (similar to procedures used to treat wet macular degeneration), or a procedure known as vitrectomy, during which blood is removed from the vitreous of the eye with a needle and replaced by saline solution. Many people experience improved vision after these procedures, but they do not cure diabetic retinopathy. The risk of new bleeding and vision loss remains.[19]

Functional implications of diabetic retinopathy, like glaucoma, vary depending on early diagnosis and severity of the disease. Some individuals with mild retinopathy may not need to make adaptations in their performance patterns, whereas others may need to learn adaptive techniques to compensate for vision loss to continue to perform activities of daily living (ADL) safely and independently. Many elders who have advanced diabetic retinopathy experience decreased contrast sensitivity, poor night vision, and fluctuating, blurry or spotty vision. Some elders may eventually need to learn nonsighted techniques for all ADL. COTAs working with elders who have diabetic retinopathy should be aware of specific interventions for this diagnosis (Box 15-3).

VISUAL DYSFUNCTION AFTER NEUROLOGICAL INSULT

The discussion of visual impairments in elders thus far has focused on impairments as a result of ocular conditions. However, the visual system is not composed of the eyeballs alone. To perceive visual information, the data must travel through a complex nervous system and must be processed by appropriate cerebral centers. In addition, effective control of eye movements depends on proper impulses from the brain. This includes feedback from areas that monitor body and head position and movement.[26] Thus, successful adaptation to the environment through the visual sense requires the proper functioning of both ocular and neurological components (Box 15-4).

BOX 15-3

> ### Intervention Gems for Individuals with Diabetic Retinopathy
>
> Diabetic retinopathy often causes blurriness, fluctuations in vision, and may sometimes result in either central or peripheral field loss.
> - Medication management may require referral to a diabetes educator. Consider talking glucometers, pre-filled syringes, syringe magnifiers, insulin "pens," large print logs for recording blood glucose readings, insulin dosage counters, and other adaptive equipment.
> - Increase contrast in environment, printed materials, writing materials, and on computer screen.
> - Control glare with yellow, amber, or light plum tinted glasses, lighting placement, and limiting reflective surfaces in environment (see Box 15-8).
> - Neuropathy can cause loss of sensation in extremities. Special attention to safety during kitchen and bathroom activities is an essential component of training. Adaptive equipment for kitchen tasks include knife guards that slip over the fingers of the hand that holds the item to be cut, long oven mitts, oven rack guards, oven rack pulls, long handled tongs, can openers that produce a smooth edge, and nonslip cutting boards.
> - Magnification or large print materials may make reading, writing, and other near tasks easier.
> - Vision substitution—talking books, scales, microwaves, glucometers, and other devices offer options for completing ADL with decreased vision.

BOX 15-4

> ### Intervention Gems for Individuals with Neurological Visual Impairments
>
> It is essential for the COTA to have as complete a picture as possible of the visual, cognitive, and physical deficits of the elder with neurological visual impairment because they will affect interventions and functional outcomes.
> - Train elders and family/caregiver about the functional implications of visual field loss for safety and ADL performance—make sure they understand how much of the environment the elder may not see or be aware of.
> - For left-sided visual field loss, train the elder to turn head and eyes toward the "missing" side or area when beginning any activity and more frequently throughout the activity.
> - Train the elder to increase visual search organization and scanning patterns beginning with horizontal left to right, right to left, vertical top to bottom, and circular patterns.
> - Use activities that widen boundaries of visual search, and encourage use of appropriate search strategies in a variety of environments: searching for objects/signage on a wall or vacuuming to use left-to-right vertical search.
> - Intervention techniques for left-to-right horizontal pattern: dominoes, card search, sweeping, wiping off a counter, and looking for items on a shelf.
> - Intervention techniques for left-to-right vertical pattern: reading columns in sports scores or financial pages, reading ingredients in a recipe, and writing a grocery list.
> - Intervention techniques for circular patterns: puzzles, walking search, checkers, sorting coins, buttons, sorting laundry, looking for item in refrigerator, grocery store advertising circular.
> - Outline doorways, edges of furniture, and closets on side of visual deficit with bright colored tape for visual cue to scan for.

Causes of brain insult can include trauma, cancer, multiple sclerosis, and cerebrovascular accidents (CVA) or strokes. The vision system is vulnerable to strokes and other types of brain insult.[27] A host of visual disorders can result from brain insult, including visual field disorders, reduced visual acuity, reduced contrast sensitivity, problems with stereopsis (depth perception), difficulty adapting to changes in light conditions, visual spatial disorders, and oculomotor dysfunction.[28]

WARREN'S HIERARCHY FOR ADDRESSING VISUAL DYSFUNCTION

Because of the complexity of the visual system, a framework for evaluation and intervention of visual impairments, whether ocular or neurological in nature, may be helpful. Warren[27] suggests a developmental model that conceptualizes vision abilities in a hierarchy (Figure 15-3). The abilities at the bottom form the foundation for each successive level. Higher level abilities depend on the complete integration of lower level abilities for their development.

The highest visual ability in this model is visual cognition. Visual cognition is the ability to mentally manipulate visual information and integrate it with other sensory information to solve problems, formulate writing, and solve mathematical problems.[27]

Visual memory is the ability directly below visual cognition in Warren's model. Visual cognition depends on visual memory because mental manipulation of a visual stimulus requires the ability to retain a mental picture.[29]

To store a visual image, individuals must be able to recognize a pattern. Pattern recognition, the next ability level, involves identification of the salient features of an object.[30,31] An individual must not only be able to identify the holistic aspects of an object such as its shape and

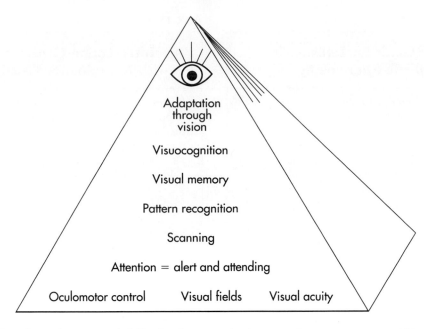

FIGURE 15-3   Hierarchy of visual perceptual skills development in the central nervous system. *(Adapted from Warren, M. L. (1993). A hierarchical model for evaluation and treatment of visual perceptual dysfunction in adult-acquired brain injury, part 1. American Journal of Occupational Therapy, 47, 42-54.)*

contour, but also specific features of an object such as its color detail, shading, and texture.

The ability to scan the environment is necessary for effective pattern recognition. Scanning, therefore, is the fundamental ability required for pattern recognition. The eye must record systematically all of the details of a scene and follow an organized scan path.[27]

The ability directly below scanning is visual attention. Engagement of visual attention is necessary for proper scanning to occur. If individuals are not attending to visual stimuli in a specific space, they will not initiate scanning into that area. A classic example is the elder with a CVA with left hemi-neglect who requires constant cueing to scan to the left to avoid colliding with objects.[27]

Visual attention and all of the higher level abilities depend on three primary visual abilities that form the foundation for all vision functions: oculomotor control, visual fields, and visual acuity. Oculomotor control enables efficient and conjugate eye movements, which ensure the completion of accurate scan paths and "teaming" of the eyes for binocular vision. The visual field is the extent of view that a person has in front of each eye. Visual acuity describes the sharpness or clearness of vision.[27] Table 15-2 addresses performance skill deficits of all of the discussed visual pathologies, and Box 15-5 is a screen that addresses performance skills with areas of occupation.

PRINCIPLES OF INTERVENTION

When an occupational therapy (OT) visual screen reveals deficits affecting ADL, the client should be referred to an

BOX 15-5

Vision Guided Occupational Survey/Profile

The following is difficult because of my vision loss:
Appliance dial
Cleaning
Cooking
Computer
Cutting/slicing
Crafts
Dressing
Driving
Eating
Grooming
Identifying money
Keys/outlets
Managing finances
Medications
Recognizing faces
Sewing/needlework
Shopping
Social activities
Spiritual participation
Sports/fitness
Telling time
Telephone use
Television
Walking/outdoors/indoors
Other_____

TABLE 15-2

Ocular Pathology Related Functional Performance Skills Deficits with Areas of Occupation

Pathology	Near distance	Intermediate	Far distance	Eye/hand	Mobility
ARMD	Reading continuous print, spot reading	Sewing, knitting, needlework, crafts, computer, handyman tasks	Driving, TV, sporting events	Writing, crafts, sports, musical instruments	Driving, curbs, and steps in low light
Glaucoma	Decreased vision in low light, difficulty with very fine print or poor contrast materials, sensitive to glare	Difficulty finding objects on shelf, difficulty with crafts, computer screens with poor contrast materials	Driving, TV, sporting events, decreased field, depth perception	Sports, crafts, musical instruments	Driving, ambulating on unfamiliar or changing surfaces, steps, difficulty seeing obstacles in peripheral fields
Diabetic retinopathy	Fluctuating/blurry vision may make continuous print reading, regular print difficult	Needlework, crafts, computer, handyman tasks	Driving, TV sporting events, decreased depth perception	Writing, sports, craft, musical instruments	Driving, curbs and steps in low light
Cataract	Decreased or blurry vision for fine detail, in low light/poor contrast, change in color perception	Needlework, crafts, computer, handyman tasks	Driving, sporting events	Crafts, fine needlework, sports, musical instruments	Driving, curbs and steps in low light
CVA/TBI	Hemianopsia or hemi-inattention, may groom or dress only one side, difficulty reading continuous print	Difficulty locating objects on shelf or in part of the room	Driving, sporting events, visual field deficits, depth perception	Writing, self-feeding, crafts, sports, musical instruments	Driving, ambulating, obstacles in area of field deficit, steps and curbs

ophthalmologist or optometrist to obtain a comprehensive visual examination. If available records and clinical observation indicate that the client's visual impairment is caused by an ocular disease, it would be best to refer the client to a low vision specialist (see later discussion of professionals for collaboration). If, conversely, diagnostic and clinical information indicate that the client's visual impairment is caused by a neurological insult such as head injury or stroke, a consultation with a neuro-ophthalmologist or neuro-optometrist is recommended. If either of these scenarios is not possible, a consultation with a trusted ophthalmologist would be the next choice. Ideally, a good working relationship should be established with low vision specialists and neuro-ophthalmologists in the area to facilitate the speed of referral and communication between professionals.

The information provided by an ophthalmologist or optometrist may vary, depending on the condition and the professional's area of specialty. A report from these professionals typically includes many of the following visual functions: visual acuity, visual field, contrast sensitivity function (the ability to distinguish subtle gradations in contrast between an object and its background), and oculomotor control. Reports may also include intraocular pressure (the pressure inside the eyeball), best correction for eyeglass prescription, dates and description of any ocular surgeries or procedures, current prescribed ophthalmic medications, and the general heath of ocular structures. Low vision specialists often also make recommendations for special optical devices to access printed materials, computer screens, or detailed eye-guided handiwork if visual acuity cannot be corrected to a functional range. This information and that gathered during the OT evaluation are invaluable in guiding intervention. Box 15-6 is a screening form for the sensory perceptual skill of vision. The following discussion addresses general interventions for many of the deficits that accompany visual loss such as decreased visual acuity, visual field loss, oculomotor dysfunction, reduced contrast sensitivity, and impaired visual attention and scanning.

DECREASED ACUITY

The input of an eye care specialist is crucial in addressing reduced acuity. Some elders are simply in need of an updated eyeglass prescription. In the case of a head injury or stroke, acuity may be reduced initially but often resolves spontaneously in a few months. (See Chapter 19 on the effects of traumatic brain injury [TBI]/stroke [CVA] for a

BOX 15-6

Sample Screening Form for the Sensory Perceptual Skill of Vision

- Do you have trouble seeing?
- Is part of your visual field missing, blurry, or dark?
- Does your vision fluctuate?
- How long have you experienced this difficulty?
- Has your eye doctor diagnosed or treated you?
- When was your last eye examination?
- Which eye is most affected?
- Can you see newsprint, headlines, computer screen, details on a TV screen, faces, food on your plate?
- Do you drive?
- Can you see traffic signals and street signs?
- Does glare bother you?
- Can you see curbs, steps, and changes in floor surfaces?
- Have you ever fallen because of your vision?

Adapted from Kern, T., & Miller, N. D. (2005). Tools for occupational therapists who work with people with low vision: Vision screening checklist. In M. Gentile (Ed.). Functional Visual Behavior in Adults: An Occupational Therapy Guide to Evaluation and Treatment Options, pp. 139-140. Bethesda, MD: AOTA Press.

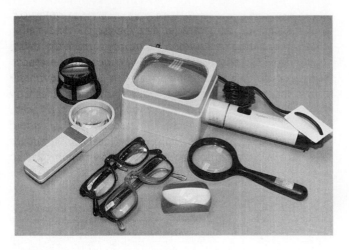

FIGURE 15-4 Some common optical aids used by individuals with low vision.

full discussion of more subtle deficits on acuity and intervention.) Reduced acuity secondary to ocular diseases, such as macular degeneration, cannot be improved through a change in eyeglass prescription. Recommendations for special optical devices may be made in this case. Diabetic retinopathy often not only causes reduced acuity, but also causes fluctuating acuity. It is important to follow the advice of the eye care specialist when planning intervention related to acuity.

As mentioned earlier, one method to compensate for reduced acuity is to use special optical devices to magnify or enlarge print (Figure 15-4). It is recommended that OTRs and COTAs receive specialized training in optical devices before attempting to train individuals in their use. (See listed resources for courses geared to OTRs and OTAs.) There are many unique concepts and techniques involved in the proper use of these devices, and elders typically require very clear instructions and encouragement to become proficient in their use. Other examples of using enlargement to compensate for decreased acuity are the use of large print materials and writing larger letters with a felt tip pen.

When an elder has decreased acuity, there are other techniques to help maximize function such as the use of proper illumination, reduction of pattern and clutter in the environment, and the use of organizational systems. Proper lighting is usually critical for optimal performance. However, some individuals may be photophobic or sensitive to light, which presents a challenge in finding appropriate lighting. Good, general room lighting (ambient lighting) is necessary for ease and safety in ambulating. Task lighting sources such as a gooseneck lamp or movable track lighting is recommended for fine-detail or low-contrast tasks such as reading, sewing, handyman work, or crafts. Proper positioning of a lamp must be considered to avoid glare. Directing the light from behind the shoulder of the better-seeing eye so that the light source does not create glare often works best. Task lighting with a gooseneck lamp can be positioned closer to the reading material, even in front of it as long as the bulb is not exposed and the shade directs the light downward, concentrating it on the material to be illuminated. Position the light source opposite the dominant hand to avoid shadows when writing.

Patterned backgrounds and clutter in the environment tend to "camouflage "objects that an elder is seeking (Figure 15-5). This can be remedied by using solid colors for background surfaces such as bedspreads, place mats, tablecloths, rugs, and furniture coverings. Care should be taken to reduce clutter where possible by limiting the number of objects in the environment and arranging the remaining objects in an orderly fashion. Once the environment is rearranged and simplified, every effort should be made to keep it organized.

There are many national and local services available for those with impaired visual acuity (and other visual impairment). Most of these services are free of charge. They can be found by contacting local state services for the blind and visually impaired (search state government website). The American Foundation for the Blind and The Lighthouse are examples of services that provide books and magazines to individuals free of charge (see Appendix). There are also catalogs that offer low-tech adaptive devices for the visually impaired such as talking clocks, large print playing cards and bingo cards, and a variety of other devices for ADL (see Appendix).

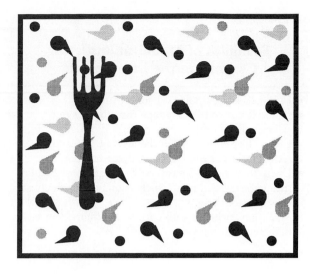

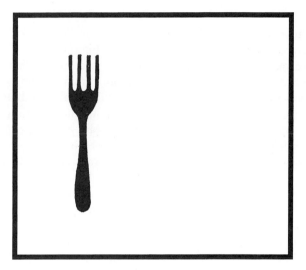

FIGURE 15-5   A patterned background can make it difficult to locate objects.

VISUAL FIELD LOSS

Elders who have a visual field loss may be taught to compensate for this loss in daily activities. The first step, however, is to increase the elder's awareness of the visual field loss. Having accurate information on the extent and location of the field loss is critical for teaching elders proper methods of compensation. The exact type and scope of visual field loss will vary depending on the cause of the disorder or disease and on individual presentation. In general, those with ocular conditions experience relatively "spotty types" of field loss, whereas those with a neurological disorder exhibit more uniform or extensive field loss. Of course, there are definitely exceptions to this rule because some ocular conditions can lead to an extensive and even total loss of visual field. Small, concentrated areas of visual field loss also have been found in those with head injuries.[32]

Elders who have central field loss, such as that seen with macular degeneration, must learn to compensate by directing their gaze off-center of the target (either slightly above, below, or to the side of) rather than directly at the target. This technique, called *eccentric viewing*, enables the individual to place the target outside of the blind spot so that it can be seen. This usually requires professional assistance to identify the best area for eccentric viewing, sometimes referred to as the *preferred retinal locus* or *PRL*.[33] Additional training and a conscious effort are required on the elder's part to override the natural tendency to direct the fovea, the most central area of the retina to the target and instead place the PRL in line with the target. Central field loss usually affects fine-detail tasks but does not significantly interfere with mobility. Those with more peripheral field loss typically require intervention aimed at increasing safety and independence with mobility skills. Elders with a homonymous hemianopsia occurring after a stroke may be taught to compensate for this loss of half the visual field by systematically training them to turn the head and scan into the impaired field during functional activities such as reading, shopping, and mobility.[34,35]

OCULOMOTOR DYSFUNCTION

Intervention for oculomotor dysfunction is likely one of the most complex areas for beginning practitioners to comprehend and implement effectively. It is highly recommended that the entry level COTA attend continuing education seminars, develop a mentoring relationship, and establish service competency in this area before attempting any of the intervention strategies suggested. It is also strongly recommended that therapists and assistants work under close supervision of an optometrist or ophthalmologist when treating oculomotor impairments. Oculomotor impairments are seen in individuals who have experienced some type of neurological insult. Ocular conditions do not affect the muscular or neural mechanisms that control eye movements.

A strabismus, or misalignment of an eye,[14] is often seen as a result of extraocular muscle weakness after a stroke or other neurological insult. This misalignment of the eyes results in diplopia, or double vision. The primary intervention methods used to address diplopia include occlusion, eye exercises, application of prisms, and surgery.[35]

Occlusion is essentially the "patching" of an eye to eliminate the double image.[14] Care must be taken to follow an occlusion protocol that optimizes the elder's comfort and reduces the likelihood of developing contractures in the muscles opposite the weak ones. Occlusion should not be carried out by simply patching the affected eye during all waking hours because this does nothing to encourage the use of the weak muscles. The protocol is typically directed by an ophthalmologist or optometrist.

Eye exercises can be used in conjunction with occlusion to help strengthen the affected muscles. One basic method would be to patch the unaffected eye and have the client track an object through all ranges of motion.[35] Optometrists may suggest additional exercises to be carried out under their direction.

Another strategy to treat diplopia is the application of prisms.[14] Prisms are sometimes prescribed and used to create a single image in the primary direction of gaze. The prism displaces the image to one side, causing the disparate images created by the strabismus to overlap and fuse into a single image. The prism can be permanently ground into the client's eyeglass lens or can be temporarily applied to the eyeglass lens using press-on prisms. If the strabismus is resolving, the elder should be gradually weaned off of the prism by reducing its strength over time.[14] An ophthalmologist or optometrist determines the strength of the prism and directs the intervention.

In some specific cases, surgery to correct the strabismus may be warranted.[35] This is further testimony to the necessity of consulting with appropriate eye care professionals to obtain optimal intervention for the individual. In most cases, the general approach to the surgery is to make the action of one or more eye muscles weaker or stronger by changing its attachment position. This is done by an ophthalmologist who is specially trained in strabismus surgery.[35]

REDUCED CONTRAST SENSITIVITY

Contrast sensitivity may be affected by both ocular and neurological conditions. This function is different than visual acuity, which reveals only the size of high contrast black and white letters that the individual is capable of seeing. Contrast sensitivity is the capacity to discriminate between similar shades.[10] In daily life, good contrast sensitivity is necessary to see a gray car on a cloudy day, to detect unmarked curbs and steps, and to distinguish subtle contours on people's faces to recognize them. Deficits in contrast sensitivity are typically addressed through environmental adaptation. For persons with low contrast sensitivity, the world often loses its definition. The primary technique to compensate for this deficit is to simply add contrast to the environment whenever possible. Many items used in daily activities can be changed to add more contrast and definition (Box 15-7). Proper illumination (as described earlier under "Decreased Acuity") is also helpful in enhancing contrast. Some individuals find that full-spectrum lighting, either incandescent or fluorescent, provides the best contrast-enhancing illumination. Color filters that may be worn over prescription lenses or alone can also enhance contrast. Light yellow, medium yellow, and light or medium plum are the colors most frequently used to enhance contrast.

IMPAIRED VISUAL ATTENTION AND SCANNING

Deficits in attention and scanning are seen in those with neurological involvement, not commonly in those with

Examples of Modifications Using Contrast in the Environment

- Use a black felt tip marker for writing.
- Add strips of contrasting tape (usually orange or yellow is best) to the edge of steps.
- Use a white coffee cup so the level of coffee can be seen against the white background when pouring.
- Use a black and white reversible cutting board and slice light-colored items, such as onions, on the black side and vice versa.
- Mark light switches with contrasting fluorescent tape to increase visibility.

ocular conditions. One type of impairment in this area is hemi-inattention, or hemi-neglect. This refers to a lack of awareness of one half of a person's visual space. Neglect of the left half of visual space is more common, but right hemi-neglect is occasionally seen.[36] Individuals with hemi-inattention are not able to take in visual information in the orderly, sequential, and comprehensive pattern needed to safely complete many daily activities. Grooming, meal preparation, and functional mobility (especially driving) are common examples of ADL affected. Initial intervention of deficits in visual attention and scanning often involves increasing the elder's awareness of the deficit followed up with appropriate compensation or remediation techniques, or both. Research has shown that individuals with left visual neglect may be trained to reorganize their scanning strategies by beginning the scan path in the impaired space.[37] This is accomplished through intervention strategies similar to those described earlier in treating homonymous hemianopsia. Activities are used that require and encourage a systematic left-to-right scan pattern with a visual anchor (such as a red line or ruler) placed to the left (or right as appropriate) as a visual cue, if necessary. There is some evidence that the effects of this training on patients with hemi-inattention may be task-specific and may not generalize to overall ADL function.[38,39] The presence of hemi-neglect also has been associated with poor rehabilitation outcome.[40-42]

HIGHER LEVEL VISUAL-PERCEPTUAL DEFICITS

Warren's[27] proposed intervention for higher level visual deficits includes addressing the foundation visual skills that may affect these areas, education of the patient to increase awareness of the deficit, and instruction in the use of compensatory strategies for the deficit. (See Warren[27] for a more detailed description of these techniques.) Refer to Box 15-4, Intervention Gems for Individuals with Neurological Visual Impairment.

SETTINGS IN WHICH VISUAL IMPAIRMENTS ARE ADDRESSED

Low-vision rehabilitation is becoming a specialty field for OTRs. OTRs may provide rehabilitation for diagnoses related to visual impairment when prescribed by an ophthalmologist, optometrist, or other physician (as of this writing, regulations vary by state). OTRs work in conjunction with other trained professionals to provide comprehensive services to individuals with vision impairments. The majority of individuals treated in low-vision clinics have impairments caused by ocular pathologies. Macular degeneration accounts for 60% of low-vision cases,[14] whereas glaucoma and diabetic retinopathy are ranked second and third, respectively.[43] For this reason, the term *low vision* is typically associated with visual impairments caused by ocular diseases. However, individuals with visual impairments secondary to neurological insult also may seek intervention in some low-vision clinics.

Because visual impairments are a common result of neurological insult and because ocular diseases are relatively common in the elderly, COTAs working in any geriatric or neurorehabilitation setting should be well educated in visual dysfunction and intervention techniques. Settings may include inpatient and outpatient rehabilitation, subacute rehabilitation facilities, long-term care facilities, and home health agencies.

COTAs working with elders with visual impairments must have specialized training in areas such as optics and use of optical devices, eccentric viewing techniques, blind techniques for ADL, and vision enhancement techniques for ADL, as well as a good working knowledge of the extensive adaptive equipment available for low-vision clients. They also must possess a good understanding of available resources to direct clients to appropriate support groups and other services.

There are many other low-vision rehabilitation professionals with whom the COTA can collaborate to provide the best functional outcomes for their clients. Orientation and mobility specialists address travel needs directly related to vision loss. They typically hold master's degrees and have a wealth of knowledge in this area. The goal of their services is to develop independent travel skill within the client's home, neighborhood, or community. These specialists may work in many settings, including public school systems, private agencies, and state-supported programs.

Rehabilitation teachers are professionals who are trained at the university level to address ADL that have been affected by visual impairment. They provide instruction in using adaptive techniques or adaptive equipment to increase independence in areas such as communication, household management, self-care, and other ADL. Rehabilitation teachers may work in private agencies, itinerant state services, residential schools, and independent living centers. The areas addressed and the knowledge base of these professionals may overlap at times with OT professionals. As long as there is open communication and collaboration, each profession will likely learn valuable techniques from the other, and the client will receive an optimal rehabilitation program.

Ophthalmologists and optometrists specializing in low vision ensure that comprehensive low-vision services are provided. They evaluate the client's visual function and prescribe optical devices and training to compensate for vision loss. They may see low-vision clients in their own broader-based private practice, or they may work in low-vision clinics. (For more information regarding a program using ophthalmology and OT to provide low-vision rehabilitation in an outpatient rehabilitation setting, see Warren.[44])

CONCLUSION

Visual impairments in elders may result from either ocular or neurological pathology. Normal physiological changes that may occur with aging include shrinkage of the peripheral field, increased time required to recover from glare, difficulty with light and dark adaptation, increased need for illumination, loss of elasticity in the lens, and yellowing of the lens. The most common ocular diseases that may occur in elders are macular degeneration, cataracts, glaucoma, and diabetic retinopathy. Elders are also at risk for CVAs, which may disrupt any of several neurological components necessary for effective visual functioning.

COTAs can play vital roles in helping elders with visual impairments learn to function as independently as possible. COTAs can provide sources for information about vision loss to help elders understand the specifics of their eye conditions. Encouraging elders to gain knowledge about their eye conditions can be an empowering first step in the process of rehabilitation. COTAs may collaborate with OTRs to provide training to compensate for vision loss in daily activities. COTAs can provide training in community resources and collaborate with other members of the intervention team to provide referral to appropriate agencies and service providers to facilitate community reintegration. Finally, COTAs may collaborate with elders, family members, and/or caregivers to make environmental adaptations, to enhance independence, and to do these safely (Box 15-8).

The loss of vision in elders is a common occurrence, whether it results from the natural aging process, ocular disease, or disruption of neurological components. Vision loss has significant functional implications and can complicate the elder's rehabilitation process with other physical impairments. This emphasizes the need for COTAs to familiarize themselves with the causes and types of vision loss and effective intervention techniques, whether they are working in general rehabilitation centers or acute care hospitals.

BOX 15-8

Environmental Adaptation Basics

- Increase relative object size—Large print, bold labels, or large-sized objects.
- Lighting—increase ambient and task lighting; add gooseneck lamps for task lighting where activities are completed.
- Color—light colors for walls and ceilings to reflect and increase light; bright colors for tools and everyday objects to make them stand out.
- Contrast—floor, walls, counters, furniture, hardware, switch-plates, and doorknobs should contrast with each other.
- Reduce clutter—limit the number of objects on counters and tabletops, limit bold patterns to decrease "visual clutter," and clear pathways between rooms and around furniture and exits.
- Reduce glare by eliminating bare bulbs, reflective surfaces, using matte finishes and using light filtering window coverings and lampshades.
- Texture—use bumpy or rough textured paint, tape or self-adhesive dots to label settings, or define edges and surface changes. Train elders to notice changes in the feel of carpet versus hard surfaced floors.
- Audio substitution—use talking clocks, kitchen scales, timers, and other items to substitute for vision when performing ADL tasks.

CASE STUDY

Mark is a 67-year-old widower who lives alone and following an amputation below the right knee was just admitted to the rehabilitation unit where you work. He has diabetes mellitus and has had many complications of the disease, including the peripheral vascular disease that led to his amputation and diabetic retinopathy. Mark states that he did not manage his condition well in the past but wants to do everything he can now to keep these complications from getting any worse. He states that he finds it difficult to see the numbers and lines on his syringes when drawing his insulin. He also has some trouble seeing the blood sugar reading on his glucometer. He needs to check his blood sugar three times a day with this machine and adjust his insulin dosage accordingly. The OT visual screen reveals that Mark has moderately decreased visual acuity and decreased contrast sensitivity.

Mark has good upper body strength and uses his walker well on the unit. He will need to use the walker at discharge while waiting for his leg to heal before being fitted for a prosthesis. Fortunately, you will be able to conduct a home evaluation to make recommendations before discharge.

■ CASE STUDY QUESTIONS

1 What are some specific areas of concern or potential hazards that you would look for on Mark's home evaluation visit?
2 What are some recommendations you could make to address these concerns and improve safety and ease of functioning in Mark's home?

3 You would like to increase Mark's independence in his diabetic management, but you do not know what techniques or adaptive equipment is available to accomplish this. Where could you turn for help? What assistive technology might you inquire about to help Mark complete his diabetic care?

■ CHAPTER REVIEW QUESTIONS

1 What are some natural age-related changes in the eye, and what implications do they have for function?
2 What are the three primary ocular conditions that account for the majority of referrals to low-vision rehabilitation clinics?
3 Which ocular conditions could potentially lead to total blindness?
4 What are some possible vision problems after a stroke or other neurological insult?
5 What are the primary vision abilities described in Mary Warren's hierarchy that form the foundation for all other vision abilities?
6 Name three environmental adaptation strategies that could be used for clients with the primary ocular conditions most commonly encountered with elders.
7 Name three other professionals and two community or state agencies with whom the COTA could collaborate regarding a low-vision client.

REFERENCES

1. American Occupational Therapy Association, 2008. Occupational therapy practice framework: Domain and process, 2nd ed. American Journal of Occupational Therapy 62, 625-683.
2. American Foundation for the Blind, 2002. Facts about aging and vision [WWW page]. URL http://www.afb.org/info_documants.asp?kitid=8&colletionid=2 and http://www.afb.org/info_document_view.asp?documentid+1809.
3. The Lighthouse, Inc., 1995. The Lighthouse national survey on vision loss: The experience, attitudes, and knowledge of middle-aged and older Americans. Lighthouse, New York.
4. Warren, M.L., 1998. The Brain Injury Visual Assessment Battery for Adults Test Manual. visABILITIES Rehab Services, Lenexa, KS.
5. Center on an Aging Society, 2002. Visual impairments data profile, no.3 [WWW page]. URL http://ihcrp.Georgetown.edu/agingsociety/pdfs/visual.pdf.
6. American Foundation for the Blind, 1999. Fact sheet: Statistics and sources for professionals [WWW page]. URL http://www.afb.org/info_document_view.asp?documentid=1367.
7. Friedman, D.B., 2004. Psychosocial factors in vision rehabilitation. In: Albert, D.M., Jakobiec, J.A. (Eds.), Principles and Practice of Ophthalmology, vol. 5. WB Saunders, Philadelphia.
8. Kubler-Ross, E., 1969. Death and Dying. Macmillan, New York, pp. 11-138.
9. Perski, T., n.d. The five-stage process of becoming a successful low vision patient. Retrieved from http://www.blindness.org/coping/resource/detail?res=1&id=20. Retrieved 09/14/2004
10. Mogk, L.G., 2000. Eye conditions that cause low vision in adults. In: Warren, M. (Ed.), Low Vision: Occupational Therapy Interventions with the Older Adult: A Self-Paced Clinical Course

from AOTA. American Occupational Therapy Association, Bethesda, MD.

11. Bennett, S.H., 1992. Low vision: Clinical aspects and interventions. In: Rothman, J. Levine, R. (Eds.), Prevention Practice Strategies for Physical Therapy and Occupational Therapy. WB Saunders, New York, pp. 258-269.

12. Christenson, M.A., 1995. Environmental design, modification, and adaptation. In: Larson, K.O., Stevens-Ratchford, R.G., Pedretti, L., Crabtree, J.L. (Eds.), ROTE: The Role of OT with the Elderly, 2nd ed. AOTA Press, Bethesda, MD.

13. Scheiman, M., 2002b. Review of basic anatomy, physiology, and development of the visual system. In: Scheiman, M. (Ed.), Understanding and Managing Vision Deficits: A Guide for Occupational Therapists. Slack, Thorofare, NJ, pp. 9-15.

14. Scheiman, M., 2002a. Management of refractive, visual efficiency, and visual information processing disorders. In: Scheiman, M. (Ed.), Understanding and Managing Vision Deficits: A Guide for Occupational Therapists. Slack, Thorofare, NJ, pp. 117-162.

15. Lighthouse International, 2009. The Ageing Eye.[WWW page]. URL http://www.lighthouse.org.

16. NEI, 2002. Age Related Eye Disease Study—Results.[WWWpage]. URL http://www.nei.nih.gov/amd/.

17. American Foundation for the Blind, 1999a. Fact sheet: Cataracts [WWWpage]. URL http://www.afb.org/info_document_view.asp?documentid=193.

18. American Foundation for the Blind, 1999b. Fact sheet: Visual impairment and age-related macular degeneration [WWWpage]. URL http://www.afb.org/info_document_view.asp?documentid=202.

19. Scheiman, M., Scheiman, M., Whittaker, S., 2006. Low Vision Rehabilitation: A Practical Guide for Occupational Therapists. Slack, Thorofare, New Jersey.

20. Mogk, L.G., Mogk, M., 2003. Macular Degeneration: The Complete Guide to Saving and Maximizing Your Sight. Random House, New York.

21. Jackson, M.L., Bassett, K., Nirmalan, P.V., Syre, E.C., 2007. Contrast sensitivity and visual hallucinations in patients referred to a low vision rehabilitation clinic. British Journal of Ophthalmology 91 (3), 296-298.

22. American Foundation for the Blind, 1999c. Fact sheet: Visual impairment and glaucoma [WWWpage]. URL http://www.afb.org/info_document_view.asp?documentid=705.

23. Jose, R.T., 1985. The eye and functional vision. In: Jose, R.T. (Ed.), Understanding Low Vision. American Foundation for the Blind, New York, pp. 3-42.

24. Bennett, S.H., 1991. Visual changes associated with aging: Influence on practice. Occupational Therapy Practice 3 (1), 12.

25. Bennett, S.H., 1992. Low vision: Clinical aspects and interventions. In: Rothman, J. Levine, R. (Eds.), Prevention Practice Strategies for Physical Therapy and Occupational Therapy. WB Saunders, New York, pp. 258-269.

26. Zoltan, B., 2006. Vision, Perception, and Cognition: A Manual for the Evaluation and Treatment of the Adult with Acquired Brain Injury, 4th ed. Slack, Thorofare, NJ.

27. Warren, M.L., 1993. A hierarchical model for evaluation and treatment of visual perceptual dysfunction in adult acquired brain injury, part 1. American Journal of Occupational Therapy 47, 42-54.

28. Kerkhoff, G., 2000. Neurovisual rehabilitation: Recent developments and future directions. Journal of Neurology, Neurosurgery, and Psychiatry 68, 691-706.

29. Ratcliff, G., 1987. Perception and complex visual processes. In: Meier, M.J., Benton, A.L., Diller, L. (Eds.), Neuropsychological Rehabilitation. Guilford, New York.

30. Julesz, B., 1981. Texton, the elements of texture perception and their interactions. Nature 290 (12), 91.

31. Julesz, B., 1985. Preconscious and conscious processing in vision. In: Chagas, C., Gattass, R. (Eds.), Pattern Recognition Mechanisms. Experimental Brain Research 11 (Suppl 11), 333.

32. Willliams, T.A., 1995. Case report: Low vision rehabilitation for a patient with traumatic brain injury. American Journal of Occupational Therapy 49 (9), 923-926.

33. Fletcher, D.C., Suchard, R.A., 1997. Preferred retinal loci relationship to macular scotomas in low-vision population. Ophthalmology 104 (4), 632-638.

34. Kerkhoff, G., Munbinger, U., Meier, E., 1994. Neurovisual rehabilitation in cerebral blindness. Archives of Neurology 51, 474-481.

35. Warren, M.L., 1998. In The Brain Injury Visual Assessment Battery for Adults Test Manual. visABILITIES Rehab Services, Lenexa, KS.

36. Diamond, R., 2001. Rehabilitative management of post-stroke visuospatial inattention (review). Disability and Rehabilitation 23 (10), 407-412.

37. Weinberg, J., Diller, L., Gordon, W.A., Gerstman, L.J., Lieberman, A., Lakin, P., 1979. Visual scanning training effect on reading-related tasks in acquired right brain damage. Archives of Physical Medicine and Rehabilitation 60, 479-486.

38. Gordon, W.A., Hibbard, M.R., Egelko, S., Diller, L., Shaver, M.S., Lieberman, A., et al. 1985. Perceptual remediation in patients with right brain damage: A comprehensive program. Archives of Physical Medicine and Rehabilitation 66, 353-360.

39. Wagenaar, R.C., Van Wieringen, P.C.W., Netelenbos, J.V., Meijer, O.G., Kuik, D.J., 1992. The transfer of scanning training effects in visual inattention after stroke: Five single-case studies. Disability and Rehabilitation 14, 51-60.

40. Fullerton, K.J., Mackenzie, G., Stout, R.W., 1988. Prognostic indices in stroke. Quarterly Journal of Medicine 250, 147-162.

41. Kalra, L., Perez, L., Gupta, S., Wittink, M., 1997. The influence of visual neglect on stroke rehabilitation. Stroke 28, 1386-1391.

42. Kaplan, J., Hier, D.B., 1982. Visuospatial deficits after right hemisphere stroke. American Journal of Occupational Therapy 36, 314-321.

43. Stuen, C., 1996. New concepts and treatments. Vision and Aging New 8 (1), 8.

44. Warren, M.L., 1995. Providing low vision rehabilitation services with occupational therapy and ophthalmology: A program description. American Journal of Occupational Therapy 49, 877-884.

Working with Elders Who Have Hearing Impairments

SHARON STOFFEL AND JESSICA HATCH

KEY TERMS

sensorineural hearing loss (sensory, neural, mechanical), conductive hearing loss, cochlear implants, tinnitus, hearing aid, assistive listening device, audiologist

CHAPTER OBJECTIVES

1. Describe sensorineural and conductive hearing losses.
2. Describe ways that slow, progressive changes in the auditory system interfere with occupations that require communication.
3. List environmental modifications that reduce background noise in homes and institutions.
4. Describe possible safety recommendations for home and institutional environments where hearing-impaired elders reside.
5. Describe the effect of age-related hearing loss on socialization, communication, and travel and its possible contribution to feelings of isolation for hearing-impaired elders.
6. List suggestions for improving communication with hearing-impaired elders.
7. Describe possible behaviors that may indicate hearing impairment.

The voice of a loved one, the chimes of a grandfather clock, a violin concerto—these are sounds many people not only enjoy, but also take for granted. For elders who have hearing impairments, these sounds may be either misinterpreted or missed altogether.

Hearing impairments may also be associated with the reduced ability to hear warning signals, ambulation difficulties, and difficulties with instrumental activities of daily living (IADL), balance problems, and increased incidence of falls.[1-3] Hearing impairments can contribute to social isolation. Safety related to hearing impairments may become a concern when elders are unable to hear alarms and other warning signals.[4]

Among the elderly, hearing loss is the third most prevalent chronic condition following arthritis and hypertension.[5] In the United States by the year 2050, 52.9 million people are expected to have hearing loss.[6] Although persons of all ages experience hearing impairments, in terms of a health disparity, elders are a primary concern.[7] Approximately one-third of elders between ages 65 and 74 years experience hearing loss. This percentage increases to 47% for those older than 75 years.[8] Furthermore, some studies indicate that 85% to 90% of nursing home residents have hearing impairments that limit function.[4]

Even though hearing impairments are more prevalent than vision loss, they are often more difficult to distinguish. Changes in hearing are often subtle and occur gradually. Many elders with significant hearing losses often wait as long as 5 years before seeking assistance with their hearing.[9] Elders, family members, and health care personnel may not recognize hearing losses. Some may accept the loss as an inevitable and unalterable aspect of aging.

According to the Occupational Therapy Practice Framework: Domain and Process (2nd ed.) hearing is addressed in the client factors table as a body function under the sensory functions and pain category, and auditory is listed in the performance skills table as a sensory perceptual skill.[10] Hearing loss can have a profound effect on engagement in occupations and activities of daily living (ADL). Certified occupational therapy assistants (COTAs) have the opportunity to diminish the impact of hearing loss on functional performance by becoming educated about hearing loss. Learning accommodations that may benefit the patient can make working with hearing impaired individuals easier and improve performance in functional tasks.[11]

Because elders seldom seek assistance or plan interventions to enhance their hearing, COTAs must be able to distinguish the various types of hearing impairments. In addition, COTAs should be aware of interventions, services, devices, and activities that can enhance occupational performance for elders who are hearing impaired.

This chapter provides an overview of the most common types of hearing losses that affect elders. The possible psychosocial effects that a hearing impairment may have on elders, their families, and their friends also are addressed. Rehabilitation considerations are discussed, including communicating with an elder who has a hearing impairment, methods for modifying home, public spaces, and institutional environments, and recommendations for assisting elders in the use of hearing aids and assisted listening devices (ALD).

HEARING CONDITIONS ASSOCIATED WITH AGING

If any hearing loss is suspected, individuals should visit their primary care physician (PCP) to be screened and/or treated for any other underlying pathological processes.[5] The term *presbycusis* is often used when diagnosing elders with hearing loss. According to the National Institute on Deafness and Other Communication Disorders (NIDCD),[12] the term *presbycusis* is the gradual loss of hearing as an individual grows older. Generally, hearing losses are divided into the three following areas: sensorineural, conductive, and mixed. These conditions may affect one or both ears.

The most common type of presbycusis or hearing loss in elders is the result of sensorineural damage to the hearing organ itself or to the peripheral or central nervous system (or both).[12] Although elders rarely have just one type of sensorineural loss, the most common type of loss is caused by hair cell damage or loss of the sensory hair cells of the cochlea. As individuals age, these hair cells are slowly lost, and the ability to hear high-frequency sounds is diminished. One of the most frustrating and handicapping aspect of this loss is the ways sounds are changed or distorted. Although the elder may hear someone speaking, the signals that allow him or her to understand what is being said are not clear. Such losses can have serious consequences in both social and therapeutic settings. For example, at a party someone may say, "How are you?" and the elder may respond, "Eighty-one." An elder in a clinic setting who is asked to hand the COTA a "dime" may respond with the correct "time." Such responses often raise questions about mental status and often lead to a loss of confidence in interacting with others.[12,13] In such situations, the COTA should seek assistance to rule out the presence of sensorineural loss before questioning the elder's orientation or ability to follow directions. If proper audiological services are not available, the elderly individual can experience decreased mobility, social isolation, and increased cognitive decline.[14] In addition, because women's voices are usually higher pitched than men's, female COTAs must understand that their voices could contribute to decreased comprehension by elders.

Elders living in areas with low exposure to loud or high-pitched noise levels may experience less sensorineural hearing loss than those living in noisy, industrial areas. Although those with better overall health seem less likely to experience this type of loss, some sensorineural loss eventually affects elders regardless of environmental conditions. However, continued exposure to loud noises for long periods may cause permanent damage.[15] For instance, current research indicates that 15% of college graduates exhibit hearing loss equal to or greater than that of their parents due to exposure to high volume MP3 music players.[16]

Three types of sensorineural hearing loss have been identified: sensory, neural, and mechanical.[13,15] Sensory loss is caused by atrophy and degeneration of the hair cells at the base of the basilar membrane. It produces a loss of high-frequency sounds but does not interfere with the discrimination of speech. Neural loss is caused by the loss of auditory nerve fibers. It affects the ability to distinguish speech sounds, especially in the higher frequencies, but does not affect the ability to hear pure tones. Mechanical loss is characterized by the degeneration of the vibrating membrane within the cochlea. This type of loss leads to the gradual impairment of hearing in all frequencies. In situations where several sounds in various frequencies are present at the same time, the ability to distinguish between the sounds becomes increasingly difficult. Table 16-1 lists common hearing conditions of elders.

A sensorineural hearing loss may be unnoticed in the early stages because the high-frequency tones that are initially lost are above the functional range used in most environments. As the condition progresses, elders may notice that they cannot hear the ringing of the telephone, the buzz of the doorbell, the ticking of a clock, or the water dripping from a faucet. With further progression, the sounds of certain consonants such as s, z, t, f, and g become increasingly difficult to distinguish. Eventually, elders may strain to hear and understand conversations and one-syllable words.[13,15]

A second hearing condition, conductive hearing loss, results in an inability of the external ear to conduct sound waves to the inner ear. Conductive hearing losses may be related to the buildup of cerumen (earwax), fluid accumulation in the middle ear from eustachian tube dysfunction, or an upper respiratory infection. These conductive problems often can be corrected by cleaning the ear, administering medications, or performing surgery. Hearing aids may be effective for persons who have an untreatable or residual conductive hearing loss. A hearing aid amplifies incoming sound and requires functioning hair cells and an intact nerve to transmit the sound to the central auditory pathways. For older adults whose residual hearing is greatly limited because of an absence of hair cells, cochlear implants may be considered.[4] Cochlear implants are appropriate when only minimal or no benefit is possible when a conventional hearing aid is used. Cochlear implants are prosthetic replacements for the functions of the lost hair cells by converting mechanical energy (sound waves) into electrical energy capable of exciting the auditory

TABLE 16-1

Common Hearing Conditions of Elders

Condition	Cause	Symptoms
Sensorineural losses	Atrophy and degeneration of the hair cells at the base of the basilar membrane	Loss of high frequency sounds; condition does not interfere with speech discrimination
Neural	Loss of auditory nerve fibers	Condition affects ability to distinguish speech sounds in higher frequencies; does not affect ability to hear pure tones
Mechanical	Degeneration of the vibrating membrane within the cochlea	Condition leads to gradual loss of hearing in all frequencies; ability to distinguish sounds becomes increasingly difficult
Conductive hearing loss	Inability of the external ear to conduct sound waves to the inner ear; may be related to buildup of earwax, fluid accumulation in the middle ear, or upper respiratory infection	Condition can often be corrected by cleaning the ear, medications, or surgery; hearing aids or cochlear implants may be considered
Tinnitus	May be related to conductive or sensorineural loss, Ménière's, otosclerosis, presbycusis, earwax buildup, lesions, or fluid in middle ear	Buzzing, ringing, whistle, roar in ears, most noticeable at night; may be necessary to rule out underlying conditions before implementing interventions designed to symptoms

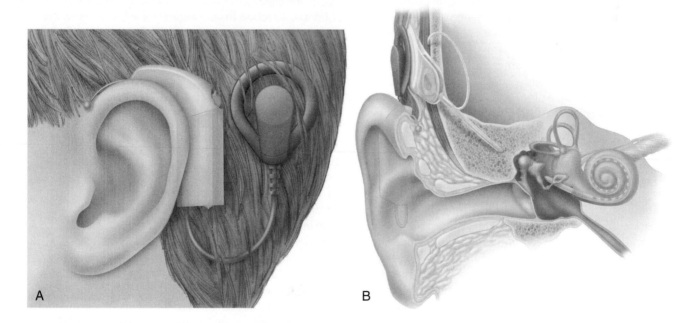

A   B

FIGURE 16-1   Cochlear implant. A, External placement. B, Internal placement. *(Courtesy of Cochlear Ltd, Englewood, CO.)*

nerve. Cochlear implants are placed within the inner ear. They bypass the hair cells of the cochlea and directly stimulate the endings of the auditory nerve. The system consists of an external microphone, processor, and transmitter, and an internal receiver–stimulator and electrode. Figure 16-1 shows the external (Figure 16-1, A) and internal (Figure 16-1, B) placements for a cochlear implant.

Tinnitus is a subjective auditory problem consisting of a ringing, whistling, buzzing, or roaring noise in the ears. Tinnitus may occur as part of a conductive or sensorineural hearing loss. It may also be associated with Ménière's disease, otosclerosis, sensorineural loss, an accumulation of cerumen pressing on the eardrum, tympanic membrane lesions, and fluid in the middle ear. Medications such as the doses of aspirin prescribed for arthritis or other medical conditions can be additional contributing factors.[15] Before planning interventions to mask the symptoms of tinnitus, possible underlying conditions such as cardiovascular disease, anemia, and hypothyroidism should be ruled out by a physician.

Tinnitus is often most noticeable at night when other noises are reduced. Ear or masking of environment noises may be an effective strategy. A radio, tape recording, or appropriate hearing aid may mask the tinnitus so the individual can fall asleep. Other therapeutic interventions may include relaxation techniques and biofeedback.[2,15]

PSYCHOSOCIAL ASPECTS OF HEARING IMPAIRMENTS

Even though much information about the environment is learned through the sense of hearing, the importance of hearing during travel, while working, and in personal and social situations often goes unnoticed. Some researchers suggest that when hearing loss is the only loss elders experience, they can adjust well.[13] Others suggest that a hearing loss may lead to isolation and even paranoia.[2,17] Unfortunately, many elders experience other losses or lifestyle changes at the same time hearing loss occurs. Retirement may lead to a loss of role identity, income, and social contacts. Adjusting to the death of a spouse or undergoing changes in vision or mobility may take priority over a loss of hearing. Elders who are predisposed to loneliness or have difficulty in initiating or maintaining relationships may become more isolated or avoid interpersonal relationships if they experience a hearing loss. This can result in an increased sense of loneliness or isolation, especially if the hearing impairment is associated with other losses.[13] Early assessment of a perceived hearing loss and recommendations for adaptations may help reduce an elder's sense of loneliness.

The elder with a hearing loss often guesses at or misses the content of conversations, is reluctant to ask for clarification, or is embarrassed when mistakes are made because of a misunderstanding. This can occur when an elder with a hearing impairment is traveling. Studies involving elderly airline travelers have found that misunderstanding or not hearing overhead paging information has resulted in missed flights.[18] Hearing changes also make it difficult to detect and understand speech in crowded and stressful situations. Limited hearing may decrease an elder's sense of security and increase feelings of vulnerability, making travel more difficult. As a result, some elders may either limit their travel or stop engaging in that occupation.[2]

Communication can be exhausting for elders with a hearing impairment. For example, an 85-year-old man registering for occupational therapy (OT) interventions at a rehabilitation clinic will likely be embarrassed if he misinterprets the receptionist's request for his address as a request to undress. He may also experience isolation if his accompanying family member interrupts and answers all remaining questions. Repeated frustrating and embarrassing experiences can contribute to feelings of vulnerability, insecurity, and doubts related to self-esteem that can lead to withdrawal from travel, social, cultural, and family contacts.

Some elders with hearing impairments may hear well at home and only struggle to hear in other social settings. Others may be isolated not only from family and friends but also from the broader world because they cannot get information from television, radio, movies, and even telephone conversations. Elders may become increasingly frustrated as family, friends, and even health care workers begin to make decisions for them.

An age-related hearing loss may only further complicate the effects of illnesses and mental health conditions such as Alzheimer's disease. Hearing loss in elders can lead to or exacerbate paranoid ideas, suspicions, and loss of contact with reality, and related tendencies.[13] Corso[19] stated that a hearing loss can magnify previously existing paranoid personality attributes. Continued expression of suspicions, hostilities, and accusations of lying may result in friends and family members avoiding the hearing-impaired elder.

REHABILITATION AND THE HEARING-IMPAIRED ELDER

Hearing loss usually accompanies other conditions and should be considered in intervention to facilitate a successful experience. Interventions based on the Occupational Therapy Practice Framework (2nd ed.)[10] address areas of occupations that have value and meaning for elders.

Managing hearing loss is about much more than the simple provision of a hearing aid. Rehabilitation for the hearing-impaired individual examines the individual's participation in a variety of activities and functions.[20] The effectiveness of rehabilitation for maximizing occupational independence is based on many factors. Those related to hearing loss may include age-related changes at the time of onset of the hearing impairment, such as vision and mobility losses, retirement, death of a spouse, and loss of clearly defined life roles. Other factors include the severity and rapidity of the loss, the degree of residual hearing, the presence of other medical conditions, and the involvement of the individual and family members in the rehabilitative process.

COTA and registered occupational therapist (OTR) teams may work together along with others on the treatment team to identify elders who have hearing impairments through an observation of behaviors (Box 16-1). The Self-Rating Hearing Inventory also can be an effective tool for assessing the effects of a hearing impairment on perceived occupational performance.[21] The American Academy of Otolaryngology–Head and Neck Surgery has developed a 5-minute hearing test to determine the need for a referral to a hearing specialist (Figure 16-2). Beyond the scope of therapy practice for more profound hearing losses, a consultation and referral to a hearing specialist regarding the use of a hearing aid, individual or computerized training in speech reading (lip reading), and instruction regarding the use of an ALD may be needed. In addition, referrals for accessing both formal and informal

Five-Minute Hearing Test

	Almost always	Half of the time	Occasionally	Never
1. I have a problem hearing over the telephone.				
2. I have trouble following the conversation when two or more people are talking at the same time.				
3. People complain when I turn the TV volume too high.				
4. I have to strain to understand conversations.				
5. I miss hearing some common sounds like the phone or doorbell ringing.				
6. I have trouble hearing conversations in a noisy background such as a party.				
7. I get confused about where sounds come from.				
8. I misunderstand some words in a sentence and need to ask people to repeat themselves.				
9. I especially have trouble understanding the speech of women and children.				
10. I have worked in noisy environments (jackhammers, assembly lines, jet engines).				
11. Many people I talk to seem to mumble (or don't talk clearly).				
12. People get annoyed because I misunderstand what they say.				
13. I misunderstand what others are saying and make inappropriate responses.				
14. I avoid social activities because I cannot hear well and fear I'll reply improperly.				
To be answered by a family member or friend: 15. Do you think this person has a hearing loss?				

Scoring
To calculate your score, give yourself 3 points for every time you checked the "Almost always" column, 2 for every "Half of the time," 1 for every "Occasionally" and 0 for every "Never." If you have a blood relative who has a hearing loss, add another 3 points. Then total your points. The American Academy of Otolaryngology–Head and Neck Surgery recommends the following:
- 0 to 5: Your hearing is fine. No action is required.
- 6 to 9: Suggest you see an ear-nose-and-throat (ENT) specialist.
- 10 and above: Strongly recommend you see an ear physician.

FIGURE 16-2 Five-minute hearing test. (*Courtesy of the American Academy of Otolaryngology–Head and Neck Surgery, Alexandria, VA.*)

support services through public and community agencies may be beneficial. Individuals for whom none of these interventions are effective may be candidates for cochlear implants.

COTAs are involved in direct interventions for other primary reasons than for hearing impairment but regardless they should address hearing issues as they impact engagement in occupations. They may also assist in adapting environments for individuals, groups, or institutional facilities. The skills and experience of COTAs may be directed toward designing and implementing individual or institutional activities. These recommendations, intended to promote successful adaptation for hearing-impaired elders, also can assist families, friends, and institutional personnel. As always, safety is a consideration with intervention. Please refer to Box 16-2 for safety tips.

BOX 16-1

Observable Behaviors That May Indicate Hearing Loss

- Inappropriate volume increase when speaking—for example, appearing to shout while talking to a person nearby
- Turning the television or radio volume inordinately high when there is no one else in the room and no noises in the background
- Turning in a chair or turning the head to get a better hearing position when being addressed
- Consistently asking for statements to be repeated
- Not responding to verbal questions or conversation
- Responding to verbal questions only when there is accompanying visual cueing
- Looking disoriented or confused or giving inappropriate responses to questions—for example, answering "yes" to a multiple choice question
- Answering questions addressed to another person when there are several persons conversing simultaneously in the same room
- Withdrawing from social situations
- Exhibiting short attention span, which is especially apparent when two people are talking simultaneously

Adapted from Kane, R. L., Ouslander, J. G., & Abrass, I. B. (1999). Essentials of Clinical Geriatrics, 4th ed. New York: McGraw-Hill.

RECOMMENDATIONS FOR IMPROVING ELDER COMMUNICATION

Psychosocial issues associated with hearing impairments often affect family members and friends, as well as the hearing-impaired elder. Information and education about the various types of age-related hearing losses and conditions may help COTAs in assisting elders to develop coping strategies.[15] The COTA should encourage family members and friends to be involved in the education and consultation process so that conversational and environmental adaptations that encourage inclusion of the elder can be promoted.

Hearing-impaired elders may need to gain confidence in requesting adaptations that help them adjust to their hearing losses. Having elders role-play situations in which they request specific needs or adaptations may increase self-confidence for reentering social situations that they may have been avoiding.

Environmental adaptations should first center on identifying and minimizing the influence of background noises because competing background noises are considered to be a difficult listening condition.[17] With a hearing difficulty, background noises greatly limit enjoyment of conversations and often contribute to an elder's avoidance of social gatherings.[22] Common sources of background noise in institutions include music, conversations on television or of persons in the room, dishes being clanked, fans in

BOX 16-2

Safety Gems for the Hearing Impaired

- Make sure that the elder's hearing has been properly evaluated.
- Check that hearing aids are working. This would be especially important during activities requiring hearing ability for safety, such as with driving.
- Evaluate the person with a hearing deficit for fall risk. Consider balance and gait, and adapt the environment to prevent falls (e.g., remove clutter, increase lighting).
- Instruct others to be aware that approaching hearing-impaired elders from the back may startle them and may cause loss of balance.
- Encourage elders to discuss with their physicians and or pharmacists medications that may have side effects related to hearing issues, such as tinnitus.
- Encourage elders to use vision (if vision is not a problem) as a compensatory safety aid in the environment. Teach scanning of the environment.
- Problem solve with elders a safety plan for fires or other issues.
- Use visual alert alarm systems (flashing lights) for awareness that someone is at the door, or that the phone is ringing.
- For fire safety in a home or facility, consider installing visual alarms with strobe lights or vibration apparatuses. Vibrating beds or pillows can help awaken the person.

Data from National Institute on Aging. 2009. Hearing loss. Retrieved from http://www.nia.nih.gov/HealthInformation/Publications/hearing.htm; TriData Corporation. (1999). Fire risks for the deaf or hard of hearing. Retrieved from http://www.usfa.dhs.gov/downloads/pdf/publications/hearing.pdf; and White, M., Russell, D., Saisan, J., & Kemp, G. M. (2009). Senior driving safety tips, warning signs, and knowing when to stop. Retrieved from http://www.helpguide.org/elder/senior_citizen_driving.htm.

use, outside traffic, overhead intercoms in use, and ice machines in use. Personnel shifts and changes in the institutional environment may also create background noise.

COTAs can recommend environments that reduce background noise. Examples include going to restaurants during times that they are less crowded, requesting to sit in less crowded areas, or sitting away from distracting background noises such as kitchen traffic or music (Table 16-2). When traveling, to help compensate for difficulty in hearing overhead paging systems, elders can be encouraged to frequently check overhead flight monitors, or check in with airport staff, or both. Using theaters and church communities that offer ALDs that amplify specific sounds is another way to reduce interference from background noises in public spaces.

Personal environmental modifications for reducing background noise include adding carpet to floors and

TABLE 16-2

	Environmental Adaptations for the Hearing-Impaired Elder	
Problem	**Intervention**
Background noises	Add carpeting to floors, acoustical tiles to ceilings, and drapes on windows, and replace (institutional and home) wood and metal furniture with upholstered furniture.
Background noises	Hang banners from ceilings; add insulating sheetrock around kitchens, maintenance, and (institutional) mechanical areas; tighten window weather seals. In dining rooms, seat no more than four persons at a table and add padded room dividers between tables to absorb sound. On special care units, eliminate ringing telephones, televisions, and intercoms; serve meals in small groups; pass medications at times other than meal times.
Background noises	Go to restaurants at less crowded times; request to sit in areas (public places) away from music and kitchen. Seek out theaters and churches that offer listening devices to amplify specific sounds.
Communication	Position to reduce glare, add closed captioning, use assisted listening devices. Use remote controls (television, radio, music) to select programming, and alternate between music, television, and radio.

acoustical tiles to ceilings, hanging drapes on windows, hanging banners from high ceilings, and replacing wood or metal furniture with upholstered furniture. Although these recommendations are intended to help absorb sound, they also can add aesthetic appeal to a home or institution.[22]

Additional interior modifications to reduce background noise within institutions include adding insulated sheetrock around noisy areas such as kitchen, maintenance, and mechanical areas, and tightening window weather seals. COTAs can assist individuals, families, and facility administrators in weighing the benefits of certain recommendations against the expenses of purchasing them. COTAs also can point out that, in some situations, background noises may provide helpful cues to locations of activity rooms, lounges, and beauty shops.

Environmental safety issues and concerns may center on the difficulties that hearing-impaired elders may have in locating the source of sounds in their home. The inability to locate sounds may contribute to a sense of insecurity in an individual's own environment and to the possibility of auditory illusions. This can lead to a decrease in the person's safety. For instance, elders may not be able to hear alarms or people moving about around them.[15] Fire and smoke alarms tend to have high-pitched sounds that are difficult for persons with sensorineural losses to hear.[4] Adding visual cues such as flashing lights is recommended for alarms.[17] Flashing lights, lower-pitched rings, or low-toned musical chimes are also available options for telephones and doorbells. COTAs should recommend adapting telephones with volume and tone controls for persons who need these modifications. Cell (portable) phones, although convenient for some individuals, may add to the confusion and frustration for persons with hearing impairments. The ring of the phone may not be heard or the phones may be difficult to locate if needed for an emergency.[23] Putting a cell phone on a vibration setting or trying text messaging with elders who can read

the screen and have adequate finger dexterity might be a good communication option. Elders can download their own ring tone and set it on "loud" for recognition. Some cell phones can be adapted for hearing aids and for amplification of sound. Cell phones can also be adapted to be used with a TTY or Voice Carry Over devise.

Research indicates hearing loss can increase the individuals risk of falling when compared to individuals who are not hearing-impaired.[3,24] Studies indicate that instruction in ways to substitute visual cues for hearing cues reduces the incidence of falls. COTAs also should make family members and health care providers aware that approaching hearing-impaired elders from the back and talking to and touching them may startle them and possibly cause them to lose balance. COTAs should recommend that hearing-impaired individuals be approached from the front, where visual contact can be made before beginning a conversation or expecting a response to a question.

To enhance conversations in areas where groups gather, COTAs should recommend that hearing-impaired individuals stay away from windows and plaster walls. Standing or sitting near soft materials that absorb sound, such as draperies, bookshelves, and upholstered furniture, also is recommended. Sitting in high-backed, upholstered chairs can help shield background noise. Focusing on the speaker's lips during conversation can help increase comprehension. If an individual has more impairment in one ear than the other, the individual can find the position that maximizes hearing with the unaffected ear.[13]

For family members and friends who want to improve communication with hearing-impaired elders, COTAs should recommend that they position themselves in the elder's field of vision and get the elder's attention before speaking. While conversing, they should look directly at the elder, reduce the rate of speech, and speak distinctly with a low tone. Additional recommendations include asking the elder to repeat what was said and providing written instructions to reinforce verbal directions. COTAs should stress that a hearing impairment does not reduce an individual's intelligence. Accommodations for the hearing impairment should not be over exaggerated or simplified to the point that elders with hearing loss feel that their intelligence or judgment is in question.

Because sensorineural hearing loss and its corresponding reduction in the ability to hear high-pitched sounds is the most common hearing disorder in elders, lowering the voice is especially important for women who address hearing-impaired elders. Increasing volume only increases tone and contributes to personal and social embarrassment (Box 16-3).

In restaurants and institutional dining rooms, seating no more than four persons at a table so eye contact can be easily made can enhance the social aspects derived from conversations during meals. In larger dining rooms, padded room dividers between tables can absorb sounds from surrounding tables. General recommendations regarding reduction of background noises also should be considered.

The effects of glare on the visual and nonverbal cues that enhance auditory communication should be considered when speaking with hearing-impaired elders. Sources of glare may include windows, lights, and glass surfaces either from behind the person speaking or reflected from eyeglasses. Before beginning a conversation, the COTA,

family member, or friend should adjust blinds or shades, adjust lighting, and reposition seating arrangements as needed (see Chapter 15 for more information on visual adaptations with aging).

Entertainment through television, music, websites with sounds on the internet, and radio offers opportunities for stimulation that are not dependent on other people. When elders control the times and selections for television and radio programs and music, the cognitive stimulation can be rewarding. When televisions and radios are on constantly or programs selected are not those the elder would choose, they become an additional source of background noise rather than a source of stimulation.[4,23] Closed-captioned television is an additional option to suggest. COTAs should identify and reduce sources of glare on the screen when positioning elders for television viewing. ALDs offer a means of controlling the volume for the hearing-impaired elder without disturbing others. Adjusting the volume and sound for music for those individuals with sensorineural hearing loss requires increasing the bass and decreasing the treble. Developments in technology have made the cost of these devices quite reasonable when weighed against the potential benefits.[23] Refer to Table 16-2 for ideas for environmental adaptations.

PROVIDING ASSISTIVE HEARING DEVICES

One of the most common assistive devices for persons with a hearing impairment is a hearing aid. An audiologist assists in determining whether a hearing aid would be appropriate. If a hearing aid would be beneficial, the audiologist works with the individual to choose the type of hearing aid that will maximize the individual's hearing and understanding of speech based on the individual's type of hearing loss.[12] Additionally, the audiologist also determines whether other factors associated with aging, lifestyle, and personality are compatible with a hearing aid. COTAs may refer elders to a physician or audiologist for assessment and evaluation. Advise patients to find out whether insurance will cover the cost of a hearing aid, and tell patients to ask whether a trial period is allowed so that the product can be tried out before it is purchased. Several visits to an audiologist may be required to get everything correct so the device is comfortable and the individual is comfortable using the hearing aid.[25]

Recent improvements in hearing aid technology have made hearing aids more acceptable. The improved devices are smaller and fit in the ear and therefore are more cosmetically appealing (Figure 16-3). In addition, hearing aids dampen certain frequencies. Some evidence indicates that younger individuals report more satisfaction than do elders with hearing aids.[26-28] This increased satisfaction may result from several factors. The onset of age-related hearing loss is often gradual, and elders may have accommodated to their hearing loss over an extended period, eventually finding the sudden amplification of all sound to be invasive and disturbing. In addition, the fine

BOX 16-3

Communication Tips for Working with the Hearing Impaired

- Face the elder so that the individual can see clearly your facial features with communication.
- Speak to the elder in a well lit area. This helps the elder with a hearing impairment observe body language and facial expressions, all of which provide clues for understanding communication.
- During conversations, limit background noise by turning off the radio or television.
- In public places sit far away from the crowded or noisy areas.
- Avoid communication when chewing food.
- Speak somewhat in a louder tone than normal, but avoid shouting because that may distort speech.
- Speak at a regular rate, not faster or slower, and do not overstress sounds.
- Give the elder with hearing loss clues about the topic of conversation whenever possible.
- Try to keep statements short and simple if the elder with hearing loss is struggling to understand the conversation. Repeat sentences as necessary.

Adapted from NIDCD. (2008). Presbycusis. National Institute on Deafness and Other Communication Disorders. Retrieved from http://www.nidcd.nih.gov/health/hearing/presbycusis.asp.

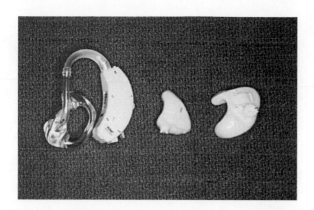

FIGURE 16-3 Hearing aids. *(From Bingham, B. J. G., Hawke, M., & Kwok, P. [1991]. Atlas of clinical otolaryngology. St. Louis, MO: Mosby.)*

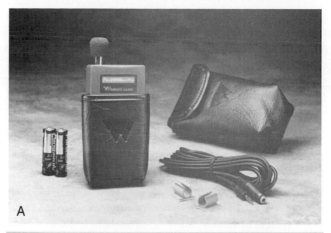

A

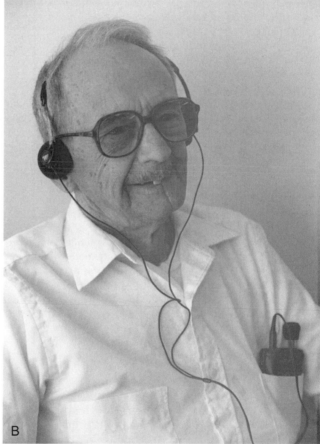

B

FIGURE 16-4 **Listening devices.** A, Certified occupational therapy assistants may need to instruct elders on maintenance of assisted listening devices such as cleaning and battery change. B, An assisted listening device helps this elder participate more fully in social interactions.

finger-and-hand dexterity required to manipulate volume and frequency controls and change batteries makes the hearing aid difficult to operate. Possible cognitive changes and short-term memory loss may affect the elder's ability to remember to turn the device on and off. The cost of replacement batteries and the elder's acceptance of new technologies are other factors to consider when determining the appropriateness of a hearing aid.[23,28] Goals for an elder who uses a hearing aid may include identifying alternative ways of operating it, building handles for tools used with the controls, changing or testing batteries with less difficulty, and learning the proper way to insert the device. (See the Appendix for additional information on hearing aids.)

Even with improved technology, hearing aids may not be effective for some individuals. For others, sound distortions may be louder with a hearing aid. When hearing aids are not effective, ALDs may be used. ALDs consist of a microphone to capture spoken sounds, an amplifier to increase sound volume, and a headset worn by the hearing-impaired person (Figure 16-4, A and B). Because the amplified sound from an ALD reaches the ear directly, background noises are reduced.[29] ALDs can augment hearing in a noisy clinic or hospital room. When an ALD is plugged into a television, the sound is amplified for the hearing-impaired person only. Use of an ALD also should be considered when visual impairment does not allow the elder to read lips or to supplement hearing loss by responding to other nonverbal cues. In addition to ALDs, there are some newer options for the hearing impaired such as computer assisted real-time transcription (CART), visual and tactile alarms, and volume controlled or caption phones.[30] COTAs can inform the elder with a hearing impairment about Telecommunications Relay Services. These services available throughout the United States allow the person to place telephone calls with the use of computers or other technology. Operators (communication assistants) facilitate these calls by converting text to voice or vice versa. There is a variety of methods available to do this type of telephone communication to meet the needs of the hearing-impaired population.[31]

CONCLUSION

As the number of elders with hearing impairments increases, the challenges and opportunities for COTAs continue to grow. The occupational performance and psychosocial and environmental issues that surround a hearing impairment demand that COTAs are informed and able to recommend appropriate interventions. COTAs can assist elders in attaining both performance and quality of life expectations by identifying limitations in hearing, referring elders for additional evaluation and intervention, and providing appropriate interventions.

CASE STUDY

Joe is an 89-year-old man who has resided at the Garden View Nursing Home for the past 7 years. His diagnoses include dementia (early stages), diabetes, congestive heart failure, and most recently an increase in hearing loss. Until recently, Joe's social history had been active and included participation in recreational activities and daily socializing with staff and other patients. At a recent care conference, the recreation director reported that Joe's participation in activity groups had decreased from nine to four groups a week. The nurse working with Joe stated that he was less social during meals and had started to sleep in the afternoons. The social worker shared her current assessments of Joe and stated that he seemed to be isolating himself from others, including his roommate. When the social worker and other staff asked him how he was doing, he seemed to have difficulty understanding the question and changed the subject to talk about the weather. The staff thought his dementia could be contributing to the confusion or perhaps to changes in the level of his hearing loss. The team recommended referrals for a professional hearing evaluation and an OT assessment. The referral for OT included an evaluation of Joe's current level of occupational functioning and suggestions for adapting his environment. In addition, staff was seeking suggestions from OT on how staff and others might interact more effectively with Joe. The OTR is a new graduate and has been at the Garden View Nursing Home for 2 months only. She has asked the COTA who has worked at the nursing home for 5 of the 7 years that Joe has been a resident at the home to assist her with the assessment.

■ CASE STUDY QUESTIONS

1 Using information from the case study and the chapter, identify why staff would think that Joe's hearing loss might have an effect on his social interaction with others.
2 Describe how Joe's recent decrease in social interaction may be influencing his mood.
3 As the long-standing COTA member of the OT department, what assistance can you provide for the OTR? For Joe?
4 Using information from the chapter, identify assessments that may be useful for Joe.
5 What recommendations would you consider to adapt Joe's environment to make it more purposeful and accommodating for him?
6 What types of assistive devices would be considered for Joe?
7 You have been asked to prepare an in-service on hearing impairments and elders and provide recommendations that will assist all staff to be more effective when interacting with those who have a hearing impairment.
    ■ How will you organize this in-service?
    ■ What information do you think would be most helpful for staff?
    ■ How will you engage the staff in the learning process?

■ CHAPTER REVIEW QUESTIONS

1 Referring to the chapter, what are some age-related hearing changes in elders?
2 How do age-related hearing impairments in elders affect their communication and socialization skills, as well as their safety?
3 How can COTAs contribute to improving communication and socialization skills in hearing-impaired elders?
4 What safety concerns should COTAs be aware of when working with an elder who has a hearing impairment?
5 What environmental modifications can COTAs suggest to reduce background noises in an elder's home?
6 What environmental modifications in an institution might be used to reduce confusion caused by hearing impairments?
7 Why might an elder prefer not to use a hearing aid?
8 Explain how a cochlear implant would improve the hearing of some elders?
9 How might a COTA use an ALD to help an elder in a clinic setting?

REFERENCES

1. Grue, E.V., Ranhoff, A.H., Noro, A., Finne-Soveri, H., Jensdóttir, A.B., Ljunggren, G., et al., 2009. Vision and hearing impairments and their associations with falling and loss of instrumental activities in daily living in acute hospitalized older persons in five Nordic hospitals. Scandinavian Journal of Caring Sciences 23 (4), 635-643.
2. Garstecki, D.C., Erler, S.F., 1998. Hearing and aging. Topics in Geriatric Rehabilitation 14 (2), 1-17.
3. Tobis, J.S., Block, M., Steinhaus-Donham, C., Reinsch, S., Tamaru, K., Weil, D., 1990. Falling among the sensorially impaired elderly. Archives of Physical Medicine and Rehabilitation 71 (2), 144.
4. Hooper, C.R., 2001. Sensory and sensory integrative development. In: Bonder, B.R., Wagner, M.B. (Eds.), Functional Performance in Older Adults. FA Davis, Philadelphia.
5. Johnson, C., Danhauer, J., Bennet, M., Harrison, J., 2009. Systematic review of physicians' knowledge of, participation in, and attitudes toward hearing and balance screening in the elderly population. Seminars in Hearing 30 (3), 193-206.
6. Kochkin, S., 2005. MarkeTrak VII: Hearing loss population tops 31 million people. Hearing Review 12 (7), 16-29.
7. U.S. Department of Health and Human Services. Office of Disease Prevention and Health Promotion, n.d. Healthy People 2010. Retrieved from http://www.healthypeople.gov/document/HTML/Volume2/28Vision.htm.
8. NIH Senior Health, 2009. Hearing loss. National Institutes of Health. Retrieved from http://nihseniorhealth.gov/hearingloss/toc.html.
9. Lichtenstein, M.J., Bess, F.H., Logan, S.A., 1991. Screening the elderly for hearing impairment. In: Ripich, D. (Ed.), Handbook of Geriatric Communication Disorders. Pro-Ed, Austin, TX.
10. American Occupational Therapy Association, 2008. Occupational therapy practice framework: Domain and process, 2nd ed. American Journal of Occupational Therapy 62, 625-683.
11. Meriano, C., Latella, D., 2007. Occupational Therapy Interventions: Function and Occupations. Slack, Thorofare, NJ.

12. NIDCD, 2008. Presbycusis. National Institute on Deafness and Other Communication Disorders. Retrieved from http://www.nidcd.nih.gov/health/hearing/presbycusis.asp.

13. Cherney, L.R., 2002. The effects of aging on communication. In: Lewis, C.B. (Ed.), Aging: The Health Care Challenge, 4th ed. FA Davis, Philadelphia.

14. Burkhalter, C.L., Allen, R.S., Skaar, D.C., Crittenden, J., Burgio, L.D., 2009. Examining the effectiveness of traditional audiological assessments for nursing home residents with dementia-related behaviors. Journal of the American Academy of Audiology 20 (9), 529-538.

15. Hooper, C.R., Bello-Haas, V.D., 2008. Sensory and sensory integrative development. In: Bonder, B.R., Bello-Haas, V.D. (Eds.), Functional Performance in Older Adults. FA Davis, Philadelphia.

16. Vogel, I., Brug, J., van der Ploeg, C., Ratt, H., 2009. Strategies for the prevention of MP3-induced hearing loss among adolescents: Expert opinions from a Delphi study. Pediatrics 123 (5), 1257-1262.

17. Bance, M., 2007. Hearing and aging. Canadian Medical Association Journal 176 (7), 925-927.

18. Canadian Transportation Agency, 1997. A look at barriers to communication facing persons with disabilities who travel by air [WWW page]. URL http://www.cta-otc.gc.ca/air-aerien/mdex_e.html.

19. Corso, J.F., 1990. Sensory-perceptual processes and aging. In: Schaie, K.W., Eisdorfer, C. (Eds.), Annual Review of Gerontology, 2nd ed. Springer, New York.

20. Howarth, A., Shone, G.R., 2006. Ageing and the auditory system. Postgraduate Medicine 82 (1), 166-171.

21. Janken, J.K., Cullinan, C.L., 1990. Auditory, sensory, and perceptual alteration: Suggested revision of defining characteristics. Nursing Diagnosis 1 (4), 147.

22. Christenson, M.A., Taira, E., 1990. Aging in the Designed Environment. Haworth Press, New York.

23. Stach, B.A., Stoner, W.R., 1991. Sensory aids for the hearing impaired elderly. In: Ripich, D. (Ed.), Handbook of Geriatric Communication Disorders. Pro-Ed, Austin, TX.

24. Kulmala, J., Viljanen, A., Sipilä, S., Pajala, S., Pärssinen, O., Kauppinen, M., et al. 2009. Poor vision accompanied with other sensory impairments as a predictor of falls in older women. Age and Ageing 38, 162-167

25. National Institute on Aging, 2009. Hearing loss. Retrieved from http://www.nia.nih.gov/HealthInformation/Publications/hearing.htm.

26. Kane, R.L., Ouslander, J.G., Abrass, I.B., 1989. Essentials of Clinical Geriatrics, 4th ed. McGraw-Hill, New York.

27. Rieske, R.J., Hostege, H., 1996. Growing Older in America. McGraw-Hill, New York.

28. Stoneham, M.A., 1994. Technology and disability. Andover Medica 13 (1), 47.

29. American Speech-Language-Hearing Association, 2009. Hearing assistive technology. Retrieved from http://www.asha.org/public/hearing/treatment/assist_tech.htm.

30. Hearing Loss Association of America, n.d. Assessability. Retrieved from http://www.hearingloss.org/advocacy/accessibility.asp.

31. Federal Communications Commission, n.d. Telecommunications Relay Services. Retrieved from http://www.fcc.gov/cgb/consumerfacts/trs.html.

17

Strategies to Maintain Continence in Elders

KRIS R. BROWN AND JESSICA HATCH

KEY TERMS

urinary incontinence, fecal incontinence, behavioral techniques,
environmental modifications

CHAPTER OBJECTIVES

1. Determine the prevalence and cost associated with incontinence.
2. Indicate common causes of incontinence.
3. Review the normal anatomy and physiology of urination and defecation.
4. Identify the different types of urinary and fecal incontinence.
5. Explain the effect of the Omnibus Budget Reconciliation Act in dealing with the problem of incontinence in nursing homes.
6. Specify the role of each team member, emphasizing the importance of an interdisciplinary approach.
7. Identify the certified occupational therapy assistant's (COTA's) role in the management of incontinence.
8. List suggestions for the management of incontinence.

Sara is a COTA who has been treating Mrs. Smith since her arrival at the nursing home 2 months earlier following a stroke. Sara works with Mrs. Smith both morning and after lunch. To start each afternoon session, per Mrs. Smith's usual routine, Sara assists Mrs. Smith with going to the restroom. However, the past few sessions that Sara has worked with Mrs. Smith, Sara has noticed that Mrs. Smith has been incontinent each time. When Sara questions Mrs. Smith about it, Mrs. Smith states, "I just can't seem to get to the bathroom in time, and lately no one has been helping me go before lunch like they used to do." Additionally, Sara observes that Mrs. Smith's bathroom door is always closed and blocked shut by the bedside table, making access to the restroom difficult. Oftentimes, her call light is not within reach.

Sara is concerned about the noticeable increase in Mrs. Smith's incontinence. She feels that, as a COTA, it is her responsibility to educate both Mrs. Smith and the nursing staff on some tips that may help Mrs. Smith decrease her incontinence episodes. As a result, Sara has begun working with the nursing staff to create a timed voiding schedule for Mrs. Smith. Sara has also made a checklist that reminds nursing staff of simple ways to reduce some of the environmental barriers contributing to Mrs. Smith's incontinence. After implementing a few simple techniques and educating both Mrs. Smith and the nursing staff on some simple tips regarding incontinence, her episodes of incontinence have decreased.

Incontinence of urine and stool is a common problem many elders face. Bowel and bladder management, toilet hygiene bowel, as well as other areas of related occupations are discussed in the Occupational Therapy Practice Framework (2nd ed.)[1] Incontinence is often considered part of the normal aging process and is therefore accepted but not treated. Society's acceptance of this condition is manifested by the availability of absorbent products and high-fiber foods found in local stores. Some elders afflicted with this problem may feel ashamed and embarrassed, which may lead to psychological conditions such as depression and avoidance of social relations or activities. Other elders may think the problem will correct itself, or they may fear that it will lead to a surgical procedure. Prolonged hospitalizations are common when incontinence is left untreated. Incontinence may even be a primary reason that caregivers decide to place elders in long-term care facilities.

During the normal aging process, bladder capacity and the ability to delay urination and defecation decrease. These changes can increase the risk for incontinence, especially with medical conditions such as pneumonia and chronic heart failure. Often, fecal incontinence results from changes in sphincter musculature and hormonal imbalances.

URINARY AND FECAL INCONTINENCE

Prevalence

The prevalence of urinary incontinence in the nursing home setting has been reported to range from 22% to 90%, with the average near 56%.[2] For non-institutionalized

241

older adults, the range is 15% to 38%.[3] In general, women are twice as likely as men to experience this problem.[3] Additionally, urinary incontinence is thought to be widely underdiagnosed and underreported.[4]

Cost

In the United States, the estimated total annual cost of managing urinary incontinence is $16.3 billion per year. For the elderly in nursing homes managing urinary incontinence is estimated at 5.34 billion dollars per year.[5] In other words, cost of incontinence is approximately $10,000 per patient each year.[6] This cost can be itemized to include routine care such as labor, supplies, laundry, and diagnostic and medical evaluation; treatment such as surgery and pharmacy and drug costs; incontinent consequences such as skin erosion, urinary tract infection, and falls; and added admissions resulting from incontinence.[2]

Private insurance companies and government programs will usually pay for only urodynamic evaluation, surgical procedures, catheterization,[7] and sacral nerve stimulation.[8] Consequently, management of incontinence is routine care. Elders and their families may feel financially strained if incontinence is the only reason for institutionalization. Therefore, poor reimbursement encourages management of incontinence rather than determination of the underlying problem and provision of the most effective intervention.

ANATOMY AND PHYSIOLOGY

The anatomic structures of the male lower urinary tract primarily responsible for normal urination include the bladder neck, prostate gland, pelvic floor musculature, and urethra. In women, the structures include the bladder neck, proximal urethra (internal sphincter), and the pelvic floor muscles that provide the strength needed to maintain the pelvic floor tone and urethra resistance.

The bladder fills and empties. The normal bladder capacity averages about 500 ml. The urinary bladder can normally hold between 250 and 350 ml of urine before the individual feels the urge to void. As the urinary bladder reaches its holding capacity, the bladder becomes strong enough to activate the stretch receptors, which, in turn, send a message to the nervous system, the pelvic floor and sphincter sense the increased pressure, and the individual feels the urge to void.[9] The urethra then relaxes, allowing the bladder to empty.

The anatomical structures involved with normal defecation include the pelvic floor muscles, anal sphincter mechanisms (internal and external), colon, rectum, and anal canal. A stool of an appropriate consistency is delivered to the rectum and anal sphincter through the gastrointestinal (GI) tract and colon. The normal sensory system acknowledges that the rectum is filling and alerts the structures of the type of rectal content (that is, solid, liquid, or gas). Once the stool passes the rectum, the internal sphincter relaxes, allowing the stool to pass.

ETIOLOGY

Causes of urinary and stool incontinence may be pathological, anatomical, or physiological. The most common potential causes of urinary incontinence are transient or reversible. These include delirium, infection such as symptomatic urinary tract infection or vaginitis, excessive urine production, and psychological factors such as depression.[9] Hypercalcemia, hyperglycemia, diabetes insipidus, chronic heart failure, lower extremity venous insufficiency, and drug-induced ankle edema are other causes of transient incontinence.[8]

Pharmaceutical causes of transient incontinence are sedative hypnotics (that is, benzodiazepines); diuretics, leading to polyuria; calcium channel blockers; anticholinergic agents (that is, antihistamines, antidepressants, antipsychotics, antiparkinsonian agents, and alpha-adrenergic agents); sympathomimetics; and sympatholytics. Potential causes of fecal incontinence include abnormal delivery of feces to the rectum, which may be drug-induced, metabolic, or caused by infection; sphincter dysfunction from trauma, diabetes mellitus, or inflammation; reduced rectal compliance such as rectal ischemia or fecal impaction; and anatomical derangement such as from a tumor or from third-degree hemorrhoids or injury. Other causes of fecal incontinence include muscular and neuromuscular disorders such as congenital or hereditary myopathy, behavioral and developmental dysfunction such as mental retardation or psychiatric disorders, and neurological impairment such as with the central nervous system, spinal system, or peripheral nervous system.[2]

TYPES OF URINARY INCONTINENCE

Urge or Urgency Incontinence

Elders commonly have a combination of types of urinary incontinence. Urgency urinary incontinence (UUI) is defined as the involuntary leakage of urine accompanied by a sudden urgency to have to go to the bathroom.[9] Elders may experience a massive and sudden loss of urine without warning and often strain to empty the bladder. This type of urge incontinence is common at night and is referred to as *nocturnal incontinence*. Urge incontinence may also occur when elders hear water trickling or when they drink small amounts of water. Uncontrolled contraction of the detrusor (bladder muscle), a condition that is also referred to as *neurogenic detrusor overactivity*, may be part of the problem.[9]

Stress Urinary Incontinence

Stress urinary incontinence (SUI) is considered more prevalent in women than in men. Elders with stress incontinence experience uncontrolled loss of urine when intra-abdominal pressure is placed on the bladder. This type of incontinence can occur while coughing, laughing, sneezing, exercising, bending, lifting a heavy object, or arising from a chair.[9] A child sitting on an elder's lap may place sufficient pressure on the elder's bladder, which can lead to incontinence. Stress incontinence is usually caused by weakened pelvic floor musculature as a result of the childbirth process in women, or a weakened or damaged sphincter mechanism. In men, stress incontinence is often the result of a radical prostatectomy performed for the treatment of prostate cancer.[4]

Overflow Incontinence

An individual with overflow incontinence experiences frequent or constant dribbling of urine, voiding only small amounts at a time. The bladder is always full, and the elder is never able to completely empty it. The elder cannot sense its fullness. The cause is often an underactive detrusor muscle. In men this type of incontinence is common when there is a blockage in the bladder, such as an enlarged prostate.[9]

Mixed Incontinence

Mixed urinary incontinence (MUI) is a combination of urge and stress incontinence. In other words, there is involuntary leakage in conjunction with a sense of urgency and increased bladder pressure. Approximately 80% of urinary incontinence cases are in this category.[9]

Functional Incontinence and Other Types

Functional incontinence is related to impaired cognitive functioning and mobility. With functional incontinence, lower urinary tract function is intact, but decreased cognitive functioning prevents individuals from recognizing the need to use the restroom or decreased mobility impacts the ability to reach the restroom in time.[4] This type of incontinence often warrants occupational therapy (OT) intervention to help with environmental and other adaptations. Other types of incontinence, which are not as common, include reflex incontinence, detrusor instability, and iatrogenic incontinence. Reflex incontinence is a storage and emptying problem resulting from a spinal cord lesion. Detrusor instability is common in individuals diagnosed with dementia. With this type of incontinence, the bladder contracts before it is full. Iatrogenic incontinence is caused by an outside medical intervention or treatment such as a new medication.[4]

FECAL INCONTINENCE

Fecal incontinence is often a result of problems with the GI tract and colon. GI problems cause changes in the consistency and volume of stools, leading to problems such as diarrhea and constipation.[4] Diarrhea is defined as "the frequent passage of loose, watery stools."[10] Associated symptoms are abdominal pain and cramping. Diarrhea can be a symptom of problems such as dietary intolerance, malabsorption syndromes, inflammatory bowel disease, fecal impaction, gastroenteritis, and GI tumors.

An individual with constipation will complain of abdominal pain and fullness in the rectum. Defecation usually occurs infrequently, and consistency of the stool is hard and dry. Constipation can result from intestinal obstruction, diverticulitis, tumors, dehydration, lack of exercise, and a poor diet.

OMNIBUS BUDGET RECONCILIATION ACT AND RELATED RESEARCH

The Agency for Healthcare Policy and Research, currently referred to as the Agency for Healthcare Research and Quality (AHRQ), was created as a result of the Omnibus Budget Reconciliation Act (OBRA) to conduct research on diseases and disorders. The following are the initial guidelines for information on urinary incontinence developed as a result of studies conducted by the AHRQ panel:

1. Improve education and dissemination of urinary incontinence diagnosis and treatment alternatives to the public and to health care professionals
2. Educate the consumer to report incontinence problems once they occur
3. Improve the detection and documentation of urinary incontinence through better history taking and health care record keeping
4. Establish appropriate basic evaluation and further evaluations
5. Reduce variance among health care professionals
6. Encourage further biomedical, clinical, and cost research on prevention, diagnosis, and treatment of urinary incontinence in the adult[11]

This special panel concluded that most elders were improperly diagnosed for urinary incontinence and ineffectively treated. Both urinary and fecal incontinence are areas that surveyors look at closely during their annual inspections because of the secondary complications such as skin erosion and falls associated with these problems. For COTAs working in nursing home practice with the Minimum Data Set (MDS) Version 3.0 bladder and bowel are addressed in *Section H.* (Figure 17-1). *Section G* of the MDS includes the functional status of toileting for which therapists may provide input. Refer to Chapter 6 for more information on the MDS According to OBRA guidelines, the goal with incontinence is to encourage the nursing home staff to use a rehabilitative model.[12]

More recently, in 2005, the Centers for Medicare and Medicaid Services (CMS) came out with new surveyor guidance regarding long-term care on urinary incontinence. The purposes of all of these guidelines are intended to help with the diagnosis, assessment, and management of urinary incontinence so that individuals can benefit from early screening and intervention.[9]

INTERDISCIPLINARY TEAM STRATEGIES

Only half of elders residing in the community actually relate incontinence problems to their physicians to receive

Resident _____   Identifier _____   Date _____

Section H — Bladder and Bowel

H0100. Appliances

↓ Check all that apply

☐ A. **Indwelling catheter** (including suprapubic catheter and nephrostomy tube)

☐ B. **External catheter**

☐ C. **Ostomy** (including urostomy, ileostomy, and colostomy)

☐ D. **Intermittent catheterization**

☐ Z. **None of the above**

H0200. Urinary Toileting Program

Enter Code ☐ A. **Has a trial of a toileting program (e.g., scheduled toileting, prompted voiding, or bladder training)** been attempted on admission/reentry or since urinary incontinence was noted in this facility?
- 0. **No** → Skip to H0300, Urinary Continence
- 1. **Yes** → Continue to H0200B, Response
- 9. **Unable to determine** → Skip to H0200C, Current toileting program or trial

Enter Code ☐ B. **Response** - What was the resident's response to the trial program?
- 0. **No improvement**
- 1. **Decreased wetness**
- 2. **Completely dry** (continent)
- 9. **Unable to determine** or trial in progress

Enter Code ☐ C. **Current toileting program or trial** - Is a toileting program (e.g., scheduled toileting, prompted voiding, or bladder training) currently being used to manage the resident's urinary continence?
- 0. **No**
- 1. **Yes**

H0300. Urinary Continence

Enter Code ☐ **Urinary continence** - Select the one category that best describes the resident
- 0. **Always continent**
- 1. **Occasionally incontinent** (less than 7 episodes of incontinence)
- 2. **Frequently incontinent** (7 or more episodes of urinary incontinence, but at least one episode of continent voiding)
- 3. **Always incontinent** (no episodes of continent voiding)
- 9. **Not rated,** resident had a catheter (indwelling, condom), urinary ostomy, or no urine output for the entire 7 days

H0400. Bowel Continence

Enter Code ☐ **Bowel continence** - Select the one category that best describes the resident
- 0. **Always continent**
- 1. **Occasionally incontinent** (one episode of bowel incontinence)
- 2. **Frequently incontinent** (2 or more episodes of bowel incontinence, but at least one continent bowel movement)
- 3. **Always incontinent** (no episodes of continent bowel movements)
- 9. **Not rated,** resident had an ostomy or did not have a bowel movement for the entire 7 days

H0500. Bowel Toileting Program

Enter Code ☐ **Is a toileting program currently being used to manage the resident's bowel continence?**
- 0. **No**
- 1. **Yes**

H0600. Bowel Patterns

Enter Code ☐ **Constipation present?**
- 0. **No**
- 1. **Yes**

FIGURE 17-1 Minimum Data Set (MDS; 3.0) form section H. Form is used by nursing staffs to rate incontinence. (*From Nursing Home Quality Initiatives, Centers for Medicare & Medicaid Services. Baltimore, MD, 2010, US Department of Health & Human Services.*)

treatment.[9] When the problem is reported, many health care professionals treat incontinence as a disease rather than determine the underlying cause, often attributing the incontinence to old age or normal body changes. However, incontinence should never be considered normal.[9]

Health care providers involved in the treatment of incontinence in elders include urologists, gynecologists, psychiatrists, nurses, psychologists, social workers, dietitians, pharmacists, and enterostomal therapists (ET nurses). Other health professionals include OT practitioners and physical and speech therapists. All members of this team work together to determine the most effective plan of care, and each provides a unique role in the interdisciplinary team.

Physicians begin care of elders with incontinence by taking a thorough medical history, performing a physical examination, and scheduling laboratory tests. They may refer the client to a specialist such as an urologist or gynecologist, if the problem is recurrent. However, a conservative approach is usually initiated. The primary preference is the use of behavioral techniques followed by pharmacological approaches. Because of potential complications, surgery is considered the last resort. Surgery for stress incontinence in women, which requires repositioning the bladder neck, has a success rate of 69% to 94%, depending on the type of procedure.[2] The success rate of surgery in men with overflow incontinence, which requires removal of the cause of blockage, is similar.[8,13] Surgery for fecal incontinence is indicated for traumatic, idiopathic, neurogenic, congenital, and medical problems. Surgery may consist of a sphincter repair, gracilis muscle transfer, and artificial anal sphincter placement.[2]

Medications are often prescribed to improve incontinence by treating infection, replacing hormones (estrogen), decreasing abnormal bladder contractions, and tightening sphincter muscles. This type of treatment is effective primarily with urge incontinence resulting from detrusor hyperactivity. Anticholinergics such as atropine, antispasmodics, tricyclic antidepressants, and calcium channel blockers are the drugs commonly prescribed. Antidiarrheal agents such as loperamide and fecal softeners and lubricants are common medications used to treat problems with defecation.[2]

The dietitian can determine hydration or nutrition patterns in the elder's diet that may be contributing to both urinary and stool incontinence. Recommendations such as a high-fiber diet[2] and liquid intake of 48 to 64 oz per day help maintain proper functioning of the bowel and bladder.[3,14] Caffeine intake should be limited because it acts as a diuretic.

A nurse should complete a bowel (Figure 17-2, A) and bladder (Figure 17-2, B) profile indicating the length of time that incontinence has been present and the frequency and timing of episodes. The nurse usually initiates behavioral approaches.

Social service specialists and psychologists are important in determining the family dynamics and support available to elders. They may help determine the effect that incontinence has on the involvement of elders in social activities and relationships. They may also provide counseling to assist elders in expressing feelings about their incontinence problems.

Speech and language therapists are involved in evaluating elders' abilities to communicate either verbally or nonverbally to make their needs known in a timely and effective manner. These professionals assist elders in compensating for impaired communication by providing instruction in the use of gestures and communication aids. Specific training is also provided to the caregiver to ensure proper carryover.

Physical therapists are involved in completing a comprehensive musculoskeletal and functional mobility assessment to ascertain range of motion, muscle strength, bed mobility, sitting balance, and gait. The treatment provided by physical therapists may also include teaching and instruction on the use of an assistive device such as a walker, cane, or brace to improve the elders' abilities to ambulate to the bathroom. Caregiver training by physical therapists may include the proper use of a mechanical lift or sliding board with transfers or encouraging elders to carry over a program involving range of motion and strengthening exercises. Electrical stimulation to strengthen the muscles in stress incontinence, biofeedback, and Kegel exercises may all be part of the physical therapy intervention. These approaches also may be applied by the COTA with demonstrated competency and according to any state licensure guidelines.

COTAs work closely with the other disciplines to determine the cause of incontinence and to develop an effective intervention plan. Understanding how incontinence fits in with the Occupational Therapy Practice Framework (OTPF) can be helpful in recognizing the role of COTAs with incontinence. According to the OTPF: Domain and Process (2nd ed.) bowel and bladder management and toileting hygiene are areas of occupations, or more specifically activities of daily living (ADL).[1] COTAs have a responsibility to their patients to address ADL that are pertinent to them.

The following intervention techniques can be provided by members of the treatment team, including COTAs, to help increase voiding, thus leading to increased independence in ADL.

Timed Voiding and Habit Training

Timed voiding and habit training consist of establishing a fixed schedule that requires the client to void every 2 hours. Toileting is adjusted according to the client's normal pattern and is determined after approximately 2 weeks of monitoring. To make timed voiding easier, associate the schedule with certain parts of the elder's daily routine, such as before/after a meal, or activity.[9] Attempts are made to increase the intervals between voiding. This habit training often is used in the nursing home setting and is successful with neurologically impaired residents.

Prompted Voiding

Prompted voiding is commonly used in the nursing facility and is recommended for frail or cognitively impaired individuals. Caregivers are responsible for documenting whether the client is wet or dry on a regular basis, usually every 1 to 2 hours. Caregivers are encouraged to ask whether elders have a need to void.

Date and Time	Stimulus to evacuation (digital, suppository, or none)	Response (amount and consistency of stool)	Incontinent episodes (time, amount, and type of leakage)

A

Name_____ Date _____

Time toilet is offered	Leakage (yes or no)	Was client aware of urge? (yes or no)	Did client void? (yes or no)	Comments
0800				
1000				
1200				
1400				
1600				
1800				
2000				

B (2200 and so forth)

FIGURE 17-2 Sample recording charts. A, A diary of bowel function. B, A diary of bladder function. *(From Doughty, D. B. (2006). Urinary and Fecal Incontinence Nursing Management. St. Louis, MO: Mosby.)*

Bladder Training

Bladder training is recommended as a first step with stress, urge, and mixed incontinence.[2] While some studies have shown a 10% to 15% improvement rate in urinary continence using bladder training,[8,13] a recent Cochrane review of the literature was able to conclude only that bladder retraining may be a beneficial intervention for urinary incontinence.[2] The goal of bladder training is to decrease the frequency of voiding and lengthen the intervals between voiding. Caregivers instruct elders to resist the urge to urinate and to follow a planned time schedule rather than to respond immediately to the urge.

Biofeedback

Biofeedback offers elders visual and auditory information to teach voluntary control of certain functions. Most elders are taught to relax the detrusor and abdominal muscles while contracting the sphincter muscle. An improvement rate of 20% to 25% in urinary incontinence has been noted for individuals using this technique.[8] A 70% to 90% success rate is reported with fecal incontinence.[15]

Pelvic Floor Exercise

Pelvic floor exercises are also known as Kegel, or childbirth, exercises. Kegel exercises are commonly used and have a 30% to 90% success rate in women with stress incontinence.[8,13] Elders are taught to relax the abdominal muscles while contracting the pelvic floor muscles. After assistance is given to identify the correct muscles, elders are told to complete a minimum of 60 contractions of the pelvic floor muscles per day working up to 150 contractions per day, if possible.[3] This technique is commonly used to improve fecal incontinence and increase muscle tone in the pelvic floor to prevent stool leakage.[2] Physical and occupational therapists can initiate these exercises.

ENVIRONMENTAL ADAPTATIONS

The ability to be continent resides heavily on being able to reach the restroom or commode. Often there are environmental barriers that contribute to incontinence. Many residents in long-term care facilities experience incontinence simply because of the inability to obtain help with toileting in a timely fashion. In most cases, changes in the physical environment must be initiated by caregivers.[2] When considering problems with functional mobility, COTAs are encouraged to look at the elder's environment to determine whether modifications are necessary to facilitate independence and to ensure safety while toileting (Box 17-1). COTAs should make recommendations for improvement where required (Table 17-1). (See Chapter 14 for more information on fall prevention.)

Many environmental modifications can be made in the bathroom. For example, grab bars can be mounted either

BOX 17-1

Considerations for Environmental Adaptations to Help with Incontinence
1. Does the client need or use side rails to assist with bed mobility?
2. Is the call light easily accessible to the client?
3. Is the height of the bed appropriate for safe transfers?
4. Is the client restrained in bed or in the wheelchair, which would limit mobility to the bathroom?
5. Is there adequate lighting to and from the bathroom? (A 60-year-old elder requires three times brighter lighting than a 20-year-old adult.)
6. Are there any obstacles or clutter that would interfere with safe mobility?
7. Is the client able to manage the door leading into the bathroom?
8. Are the floors highly waxed, which could cause a fall?
9. Is the doorway leading into the bathroom wide enough to allow proper clearance for a wheelchair or walker?
10. Is the height of the toilet appropriate?
11. Are there any grab bars or support to assist with a transfer to the toilet?

TABLE 17-1

Environmental and Safety Adaptations to Help with Incontinence	
When implemented appropriately, the following safety adaptations are ideas that may be used to make it easier for the elders to maneuver around in their environment.	
Room	**Safety Adaptations**
Bedroom, room in an institution	Keep the walkways clear and free of clutter. Provide adequate lighting. Install handrails leading to the bathroom. Place a commode near the bed. Make a urinal or bed pan available. Adjust the height of the bed. Add side rail to the bed for ease with transfers.
Bathrooms	Add a nightlight to increase visibility with mobility. Use a contrasting color toilet seat. Add any combination of a toilet safety frame, elevated toilet seat, and grab bars to facilitate independence and ensure safety with transfers and clothing management. Eliminate throw rugs or bath mats. Add a nonskid material (Dycem) in front of the toilet or commode. Suggest that the client wear clothing that is easily removed such as Velcro or elastic waistband pants.

Data from Miller, C. (2009) *Nursing for Wellness in Older Adults*, 5th ed. Philadelphia: Lippincott Williams & Wilkins.

in a 45-degree horizontal fashion to assist in pushing up or in a vertical position to facilitate pulling up. The length of the bars should be between 24 and 36 inches on the back wall and 42 inches on the side wall.[16]

Physical restraints can sometimes be used by caregivers in nursing facilities to prevent individuals from falling out of bed or the wheelchair. However, the use of a restraint may cause increased agitation for many reasons, including elders being unable to take care of bathroom needs if call lights are not answered in a timely manner. Because of the original OBRA law, the use of restraints is carefully monitored. Restraints are recommended only to encourage more functional independence, to decrease the risk for a life-threatening medical problem, or to promote a better anatomical seating position that is minimally restrictive.[17] OBRA protects the rights of elders to freedom of movement and access to the body. COTAs must work closely with other staff members in deciding on a restraint program that allows the client to remain continent while minimizing the use of restraints (see Chapter 14).

CLOTHING ADAPTATIONS AND MANAGEMENT

Clothing management before and after toileting is a functional independence measure. This measure is often used to evaluate toileting and bowel and bladder management at admission to and on discharge from inpatient rehabilitation facilities.[18] COTAs can help elders improve clothing management by providing activities that use fine motor coordination, such as increasing dexterity with manipulation of zippers or buttons. Range of motion and strengthening exercises may facilitate pulling pants over the feet and hips. Another option is to suggest that elders wear clothing that can be easily manipulated, such as clothing with Velcro or elastic waistbands.[3]

ADAPTATIONS FOR CLIENTS WITH FUNCTIONAL INCONTINENCE

An increased incidence of incontinence is often seen in elders with dementia. In addition to an inability to manage their clothing, these elders also have difficulty locating the bathroom and toilet. Some may have problems with their strength, coordination, range of motion, and sense of balance, which affect their abilities to toilet in a timely and safe manner. They may be seen urinating and defecating in inappropriate places. This level of functioning is described by Allen and colleagues[19] as Allen Cognitive Level 3 (see Chapter 7 for more information on this theory). Elders with dementia might perform part of the toileting task but become confused at some point and require verbal or physical assistance, or both, to continue. COTAs can encourage maximal functioning by determining what tasks the client can do and by training caregivers to assist with only those tasks that become difficult.

Impaired functional mobility of elders can be addressed by COTAs in conjunction with physical therapy. The goal is to improve functional mobility skills and train caregivers to provide the proper physical and verbal cues needed for elders to become successful with safe mobility.

PREVENTION OF SKIN EROSION

One of the secondary effects of incontinence mentioned earlier is skin erosion. Caregivers must be educated on a bowel and bladder program, a repositioning schedule, and proper wound care. Skin integrity may be improved by placing a special mattress on the bed or an incontinence cushion on the sitting surface.

Nutrition is extremely important in wound healing. COTAs must consider elders' abilities to feed themselves. Elders may need to learn how to use adaptive equipment to aid this procedure. Elders must be able to obtain and drink fluids to maintain hydration.

CASE STUDY

Ricardo was recently admitted to a skilled nursing facility (SNF) from his home, where his aging partner Paul was attempting to care for him. Ricardo's urinary and bowel incontinence was becoming burdensome, and with little support and inconsistent in-home services, the daily routine had become too much for Paul. The situation was also causing a strain on their relationship.

On admission to the SNF, Ricardo was diagnosed with early-stage Alzheimer-type dementia, rheumatoid arthritis, and long-term low back pain. In addition, Ricardo had the beginning of a pressure sore forming on his coccyx. The nursing home physician reviewed Ricardo's medical history and performed a physical examination. He determined that Ricardo's incontinence was not caused from medications, but rather was related to the Alzheimer's disease process and pain associated with movement. OT and physical therapy were ordered to evaluate and provide appropriate intervention for Ricardo.

The findings from the OT evaluation were as follows:

1   Working memory deficits
2   Limited mobility and ambulation secondary to pain
3   Limited upper extremity range of motion
4   Weakness in the upper extremities
5   Ability to follow simple two-step directions

Josie, the COTA at the SNF, was assigned to provide OT treatment five times a week. She was to assess bed and wheelchair positioning, adaptive equipment needs, fine motor skills, and toileting tasks and transfers. It was determined through the interdisciplinary team process that nursing would assist with pain management, including appropriate medications. Nursing would also implement scheduled toileting and begin intervention to heal the pressure ulcer. The dietitian would provide suggestions for a proper diet, intake, and suggest nutritional supplements to promote healing of the pressure ulcer. Physical therapy would address bed mobility, sitting and standing balance, and safe ambulation.

By the end of the first week of intervention, Josie recommended a higher bed to ease Ricardo's transfer process and to decrease the amount of pain associated with transfers. A bedside commode was placed in Ricardo's room until his ability to ambulate to the bathroom in his room could be evaluated. Because of his dementia, Ricardo was unable to complete pericare; however, with verbal cueing he was able to assist with clothing management before and after toileting. Josie also recommended a pull-up incontinent undergarment to be used because Ricardo was able to assist with clothing management. She also provided positioning equipment for the bed and wheelchair to assist in the healing of and prevention of further pressure ulcers. This included a bed wedge to help Ricardo maintain side-lying during scheduled turning when in bed and a gel cushion with a coccyx cut-out for his wheelchair to decrease heat and shear.

Paul began to make regular visits, and the social worker helped them adjust to the changes in their lives.

◼ **CASE STUDY QUESTIONS**

1 Why would a pull-up incontinence product be the most appropriate recommendation for Ricardo?
2 What is the advantage of using a gel cushion?
3 List three possible reasons why a pressure ulcer was developing before Ricardo's admission to the SNF.
4 Identify two reasons why an elder in Ricardo's situation benefits from scheduled turning.
5 Why would Ricardo's incontinence cause strain on his relationship with his partner Paul?
6 Why is timely pain medication helpful?
7 Identify one reason why improved nutrition is important in Ricardo's situation.

◼ **CHAPTER REVIEW QUESTIONS**

1 List the members of any incontinence team.
2 Describe how OBRA has affected the management of incontinence in the nursing facility.
3 Discuss whether urinary and fecal incontinence are part of the normal aging process.
4 What type of incontinence is more prevalent in women?
5 Describe the effect of incontinence on nursing home placement.
6 Which behavioral technique is commonly used for incontinence training with an elder who has dementia?
7 What are some of the secondary complications associated with incontinence?
8 What is the role of the COTA in the management of incontinence?
9 What are some environmental modifications that can improve continence?
10 Discuss the various ways that incontinence can be addressed by using Table 17-1, areas of occupation in the OTPF.[1] Consider beyond the categories of bowel and bladder management and toilet hygiene to other categories that could be related to incontinence.

REFERENCES

1. American Occupational Therapy Association, 2008. Occupational therapy practice framework: Domain and process, 2nd ed. American Journal of Occupational Therapy 62, 625-683.
2. Doughty, D., 2006. Urinary and Fecal Incontinence, 3rd ed. Mosby, St. Louis, MO.
3. Miller, C., 2009. Nursing for Wellness in Older Adults, 5th ed. Lippincott Williams & Wilkins, Philadelphia.
4. Smeltzer, S., Bare, B., Hinkle, J., Cheever, K., 2009. Brunner and Suddarth's Textbook of Medical-Surgical Nursing, 12th ed. Lippincott Williams & Wilkins, Philadelphia.
5. Palmer, M., 2008. Urinary incontinence quality improvement in nursing homes: Where have we been? Where are we going? Urologic Nursing 28 (6), 439-444, 453.
6. Fink, H., Taylor, B., Tacklind, J., Rutks, I., Wilt, T., 2008. Treatment interventions in nursing home residents with urinary incontinence: A systematic review of randomized trials. Mayo Clinic Proceedings 83 (12), 1332-1343.
7. Hu, T.W., 1990. Impact of urinary incontinence on health-care costs. Journal of the American Geriatric Society 38 (3), 292-295.
8. U.S. Department of Health and Human Services, 1999. Urinary incontinence in adults. U.S. Department of Health and Human Services, Rockville, MD.
9. Newman, D., Wein, A., 2009. Managing and Treating Urinary Incontinence. Health Profession Press, Baltimore, MD.
10. Mosby's Dictionary of Medicine, Nursing, and Health Professions, 7th ed. 2006. Mosby, St. Louis, MO.
11. Hood, F.J., 2002. Coverage of urinary incontinence. Southern Medical Journal 95 (2), 198-201.
12. NovaCare, Inc., 1993. OBRA guidelines for occupational therapy and physical therapy clinicians. (Pamphlet). King of Prussia, PA.
13. Centers for Medicare and Medicaid Services, 2001. Deficiency decision-making and severity scope determination (draft). Centers, Baltimore, MD.
14. Beers, M., Berkow, A. (Eds.), 1997. The Merck Manual of Diagnosis and Therapy, 17th centennial ed. Merck & Co, Whitehouse Station, NJ.
15. Blaivas, J.G., Romanzi, L.J., Heritz, D.M., 1998. Urinary incontinence: Pathophysiology, evaluation, treatment, overview, and nonsurgical management. In: Walsh, P.C., Retik, A.B., Vaughan Jr., E.D., Wein, A.J. (Eds.), Campbell's Urology. WB Saunders, Philadelphia, pp. 1007-1036.
16. Schmitz, T., 2001. Environmental assessment. In: O'Sullivan, S.B. (Ed.), Physical Rehabilitation: Assessment and Treatment, 4th ed. FA Davis, Philadelphia.
17. Health Care Financing Administration, 1995. Omnibus Budget Reconciliation Act. Administration, Baltimore.
18. Uniform Data System for Medical Rehabilitation, 2001. Guide for the uniform data set for medical rehabilitation (Adult FIM). Uniform Data System for Medical Rehabilitation, Buffalo, NY.
19. Allen, C., Earhart, C., Blue, T., 1992. Occupational Therapy Treatment Goals for the Physically and Cognitively Disabled. American Occupational Therapy Association, Rockville, MD.

18

Dysphagia and Other Eating and Nutritional Concerns with Elders

DEBORAH L. MORAWSKI, TERRYN DAVIS, AND RENÉ PADILLA

KEY TERMS

oral intake, undernourishment, malnutrition, dehydration, institutionalized, nutrition, hydration, bolus, velum, compensations, dysphagia, aspiration pneumonia, positioning, alternative means, contraindicated

CHAPTER OBJECTIVES

1. Discuss the increased incidence of swallowing, eating, and nutritional problems occurring with elders.
2. Identify the basic anatomical structures related to swallowing and the swallow sequence.
3. Relate the physiological changes and the onset of increased age-related medical conditions with the increased incidence of swallowing problems.
4. Identify intervention strategies and precautions for improving oral intake and nutrition.
5. Discuss the roles of the team members and the importance of teamwork in addressing swallowing and nutritional concerns.
6. Relate ideas for managing different types of feeding problems.
7. Discuss the psychological and ethical concerns that are present when swallowing problems develop.

Eating is essential for survival, is a basic activity of daily living (ADL), and often a very meaningful area of occupation.[1] As the elder population continues to increase, the incidence of swallowing, eating, and nutritional problems is increasing. Death and illness resulting from impaired oral intake are now considered major health problems of elders.[2]

Most elders have at least one chronic medical condition, and many have multiple conditions. These conditions include arthritis, hypertension, heart disease, hearing impairments, orthopedic impairments, sinusitis, diabetes, and vision impairments. These chronic conditions can influence elders' abilities to effectively and independently perform ADL, such as eating, self-care, transfers, going outside, and instrumental activities of daily living (IADL), such as meal preparation, shopping, money management, and housework. The need for individuals to receive help increases with age.[3] When such help is unavailable, this lack of assistance can lead elders to social isolation and depression, which may lead to decreased oral intake. In addition, many elders often take multiple medications, which may affect oral intake.[4] This decrease in oral intake can result in undernourishment, malnutrition, and dehydration.

Among institutionalized elders, the prevalence of undernourishment and malnutrition may be as high as 80%. This high prevalence may be explained by the increased numbers of elders who need assistance with feeding and the lack of sufficient staff to assist them. In nursing homes, government statistics show that 23% of residents are reported to need total feeding assistance and 45% require some feeding assistance. In these settings, it has been reported that a nursing assistant may feed from 5 to 20 individuals an hour, with research showing that it may take up to 40 minutes for a nursing home resident to complete a meal.[5]

These statistics clearly reflect the growing need for occupational therapy (OT) involvement with elders to help them maintain optimal independence in a home, hospital, or nursing home setting. OT assistance may include training in self-feeding, safe swallowing, positioning, mobility, meal preparation and cleanup, shopping, money management, provision of assistive equipment, and caregiver and nursing instruction. All of these activities are essential for elders to adequately maintain nutrition and hydration.

THE ROLE OF THE CERTIFIED OCCUPATIONAL THERAPY ASSISTANT

The certified occupational therapy assistant (COTA) works in partnership with a registered occupational therapist (OTR) to collect data to identify the strengths and weaknesses of elders and establish and implement intervention plans to attain their goals. Ongoing assessment and communication between the COTA and the OTR are necessary for program and goal changes. The COTA is involved in individual and group intervention and in staff and caregiver instruction. Providing quality care is the function of the entire health care team. The amount of involvement of the COTA with elders with swallowing problems depends on the COTA's level of experience. An entry-level COTA may work on activities that reinforce good nutrition and hydration such as meal preparation, money management, shopping, oral-facial exercises, instruction in assistive devices, and energy conservation during activities. An experienced COTA who has demonstrated competence in this area may participate in videofluoroscopic swallow studies and assist tracheostomized and ventilator-dependent elders with self-feeding and swallowing. It is recommended that the COTA review the article "Specialized Knowledge and Skills in Feeding, Eating, and Swallowing for Occupational Therapy Practice," developed by the American Occupational Therapy Association.[6]

NORMAL SWALLOW

The swallow response requires a rapid interplay between the brain, 6 cranial nerves, 48 pairs of muscles, the salivary glands, and cartilaginous structures (Figure 18-1). The COTA working with elders who have dysphagia must clearly understand the anatomy and physiology of swallowing.[7]

Four phases of swallowing have been defined: oral preparatory, oral, pharyngeal, and esophageal (Figure 18-2, A to E).[8]

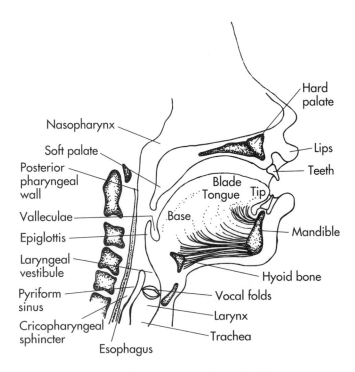

FIGURE 18-1   Oral structures and mechanisms at rest.

1. Oral preparatory phase: The oral preparatory phase includes seeing, smelling, reaching for the item, bringing it to the mouth, and putting it in the mouth. Once the item is placed in the mouth, the lips close to maintain a seal, and the tongue and cheek muscles move the bolus (that is, the food or liquid) around the mouth in preparation for swallowing. The base of the tongue and the velum (soft palate) also make a seal to prevent the bolus from entering the pharynx prematurely. Saliva mixes with the bolus to aid in swallowing. Taste, temperature, and texture receptors of the tongue also play a part in preparing for the action of swallowing.

2. Oral phase: The oral phase occurs once the bolus is prepared and formed by the tongue. The bolus is then propelled by the tongue to the back of the mouth and over the base of the tongue.

3. Pharyngeal phase: The pharyngeal phase occurs when the bolus passes over the base of the tongue and enters the pharynx. At this time, the soft palate elevates to seal the entrance to the nose, the hyoid bone and larynx elevate upward and anteriorly, the vocal folds close, the epiglottis tilts downward, and the cricopharyngeal sphincter opens to allow the bolus to enter the esophagus.

4. Esophageal phase: The esophageal phase occurs when the bolus passes into the esophagus and is propelled to the stomach.

Changes of Swallowing Structures

When individuals eat and swallow, the oral and pharyngeal structures adapt easily to different liquid and food consistencies and to the texture, temperature, and volume of the bolus. These structures also adapt to the different positions that the head and body may assume while swallowing. As individuals age, changes in these swallowing structures occur naturally.[2] Individuals develop compensations to these changes spontaneously and often unknowingly. These compensations allow them to eat safely and efficiently, such as with smaller bites, longer chewing time, and softer food.[8] However, if individuals also develop a medical or neurological disorder, these compensations may no longer be effective and may result in increased swallowing problems (Table 18-1).[9,10] In addition to understanding the physical changes that occur, COTAs must be aware of the psychological effect of swallowing problems on individuals who can no longer eat as they once did. COTAs should acknowledge elders' and caregivers' feelings about certain types of liquids or favorite foods being eliminated from their daily diet.

ETIOLOGY OF DYSPHAGIA

Dysphagia is the inability to swallow. This condition is often seen in elders and may have a variety of causes. These causes may be neurological (for example, from a cerebrovascular accident, brain tumor, or head injury),

252

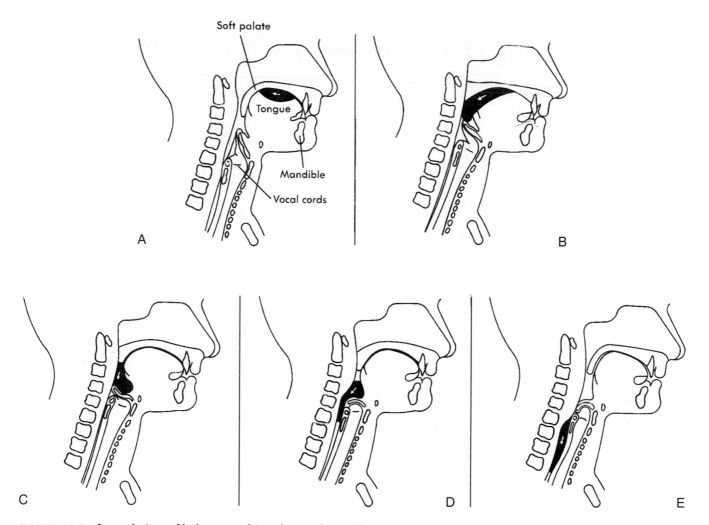

FIGURE 18-2 Lateral view of bolus propulsion during the swallow. A, Oral preparation of the bolus and voluntary initiation of the swallow by the oral tongue. B, Bolus moves from oral cavity to pharynx, pharyngeal swallow is triggered. C, Bolus enters the valleculae and the airway is protected. D, The tongue base retracts to the anteriorly moving pharyngeal wall. E, Bolus enters the cervical esophagus and cricopharyngeal area. *(From Logeman, G. [1998]. Evaluation and Treatment of Swallowing Disorders, 2nd ed. Austin, TX: Pro-Ed.)*

neuromuscular (for example, from Parkinson's disease, multiple sclerosis, or amyotrophic lateral sclerosis), dementia (such as with Alzheimer's disease), multi-infarct structural (for example, from cancer), and systemic (for example, from diabetes, rheumatoid arthritis, and scleroderma). Dysphagia may also result from prolonged illnesses or from the side effects of medications. If swallowing problems are not identified, they can result in aspiration pneumonia, malnutrition, dehydration, and death.[8,11]

INTERVENTION STRATEGIES

Elders achieve a sense of empowerment, control, and motivation when they are successful at self-feeding and swallowing. To achieve this success, COTAs should implement individually planned interventions to resolve swallowing problems and promote functional self-feeding. The COTA must first establish a therapeutic relationship with the elder. This will enhance the interventions affecting empowerment and quality of life during mealtime. Intervention of swallowing disorders entails focusing attention on every aspect of the mealtime experience, including preparation, the dining environment, positioning of the elder, assistive devices, direct intervention, dietary concerns, precautions, and caregiver training (Box 18-1).

Environmental Concerns

In American society, people usually eat three meals each day, or about 1,092 meals each year, excluding snacks. Eating is a vital part of social participation[1] and greatly adds to the quality of an individual's life. To promote an enjoyable dining experience, pleasant surroundings and personal comfort should be provided to elders during meals. Aesthetics of the dining area should include

TABLE 18-1

	Age-Related Swallowing Changes	
Swallowing phase	**Healthy elder**	**Frail elder**
Oral preparatory	Vision may be declining. Sense of smell and taste decrease and may result in decreased intake. Elder may be missing teeth and need to wear full or partial dentures and require more time to chew food.	Cognitive impairment (poor memory and decreased attention may exaggerate the influence of normal aging changes). Isolation and depression result in decreased food intake and weight loss. Decreased endurance may interfere with chewing and result in slow eating and low intake. Missing teeth and poor-fitting dentures may result in slow eating and poor intake.
Oral	Tongue and lip muscles atrophy, and elder may take smaller bites and require softer food. Elder may require longer time to form bolus in mouth.	Decreased strength in lips and tongue and jaw muscles may result in drooling, decreased chewing, and problems moving the bolus in the mouth.
Pharyngeal	Phase becomes mildly prolonged. Muscle tone decreases and may delay clearing of food residuals. Bolus moves more slowly through the pharynx. Upward movement of hyoid and larynx becomes delayed. Epiglottis may become smaller and move more slowly. Cricopharyngeal sphincter remains open for shorter time.	Time of passage of bolus increases. Structures move more slowly and may put elder at greater risk for aspiration.
Esophageal	Decreased strength of muscles results in increased time for passage of bolus to stomach.	Increased time needed for bolus to reach stomach. Food contents may reflux from stomach and reenter esophagus and pharynx.

Adapted from Cherney, L. (2004). *Clinical Management of Dysphagia for Adults and Children*, 2nd ed. Rockville, MD: Aspen.

tablecloths, centerpieces, flowers, and cleanliness. If elders are institutionalized, food items should be taken off serving trays and put directly on the table to help establish a homelike atmosphere. Deficits in visual acuity, light sensitivity, and color perception are common in elders. Poor lighting can greatly exaggerate these problems; therefore, insufficient light and glare should be avoided. Natural light without glare or soft, diffused overhead lighting is best. A quiet, calm environment excludes television but may allow for age-appropriate dining music. Television may be distracting and detract from social interaction. Compatible table mates in small groups around a table can add to a positive dining experience (Figure 18-3). COTAs and other service providers should maintain a therapeutic attitude by allowing elders plenty of time to eat a meal. Lengthy waiting periods before being served may decrease the elder's interest in food and may increase fatigue. The table height should be between 28 and 30 inches to accommodate both regular chairs and wheelchairs. The distance between the table surface and an elder's mouth should be between 10 and 15 inches.[12] Adopting these suggested environmental factors can help provide a pleasurable experience during mealtime and possibly assist elders to increase their food and fluid intake.

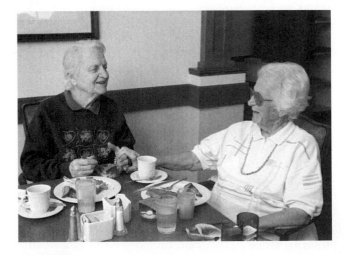

FIGURE 18-3 Compatible table mates can make dining a pleasurable experience.

Positioning Techniques

COTAs must have knowledge of proper positioning techniques with elders who have dysphagia. Proper positioning is important for effective and safe swallowing, correcting mechanical problems with swallowing, and

BOX 18-1

Preparation Checklist for Dysphagia and Self-Feeding Interventions

1. Collect information.
   - Evaluate dysphagia.
   - Review medical chart.
   - Consult nursing staff.
   - Assess changes in medical status.
   - Assess changes in diet.
2. Inform elder.
   - Give evaluation results.
   - Recommend intervention.
   - Discuss intervention goals with client.
   - Provide input.
3. Create environment.
   - Ensure that environment is positive and appropriate.
   - Ensure that environment is conducive to eating.
4. Ensure proper fit.
   - Eyeglasses
   - Hearing aides
   - Partial and full dentures
5. Assess.
   - Arousal and alertness
   - Safety for eating
6. Position safely.
   - Trunk
   - Lower extremities
   - Upper extremities
   - Head
   - Height of table surface
7. Complete oral preparation as prescribed by the OTR.
   - Have client perform oral exercises.
   - Have client perform sensory stimulation.
   - Have client perform tone facilitation or reduction techniques.
8. Check food tray.
   - Correct diet consistency.
   - Provide needed assistive equipment.

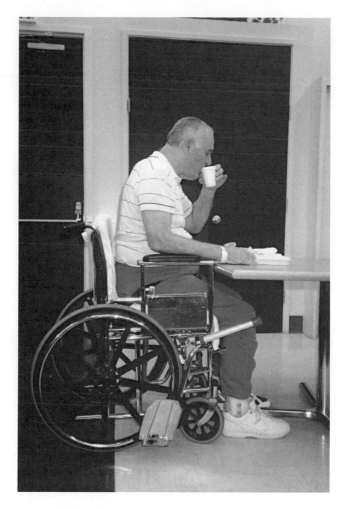

FIGURE 18-4   This gentleman is correctly positioned in his wheelchair for self-feeding. This position promotes dynamic trunk movement. *(From Community Hospital of Los Gatos, CA, 1996.)*

increasing dining pleasure. The trachea, or airway, is next to the esophagus, which is the food pipe. Safe positioning can prevent food from entering the trachea, avoiding aspiration. Proper positioning of elders also increases alertness, normalizes muscle tone, provides comfort, and helps with digestion, while allowing dynamic movement for self-feeding.

The preferred seating position for mealtime is sitting in a dining room chair with armrests rather than sitting in a wheelchair. A wheelchair, however, is preferable to a geriatric chair, which is preferable to sitting up in bed. COTAs should transfer an elder to a regular chair if the elder can possibly sit in one. If optimal posture cannot be obtained in a regular chair, use of a wheelchair may be necessary (Figure 18-4). The elder's head, neck, trunk,

and hips should be aligned. First, the pelvis should be positioned in neutral with a slight anterior tilt. The elder should have an erect posture and sit symmetrically with weight distributed equally on each hip. Second, the elder's head should be positioned in midline with the chin slightly tucked. Both upper extremities should be fully supported on a table or lap tray of appropriate height. Finally, the lower extremities should be in a weight-bearing position. Hips and knees should be flexed 80 to 90 degrees, with ankles in neutral position under the knees and the feet flat on the floor. If the feet do not reach the floor, a stool or wheelchair footrest should be used to provide a secure base of support.

If feeding in bed is essential, elders should be as close to the headboard as possible before the head of the bed is elevated to 45 degrees or more (Figure 18-5). A pillow may be placed behind the elder's back to increase upright trunk posture and hip flexion. To prevent elders from sliding down in the bed, the knees should be flexed and supported from underneath with pillows if necessary.[12]

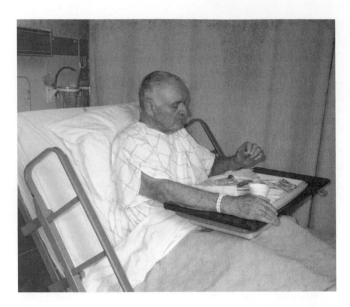

FIGURE 18-5 This gentleman is correctly positioned in bed for self-feeding. *(From Community Hospital of Los Gatos, CA, 1996.)*

As with sitting in a chair, elders should be upright and aligned symmetrically for optimal safety while eating and drinking.

Positioning devices are often required to aid elders in maintaining a straight midline for a dynamic, upright posture. Padded solid back and solid seat inserts provide better postural support that offsets the slinging seats and backs of wheelchairs. Lumbar and thoracic support can facilitate increased scapulohumeral control for self-feeding. Elders with low muscular tone may benefit from high-back wheelchairs. Wedges, lateral and forward trunk supports, headrests, pelvic belts, pillows, and towel rolls are often used to obtain proper positioning. Seating systems must be designed to correct or to accommodate postural problems while preventing skin erosion, maintaining comfort, promoting self-feeding, and providing the right position for safe swallowing.

Many variables affect elders' positioning. If an elder is sitting in a kyphotic posture, the COTA should have the elder lean back slightly so the chin is parallel to the floor. Special considerations are also needed for elders with scoliosis, depending on the curvature of the spine. Elders with a hemiplegic arm should have the arm placed on the table. The arm/hand should be incorporated as a gross stabilizer during meals. Those elders who have recently had a lower extremity amputation may also have special positioning needs. COTAs also must consider poor sitting tolerance. Elders with back pain or low endurance need to complete their meal within the time limitations of their upright tolerance. The lower extremities may need to be elevated when sitting up in a chair if edema is present, which often occurs as a result of congestive heart failure. Hearing and visual deficits should also be considered when positioning elders to increase their awareness of their surroundings and to maximize social interaction. The COTA is responsible for following through with the OTR's instructions for positioning while considering the elder's individual needs.

Assistive Devices

An abundance of options for assistive devices is available to assist elders in maintaining independence in self-feeding and safe swallowing. Some devices are prefabricated, whereas others are designed by the creative minds of the COTAs. A hole punched in the plastic lid of a cup can hold a straw and will prevent spilling for elders who have tremors or ataxia. Built-up handles can be used for joint protection or a weak grasp. A universal cuff is available for elders who have no grasp. A swivel spoon or a long-handled spoon is available to assist elders with limited range of motion. Nonslip mats or plates with suction cups can keep items from sliding on the table. Plate guards and plates with lips prevent food from spilling off of the plate. Cutout cups and straws can reduce the need for the elder to tilt the head back while drinking, thus protecting against aspiration while swallowing. Straws and cups with spouted lids can also limit the amount of each sip and are helpful for elders with severe dementia who have a sucking reflex only. Small rubber-coated spoons can help control bite size and prevent elders from hurting themselves when biting down on utensils. Rocker knives can be used for one-handed cutting. Mobile arm supports can provide stabilization and assist in hand-to-mouth movement.

Assistive devices should be issued if elders experience a decrease in function. However, elders should be encouraged toward further independence rather than to continue using assistive devices. Before assistive equipment is issued, the COTA should consult with the OTR regarding his or her recommendations.

Direct Intervention

Various feeding strategies may be used to help elders with dysphagia to feed themselves and to swallow safely. To ensure that mealtime is a pleasurable experience, the COTA should avoid making parental comments or giving parental cues (for example, use the word *napkin* rather than *bib*). A method of communication must be established with nonverbal elders so they can indicate when they are ready for another bite or drink. All team members, including family and other caregivers, should use this method consistently. Examples may be a nodding of the head or raising a finger. In addition, the COTA should sit next to the elders rather than standing over them during meals.

As noted in the preparation checklist in Box 18-1, oral exercises, sensory stimulation, and tone facilitation or reduction techniques are often needed before eating. Slow, deep pressure on facial and jaw muscles in the opposite direction to the pull of increased muscle tone may help reduce it.[13] Tongue and facial exercises can increase strength and tone for bolus manipulation. Sensory stimulation may include brushing teeth and icing the cheeks and tongue to increase oral tone and sensation. Brushing teeth also stimulates the salivary glands and helps elders with dry mouths manipulate the bolus easier. After using these necessary strategies, elders are ready to begin eating.

These and many other general strategies help elders with eating and should be enacted before food enters the mouth. Hand-over-hand guiding can provide tactile cueing while bringing food to the mouth and is especially helpful for elders with perceptual difficulties. Proximal upper extremity stabilization techniques can compensate for tremors, ataxia, and weakness. To help with weakness, elders may also use the opposite hand to assist in the movement of the dominant hand when bringing food to the mouth. The "clock method" is helpful for blind elders or for those with other visual deficits to orient them to the position of the plate, cup, eating utensils, and food in front of them. Items should be positioned consistently for this method to be most effective. Elders who are impulsive may require cues for both bite size and pacing of bites. Elders can be guided or instructed to put the eating utensil down between bites to pace the amount of food entering the mouth. Presenting elders with one food item at a time may also be helpful. Large food items should be cut into bite-sized portions. Using a spoon for liquids is often helpful. COTAs should coordinate eating with breathing for elders on ventilators or for those with other breathing difficulties. Energy conservation may also be indicated, including limiting conversation during mealtime. For elders with low endurance, alternating food textures during the meal, ordering foods that are easy to chew, and/or having six small meals available during the day may be helpful.

Several strategies may be helpful to use with elders who have severe dementia. Frequent small feedings and finger foods are useful for elders with low attention spans or who pace constantly and cannot sit still long enough to complete a meal. Decreasing environmental stimulation, maintaining consistency in feeding helpers, and reducing verbal communication during the meal may help decrease distractions and permit elders with dementia to focus longer on eating. When such elders refuse a particular food item, a helpful strategy is to place that food item on a plate of a different color, reheat it, and serve it again. With this particular elder population, COTAs should be careful that elders do not eat nonedible items placed on the table such as plants and napkins. Removing the knife from the place setting of such elders may also be necessary for safety.[14]

Several interventions may be used during the oral phase. Tongue sweeps prevent oral pocketing of food. Alternating solids and liquids helps clean the mouth and remove any food residue in the mouth, but may be contraindicated when dysphagia is present. Food should be placed in the center of the tongue. Varying food temperatures with each bite may promote a safer swallow by stimulating the mouth and increasing awareness of the bolus. Occasionally, elders with hypertonicity need food to remain at a consistent temperature to avoid increasing muscle tone. Asking elders to increase the number of times they chew a bite of food helps break down the bolus and reduce the pace of eating. Elders may need to be cued to close the lips to prevent spillage. The oral cavity should be checked for any residue after each meal. Dentures must fit well and should be thoroughly cleaned after each meal to prevent ulcers from developing in the mouth, to prevent chipping of the dentures from hardened food, and prevent risk for aspiration from food residue under the dentures.[15]

Problems during the pharyngeal phase of swallowing may require many intervention strategies. Elders should be given sufficient time to swallow between bites. COTAs should learn to observe and palpate swallowing and be able to recognize delays in the swallow response. These skills help in the ongoing assessment of elders. Individuals with hemiplegia may benefit from turning the head toward the hemiplegic side or tilting the head toward the non-hemiplegic side to protect the airway while swallowing.[16] Elders should be checked for voice clarity after a swallow to make sure that there is no food or liquid residual on the vocal folds.[17] Coughing or clearing the throat followed by a dry swallow may help eliminate a wet-sounding voice after a swallow. Multiple swallows after each bite may also be encouraged. The COTA should work closely with the OTR when feeding elders with tracheostomies. If approved by the physician, the tracheostomy may or may not be plugged, and the cuff can be deflated during feeding to increase air pressure for a stronger swallow.

Several advanced techniques, including the supraglottic swallow, Valsalva maneuver, and Mendelsohn maneuver, may be required, for which close instruction and supervision from the OTR is essential.[8] Advanced training is necessary for the implementation of these strategies, and the COTA should demonstrate competency in their application because they are not entry-level skills. Because of the wide range of individual dysphagia problems, the strategies presented here can be modified as necessary. When interventions are planned and carried out with the elder's quality of life in mind, as well as his or her safety while swallowing, the elder's motivation for food intake and sense of empowerment will prevail.

Dietary Concerns

Research into the nutritional needs of elders has increased as the elderly population grows.[17-19] COTAs should understand elders' nutritional requirements. Elders often prefer to eat softer, sweeter, and easy-to-prepare foods, and also often drink less fluids. These habits may result in the elder becoming undernourished or malnourished. If elders become ill and are institutionalized, undernourishment or malnutrition can lead to other health problems and delay recovery.

Physiological changes occur slowly over time in all body systems as people age. These changes are influenced by past nutritional habits, life events, illnesses, genetic traits, and socioeconomic factors.[20] Sensory changes may include a decline in sight and peripheral vision, hearing, smell, and taste.[21] Although the losses are neither total nor rapid, they can affect nutritional intake and health status. For example, loss of visual acuity may lead to less activity or a fear of cooking, especially using a stove. Inability to read food prices, nutrition labels, or recipes may affect grocery shopping, food preparation, and eating. Loss of hearing may lead to less eating out or not asking questions of the waiter or store clerk. Finally, changes in smell and taste are more obvious. If food does not taste appetizing or smell appealing, elders may not want to eat it. If they must cut back on salt, sugar, or fat, they may tend not to eat.[22]

Many structural changes may also take place as people age, particularly loss of lean body mass. Muscle loss may include skeletal and smooth muscle mass that can affect the function of organs, particularly the heart. This may result in reduced cardiac capacity. Because about 72% of total body water is in lean muscle tissue, loss of total body mass also means loss of hydration.[23] Other organs often affected include the kidneys, lungs, and liver, which may result in the body's lowered ability to generate new protein tissue or in slowing the immune system's ability to produce antibodies.[24] The most significant result of the loss of lean body mass may be the decrease in basal energy metabolism because of the decline in total protein tissue. As protein tissue declines, calories are more likely to become body fat if a person's level of activity also decreases.[25] Finally, women tend to lose bone mass at an accelerated rate after menopause. Severe osteoporosis is debilitating and serious because of the risk of falls and fractures. Vertebral compression as a result of loss of hydration and/or fractures can change chest configuration which, in turn, can affect breathing, intestinal distension, and internal organ displacement.[26]

Nutrition can be a factor in all of the changes noted above. However, the slowing of the normal action of the digestive tract plus general physiological changes have the most direct effect on nutrition. Digestive secretions diminish markedly, although enzymes remain adequate. Adequate dietary fiber will maintain regular bowel function and not interfere with the digestion and absorption of nutrients, as may occur with laxative use or abuse.[26] The challenge for the elderly is to meet the same nutrient needs as when they were younger, yet consume fewer calories. Choosing nutrient dense foods (high in nutrients in relation to their calories), reducing overall fat content of the diet, emphasizing complex carbohydrates, enhancing

dietary fiber intake, assuring adequate liquid intake, and consuming a variety of food remain a priority for elders.[22] It may be important for the elder to be referred to a dietitian to obtain information about optimal nutrition and hydration that does not interfere with medications.

Diet modifications are frequently needed for elders with dysphagia. These modifications may include different consistencies of liquids (for example, thin-like water, semi-thick-like nectar, and thick-like honey) and different methods of preparing solid foods (for example, pureed, minced, chopped, and soft).[8] If oral intake is limited or impossible, elders with dysphagia may receive nutrition and hydration through alternative means (such as a nasogastric tube, a gastrostomy, a jejunostomy, or parenteral nutrition). The entire treatment team is responsible for monitoring intake and ensuring that elders consume the appropriate amounts of protein, fiber, vitamins, minerals, and fluids.[2,12] Misinterpretations regarding intake may occur when intake is being monitored if food sources are not also recorded together with calories consumed.

Food preferences, food allergies, and any diet restrictions resulting from medical conditions such as diabetes and congestive heart failure should be considered when food and liquid selections are being made with elders and their families. Cultural issues regarding food must also be considered when planning for an elder's care. Increased discussion has occurred regarding the ethical and legal issues associated with permitting elders to consume unsafe liquid or solid food consistencies or imposing alternative means for feeding. Ultimately, the physician is responsible for finalizing a decision regarding this issue with elders and their families. This issue, however, requires much input from the team regarding the benefits, risks, alternatives, and prognoses. If the decision is made to allow elders to consume unsafe food items, discontinuation of OT intervention is recommended.[27,28]

Precautions

When working with elders with feeding and swallowing problems, COTAs should consider many factors concerning the safety of oral intake. Some of these factors include level of alertness, orientation and cognitive status, positioning, general endurance, and the ability to self-feed. The presence of a delayed swallow, food pocketing, effortful chewing, coughing, choking, a runny nose, and a wet-sounding voice indicates swallowing difficulties with the food or liquid being consumed. The COTA should either discontinue the troublesome food or liquid or modify it to a safer consistency. The OTR should be informed of this as soon as possible so that the elder can be further evaluated.

Other indicators of swallowing and nutritional problems may include an increased temperature, lung congestion, and poor intake. Increased temperature and lung congestion may be a sign that the elder has aspirated food or liquid and that pneumonia is developing. Poor intake may indicate an inability to swallow rather than a poor appetite. All personnel working with elders with possible swallowing problems must be aware of these indications and be trained in how to assist someone who is choking and in cardiopulmonary resuscitation in the event that an elder chokes.

Many elders receive medications for various conditions. Medications must be taken with the correct liquid or semisolid consistency. More than 1 oz (30 ml) liquid should be taken after each pill to ensure adequate transport to the stomach. Elders should be sitting up and should be prevented from reclining for 20 minutes after a meal or after taking medication to ensure the safe passage of the food or pill to the stomach. Pills should be taken as specified by the physician. COTAs should consult with the physician or pharmacist to check whether the pills can be halved or crushed because some pills work through time release and crushing them may result in too much medication being absorbed at once. Nursing staff should be present while the medications are taken to ensure that swallowing has actually occurred.

Many elders are at greater risk for aspiration when using straws and taking serial swallows with liquids. The OTR should alert the COTA if an elder is safe to drink fluids in these ways. Many elders who are impulsive require close supervision to prevent overfilling the mouth or eating too fast, activities that may result in choking. The COTA should gain extensive knowledge and experience with the swallowing process before attempting to work with elders who have tracheostomies or are on ventilators. Again, service competency in this should be established with the OTR before the COTA implements any intervention.

Nursing/Caregiver Instruction

COTAs have a vital role in training caregivers to assist elders with self-feeding and dysphagia management. Caregivers may include spouses, partners, family members, friends, hired attendants, and other health care workers such as nurses and nurse's aides. COTAs must consider the caregiver's culture and lifestyle when making decisions about the most beneficial type of teaching technique to use. Some individuals learn best through observing the COTA. Others may learn best by doing it themselves under the direction of the COTA, and others may perform best with verbal instruction. Written information and instructions should be provided to elders and caregivers whenever possible. In general, all of these techniques should be used with each caregiver to assure the best follow-through. COTAs must be aware of their verbal tone when teaching the caregiver, taking care not to sound condescending.

The education of caregivers must include training in many aspects of self-feeding and swallowing. First, caregivers should understand the feeding strengths and weaknesses of elders. The need for quality time during the meal and for presentation of a positive attitude to promote elder motivation and independence should be stressed. Thorough instruction should be given on proper body mechanics required by caregivers when assisting elders with feeding. Additional instruction should be provided regarding safe positioning, environmental concerns, use and care of assistive equipment, specific intervention techniques, appropriate verbal and nonverbal cueing, dietary modifications, and signs of possible food or liquid aspiration. Caregivers may take some time to develop good observation and problem-solving skills. Caregivers must understand the importance of communicating any problems or changes in an elder's status to the appropriate team member. Caregivers should also be familiar with choking prevention maneuvers and emergency suctioning procedures. Problem solving together with caregivers is useful when dealing with elders who have difficult feeding behaviors. COTAs may share with caregivers their anecdotal successful experiences in cueing and obtaining desirable behaviors and eliminating undesirable ones with a particular elder.

An integral part of caregiver training is monitoring the food and fluid intake of elders, together with considering nutritional value and maintaining a modified diet. Family and friends may occasionally present a problem by not complying with the dietary restrictions of their loved one. The possible negative consequences of not following through with the prescribed feeding program should be stressed. COTAs should work with dietitians and caregivers in helping families plan meals. COTAs may also ask the caregivers of institutionalized elders to bring a meal from home and modify it with the assistance of a COTA.

Instructing caregivers on the swallowing and self-feeding protocols set up for elders helps COTAs promote continuity and quality of care. Caregivers should be integrated as soon as possible in the intervention and care of elders. Training several family members and nursing staff helps spread the responsibility of assisting elders during the meal. As with any intervention given to elders, all training of caregivers should be thoroughly documented. By fulfilling these principles, the COTA abides by the Code of Ethics developed by the AOTA.[29]

Ideas for Managing a Feeding Program

Residents of skilled nursing facilities who are fed in their rooms are frequently positioned poorly, spend most of their day in bed, are often rushed, and often cannot finish their meals. Consequently, their intake, nutrition, and body weight decrease.[18,19] A well organized facility-wide feeding program helps get elders out of bed, changes their environment, provides social stimulation, ensures good nutrition and hydration, and increases safety. This type of program also helps maximize their functional abilities and enhances the quality of the mealtime for institutionalized elders. Although many feeding program formats designed for a variety of settings are available, the following is a generic program that requires adjustments to fit the needs of particular elders and particular facilities.

An interdisciplinary approach is the most beneficial in a feeding program. Usually the elder, the OTR, COTA, speech and language pathologist, dietitian, kitchen staff, physician, nursing staff, and family are involved. The physical therapist may also be included to assist with positioning, and the respiratory therapist may be included to assist with issues of pulmonary hygiene or coordination of tracheostomy or ventilator equipment. Elders with self-feeding and dysphagia difficulties are evaluated and referred to a dining group by the OTR or the speech and language pathologist, or both. These elders then are placed in one of several groups organized by the amount of assistance they require. The ratio of elders to COTAs varies depending on the needs of the group. COTAs should always have a group size that can be safely managed. A written protocol should exist that includes information on the purpose of the program and the format, staffing, size, and site of the group. There also should be criteria for referral to, continuation in, and discharge from the program. Timelines, goals, and responsibilities of the COTA or other leader should be made explicit, and documentation and equipment protocols should be explained. There should also be an established system to maintain communication with the entire team to ensure a successful program.

The feeding program should address all meals. In some settings, COTAs are unable to be present at each meal. In other settings, a COTA may not be needed to assist higher-level groups that require minimal assistance or supervision. In these situations, nursing aides, restorative aides, family members, and volunteers may be best used. However, before volunteers are used in this capacity, the guidelines from regulatory agencies should be consulted. For all individuals to perform effectively and safely, they must receive formal training on leading groups, on therapeutic interventions, and on safety.

CASE STUDY

Eric is a 68-year-old, right-hand dominant man who experienced a left cerebrovascular accident and now has right hemiplegia. He has impaired movement and sensation on the right side. In addition, he has apraxia, aphasia, right hemianopsia, and right neglect. One week after his stroke, Eric was transferred to a skilled nursing facility's rehabilitation unit.

A dysphagia evaluation and videofluoroscopy were done and the following observations were noted: decreased muscle tone with impaired movement and sensation of the face, tongue, and soft palate on the right side, resulting in facial droop, poor lip seal, minimal drooling and food spillage, slurred speech, and a nasal quality to his speech. The videofluoroscopy revealed impaired oral control of the bolus and spillage of food and liquid into the pharynx before the swallow was initiated. Initiation of the swallow was delayed up to 5 seconds. Residual pooling was observed in the valleculae and pyriform sinuses after the swallow. Spontaneous clearing of the throat with additional swallows was impaired. Eric required verbal cueing to initiate clearing swallows. Aspiration into the trachea was observed while Eric swallowed thin and semi-thick liquids by spoon and thick liquids by cup and a mixed consistency bolus (liquid and solid combination, such as soup). Eric did cough spontaneously when aspiration occurred. He had difficulty chewing dry, hard solids and did better with moist, soft solids and semisolids, although oral pocketing and spillage from the mouth was observed with these consistencies. When Eric used the compensation method of turning his head to the right, decreased pooling in the right valleculae and pyriform sinus resulted.

Therapeutic recommendations included one-on-one assistance at meals for self-feeding and a modified diet of thick liquids by spoon. Semisolids and minced, soft solids with no mixed consistencies also were recommended. Further suggestions were to provide verbal and tactile cues for Eric to turn his head to the right side during the initial swallow and to follow up the initial swallow with two dry swallows. In addition, Eric's caloric and fluid intake were to be closely monitored.

Before the meal, the COTA reviewed the chart for any recent orders and nursing and therapy progress notes to understand how the elder's day had gone thus far. The COTA arranged to meet Eric's family in the dining room for them to observe this meal. When Eric arrived in the dining room, the COTA observed that he was not sitting erect in his wheelchair and that he needed to be repositioned. When Eric was sitting erect, the COTA brought him to the table, locked the wheelchair, positioned Eric's feet on the floor, and placed his hemiplegic arm forward on the table.

Before the meal the COTA directed Eric through several oral-facial exercises. Icing also was used to increase tone and sensation in his right cheek and throat. The COTA iced the outside of Eric's mouth with ice wrapped in a washcloth and then iced the inside of his cheeks and tongue with a cold metal spoon that was dipped in a cup of ice. Icing also would be done on the cheek, the anterior part of the neck, and inside his mouth on the right side during the meal.

When the tray with Eric's meal arrived, the COTA checked to ensure that the consistencies of both solids and liquids were correct. The liquid on the tray was semi-thick, therefore the COTA thickened it with a thickening agent. No other modifications were needed. A plate guard was put on the plate to prevent food from spilling.

Because Eric requires assistance with tray setup and self-feeding, the COTA guided Eric's left hand (non-hemiplegic) using the hand-over-hand method to remove the container lids, butter the bread, cut the food with the rocker knife, and bring the food to his mouth. When Eric was able to integrate the movement and its rhythm and was able to feed himself independently, the COTA stopped providing hand-over-hand guiding. However, when Eric moved too quickly and took too large a bite, the COTA resumed the guiding. When Eric drooled, the COTA guided him to wipe his face with a napkin. With each bite the COTA directed Eric to double swallow and felt Eric's throat for the swallow. The COTA asked Eric to speak occasionally to check his vocal quality, and when it was wet-sounding, the COTA asked Eric to clear his throat. Whenever Eric was unable to clear his throat, the COTA asked him to dry swallow. Finally, the COTA periodically checked Eric's mouth for food pocketing and directed him to clear residuals in his right cheek by using his tongue or left index finger.

After the meal, the COTA guided Eric to use a toothette to clean his oral cavity of the food residue. The COTA instructed

Eric to remain upright for at least 20 more minutes. A nurse then arrived with medications, which were crushed and mixed with the thick liquid and given to Eric with a spoon. After he swallowed the medication, Eric was given additional thick liquid by spoon to ensure that the medication passed to the stomach.

The COTA then asked the family if they had any questions and provided them with additional instructions. Finally, the COTA documented what and how much Eric ate; the level of assistance that was required; how long it took to complete the meal; the presence of any coughing, wet-sounding voice, or choking; and the food consistency given to him when these events occurred. In addition, the COTA documented all instructions given to the family.

As Eric progressed during meals, he needed less and less hand-over-hand guiding and verbal instruction from the COTA. The COTA began supervising family members as they assisted Eric with meals. Eric progressed to a group dining situation, and when Eric seemed to have a little problem with a wet-sounding voice, food pocketing, follow-through with compensatory techniques, duration of the meal, caloric intake, and spiking temperatures, the COTA requested that the OTR reevaluate him. A follow-up videofluoroscopy was done to rule out aspiration of thin liquids and mixed consistencies, and it showed that Eric had improved but still had impaired oral control of the bolus and pooling in the pharynx. However, Eric now clears this pooling spontaneously, no aspiration is noted, and these items were added to his diet.

Because Eric can now set up his tray with minimal assistance, cut the food with a rocker knife, bring the food to his mouth, eat slowly, and check for pocketing independently, he no longer requires OT supervision at meals.

CHAPTER REVIEW QUESTIONS

1 What is the definition of dysphagia?
2 What are the four phases of swallowing?
3 What are the three liquid consistencies?
4 Name four signs that may indicate the presence of swallowing problems.
5 Name three common changes that occur during the phases of swallowing as an individual ages.
6 Identify at least two psychological issues that may have an effect on oral intake.
7 Explain why the COTA should be concerned about nutritional balance and amount of oral intake.
8 Why is the dining environment important for nutritional intake?
9 What should the COTA do if an elder coughs continuously during a meal?
10 Describe how an individual's body should ideally be positioned during a meal.

REFERENCES

1. American Occupational Therapy Association, 2008. Occupational therapy practice framework: Domain and process, 2nd ed. American Journal of Occupational Therapy 62 (6), 625-683.
2. Ney, D., Weiss, J., Kind, A., Robbins, J., 2009. Senescent swallowing: Impact, strategies, and interventions. Nutrition in Clinical Practice 24 (3), 395-413.
3. Administration on Aging, 2008. A Profile of Older Americans: 2008. U.S. Department of Health and Human Services, Washington, DC.
4. Hays, N., Roberts, S., 2006. The anorexia of aging in humans. Physiology & Behavior 88 (3), 257-266.
5. Schnelle, J., Bertrand, R., Hurd, D., White, A., Squires, D., Feuerberg, M., et al., 2009. The importance of standardized observations to evaluate nutritional care quality in the survey process. Journal of the American Medical Directors Association 10 (8), 568-574.
6. American Occupational Therapy Association, 2007. Specialized knowledge and skills in feeding, eating, and swallowing for occupational therapy practice. American Journal of Occupational Therapy 61, 686-700.
7. McFarland, D., 2008. Netter's Atlas of Anatomy for Speech, Swallowing, and Hearing. Mosby, St. Louis, MO.
8. Murray, T., Carrau, R., 2006. Clinical Management of Swallowing Disorders. Plural, San Diego, CA.
9. Cherney, L., 1994. Clinical Management of Dysphagia for Adults and Children. Aspen, Rockville, MD.
10. Cook, I., 2009. Oropharyngeal dysphagia. Gastroenterology Clinics of North America 38 (3), 411-431.
11. Puisieux, F., D'andrea, C., Baconnier, P., Bui-Dinh, D., Castaings-Pelet, S., Crestani, B., et al., 2009. Swallowing disorders, pneumonia and respiratory tract infectious disease in the elderly. Revue Des Maladies Respiratoires 26 (6), 587-605.
12. Dewing, J., 2009. Prioritising mealtime care, patient choice, and nutritional assessment were important for older in-patients' mealtime experiences. Evidence-Based Nursing 12 (1), 30.
13. Hägg, M., Anniko, M., 2008. Lip muscle training in stroke patients with dysphagia. Acta Oto-Laryngologica 128 (9), 1027-1033.
14. Amella, E., Grant, A., Mulloy, C., 2008. Eating behavior in persons with moderate to late-stage dementia: Assessment and interventions. Journal of the American Psychiatric Nurses Association 13 (6), 360-367.
15. Haidary, A., Leider, J., Silbergleit, R., 2007. Unsuspected swallowing of a partial denture. American Journal of Neuroradiology 28 (9), 1734-1735.
16. Singh, S., Hamdy, S., 2006. Dysphagia in stroke patients. Postgraduate Medical Journal 82 (968), 383-391.
17. Foley, N., Martin, R., Salter, K., Teasell, R., 2009. A review of the relationship between dysphagia and malnutrition following stroke. Journal of Rehabilitation Medicine 41 (9), 707-713.
18. Walton, K., Williams, P., Bracks, J., Zhang, Q., Pond, L., Smoothy, R., et al., 2008. A volunteer feeding assistance program can improve dietary intakes of elderly patients—a pilot study. Appetite 51 (2), 244-248.
19. Wright, L., Cotter, D., Hickson, M., 2008. The effectiveness of targeted feeding assistance to improve the nutritional intake of elderly dysphagic patients in hospital. Journal of Human Nutrition and Dietetics 21 (6), 555-562.
20. Thomas, D., 2007. Nutritional requirements in older adults. In: Morley, J., Thomas, D. (Eds.), Geriatric Nutrition. CRC Press, Boca Raton, FL, pp. 103-122.
21. Schiffman, S., 2009. Sensory impairment: Taste and smell impairment in aging. In: Bales, C., Ritchie, C. (Eds.), Handbook of Clinical Nutrition and Aging, 2nd ed. Humana Press, New York, pp. 77-98.
22. Chernoff, R., 2006. Geriatric Nutrition: The Health Professional's Handbook, 3rd ed. Jones & Bartlett, Sudbury, MA.
23. Thomas, D., Morley, J., 2007. Water metabolism. In: Morley, J., Thomas, D. (Eds.), Geriatric Nutrition. CRC Press, Boca Raton, FL, pp. 131-136.
24. Morley, J., 2007. The role of nutrition in the prevention of age-related diseases. In: Morley, J., Thomas, D. (Eds.), Geriatric Nutrition. CRC Press, Boca Raton, FL, pp. 29-44.

25. Drozdowski, L., Iordache, C., Woudstra, T., Thompson, A., 2009. Lipid absorption in aging. In: Watson, R. (Ed.), Handbook of Nutrition and the Aged, 4th ed. CRC Press, Boca Raton, FL, pp. 113-148.

26. Omran, L., Aneed, W., 2007. Nutrition and gastrointestinal function. In: Morley, J. Thomas, D. (Eds.), Geriatric Nutrition. CRC Press, Boca Raton, FL, pp. 451-468.

27. Groher, M.E., 1990. Ethical dilemmas in providing nutrition. Dysphagia 5, 102-109.

28. Vesey, S., Leslie, P., Exley, C., 2008. A pilot study exploring the factors that influence the decision to have PEG feeding in patients with progressive conditions. Dysphagia 23 (3), 310-316.

29. American Occupational Therapy Association, 2005. Occupational Therapy Code of Ethics. American Journal of Occupational Therapy 59, 639-642.

chapter 19

Working with Elders Who Have Had Cerebrovascular Accidents

DEBORAH L. MORAWSKI AND RENÉ PADILLA

KEY TERMS

cerebrovascular accident, aphasia, midline alignment, muscle tone, hypotonicity, hypertonicity, subluxation, shoulder-hand syndrome, hemiplegia, transfers, edema, weight bearing, functional activities

CHAPTER OBJECTIVES

1. Discuss cerebrovascular accidents by describing the major features of strokes affecting the main arteries of the brain.
2. Discuss at least three considerations in the occupational therapy evaluation of elders who have had a stroke.
3. Describe the sequence of facilitating midline alignment while elders are supine, sitting, and standing, and explain the steps to follow when transferring elders from a supine position to the edge of the bed or from a sitting to a standing position.
4. Explain precautions for handling an elder's hemiplegic upper extremity.

Virtually every human endeavor is the result of the brain's unceasing activity. The brain is the organ of behavior, cognition, language, learning, and movement. The sophistication of the brain's circuitry is remarkable, if not baffling. Billions of neurons interact with each other to do the brain's work. To appreciate the aging process, certified occupational therapy assistants (COTAs) must have an understanding of the way the brain works.[1-3] Implications of neuropathological disorders for occupational therapy (OT) intervention with elders are described in this chapter. The many biological and behavioral changes that accompany normal aging are explained in other chapters in this book.

Effects of normal age-related changes in the nervous system vary greatly among individuals and are not generally associated with specific diseases. These changes clearly have little detrimental effect on many elders. Senility is not an inevitable aspect of aging. However, a number of conditions can be devastating to elders because they present serious obstacles to the process of normal, healthy aging. Some of these conditions are related to cerebrovascular accidents (CVAs). (Chapter 20 presents the issues related to Alzheimer's disease, which is another disorder affecting the brain.)

CEREBROVASCULAR ACCIDENTS

CVAs, or strokes, are lesions in the brain that result from a thrombus, embolus, or hemorrhage that compromises the blood supply to the brain. This inadequate supply results in brain swelling and ultimately in the death of neurons in the stroke area.

Strokes are the third leading cause of death in the United States and the leading cause of disability among adults. Although the incidence of CVA has decreased over the past 50 years, approximately 750,000 individuals experience strokes each year, and nearly 167,000 die as a result, making it the third leading cause of death in the United States.[4] About 4 million individuals live with varying degrees of neurological impairment after strokes.[5] The incidence of strokes increases with age, with the rate doubling every decade of life after age 55 years, and two-thirds of all strokes occur after age 65 years. Recurrent strokes account for 25% of yearly reported strokes and usually occur within 5 years.[6] Black individuals have a greater risk for disability and death from stroke than other racial and ethnic groups.[7] Men experience strokes more frequently than women until age 55 years, when the risk for women equals that for men; however, more women die of strokes at all ages.[5]

Ischemic strokes, caused by both thrombus and embolus, account for about 80% of strokes. Intracerebral and subarachnoid hemorrhagic strokes account for about 20% of strokes.[8] Mortality rates associated with stroke have been declining steadily since the 1950s and are reported to be between 17% and 34% during the first 30 days after a stroke, between 25% and 40% within the first year, and between 32% and 60% during the first 3 years. Consequently, about half of the patients with first strokes live for 3 or more years, and more than one-third of individuals live for 10 years.[7]

Risk factors for stroke can be separated into modifiable and unmodifiable. Modifiable factors are those that can be altered by changes in lifestyle or medications, or both. These factors include hypertension, carotid artery stenosis, coronary artery disease, atrial fibrillation, congestive heart failure, cigarette smoking, alcohol and other drug consumption, obesity, diabetes mellitus, and high serum cholesterol, among others. The most preventable of these risk factors is hypertension. Unmodifiable, or fixed, risk factors include prior stroke, age, race, sex, and family history of stroke. Among these unmodifiable factors, increasing age is by far the most significant because two-thirds of strokes occur in people age 65 years and older.[9]

In elders, stroke can result in various neurological deficits (Table 19-1). Neurological and functional recovery occurs most rapidly in the first 3 months after a stroke; most elders continue to progress after that time but at a slower rate.[10] For this reason, predicting functional recovery after stroke and which elders will benefit from rehabilitation are difficult. The World Health Organization proposes that the prognosis for recovery and successful rehabilitation should be indicated in the following order: (1) clients who spontaneously make good recovery without rehabilitation, (2) clients who can make satisfactory recovery through intensive rehabilitation only, and (3) clients with poor recovery of function regardless of the type of rehabilitation.[11] Other factors that complicate prediction of recovery include comorbidity and depression.

The outcome of a stroke depends greatly on which artery supplying the brain is involved (Table 19-2). Medical treatment of a stroke depends on the type, location, and severity of the vascular lesion. In the acute stages, medical intervention is focused on maintaining an airway, rehydration, and management of hypertension. Measures are often taken to prevent the development of deep venous thrombosis (DVT)—that is, blood clots that form in the veins of the lower extremities after prolonged periods of bedrest or immobility. If such clots are released, they can become lodged in the lungs and can cause death. The COTA must be alert to any sign of DVT and should request and carefully follow mobilization and activity guidelines set by the physician. Localized signs in the lower extremity that suggest the presence of DVT include abnormal temperature, change in color and circumference, and tenderness. In addition to the use of medications, elders can prevent DVTs by wearing elastic stockings and intermittent compression garments, and through early mobilization. Because of DVT and other potential complications of stroke, the COTA should check the elder's medical record and communicate with other team members before initiating each intervention session. By doing this, all team members are fully informed and can modify the interventions with the elder to best serve the elder's needs.

Bowel and bladder dysfunction is common during the initial phases of recovery from a stroke. Usually, a specific bowel and bladder program that includes fluid intake, stool softeners, and other remedies is ordered by the physician. The COTA may be involved in structuring a scheduled toileting program for the elders, which is essential for success. (Chapter 17 presents a more detailed discussion about bowel and bladder training programs.) Other complications during the early phases of recovery from a stroke may include respiratory difficulties and pneumonia caused by the decreased efficiency of the muscles involved in respiration and swallowing. Good pulmonary hygiene, use of antibiotics, and early mobilization are effective prevention measures. Dysphagia, or problems with swallowing, also must be addressed to prevent aspiration pneumonia (see Chapter 18).

OCCUPATIONAL THERAPY EVALUATION

Research evidence and expert opinion suggest that stroke rehabilitation should begin in the acute stage and continue long-term, extending several years after onset.[12-14] OT is an essential component in this rehabilitation process.[15] The COTA is an active participant in the evaluation process under the supervision of the registered occupational therapist (OTR).[16] As with any client, OT evaluation is an ongoing process that occurs during each intervention session. This is particularly true for elders who have had a stroke because they may experience many changes during the first few months of recovery. These changes may be noted especially during intervention. Although motor, visual, perceptual, sensory, and cognitive deficits may all contribute to functional impairments, the psychosocial skills and performance of elders and the environment in which they live and perform are critical

TABLE 19-1

Incidence of Neurological Deficits after Stroke

Neurological impairment	Incidence (%)
Sensory deficits	55
Dysarthria	46
Right hemiparesis	47
Left hemiparesis	37
Cognitive deficits	38
Visual-perceptual deficits	34
Aphasia	30
Bladder control	29
Hemianopsia	31
Ataxia	24
Dysphagia	13

Adapted from U.S. Department of Health and Human Services. (2009). Stroke facts and statistics. Retrieved November 19, 2009, from http://www.cdc.gov/stroke/stroke_facts.htm.

TABLE 19-2

Impairments Resulting from Cerebrovascular Accidents of Specific Arteries

Artery	Impairment
Middle cerebral artery	Contralateral hemiplegia Contralateral sensory deficits Contralateral hemianopsia Aphasia Deviation of head and neck toward side of lesion (if lesion is located in dominant hemisphere) Perceptual deficits including anosognosia unilateral neglect, visual spatial deficits, and perseveration (if lesion is located in non-dominant hemisphere)
Internal carotid artery	Contralateral hemiplegia Contralateral hemianesthesia Homonomous hemianopsia Aphasia, agraphia, acalculia, right/left confusion, and finger agnosia (if lesion is located in dominant hemisphere) Visual-perceptual dysfunction, unilateral neglect, constructional dressing apraxia, attention deficits, topographic disorientation, and anosognosia (if lesion is located in non-dominant hemisphere)
Anterior cerebral artery	Contralateral hemiplegia Apraxia Bowel and bladder incontinence Cortical sensory loss of the lower extremity Contralateral weakness of face and tongue Perseveration and amnesia Sucking reflex
Posterior cerebral artery	Homonomous hemianopsia Paresis of eye musculature Contralateral hemiplegia Topographic disorientation Involuntary movement disorders Sensory deficits
Cerebellar artery	Ipsilateral ataxia Nystagmus, nausea, and vomiting Decreased touch, vibration, and position sense Decreased contralateral pain and thermal sensation Ipsilateral facial paralysis
Vertebral artery	Decreased contralateral pain, temperature, touch, and proprioceptive sense Hemiparesis Facial weakness and numbness Ataxia Paralysis of tongue and weakness of vocal folds

components of any OT assessment. In addition, the assessment should always consider elders' performance skills, past performance patterns, occupational contexts, values, beliefs, and spirituality, not just their deficits.[17] Assessment of performance skills (motor and praxis skills, sensory-perceptual skills, emotional regulation skills, cognitive skills, and communication and social skills) is done simultaneously during the performance of an activity. Although the evaluation of each discrete area may be conducted separately, the interaction of these skills and their effects on occupational participation are of primary importance to OT.[17] Typical impairments are discussed in the section on intervention, but areas of necessary assessment for COTAs are discussed in the following paragraphs.

In the context of motor assessment, the COTA must have an understanding of the elder's ability to maintain the body in an upright position and in the midline against gravity (postural reactions). To do this, the COTA must observe the elder's degree of hypertonicity or hypotonicity, the presence of abnormal movement patterns, primitive reflexes, righting and protective reactions, equilibrium, coordination, and range of motion. The COTA should remember that all of these performance skills may be, and often are, affected by posture and endurance, and that the optimal assessment will occur when elders are upright and not too fatigued. Alignment of the trunk, pelvis, and shoulder girdle, and any voluntary motor control should be noted. Assessment of strength has limited benefit in the presence of hypotonicity or hypertonicity and can possibly increase the degree of hypertonicity.[18]

The sensory assessment should include the evaluation of light touch, pressure, pain, temperature, stereognosis, and proprioception. The visual and perceptual areas to be assessed include tracking (smooth pursuits), visual fields, inattention to the right or left sides, spatial relations, figure ground, motor planning, and body scheme. In addition, elders may have other visual impairments that may affect their performance (see Chapter 15 for a review of this topic). Cognitive skills often assessed include attention, initiation, memory, planning, organization, problem solving, insight, and judgment. The ability to do calculations and make abstractions may also be tested. COTAs should remember that posture can have a significant effect on sensory, visual, perceptual, and cognitive functioning, and the assessment of these areas should occur when elders are upright.

Assessment of swallowing ability and safety is crucial for all elders who have experienced a stroke. Swallowing is a complex behavior that results from the simultaneous performance of motor, sensory, perceptual, and cognitive skills, and deficits in any of these areas may result in elders being at a greater risk for aspirating food into the lungs and subsequent development of pneumonia (see Chapter 18 for a review of this topic).

Depending on the elder's ability to communicate, an evaluation of psychosocial skills of elders may need to be completed by interviewing their family or other significant people. Knowledge of the occupations or pursuits that the elder was involved in before the stroke and of the elder's values and interests is crucial in the selection of intervention strategies. Occupational task considerations should be made at every stage of OT intervention.

OCCUPATIONAL THERAPY INTERVENTION

The long-range goal of OT intervention for dysfunction caused by stroke is to facilitate maximal participation in all contexts of the elder's life. To reach this goal, intervention is focused on the restoration of neuromuscular, visual-perceptual-cognitive, and psychosocial skills that support the elder's ability to perform self-care and engage in all areas of occupation. The degree to which each of these areas is emphasized is determined by the previous physical and social environments of elders and their plans after hospitalization. Because each elder's context is unique, the OT intervention plan is tailored specifically to that individual. By recognizing all of these areas of an elder's being, the COTA is adhering to the Occupational Therapy Code of Ethics.[19]

CASE STUDY

The need for tailored intervention programs is illustrated by the cases of Rose and Maria. Both women are in their late seventies and had strokes that have left them with a hemiplegic right side and difficulty verbally expressing themselves (aphasia).

Their visual, perceptual, and cognitive skills appear to be intact. Rose is a widow and lives in a senior community that provides one meal a day and assists her with laundry and cleaning. Her two sons live in other states. Maria lives at home with her husband and 2 of her 8 adult daughters; 10 grandchildren, whose ages range from ages 3 to 18 years, also live in her home. Both Rose and Maria want to return to their previous living environments. The OT program for both women will address all their needs, but the emphasis in Rose's program will be on self-care, meal preparation, and light home management tasks because she must be independent in these areas to maintain her apartment at the senior community. Maria, however, is counting on family assistance for her self-care and is more interested in cooking again for her extended family; therefore, her program will focus more on meal preparation, light home management, and social skills. The OT programs for both women will address their neuromuscular, visual-perceptual-cognitive, and psychosocial skills, but the activities chosen as therapeutic media should reflect their life contexts.

The cases of Rose and Maria illustrate another important principle in stroke rehabilitation: The more familiar the individual is with the activities selected for intervention, the more spontaneous and unconscious are the motor, visual, perceptual, cognitive, and psychosocial reorganization; consequently, changes will last longer.[20] Conscious, attention-focused learning is often necessary in rehabilitation, especially when the likelihood of recovery is small and compensation strategies are more viable. However, these strategies may also slow the rehabilitation process because of the mental effort they require. To illustrate this, COTAs should do the following exercise with partners. Have your partner time you as you write your full name on a piece of paper using your dominant hand, then have your partner time you writing your name again, but this time with your non-dominant hand. Focus carefully on your body while you write your name and on the amount of mental control this task requires. The experience of rehabilitation after a stroke is similar to your experience of writing with your non-dominant hand. Although clients who are recovering from stroke may not be learning to use their non-dominant hand, they are relearning task accomplishment with a different body. The more these clients must concentrate on the task they are attempting, the longer it may take them to complete it. Engagement in automatic activities may take less time and may reinforce the automatic postural adjustments that support all actions. Consequently, whenever possible, the COTA should approach the intervention for stroke impairments with strategies designed to restore lost function in ways that use the learning and work experiences of elders before they experienced the stroke. Compensation strategies, particularly those related to the use of assistive equipment or alternative motor patterns, should be evaluated carefully because they require conscious attention and may create habits that may be difficult to break later.

Motor Deficits

Several sensorimotor approaches exist for the treatment of motor dysfunction resulting from stroke. Some of these include Brunnstrom,[21,22] Bobath's neurodevelopmental therapy and proprioceptive neuromuscular facilitation,[23-26] constraint-induced movement therapy,[27-29] and mirror therapy.[30-32] Regardless of the approach, the goal of intervention is to facilitate normal voluntary movement and use of the affected side of the body. Thus, normal postural mechanisms must also be developed, and abnormal reflexes and movements must be inhibited.

Although hypertonicity is often the most visible sign that a person has a motor dysfunction, this problem is best addressed in the context of postural control rather than in isolation. Abnormal tone in any extremity may drastically change depending on whether the individual is lying, sitting, or standing. Therefore, motor dysfunction should be treated when the individual is in alignment. Alignment means that the individual's pelvis is in a neutral position with no anterior or posterior tilt, that the spine is in midline alignment, and that the upper and lower extremities are in a neutral position.

The correct positioning while the elder is reclining can have a dramatic effect on muscle tone and pain, especially in the presence of shoulder-hand syndrome. (Specific issues with the hemiplegic upper extremity are discussed later in the chapter). Having elders lie on the more affected side is most helpful in inhibiting abnormal tone and pain because of the heavy pressure exerted on that side (Figure 19-1, A). However, caution must be taken to determine that the shoulder girdle is correctly aligned, the scapula is slightly abducted, and the humerus is in external rotation. The position of the bed should be rearranged (unless the elder finds the change too disorganizing) so that the elder can lie on the affected side and face the side of the bed from which transfers will occur. An added advantage of lying on the affected side is that it frees the less involved upper extremity for functional use while the elder is in this position (Figure 19-1, B).

Body alignment should also be maintained during transitional movements, such as changing from a side-lying position to sitting at the edge of the bed and back to side-lying; transferring to and from a chair, wheelchair, toilet, or car; changing from a sitting to a standing position and back to sitting; and while walking. COTAs should follow established sequential procedures when assisting elders to change from a supine position to sitting at the edge of the bed or when doing transfers (Boxes 19-1 and 19-2). In all of these circumstances, COTAs must remember not to pull on the affected upper extremity to assist elders. COTAs should assist by holding the elder from the shoulder with the COTA's hand on the elder's scapula. Pulling the arm or supporting the elder from the axilla can easily cause or worsen any shoulder pain or glenohumeral subluxation. Shoulder subluxation can occur inferiorly, anteriorly, and superiorly. Alignment of the humerus in the glenohumeral fossa is evaluated by the OTR. The COTA needs to determine whether the alignment is correct before range of motion of the shoulder. Shoulder pain is a frequent problem and can occur from malalignment of the trunk, shoulder girdle, and humerus; subluxation; adhesive capsulitis; and trauma.[33] Shoulder subluxation and pain can lead to other complications such as increased hypertonicity, contractures, edema, nerve injury, and

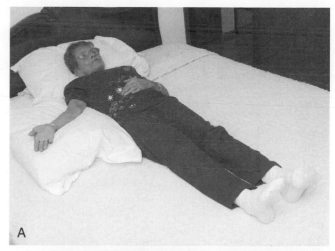

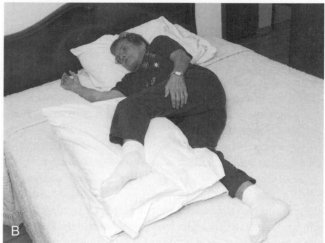

FIGURE 19-1 A, In the supine position, the trunk and upper extremities should be aligned. The hemiplegic upper extremity should be supported on pillows with the palm facing up. B, Lying on the hemiplegic upper extremity frees the less involved arm for functional use.

shoulder-hand syndrome. Before the COTA attempts any intervention for these conditions, service competency should be established with the OTR.

COTAs must pay constant attention to the elder's body alignment during sitting because this is often the elder's position during most activities, especially during the initial stages of rehabilitation. If the elder must sit fairly still for long periods, the therapist must ensure that the elder's pelvis is in a neutral position and is as far back in the chair as possible. Hips should be flexed at no more than 90 degrees. Greater hip flexion will cause posterior pelvic tilt and lumbar and thoracic spine flexion, inhibiting breathing and active upper extremity control and requiring greater cervical spine extension for the person to look straight ahead. Placing a folded towel or thin pillow in the small of the back to maintain alignment may be helpful. However, too thick a pillow or support can push the lumbar spine into hyperextension, causing anterior pelvic

BOX 19-1

Sequential Procedures for Changing from a Supine Position to Sitting at Edge of Bed

1. Plan to have elder exit bed toward hemiplegic side.
2. Gently provide passive abduction to hemiplegic scapula, and extend hemiplegic arm at side of body so that humerus is in external rotation and palm is facing up; an alternative is to have elder clasp hands and hold arms in 90-degree flexion with straight elbows and roll toward side of bed.
3. Have elder hook less affected leg under hemiplegic ankle, and slide both legs toward edge of bed.
4. Have elder roll on to hemiplegic side, facing side of bed.
5. Have elder cross less affected upper extremity in front of body and place on bed at a level slightly below chest.
6. As the elder lowers legs at the side of the bed, have elder push up with less affected hand and hemiplegic elbow (if able).
7. Once sitting at edge of bed, have elder scoot forward by alternating weight bearing on each thigh and scooting the free thigh forward until both feet are flat on floor.

BOX 19-2

Sequential Procedures for Transfers

1. If transferring from the wheelchair to another chair, toilet, or bed, place wheelchair at no more than 45 degrees (perpendicular) from destination surface; elder should transfer toward hemiplegic side whenever possible.
2. Make sure wheelchair is locked and footrests and armrests are out of the way.
3. Place both feet flat on floor.
4. Have elder sit upright so back is not against back rest.
5. Have elder scoot forward to front edge of chair by alternately shifting weight onto one thigh and scooting other thigh forward; do not permit elder to push off back of chair using back extension because this will increase abnormal muscle tone throughout the body.
6. Position elder's feet so tips of toes are directly below knees; make sure feet remain flat on floor; if ankle dorsiflexion is limited, toes may be placed somewhat anterior to knees.
7. Have elder lean forward until shoulders are directly above knees.
8. Have elder push off from knees with both hands, if elder is able.
9. As elder leans forward, have elder stand up; if unable to stand up fully, guide elder's body toward target chair, toilet, or bed while elder is partially weight bearing on both feet.

---

tilt and encouraging the elder to use back extension as the primary means of posture control. When back hyperextension is the base from which the elder begins movement in the extremities, hypertonicity throughout the body is likely to increase.

Another concern when the elder is in the sitting position is lateral pelvic tilt, or lateral flexion of the spine. Because of sensory and tone changes, half of the trunk muscles may not be working well; consequently, the other side of the trunk may be overworking. The resulting misalignment causes the spine to flex toward one side. Because of this lateral flexion, the spine is no longer in midline, and weight bearing on the elder's thighs is unequal. A pelvic tilt upward toward one side results in the shortening of the trunk on the same side and elongation of the trunk on the opposite side. Weight bearing occurs primarily on the side of the elongated trunk. The COTA must help to actively or passively align the spine toward the midline, rather than to simply build up one side of the sitting surface.

When pelvic and spine alignment are achieved, the COTA can focus on placing the feet flat on the floor or on footrests so that knee flexion and ankle dorsiflexion of no more than 90 degrees are present. The COTA should take care that the femurs are in neutral rotation (that is, there is no external or internal rotation) and that there is little or no hip abduction or adduction. Thus, the heels will be resting directly below the knees, and the knees will

be aligned with the hips. Unless the elder is being pushed in a wheelchair, both feet should be placed on the floor so that they bear weight more evenly. Consequently, hemi-wheelchairs, the seats of which are slightly lower than standard wheelchairs, are recommended so that the elder's feet can comfortably reach the floor. The use of a padded seat and backboards placed in the wheelchair also improves the elder's sitting position and midline orientation, thus preventing the problems that may occur from poor positioning in a wheelchair.

After attending to the pelvis, spine, and lower extremities, the COTA can align the elder's hemiplegic upper extremity. The strategies for positioning are similar for both hypotonic and hypertonic arms. The elder should be placed in front of a table or outfitted with a full or half lapboard so that the hand can be placed face down on a flat surface to benefit from the normalizing effects of weight bearing. To accomplish this, the COTA should ensure that the elder's scapula is slightly abducted, the shoulder is flexed so the elbow is anterior to the shoulder, the humerus is in neutral or slight external rotation, the elbow is resting lightly on the lapboard to provide support for the shoulder, the forearm is pronated and positioned away from the trunk, and the hand is resting on the support surface. This permits the hand to bear weight normally. The normal weight-bearing surface of the hand includes the lateral external surface of the thumb, fingertips, lateral border of the hand, and thenar and hypothenar eminences. The COTA should maintain the arch formed by the metacarpophalangeal joints so that the hand is not flattened. The hand should not be fastened in any way to the lapboard except in extreme cases in which clear evidence indicates that the elder may otherwise be hurt. Restricting normal, spontaneous weight bearing inhibits normalization of muscle tone. In cases of extreme hypertonicity in the hand, the COTA can place a soup bowl or a ball cut in half face down on a square of nonslip material on the lapboard, thus permitting some weight bearing against a hard surface (Figure 19-2). However, the elder's hand should never be placed on nonslip material. Such material can contribute to shoulder pain or subluxation because the hand cannot move when repositioning of the shoulder or body occurs. Caution must be used when a lapboard is used with an elder because it may be considered a form of restraint unless the elder is independently able to remove it. (See Chapter 14 for a detailed discussion on this topic.)

During intervention sessions that do not require sitting for long periods, the elder should sit in a chair, on a stool, or at the edge of a mat. The concerns with alignment in this position are similar to those described earlier for sitting, but the focus of intervention will be on the elder moving into and out of alignment while participating in activities. Sitting on a stool or at the edge of the mat forces active trunk control because there are no back or armrests for support, and the base of support under the thighs is reduced. Concerns regarding lower extremity placement are the same as described previously. However, as the

elder's ability to control the trunk increases, the height of the mat can be increased, thus gradually increasing and challenging the amount of active weight bearing on the lower extremities. This gradation prepares the elder for the trunk and postural control required during standing activities. If the elder has little or no active movement of the hemiplegic upper extremity, the elder should position the limb on a table, following similar guidelines as those described previously. As the height of the mat increases, so should the height of the table or surface that supports the hand.

Although standing and ambulation training does not traditionally fall into the realm of OT, it should be considered a transitional movement that permits elders to perform and maneuver from one task or occupation to another. For example, elders may need to ambulate from the bed to the bathroom and stand to complete toileting tasks, or ambulate from the sink to the stove to the refrigerator and stand to complete a meal preparation task. Consequently, COTAs should assist in maintaining alignment in the same way as described previously. During standing and ambulation, the person's midline shift toward the less affected side is most obvious. This is often accentuated when elders are taught to walk using a broad-based cane, and they establish the habit of maintaining the midline in the middle of the less affected side rather than in the middle of the body. Because there is less motor control or less sensory feedback, elders may hesitate to bear weight equally on each leg as they stand or take a step. The COTA should coordinate intervention with the registered physical therapist to understand what standing and ambulation pattern to reinforce with elders during OT intervention.

Special attention should be given to the hemiplegic upper extremity. This extremity should be purposefully included in any activity early during the course of intervention, even if little or no active motor control is present, because this will keep the elder's attention on the extremity and will reduce its neglect and the development of learned nonuse.[27,29] Before any active or passive motion is expected of the elder, the COTA must first passively mobilize the elder's scapula to ensure that it glides when the arm is moved. The scapula may not glide sufficiently or may stop altogether because of muscle paralysis or hypertonus. Consequently, the COTA should never flex or abduct the shoulder of elders more than 90 degrees unless the COTA can be sure that the scapula is gliding properly. If elders do not have active scapular control, the COTA can passively move the scapula while ranging the shoulder. When the shoulder is flexed more than 90 degrees, the scapula glides downward on the posterior wall of the rib cage. In addition, the inferior border, or angle, of the scapula rotates slightly upward. When the shoulder is abducted more than 90 degrees, the scapula glides toward the vertebral column and the inferior border rotates slightly downward.

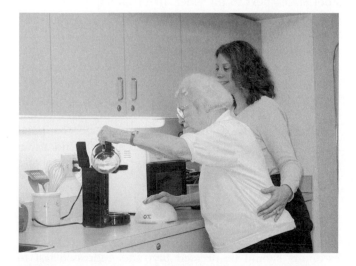

FIGURE 19-2   In cases of hypertonicity, the hemiplegic hand can be placed on an inverted soup bowl or ball cut in half to bear weight more comfortably.

If elders have minimal or no active movement in the hemiplegic upper extremity, they should be instructed to move it by holding their hands together in one of two ways. If the elder has any active movement in the hand, clasping the hands with the thumb of the hemiplegic hand on top is recommended. If there is no movement in the hand, the uninvolved hand should be placed on the ulnar side of the hemiplegic wrist and hand and the uninvolved thumb in the palm of the hemiplegic hand. This method will protect the small joints of the hemiplegic hand and will maintain the arches in the palm. While holding onto the hands using either method, elders should be instructed to extend the elbows and hold the shoulders flexed at approximately 90 degrees. With the arms in this position, elders can go from a supine to a side-lying position, from a sitting to a standing position, or they can hold on to the knee of the hemiplegic lower extremity to cross it during dressing and bathing and during other functional activities. The COTA's imagination and creativity are essential in assisting elders to use this two-hand technique to perform numerous functional activities such as picking up a mug to drink and mixing a cake. In addition, elders can flex or abduct the hemiplegic shoulder themselves by guiding the arm when the hands are held together. This bilateral integration assists with normalizing tone and encourages elders to actively care for the hemiplegic upper extremity.[23]

Elders may develop shoulder-hand syndrome if the hemiplegic upper extremity is not managed appropriately. This syndrome is characterized by swelling or edema that is usually observed in the hand but may also be present in the forearm and upper arm, tenderness, loss of range of motion, and vasomotor degradation. Pain and subluxation of the glenohumeral joint may not necessarily be present. The COTA should address all of these problems immediately to avoid irreversible atrophy of bones, skin, and muscles.[23] The swelling is best decreased by filling a bucket or pail two-thirds full with crushed ice and adding cold water to the level of the ice. Elders should sit, while maintaining good alignment, with the bucket in front of them, which is placed on the floor, and should lean forward to place the hemiplegic hand and wrist in the water. The edematous hand should be kept in the water for 3 to 5 seconds, and this process should be repeated three times. The COTA should dry the hand gently with a towel. The COTA should ask the elder to flex the fingers, if possible, or the COTA should provide gentle passive ranging of the fingers and hand. The whole procedure should be done repeatedly during the day until swelling subsides. While the COTA is providing the range of motion exercise, retrograde massage while the limb is elevated can also be done, and a simple cock-up splint can be used to hold the wrist in extension (no more than 30 degrees) to help reduce the buildup of fluid in the hand when elders are not receiving therapy (Figure 19-3). Swelling also occurs from decreased muscle activity to move the fluid from the limb, dependent positioning, and trauma.

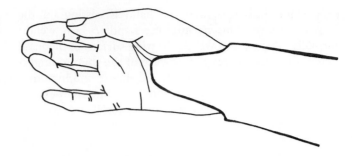

FIGURE 19-3   A modified cock-up splint holds the wrist in slight extension and helps reduce fluid buildup in the hand.

COTAs can use graded activities to facilitate voluntary control of an elder's hemiplegic upper extremity. Such activities should be geared toward developing control in a progression from shoulder to elbow to hand. Elders may develop control in the hand before the more proximal parts of the arm. Despite the apparent control in the hand, the COTA should first facilitate active movement in the shoulder by engaging elders in activities that emphasize the body moving on the arm while the hand is maintained in weight bearing. The weight-bearing surface of the hand is limited to the lateral surface of the thumb, the thenar eminences, and the fingertips. In this position the palm of the hand is free and not in contact with the weight-bearing surface. Weight bearing on the hand does not need to be forceful, and elders should never have the hand completely flattened. Placing weight on a flat hand can lead to loss of the normal and functional arches of the hand and, consequently, can interfere with elders' abilities to develop grasp later. Placing weight on the hand can be done in both sitting and standing positions. In a sitting position, for example, an elder's affected hand can be placed in a weight-bearing position on the table or on a stool placed next to the elder. In a standing position, the elder should be taught to place the affected hand on a weight-bearing surface such as a table or countertop while performing functional tasks, such as putting away dishes or groceries or folding laundry (Figure 19-4). As control of the shoulder increases, activities should be introduced that emphasize free movement of the hemiplegic extremity on the more stable part of the body. During all of these activities, the COTA should continue to ensure that good body alignment is maintained and that elders are not using abnormal movements in one part of the body to obtain control in another.

COTAs should instruct elders in proper one-handed dressing techniques to protect the hemiplegic upper extremity and to avoid falling. Dressing should be done while sitting in a chair and, in general, the hemiplegic extremity should be dressed first and undressed last to avoid pulling on it or twisting it unnecessarily. Front-buttoned shirts or blouses are easiest to don by first dressing the hemiplegic arm and then draping the shirt over

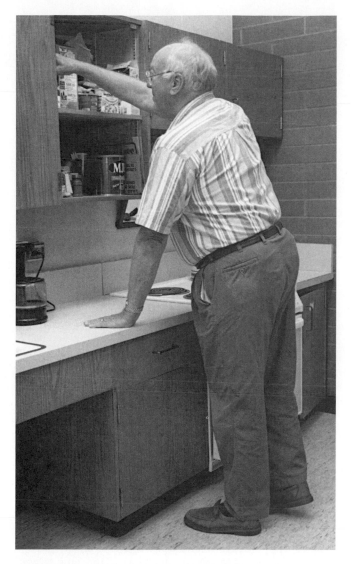

FIGURE 19-4   Bearing weight on the hemiplegic hand can be done while standing at a counter.

the shoulders by holding on to the shirt collar with the other arm. When the shirt is draped over the opposite shoulder, the elder can reach into the sleeve with the unaffected arm. This procedure is reversed when taking the shirt off. The process is similar when putting on pants, with the exception that the elder should cross the hemiplegic leg over the opposite leg to dress the hemiplegic leg first. If the elder is able to stand to pull up the pants, the elder may do so when both legs are clothed. If standing is not possible, the elder can shift weight to each side while sitting in the chair and gradually can pull the pants up over the buttocks.

All of the principles mentioned previously should be considered when training elders in functional activities or selecting assistive equipment. Although progress may seem slower at the beginning, following these principles can make a marked difference in the quality of movement

that elders develop. When tasks are too difficult, elders are more likely to use abnormal movement patterns, become fatigued quickly, and become discouraged. The COTA must use good observation and clinical reasoning skills in selecting activities that challenge elders at the appropriate levels.

Visual-Perceptual-Cognitive Deficits

Although the motor deficits resulting from a stroke are the most easily observed, many less visible problems can severely hinder the rehabilitation process if not appropriately addressed. Depending on the type of brain lesion, the individual may have sensory disturbances that range from a total absence of sensation to a heightened perception of pain and other distorted sensations. These problems are accentuated when the individual has a body scheme disorder or difficulties planning motor actions, which is known as apraxia. Consequently, the individual has difficulty integrating and using any perceptual input from the hemiplegic side. Visual–perceptual deficits common in strokes include hemianopsia, poor figure ground perceptions, and difficulty with spatial relationships. Unilateral neglect results from a unique constellation of these symptoms when elders have no sense that the hemiplegic side of the body even exists, and they fail to visually scan toward that side.[34,35] All of these disorders should be addressed simultaneously during intervention, using bilateral functional activities that encourage the use of the hemiplegic side of the body. The use of normal movement will provide repeated sensory stimulation to the hemiplegic side and relay information that will be processed in the brain and used as feedback in determining where each body part is and what it is doing. Consequently, the COTA should grade a variety of motor and sensory activities so that they maximize the elders' abilities to control movement independently and provide increased sensory input. However, the activities should not be so overwhelming that they cause withdrawal reactions or increases in abnormal tone. Various textures, smells, colors, distances, and depths can be graded during most functional activities. In addition to these remedial approaches, the COTA should teach elders to compensate for deficits by providing repeated practice in establishing habits of visually scanning the hemiplegic side and methodically protecting and integrating the hemiplegic extremities in whatever activity they may be involved.

Other areas of concern for the COTA include elders' abilities to comprehend and produce language and to plan and safely perform activities. As a result of stroke, elders may not be able to understand what others are saying, a condition known as receptive aphasia, or may not be able to produce the words they intend to utter, a condition known as expressive aphasia, or both disorders may be present, which is known as global aphasia. These disorders may also extend to nonverbal language because elders may be unable to interpret or appropriately use gestures.

Language deficits are usually treated by the speech language pathologist, but strategies must be reinforced during OT intervention. When talking to elders, COTAs should keep instructions and explanations simple and concrete and should state them in an empathetic, patient way. Demonstration is usually helpful. The best way to ensure that elders have understood the instructions is to observe their performance.[34,36]

Cognitive dysfunction is often believed to be a major cause for failure of elders to reach rehabilitation goals and must be considered, particularly when planning for discharge.[37] Safety may be compromised if elders cannot plan activities, make judgments, solve problems, or express verbally their needs for emergency care. For example, limited memory may cause elders to overmedicate themselves or not turn off the stove after cooking. Being unable to remember all of the steps involved in a task may mean that elders can often be surprised by the outcome. Elders may get stuck on a step and may be unable to determine what to do next or may neglect to realize that something dangerous could happen if an inappropriate action is taken. OT intervention, as mentioned earlier, should involve graded repetition of procedures until elders can routinely perform them safely. Emphasis should be placed on varying the context or situation in which the procedure is practiced to enhance learning.[38]

Emotional Adjustment

COTAs should consider the emotional adjustment of elders to the disability caused by the stroke. Depression, a common reaction to any catastrophic event, is one of the most undiagnosed and untreated responses to stroke.[39,40] Depression may be caused from natural grief trying to cope with the loss of function, but also may be caused by the location of the lesion in the brain, previous or family history of depression, and social functioning before the stroke. Mild or major depression can develop from 2 months to 2 years after the stroke in up to 53% of clients.[40,41] Anxiety, poor frustration tolerance, denial, anger, and emotional lability are all signs that elders are struggling to deal with the reality of their condition. COTAs must listen empathetically and supportively, while sensitively maintaining the focus on areas of realistic recovery. Permitting elders to control choices in intervention as much as possible can reinforce the sense that they can affect their environments. Although a complete recovery cannot be guaranteed, neither can a lack of recovery. COTAs must honestly explain to elders that residual limitations will probably be present, but the best chance for recovery will occur by the practice of skills. COTAs should use their creativity and ingenuity skills to help elders adapt tasks or environments that elders consider lost, thus instilling new hope and motivation in the rehabilitation process. As with any area of intervention, family and social involvement is crucial for elders to accept residual limitations and maximize their residual abilities. Ultimately,

elders must see that they can continue to be effective in some measure and can still actively pursue activities and ideals they valued highly before the stroke.

CASE STUDY

Gabriel is a 75-year-old man who recently returned home after having a left Middle Cerebral Artery stroke. He had spent three weeks in an acute care hospital followed by three weeks in a rehabilitation center. The rehabilitation team concluded that with the right supports, Gabriel would be safe at home. At the time of discharge home he had some residual weakness of the right side of his body, particularly the leg. He was able to flex the hip and knee against gravity, but continued to have the tendency to drag the foot when he walked. He still had some difficulties coordinating is right arm, and tended to ever-reach with it, on occasion knocking objects off tables, counters and shelves. The discharge report from the occupational therapists at the rehabilitation hospital indicated that Gabriel was able to feed, toilet, and dress himself independently, although on occasion became confused about the sequencing of dressing tasks.

John, an OTR, and Pam, a COTA, evaluated Gabriel as part of the home-health team and noted that Gabriel still had a slight decrease in tactile abilities with this right, dominant hand. They noted a slight droop in the right side of his face was still present, and that his lingual control toward the right side was also reduced. They confirmed that Gabriel was able to dress and toilet himself, but discovered that although he had been able to shower himself in the hospital, at home this would require transferring into an old-fashioned bathtub. This tub was higher than the standard tub in which he had been evaluated at the hospital. John and Pam determined that without grab bars for safety, Gabriel would need minimal to moderate assistance with his shower for safety.

John and Pam included an analysis of Gabriel's home and supports in their intake evaluation. Gabriel lived in a first floor apartment which had wooden floors. There were several floor rugs that Gabriel had collected in his travels. The furniture was already arranged in a way that John and Pam believed would not interfere with Gabriel's safety. They noted that Gabriel lived alone, although his younger brother visited every day and lived only a few blocks away. Up to the time of the stroke, Gabriel had been driving his car to get to the grocery store and move around in the community.

■ CASE STUDY REVIEW QUESTIONS

1 Should John and Pam conduct any additional evaluations to determine Gabriel's needs? What additional information should they consider before finalizing the intervention plan?
2 What interventions should John and Pam implement to help Gabriel continue to make gains in his neuromuscular functions?
3 What strategies should be considered to assure Gabriel's safety in the kitchen considering his remaining neuromuscular deficits?
4 What precautions should be considered given Gabriel's facial droop and limited lingual control?
5 What safety measures should be considered in Gabriel's home to assure it is a safe environment for him?
6 What alternatives for community access should be considered with Gabriel?

▍ CHAPTER REVIEW QUESTIONS

1 Sit at the edge of a bed or chair and lift up the left side of your pelvis. What happens with your spine and trunk when you do this? What occurs with the imaginary midline of the body when you sit in this position? Where on your thighs do you feel the most pressure while sitting in this position? Can you tell any difference in how your arms work while sitting this way? How would you feel after sitting in this position for 10 or 15 minutes?

2 Sitting on a firm chair, make sure that your pelvis is as far back in the chair as possible and your back is well supported. From that position, without moving forward, attempt to stand. What did you do with your arms while attempting to stand? How much work did your trunk have to do to get you to a standing position? Now repeat the activity, but first scoot to the edge of the chair before you stand. Did you notice any differences in the amount of work that your upper trunk and arms had to do to get you upright? From which position was it easier to stand?

3 Sitting at the edge of a chair with your trunk well aligned, move your feet as far forward as you can, making sure that they are flat on the floor. From that position, attempt to stand. Were you able to do so? How much work did your upper trunk and arms have to do? Return to sitting at the edge of the chair, and now attempt to stand again, but first place your feet as far back behind your knees as possible. Was standing from this position more or less difficult than your first attempt? Did you fall forward? Now return to sitting at the edge of the chair, and this time place your feet so that your toes are directly aligned below your knees and are flat on the floor. Did this help keep your midline where it should be, even during movement?

REFERENCES

1. Orrison, W., 2008. Atlas of Brain Function, 2nd ed. Thieme Medical, New York.
2. Siegel, A., Sapru, H., 2006. Essential Neuroscience. Lippincott Williams & Wilkins, Baltimore.
3. Umphred, D., 2006. Neurological Rehabilitation, 5th ed. Mosby, St. Louis, MO.
4. Kung, H., Hoyert, D., Xu, J., Murphy, S., 2008. Deaths: Final data for 2005. Centers for Disease Control National Vital Statistics Reports 50 (20).
5. Carandang, R., Seshadri, S., Beiser, A., Kelly-Hayes, M., Kase, C., Kannel, W., et al., 2006. Trends in incidence, lifetime risk, severity, and 30-day mortality of stroke over the past 50 years. Journal of the American Medical Association 295, 2939-2946.
6. Russo, A., Andrews, R., 2008. Hospital stays for stroke and other cerebrovascular diseases: Statistical brief #51. Agency for Healthcare Research and Quality, Washington, DC. Retrieved November 19, 2009, from http://www.hcup-us.ahrq.gov/reports/statbriefs/sb51.pdf.
7. Centers for Disease Control and Prevention, 2007. Prevalence of stroke—United States, 2005. Morbidity and Mortality Weekly Report 56 (19), 469-474.
8. American Heart Association, 2008. Heart disease and stroke statistics—2008 update. Author, Dallas, TX.
9. Feigin, V., Lawes, C., Bennett, D. Anderson, S., 2009. Epidemiology of stroke. In: Stein, J., Harvey, R., Macko, R., Winstein, C., Zorowits, R. (Eds.), Stroke Recovery and Rehabilitation. Demos, New York, pp. 31-44.
10. Duncan, P., Zorowitz, R., Bates, B., Küst, J., Rietz, C., Karbe, H., 2005. Management of adult stroke rehabilitation care: A clinical practice guideline. Stroke 36, e100-e143.
11. Mackay, J., Mensah, G., 2004. Atlas of Heart Disease and Stroke. World Health Organization Press, Geneva, Switzerland.
12. Bernhardt, J., Thuy, M., Collier, J., Legg, L., 2009. Very early versus delayed mobilization after stroke. Cochrane Database of Systematic Reviews, Issue 1. Art. No.: CD006187. DOI: 10.1002/14651858.CD006187.pub2.
13. Jones, S., Auton, M., Burton, C., Watkins, C., 2008. Engaging service users in the development of stroke services: An action research study. Journal of Clinical Nursing 17 (10), 1270-1279.
14. Swayne, O., Rothwell, J., Ward, N., Greenwood, R., 2008. Stages of motor output reorganization after hemispheric stroke suggested by longitudinal studies of cortical physiology. Cerebral Cortex 18 (8), 1909-1922.
15. Legg, L., Drummond, A., Langhorne, P., 2006. Occupational therapy for patients with problems in activities of daily living after stroke. Cochrane Database of Systematic Reviews, Issue 4. Art. No.: CD003585. DOI: 10.1002/14651858.CD003585.pub2.
16. Moyers, P.A., 2007. The Guide to Occupational Therapy Practice, 2nd ed. American Occupational Therapy Association Press, Bethesda, MD.
17. American Occupational Therapy Association, 2008. Occupational therapy practice framework: Domain and process, 2nd ed. American Journal of Occupational Therapy 62 (6), 625-683.
18. Kelley, R., Borazanci, A., 2009. Stroke rehabilitation. Neurological Research 31 (8), 832-840.
19. American Occupational Therapy Association, 2005. Occupational Therapy Code of Ethics. American Journal of Occupational Therapy 59, 639-642.
20. Gillen, G., Burkhardt, A., 2004. Stroke Rehabilitation: A Function-Based Approach, 2nd ed. Mosby, St. Louis, MO.
21. Sawner, K., Lavigne, G., 1992. Brunnstrom's Movement Therapy in Hemiplegia: A Neurophysiological Approach. Lippincott Williams & Wilkins, Hagerstown, MD.
22. Schabrun, S., Hillier, S., 2009. Evidence for the retraining of sensation after stroke: A systematic review. Clinical Rehabilitation 23 (1), 27-39.
23. Davies, P., 2004. Steps to Follow: The Comprehensive Treatment of Patients with Hemiplegia, 2nd ed. Springer-Verlag, New York.
24. Adler, S., Beckers, D., Buck, M., 2003. PDF in Practice: An Illustrated Guide, 3rd ed. Springer-Verlag, New York.
25. Thaut, M., Leins, A., Rice, R., Argstatter, H., Kenyon, G., McIntosh, G., et al., 2007. Rhythmic auditory stimulation improves gait more than NDT/Bobath training in near-ambulatory patients early post-stroke: A single-blind, randomized trial. Neurorehabilitation and Neural Repair 21 (5), 455-459.
26. Hafsteinsdóttir, T., Algra, A., Kappelle, L., Grypdonck, M., 2005. Neurodevelopmental treatment after stroke: A comparative study. Journal of Neurology, Neurosurgery 76 (6), 788-792.
27. Azab, M., Al-Jarrah, M., Nazzal, M., Maayah, M., Sammour, M., Jamous, M., 2009. Effectiveness of constraint-induced movement therapy (CIMT) as home-based therapy on Barthel Index in patients with chronic stroke. Topics in Stroke Rehabilitation 16 (3), 207-211.

28. Hammer, A., Lindmark, B., 2009. Effects of forced use on arm function in the subacute phase after stroke: A randomized, clinical pilot study. Physical Therapy 89, 526-539.

29. Blanton, S., Wilsey, H., Wolf, S., 2008. Constraint-induced movement therapy in stroke rehabilitation: Perspectives on future clinical applications. Neurorehabilitation 23 (1), 15-28.

30. Dohle, C., Püllen, J., Nakaten, A., Küst, J., Rietz, C., Karbe, H., 2009. Mirror therapy promotes recovery from severe hemiparesis: A randomized controlled trial. Neurorehabilitation and Neural Repair 23 (3), 209-217.

31. Ezendam, D., Bongers, R., Jannink, M., 2009. Systematic review of the effectiveness of mirror therapy in upper extremity function. Disability & Rehabilitation 31 (26), 2135-2149.

32. Yavuzer, G., Selles, R., Sezer, N., et al., 2008. Mirror therapy improves hand function in subacute stroke: A randomized controlled trial. Archives of Physical Medicine and Rehabilitation 89 (3), 393-398.

33. Kumar, P., Swinkels, A., 2009. A critical review of shoulder subluxation and its association with other post-stroke complications. Physical Therapy Reviews 14 (1), 13-25.

34. Wolf, T., Baum, C., Conner, L., 2009. Changing face of stroke: Implications for occupational therapy practice. American Journal of Occupational Therapy 63 (5), 621-625.

35. Cappa, S., 2008. Neglect rehabilitation in stroke: Not to be neglected. European Journal of Neurology 15 (9), 883-884.

36. Bowen, A., Lincoln, N., 2007. Cognitive rehabilitation for spatial neglect following stroke. Cochrane Database of Systematic Reviews, Issue 2. Art. No.: CD003586. DOI: 10.1002/14651858.CD003586.pub2.

37. Woodson, A., 2007. Stroke. In: Trombly, C. (Ed.), Occupational Therapy for Physical Dysfunction, 6th ed. Williams & Wilkins, Baltimore, MD, pp. 1001-1041.

38. Barrett, A., Buxbaum, L., Coslett, H., Edwards, E., Heilman, K., Hillis, A., Milberg, W., Robertson, I., 2006. Cognitive rehabilitation interventions for neglect and related disorders: Moving from bench to bedside in stroke patients. Journal of Cognitive Neuroscience 18 (7), 1223-1236.

39. Schepers, V., Post, M., Visser-Meily, A., van de Port, I., Akhmouch, M., Lindeman, E., 2009. Prediction of depressive symptoms up to three years post-stroke. Journal of Rehabilitation Medicine 41 (11), 930-935.

40. National Institute on Mental Health, 2008. Preventive treatment may help head off depression following a stroke. Retrieved November 19, 2009, from http://www.nimh.nih.gov/science-news/2008/preventive-treatment-may-help-head-off-depression-following-a-stroke.shtml.

41. Fang, J., Cheng, Q., 2009. Etiological mechanisms of post-stroke depression: A review. Neurological Research 31 (9), 904-909.

20

Working with Elders Who Have Dementia and Alzheimer's Disease

CARLY R. HELLEN AND RENÉ PADILLA

KEY TERMS

Alzheimer's disease, activity-focused care, personhood, person-centered care, "therapeutic fibs," creative reality, rescuing, chaining, bridging

CHAPTER OBJECTIVES

1. Understand that elders with Alzheimer's disease (AD) are persons first; they are not their disease. Therefore, person-centered care (personalized) focuses on overall well-being, reflecting the elders' remaining strengths and abilities.
2. Describe person-centered care and personhood.
3. Gain awareness and sensitivity to the cognitive, physical, and psychosocial needs of elders with AD.
4. Describe occupation-focused care.

5. Relate suggestions to promote wellness through task simplification and modification.
6. Identify caregiving techniques, approaches, and interventions that can be used to help empower elders who have AD to participate in daily living tasks.
7. Suggest appropriate communication responses to elders with AD.
8. Problem solve antecedents and approaches to refocus unwanted behavioral responses.

Travis is a certified occupational therapy assistant (COTA) who works in a skilled nursing facility. One of his responsibilities is consulting with staff at a special care unit for persons with AD. John, the charge nurse on the unit, contacts Travis. "We are having problems with Grace. She is wandering in and out of others' rooms and taking their possessions, which is irritating the other residents. She is also having difficulty communicating her needs. Her performance with activities of daily living (ADL) functions seems variable. We are also having problems with increased agitation with Grace and all of our residents, especially at shift change. Do you have any ideas?"

Hilde is a COTA working on a subacute unit. Ruth, one of the elders, was admitted after a total hip replacement. After reviewing her chart, Hilde finds out that Ruth has a history of AD. Both Travis and Hilde can provide practical suggestions to better help these elders with AD function. This chapter provides background information about AD and occupational therapy (OT) interventions.

An estimated 5.3 million Americans have AD. AD is the sixth leading cause of all deaths in the United States, and the fifth leading cause of death in Americans age 65 and older.[1] Between 2000 and 2006, heart disease deaths decreased nearly 12%, stroke deaths decreased 18%, and prostate cancer–related deaths decreased 14%, whereas deaths attributable to AD increased 47%.[1] Every 70

seconds someone in the United States develops AD, and, by 2050, this time is expected to decrease to every 33 seconds.[2] Over the coming decades, the "baby-boom" population is projected to add 10 million people to these numbers. In 2050, the incidence of AD in the United States is expected to approach nearly a million people per year, with a total estimated prevalence of 11 to 16 million people.[3] The incidence of AD across the world is expected to double every 20 years so that today's figure of 35.6 million people with the disease will rise to 65.7 million by 2030 and 115.4 million by 2050, if a cure is not found.[4]

Dementia does not follow a uniform or single predictable course. The dementia syndrome includes unpredictable fluctuations in basic memory, judgment, and performance.[5] While depression, medications, and metabolic dysfunction may cause a reversible dementia, nonreversible dementia may be caused by small strokes (vascular dementia), dementia with Parkinson's disease, dementia with Lewy bodies, frontal lobe dementias, and AD.[6] Alzheimer's is the most common form of dementia and accounts for 50% to 70% of cases.[7] AD is a progressive, degenerative, and fatal disease of brain tissue that leads to memory loss and problems with thinking and carrying out daily life activities. Participation in routine occupations, using good judgment, being aware of surroundings, communicating effectively, and coping with life become more difficult as the disease progresses. Problems start gradually and become more severe over time, leading to a total disruption in performance patterns and the inability to participate in most areas of occupation.[8] Although the rate of change varies, the usual stages are mild, moderate, severe, and terminal (Table 20-1).[9]

AD can last 3 to 20 years. Most people die after 8 years, often from pneumonia or other systemic problems. Causes of AD are not known, but current research suggests the involvement of two abnormal structures called *plaques* and *tangles* as prime suspects in damaging and killing nerve cells. Plaques are deposits of a protein fragment called *beta-amyloid* that build up between nerve cells. Tangles are twisted fibers of another protein called *tau* that form inside dying brain cells. Although most people develop some plaques and tangles as they age, those with Alzheimer's tend to develop far more. The plaques and tangles tend to form in a predictable pattern, beginning in areas important in learning and memory and then spreading to other regions.[8] With the help of standardized diagnostic criteria, physicians can now diagnose AD with an accuracy of 85% to 90% once symptoms occur.[9,10] Intervention is based on the combination of medical and psychosocial support.[8] Two types of medications are often used (cholinesterase and memantine) to support communication among nerve cells and delay problems with learning and

TABLE 20-1

Four Stages of Alzheimer's Disease	
Early/mild impairment stage	Average 1 to 3 years, possibly longer Memory loss, especially with recent events Difficulty with complex cognitive tasks Difficulty with decision making and planning Decreased attention span and concentration Lack of spontaneity and lessening of initiative Impaired word-finding skills Preference for familiar settings
Mid-/moderate impairment stage	Average 5 to 7 years, possibly longer Chronic recent memory loss Difficulty with written and spoken language Tendency to ask questions constantly Tendency to experience visual-spatial perceptual problems Possible delusions, hallucinations, and agitation Increasing difficulty with familiar objects and tasks Assistance with ADL functions necessary Ability to respond to multisensory cueing Tendency to wander, pace, and rummage May get lost at times even inside the house
Late/severe impairment stage	Average 2 to 3 years Dependence on others for ADL functions Ability to respond to hand-over-hand activity Decreased interest in food Difficulty with chewing and swallowing Incontinence Decreased vocabulary Misidentification of familiar objects, persons Impaired ambulation/gait, increased falls Repetitious movement or sounds
Terminal stage	Average 3 months to 1 year Usually in bed or wheelchair Limited ability to track visually Mute or few incoherent words Little spontaneous movement Loss of appetite, severe weight loss Difficulty in swallowing Tendency to utter sounds rather than words Total dependence on others for care Possible development of contractions, skin breakdown Possible reaction to music and touch, fleeting attention span

memory.[11] Recently, concerns have been raised about the growing number of herbal remedies, vitamins, and other dietary supplements being promoted as memory enhancers or interventions for AD. Claims of their effectiveness and safety are based mostly on anecdotal evidence or on very small clinical research studies.[12] Because of unknown side effects or potentially dangerous interactions with prescribed medications, the COTA should encourage the elder and/or caregivers to consult a physician before beginning use of any alternative or complementary medicine approaches. Smith[13] reported that of the 1.7 million residents of nursing homes in the United States, more than half have AD or some other form of dementia. COTAs work with elders who have AD and related dementia in hospitals, nursing homes, assisted living facilities, adult day programs, special care units, and homes. OT intervention for these elders usually focuses on participation in the various areas of occupation by concentrating on performance skills and patterns or modifying activity demands in considerations of various client factors and, the degree possible, within the elder's context and environments.[14]

PERSON-CENTERED AND OCCUPATION-FOCUSED CARE FOR ELDERS WITH ALZHEIMER'S DISEASE

Like all human beings, elders who have AD or related dementia continue to seek meaningful participation in life. Although sometimes the behavior brought on by AD may make it appear as though they no longer are the same elders they once were, it is important to remember that they are not defined by the dementia.[15,16] Personhood, as described by Kitwood,[17] refers to one's sense of self, the "I am" within each person. Kitwood described indicators of personhood and well-being for individuals with dementia, including the assertion of desire or will, the ability to experience and express a range of emotions, initiation of social contact, self-respect, humor, creativity, and self-expression. Person-specific or person-centered care daily supports elders with dementia and enhances and promotes their sense of personhood and meaning in life.[18]

The COTA developing a therapeutic program for elders with dementia individualizes care that supports wellness, strengths, and abilities. This personalized, or person-centered, care also supports the components of activity-focused care that recognizes that all of life is an activity of being and doing or, as OT philosophy articulates it, of seeking meaning through occupation.[14] The tasks of life, therefore, are interconnected. The objectives of occupation-focused care include concentrating on abilities, not limitations; promoting the purposeful and meaningful use of time; supporting the sense of belonging; and enabling verbal and nonverbal communication skills. Occupation-focused care encourages positive behaviors and the development of interventions to refocus unwanted behaviors.[18]

Occupation-focused care redefines interventions, especially in long-term care settings and special care units. Success is achieved through augmenting the client's strengths by reframing expectations and relating to all of daily life tasks as parts of meaningful occupation. It involves the willingness to enter the client's world with sensitivity and flexibility and the provision of holistic support. In this process, the COTA must remain mindful that the goal is for the client to find meaning, not for the caregivers, staff, or OT personnel to understand such meaning.[19]

Communication: Understanding and Being Understood

Communicating with people who have AD is often challenging. As the disease progresses, verbal abilities decrease and communication continues through nonverbal gestures and sounds. Verbal and nonverbal communication reflects the same objectives: expressing thoughts and needs and supporting the elders' self-image and a sense of worth. Other objectives for communication include improving socialization, maximizing quality of life, increasing involvement in a supportive community, understanding others, and promoting safety and comfort. COTAs must care enough to listen carefully. During the early stages of AD, changes that occur in language and communication include the onset of difficulty with using nouns. Substituted words are sometimes used for the noun.[20] For example, Mary was asked to identify an object (a comb). Her response was, "Oh, honey, you know," as she ran her hand through her hair. She was unable to use the noun *comb* but the gesture denoted she knew what the object was.

Reality orientation is usually embarrassing for elders with AD because of their inability to remember and retrieve words to answer questions. One type of response that maintains the dignity of elders with disorientation is to refrain from confronting them with corrections, especially if the confrontation would increase agitation. Caregivers should use creative reality with elders by focusing on the emotions being expressed and responding appropriately by validating feelings. Improvements in orientation and subjective sense of quality of life may result from verbal cues that encourage the person to use information processing rather than factual knowledge.[21]

A strategy called *therapeutic fibs* can be used as illustrated by the following story. Jim states, "My wife is taking me home in 5 minutes." In reality, the intervention session has an additional 30 minutes remaining. Sue, the COTA, agrees with him, stating that he and his wife will soon be together and that he has a wonderful, caring wife. Sue realizes that a discussion of the amount of remaining time would increase Jim's agitation. Sue, having validated Jim's desire for his wife, can then redirect him to do a meaningful task. Elders asking for their mothers or wanting to go home may be seeking acceptance and the need to feel connected. They may also be expressing the need for safety, purposeful use of time, or the company of others. Telling them that their mother is dead or the facility is now their home can upset them. Instead, the COTA may say, "You are safe with me and I will be here today with you. If you are like your mother, she must have been wonderful. I miss my mother too; we used to have fun folding the laundry; perhaps you and I can work together." The purpose of such communication is to acknowledge the meaning or emotion behind an elder's statement.[22]

As the disease progresses, the ability to speak and understand decreases. Some elders become more intuitive, often with increased awareness of people's attitudes and the environment.[23] Therefore, caregivers should be aware of their nonverbal messages such as acting rushed, looking at the clock, sighing, or raising one's voice. In time, elders with AD lose almost all language skills, but they may still occasionally utter a perfectly appropriate statement.[24] For example, Juan talked a lot, but his words were just sounds that made no sense. When a caregiver impatiently spoke to him in an abrupt and firm tone, saying "Juan, time out; go to your room," Juan responded, "In the military, I was in solitary confinement and I can do that standing on my head." The family later confirmed that Juan had indeed been in the military and the story was true. The caregiver's "drill sergeant" tone and body posture triggered Juan's response.

People with AD need to experience acceptance and success, especially as their language skills diminish. COTAs can keep the dialogue going even when the words are few (Box 20-1).[16]

Behavior and Psychosocial Aspects

People with dementia are not "stupid"; they are forgetful and often maintain an inner wisdom. Like anyone else, they have needs and should be approached and cared for with respect. They also should have opportunities for proud and meaningful involvement. Knowledge of the elders' life story often becomes the basis for COTAs to plan and carry out therapy. A "Life Story" book can be used for this purpose. This book can include pictures with captions, lists, favorite recipes, family traditions, schools attended, and military history. Using the book is an excellent tool for connecting with elders and as an intervention to refocus difficult behaviors and to reduce agitation.[25]

The behaviors of people with dementia are often attempts to communicate. For example, increased agitation may be the client's way of communicating illness. Rapid pacing might be a sign of an inability to cope with others, escape from excessive noise, or environmental factors.[26]

Some of the typical behaviors displayed by people with AD include wandering, pacing, and rummaging or redistribution of personal belongings. Combativeness and aggression also can occur. Catastrophic reactions are explosive responses to distress.[5] These reactions result

BOX 20-1

Suggestions for Improving Communication and Connectedness

- Attract the client's attention by using touch and talking to him or her at eye level.
- Use short, simple sentences to express one thought at a time. Be willing to repeat as needed, allowing time for the elder to respond. Do not appear rushed; offer the elder your full attention. Assess and limit distractions from the environment, such as the TV, vacuum cleaners, and loud nearby conversations.[16]
- Be aware that asking questions often can be embarrassing for people with AD, who often have difficulty finding the right words for the answer. Instead, help them respond by giving as many multisensory verbal or nonverbal cues as possible. If asking a question, offer two choices. For example, ask Ella if she would like to shower before breakfast or after breakfast, showing her the towel and clean clothing that you are holding.
- Do not try to apply logic or to give long explanations. Ignore the need to be right, to argue, or to confront. At times having information written down for elders helps them focus and understand, especially when they ask the same question repeatedly. For example, providing Richard with a business type letter with his name on it that states that his apartment has been paid in full and that he has a place to spend the night helps him retain the information. Be willing to supply this letter as often as he needs for reassurance of having a place to stay.
- State requests with positive words ("Please sit here" rather than "Don't sit there").
- Listen carefully to all of the words, gestures, and facial expressions that the person uses. Validate feelings behind the words. For example, if Henry's words seem to make no sense but sound angry and upset, say, "You sound upset, Henry. I know when I feel that way I like a hug. Can I give you a hug?" However, be aware that some people are tactile defensive and become agitated when touched.
- Realize that elders with AD often respond literally to words (because the fire alarm says "pull," Hazel pulls it).
- Be aware that elders with AD often revert to their primary language. COTAs may have to learn appropriate key words in that language to encourage therapy.

from the inability to understand, interpret, and cope with real or imagined situations, people, the environment, or oneself. "Sun-downing" results from a combination of increased behavioral responses occurring in the mid-to-late afternoon. These responses often reflect physical problems such as dehydration and physical/emotional exhaustion. Screaming, yelling, and calling often reflect fear, a need for acceptance, and a lack of active participation and connectedness during the day. Other behavioral manifestations may include inappropriate sexual conduct, hitting or pushing staff or other elders, accusing or demanding speech, withdrawal from activities, and apathy. Elders with AD might also show perseveration in their actions by repetitive movement or sounds, such as wiping or patting the table surface, pulling on clothing, and shouting.[27]

Difficult behaviors are usually not done on purpose as a method of making care more difficult; rather, they are often part of the disease. At times, behaviors can be a problem to others but not to the elder.[28] For example, Betty, who lives in a special care unit, goes into other people's rooms. She looks through their closets and takes clothing and items from their drawers. This behavior suggests that Betty likes to feel in control and is "cleaning up the house." Whose problem is it? Carmen, the owner of these possessions, is angry and feels that her privacy has been invaded. The facility staff meets the challenge of working with both people in a supportive way by identifying acceptable places for Betty to rummage, such as a bureau or desk in the social center and "busy boxes" or baskets filled with safe items. Examples of items to include in a "busy box" are balls of yarn, greeting cards, small scrapbooks, car brochures, maps, catalogs, fabric pieces, and carpet samples. Having Betty participate in the purposeful activity of carrying safe items can help address her need to feel connected.

A respectful response exists for every behavior. In some cases, attempting to reason with people with AD may not work, especially if they mistake others for people whom they do not like. Logic also may not work, especially with people who are having visual or auditory hallucinations.[29] Usually, COTAs can identify the event that precipitated the unwanted behavior and make adjustments that might prevent it, stop it, or decrease the likelihood of recurrence. Three problem-solving tools can help refocus unwanted behavior: the behavioral profile, the behavioral analysis, and the behavioral observation form.

The behavioral profile is a tool used to examine the situation. COTAs can ask themselves the following thought-provoking questions: What exactly is happening? Why has the behavior happened, and what was the antecedent? Who is involved, and where is the behavior exhibited? When does the behavior usually occur? What now? (Box 20-2).

The behavioral analysis outlines the specific behavior by focusing on the client's actions and defining the antecedent or possible causes. In addition, it outlines acceptable approaches and interventions with attention to the impact on the family, environment, and activity (Table 20-2).

The behavior observation form is used to determine a behavioral pattern involving the time of day and possible antecedents. This form can help COTAs and other health

BOX 20-2

Behavior Profile
▪ WHAT exactly is happening? ▪ WHY has the behavior happened? ▪ WHAT was the antecedent? ▪ WHO is involved? ▪ WHERE is the behavior exhibited? ▪ WHEN does the behavior usually occur? ▪ WHAT now?

care workers make appropriate changes for reducing or refocusing difficult behaviors (Figure 20-1).

The challenge of identifying the source of the difficult or unwanted behavior and a solution to the problem also requires critical reasoning. The following are some questions that COTAs can ask themselves to help with the critical reasoning process: What is this behavior "saying"? Whose problem is it? What are some environmental factors that might be contributing to the behavior?

The story of Alfonso, an elder in an AD special care unit, illustrates the importance of critical reasoning in addressing difficult or unwanted behaviors. Alfonso tries constantly to go out of the door because he thinks it is time to go to work. Possible reasons for his attempts to leave include the time of day, that he sees visitors leaving with their hats and coats, and lack of involvement in meaningful activities. The staff may not be trained to redirect him when his anxiety and agitation increases, the day room may be too noisy, or he may believe that the intercom voice is calling him to the phone. The COTA might consider the following options: asking him to help with a project (he might forget his need to leave), painting the exit door the same color as the walls on either side so it appears less obvious, involving Alfonso in a meaningful activity (drawing ideas from his life story), and spending some quality time with Alfonso.

Audrey is another person in the same unit. She often becomes combative when performing ADL functions, especially showering. In fact, she strikes the COTA during an assessment of showering. The COTA considers possible causes for this behavior: Did Audrey formerly take baths, and is she unhappy with the change in her routine? Is Audrey a very private person, and is she embarrassed that someone is helping her? Did she react to the COTA's tone of voice? Is Audrey getting sick and unable to report it? Is she too tired when the shower is scheduled? Is she experiencing chronic pain such as arthritis, which may be upsetting her? Does she feel rushed? Has the showering task been simplified enough so that she can participate and feel in control? The COTA then considers the following behavioral interventions: asking Audrey to help wash down the shower, singing Audrey's favorite hymn with her while she showers, postponing the shower for another

TABLE 20-2

Problem: Pacing, or Wandering, or Both (Behavior Analysis Approach)	
Behaviors exhibited	Pacing with increases in speed, intensity, and length of time; unable to respond to normal fatigue Trying to exit area without supervision Displaying increased agitation, anxiety, frustration, pushing, or kicking Seemingly lost; packing and leaving Searching behavior for something unattainable (for example, mother) Inappropriately going into areas/rooms not their own
Possible cause or antecedent	May have feelings of fearfulness, insecurity May be reflecting on a past life role such as being in the workforce or being a parent May want to escape May be feeling out of control or sensing overmanipulation by others May be searching for something familiar or something lost May be acting consistent with former habits (always "on the go") or doing a stress-reducing activity May reflect need for self-stimulation as a method to reestablish sense of well-being May be expressing a physical need such as hunger, constipation, or illness May result from anxiety, boredom, hyperenvironmental or hypoenvironmental stimulation
Interventions with the resident	Ask what the wandering is "telling" you: whether the client is hungry, needs to void, feels uncomfortable, is really lost. Identify positive aspects of the pacing/wandering. When attempting redirection, use a calm approach with eye contact. Use distraction techniques to break up the pacing pattern (offer to sit with the elder, have a glass of juice). Monitor elders for unwanted weight loss and excessive fatigue. Monitor elders for increased risks for falls and compromised safety. Have elders wear Medic-Alert ID bracelet of Alzheimer's Association's "Safe Return" program. Take photographs for the police, if elopement is a factor. Avoid stressful situations such as excessive environmental stimulation, too many people present, or overwhelming demands. Provide regular and consistent routines with familiar staff and caregivers. Develop a "head count" system for elders at high risk for elopement.
Family/ caregiver focus	Discuss treatment approaches. Provide information on policies and procedures. Provide information such as the phone number of the local Alzheimer's Association chapter and their "Safe Return" program. Instruct not to contradict the elder's stories; instead, they should assure the elder that everything will be all right. This helps facilitate a sense of security and reduces feelings of fearfulness. Recommend to not overdramatize entrances, exits, and promises to return. Encourage walks with the elder and usage of walking areas, "discover" paths or fitness trails. Inform of possible risks for elopement even when the treatment area has a security system. Encourage use of local support groups for discussions with others.
Facility adaptations	Provide environmental changes and sensory stimulation to decrease stress and restlessness, and to increase physical well-being, gross motor skills, appetite, and healthy fatigue. Allow for environmental changes that promote purposeful ways to spend time. Remove environmental cues that suggest leaving the facility, such as coats and suitcases. Use familiar objects in rooms that facilitate a sense of comfort and security. Install Dutch doors, if permitted by regulations. Design walking areas, "discover" paths, or fitness trails within the care setting that offer safe, monitored spaces for pacing. Develop procedures to follow such as periodic unit safety checks and checks for missing persons. Provide routine orientation and escorts for new admissions. Alert visitors to facility procedures. For example, when leaving an area visitors should turn around and check that wandering elders have not followed them out of the door. Employ experienced, trained staff who know the elders. Introduce the elder to all staff, especially those near the doors (for example, switchboard operators and receptionists). Write problems/interventions on a Kardex after identifying any positive aspects from the physical activity of pacing and wandering.

TABLE 20-2

Problem: Pacing, or Wandering, or Both (Behavior Analysis Approach)—cont'd	
Activity	Support physical exercise to promote overall wellness. Offer to walk with the elder as a meaningful activity. Suggest that the elder help out by taking letters to be mailed, visiting a friend, or picking up laundry. Establish a walking club, keep track of miles walked, and provide club t-shirts. Provide supervised outings with a focus on safety and the reduction of elopement risks. Offer expressive arts that include large muscle groups and movement or dancing activities. Present routine, familiar, normalized activities that promote sense of connectedness, respect, and meaningfulness. Set up a fitness trail that includes repetitive upper and lower extremity movements such as doing pulley activities, finger climbing ladders, and deep knee bends. Train volunteers and family members to involve the elders with the trail's activities.

Name:						
Date	Time	Observed activity and behavior	Behavior			Observer
			Trigger (What started it)	Intervention (What stopped it)	Time elapsed •Before stopping •Stayed stopped	

FIGURE 20-1 Behavioral observation form.

time, and allowing Audrey to bathe with some of her clothes on or wrapping her in a bath blanket during the bathing process.

As illustrated by the preceding examples, handling the behavioral difficulties of elders who have AD can be a trial-and-error process until COTAs identify solutions that work. Each elder will respond differently. Different techniques, based on the person's abilities, can succeed one time and fail the next. Even when COTAs cannot ascertain the exact reason for the behaviors, they can try the following intervention techniques. Distraction is a helpful technique, especially if the person is agitated.

COTAs can be creative with ideas for distraction that involve the person in a meaningful activity, such as listening to music or offering a snack. Rescuing is another distraction technique: When one caregiver is in conflict with the client, a second caregiver responds by "rescuing" that person. This technique is illustrated by the following example. Sally, a nursing assistant, says to Theresa, the resident, "Don't go out the door." If Amy, the COTA, approaches Theresa in the same fashion, Theresa might feel outnumbered. Conversely, if Amy says, "Sally, Theresa and I want to be alone; please leave us," Theresa might feel "rescued" and go with Amy.

Inappropriate timing, attempts to manipulate the elder to fit a schedule, and unrealistic performance expectations can cause negative behavior such as hitting. Consequently, caregivers must be aware of the elder's mood before approaching with an ADL or social event.

INTERVENTION

Observations, Screening, and Assessment

As with any OT client, the first step in the OT process is of assessment and development of the client's occupational profile. The profile "provides an understanding of the client's occupational history and experiences, patterns of daily living, interests, values, and needs. The client's problems and concerns about performing occupations and daily life activities are identified, and the client's priorities are determined."[14] Later, the registered occupational therapist (OTR)/COTA team should analyze the elder's occupational performance to identity his or her assets, problems, or potential problems more specifically. During this phase of the evaluation, "actual performance is often observed in context to identify what supports performance and what hinders performance. Performance skills, performance patterns, context or contexts, activity demands, and client factors are all considered, but only selected aspects may be specifically assessed."[14] This helps the team identify targeted outcomes.

The OTR/COTA team may collaborate in the administration of the following evaluations among others. The Folstein Mini-Mental State is a short and simple quantitative measure of cognitive performance. This measure is a questionnaire in five areas of cognition, including orientation, registration (memory), attention, and calculation, as well as recall and language (following oral and written instructions).[30] The Global Deterioration Scale measures clinical characteristics at seven levels based on the progressive stages of AD.[31]

The Allen Cognitive Performance Tests and the Routine Task Inventory examine cognitive function through the completion of tasks.[32] The levels of function help predict behavior and effects on ADL functions. These levels range from the ability to use complex information and perform ADL functions accurately and safely to severe deficits in recognition and use of familiar objects. This assessment includes information on communication, response to tasks, and need for task simplification. It also addresses the role of the therapist during intervention. (See Chapter 7 for a more detailed explanation of these tests.)

The Cognitive Performance Test is a standardized functional assessment instrument designed for the evaluation of Allen cognitive levels.[33] Six functional tasks—dressing, shopping, making toast, making phone calls, doing laundry, and traveling—comprise the test. This test also looks at the person's abilities to process information in relation to functional performance.

The importance of the COTA being an integral part of the overall treatment team with other disciplines cannot be stressed enough.[34,35] The continuous development of dementia-specific assessments provides the treatment team with sensitive, appropriate tools that not only bring together information about the elder's challenges, but also encourage the recognition of the client's personhood and how to build on current strengths and abilities.[36,32] For example, the Person, Environment, Occupation measurement model helps determine how AD affects the function of both the person with disease and his or her family.[37]

Intervention Planning

OT for people with AD most often involves attention to participation in self-care and leisure occupations, consideration of communication and functional mobility, and careful regard for safety. Areas to address in intervention planning include decreased attention span, the inability to initiate tasks, difficulty with sequencing tasks, impaired judgment, and overall wellness. Intervention planning begins with establishing a cognitive and functional baseline and includes ability-based goals. These goals should identify functional capacity and needs to restore, maintain, or improve skills. The goals should focus on abilities and opportunities for participation in activities that support cognitive, physical, and psychosocial wellness. These goals should include interventions that enable person-centered caregiving and refocus difficult behaviors in a supportive and safe environment.

Intervention planning should include the use of assessment and observation to measure changes in functional status. The process of intervention planning includes providing and suggesting continuous modifications and adaptations of approaches, such as task simplification and cueing. The elder's life story may be used as the basis for intervention that focuses on past (and present) wisdom and experiences. Intervention planning also involves assessing all aspects of intervention support and factors that lead to negative responses, including environmental components.[38] For example, Andrew's limited attention span prohibited him from eating more than a few mouthfuls of each meal. He was seated in a large dining room with five other people at his table. Music was played on the tape deck, and the staff often talked loudly with each other. When the COTA suggested relocating Andrew to a small dining area where the tables seated two and reducing the environmental stimulation, he was able to focus on his food and complete his meal.

Intervention Implementation

OT interventions consider the effects of dementia on the elder's cognitive abilities and well-being. Success with interventions entails many crucial components, including the COTA's flexibility and creativity. Success may need to be redefined, as exemplified by Beverly, a resident of a special care unit. Beverly liked to wear a yellow floral blouse and her favorite orange and black plaid skirt. She was proud of her ability to select and dress independently, although some disapproved of her choices.

Equally important for successful intervention is the COTA's nonverbal approach. It should reflect acceptance and respect for the elder with AD. To ensure success, intervention should not place elders in situations in which their inabilities may lead to failure. For example, Clara had always been a talented knitter of lovely sweaters. Her ability to do intricate stitches became impaired as her dementia progressed. The COTA set up the stitches on large needles and helped her get started knitting squares using a basic stitch. Clara was able to knit the simple squares for a baby blanket and was delighted in the recognition of her success. This activity could be further adapted by involving Clara in winding yarn as her knitting abilities diminish.

Applying life history and experiences to functional abilities also is meaningful. For example, Sara, a 78-year-old mother of five, responds to normalization activities such as washing dishes, hanging laundry, and sweeping floors. These activities provide tactile stimulation, lower and upper body range of motion, strengthening, trunk stabilization, and fine hand motor skills.

COTAs can use their skills in analyzing activities to identify steps toward task simplification. Harry was able to dress himself independently when each item of clothing was placed on his bed in the appropriate sequence for dressing. Successful intervention also should focus on working with elders to promote active participation and collaboration. Charles had lost interest in feeding himself but accepted the COTA's suggestion to have the caregiver place a hand over his hand. That way he could continue to feed himself with assistance rather than being fed by others.

When possible, intervention should be provided in appropriate and familiar settings.[39] For example, Millie was unable to experience success with simple dressing tasks when she attempted them in the clinic. However, when the COTA arrived at Millie's bedside early each morning, Millie was able to use visual cues found in her bedroom, including the bureau and closet, to trigger self-dressing skills.

Activities of Daily Living

COTAs can make a significant contribution to the well-being of elders with AD and enhance their quality of life by supporting ADL occupations. Understanding the activity's demands, breaking down and simplifying tasks, and so on, enables these elders to become involved in performing these familiar skills. This understanding can be facilitated by using one-step commands and visual cueing, including objects or gestures. The use of the Allen's stage levels can be a helpful measure of the elder's level of functioning.[40]

Difficulties with ADL occupations associated with dementia include a decreased attention span, limited ability to follow directions, and increased length of time to complete tasks. Other difficulties include problems with sequencing, perception, and body awareness. Emotional responses of fear, paranoia, and reactions to excessive environmental stimulation that are real or imagined also can influence ADL functioning. Aggressive behavior of elders with cognitive impairments can significantly affect ADL outcomes.[22]

Modifications in the ways in which people with Alzheimer's dementia carry out daily activities can help maintain their independence longer and even regain some lost function. Further maintaining engagement in meaningful activities for longer periods of time reduces dementia-related behaviors such as screaming, wandering, and physical aggression. The consistent use of directed verbal prompts and positive reinforcement maximizes ADL functional status, particularly with feeding.[41] COTAs working on ADL functions will be most successful when they use creative problem solving. Therapy requires working with elders, not doing to or for them.[16] COTAs should do everything possible to make ADL functions meaningful. The use of distraction techniques (for example, singing and holding items such as costume jewelry, scarves, and neckties) should be part of daily care. The COTA's attitude, approach, and direct involvement are key components in supporting the elder's quality of life.

COTAs should consider the timing when working on ADL functions. Often, these decisions are based on knowing the elder and responding to nonverbal language that suggests the best and worst times for these activities. Sometimes, COTAs must come back several times because many elders with AD are sensitive to being rushed. For example, Charles appeared agitated when the COTA wanted to work on dressing skills. After several attempts the COTA decided to return later. At that time, Charles was calmer and accepting of the activity.

Assisting with ADL functions can also provide opportunities for COTAs to monitor the elder's physical well-being and safety. Elders with AD often do not report bruises, rashes, and blisters. Decreased cognitive ability and judgment, combined with an unawareness of perceptual difficulties, may lead to unsafe situations. Elders may eat dirt or plants, walk on wet floors, put their shoes on the wrong feet, forget necessary items such as glasses, misjudge a chair seat and fall, or scald themselves in the shower because they do not know how to turn on the cold water—all of these are examples of potential dangers.

When working with elders on ADL functions, COTAs should always focus on abilities by encouraging active involvement. The techniques of hand-over-hand guidance, chaining, and bridging can be used. Hand-over-hand guidance may help the elder complete the ADL task. With chaining, the caregiver begins a task by putting one hand over the elder's hand and continuing until the elder can take over and complete the task. For example, Astrid had no idea what a toothbrush was or how to use it.

However, when the COTA placed it in her hand and guided it to her mouth to start the brushing action, Astrid was able to complete the task independently. With these techniques the palmar surfaces of the hand or the surface receiving touch during a handshake can be a more "accepting" surface than the back of the hand. COTAs should establish contact with the elder's palm before moving their hand around to the dorsal surface if needed for assisting the elder during activities.

With bridging, elders who are unable to perform any part of the daily living task can focus their attention by holding the same object the caregiver is using. This technique also can help to decrease anxiety. For example, Allan could not shave. The COTA demonstrated to the caregivers a bridging technique to try with Allan. She placed a turned-on electric razor in his hand so he could feel the vibration while she shaved him with another electric razor. By holding a razor, Allan was better able to focus attention on the task.[16]

The creativity and flexibility of COTAs can promote the remaining abilities of elders and their willingness to be actively involved in daily life tasks (Table 20-3). Knowledge of the client's past routines is helpful during ADL functions.

Using Adapted Equipment

Elders with AD often refuse or misuse adapted equipment. Improper use may affect the elder's safety, especially if the item does not look familiar. For example, a plate guard may appear so strange that the elder with AD might

TABLE 20-3

Suggestions for Provision of Activities of Daily Living Support for Elders with Alzheimer's Disease	
Bathing	Know whether client prefers a bath or shower; use handheld shower head.
	If privacy is an issue, elder can bathe with some clothing on or with a bath blanket.
	If needed, elder may wash one part of the body per day until able to accept total bathing.
	Consider safety by using adaptations such as bath seats, grab bars, and floor mats.
	Create a warm and homelike bathing environment. Placing colorful beach towels on the walls can help reduce the room's echo and loud water sounds. The towels also can be used to wrap elders if they become agitated during clothing removal.
	Consider alternatives such as having a family member present to assist with bathing to help reduce the elder's anxiety.
Shaving	Use a mirror unless elders do not recognize themselves or feel that they are being "watched."
	Use a bridging technique with elders incapable of actually shaving. Have them hold an electric razor that they can see, feel, and hear while shaving them with another electric shaver.
Oral care	Use a child-sized tooth brush.
	Pretend to be brushing your own teeth and encourage elders to mirror the activity.
	Use bridging technique of asking the elder to hold an extra set of dentures while removing the elder's dentures.
	Set up a simulated dental chair and announce that the dentist has sent you to assist with dental care.
	Set up a monitor system so that presence of dentures are checked after each meal in case elders have wrapped them up in a napkin for disposal.
Dressing	Suggest clothing one size larger for dressing ease. Keep the clothes appropriate to the elder's past lifestyle.
	Use verbal and visual cues to simplify each step, and always thank the elders for helping.
	If elders become anxious, ask them to show you how the clothing items are put on.
	If possible, use washable shoes with Velcro closures.
	Use 100% cotton clothing because it does not retain the odor of urine.
	Ask the elder to sit when dressing, especially if balance is a concern.
Toileting	Be aware of elder's past toileting routines and habits.
	Use pictures of toilets with the word "toilet" on the bathroom doors.
	Determine whether the bathroom mirror prohibits elders from using the toilet because they do not recognize their image and think someone else is there.
	Be sure the toilet seat color contrasts with the floor. Change the seat or use a washable rug around the toilet base.
	Use key words to remind the elder about the task. Often, the words they used when toilet training their children work well.
	Offer the elder something (for example, a magazine) to hold or do while seated on the toilet.
	Never refer to pads for incontinence as "diapers" (use terms such as panties or shorts).
	Have different types of incontinence products available. Don't assume that a full-sized item is needed immediately. For example, a pad placed within a panty can be used if urine is leaked.
	Use suspenders to keep full-sized incontinence products in place.

TABLE 20-3

Suggestions for Provision of Activities of Daily Living Support for Elders with Alzheimer's Disease—cont'd

Eating*	Observe eating for safety problems such as overstuffing the mouth, not chewing before swallowing, and eating nonedibles (napkins, foam cups). If the elder is storing food in the mouth, check for a clear swallow. Obtain a swallowing evaluation if a problem is apparent.
	Offer the meal in a quiet area to decrease distractions and to improve attention span. If the food needs to be set up, always do that out of the elder's sight. This prevents reinforcement of the elder's inability to perform certain simple tasks.
	Provide color contrast between the food and the plate and the plate and the table.
	Avoid plastic utensils, which are easily bitten and broken.
	Obtain, if appropriate, a dietary order for variation in food textures.
	Simplify the meal by serving one item and one utensil at a time.
	If elders will not sit to eat, use finger foods or have a small bowl that can be easily carried.
	Incorporate food into a sandwich. Pureed food can be put into an ice cream cone to assist elders who want to continue self-feeding.
	If elders are not eating and no medical reasons prohibit it, use sugar or honey on the food to increase palatability.
	After a swallowing evaluation, if deemed appropriate, provide non-salty chicken or beef broth that can be poured over the food for a more "slurpy" consistency to facilitate an appropriate swallow.
	If the elder needs to be fed, bridge the task by having the elder hold a spoon or plastic cup.
	If the elder is disinterested in eating, alternate bites of hot and cold foods and sweet and nonsweet food.
	When the elder appears to stop eating or has lost all interest in food, ask the family to identify the elder's "comfort foods" to facilitate reinterest in eating.
	Foods such as mashed potatoes and gravy, pizza, and macaroni give a sense of well-being.
	If weight loss is a problem, double the elder's breakfast.
	Try to avoid commercial food supplements, if possible, by allowing time for the meal to be eaten and providing protein-enriched foods such as milkshakes.
	Sit with the elders. Have something to eat or drink to reduce elders' anxiety that you don't have anything to eat and therefore must have some of theirs.
	If elders refuse to eat because of not having money, provide a letter stating that their dues to your association (the name of your facility or place of practice) have been paid in full and meals are included in their membership.

*See discussion of dysphagia in Chapter 18 for more specific information about safe eating.

spend the mealtime trying to remove it from the plate. Sometimes, large, built-up handles on eating utensils may feel so different that clients do not use them. Reachers and other metal devices used for ADL functions can be used as weapons. Flatware with large handles and scoop dishes can be helpful because they closely resemble their ordinary counterparts. Adapting the environment by using color contrast between objects, pictures, words, labels, and arrows is often the best way to cue for successful involvement in ADL functions.

Using Activities to Promote Well-Being

Activities can be adapted for individuals and groups. The objectives of therapeutic activities are enhancing meaning, encouraging active participation, and ensuring success. All of life's activities can be used as intervention modalities. Suggestions for cognitive activities are adapted trivia games, word puzzles, rhyming games, singing of familiar songs, and reminiscence. Others include spelling games, simple crafts, clothes-sorting, cards, and Life Story "book

clubs." Suggestions for physical activities include parachute exercises; dancing; and tossing, hitting, and kicking balls and balloons. An exercise program may include the use of handheld wands, light weights, scarves, and fabrics. Psychosocial activities include parties, service projects, grooming tasks, celebrations of special days, field trips, and pet care. Worship and related spiritual activities may offer elders with dementia a sense of the familiar, well-being, and security. Recommendations for normalizing activities are folding and hanging up laundry, dusting and sweeping, sorting silverware, and shining shoes.[16]

Environment-based interventions appear to have some positive effect on reducing agitation of people with dementia. Simulations of a natural environment (e.g., use of recorded sounds of babbling brooks, birds, and other small animals; large pictures of the outdoors) during bathing reduce agitation and can improve the relationship between caregivers and the individual.[42] There is some evidence that ambient, nonvocal music has some calming effect on people with AD.[43] The OTR/COTA team should consider this intervention as part of a multisensory stimulation program or as part of the background feature of a dining room, for example. However, music selection may need to be matched to the person's taste. Because of the low cost, these types of intervention could be implemented in institutional, community, or home settings.

Communication with and Teaching Caregivers

OT intervention with elders who have AD focuses on maintaining functional abilities and preventing secondary complications. These objectives can be achieved by tailoring communication and education to caregivers. About 9.8 million family members, friends, and neighbors provide 8.4 billion hours of unpaid care for persons with AD each year. This care is estimated to make an annual contribution to the nation valued at 89 billion dollars.[44] About 60% of unpaid caregivers are wives, daughters, daughters-in-law, granddaughters, and other female relatives, friends, and neighbors. At any one time, 32% of family and other unpaid caregivers of people with AD have been providing help for 5 years or longer, and 39% have been providing care for 1 to 4 years.[45]

Caregivers benefit from a variety of techniques, including written instruction and demonstration. The instructional method of requiring a "return demonstration" allows COTAs to observe first-hand that caregivers follow through with activities. Afterward, the COTA can make necessary suggestions or corrections. As the dementia progresses, caregivers provide more and more care, until they can no longer manage their caregiving responsibilities on their own. Caring for a person with AD is often very difficult, and caregivers have high rates of anxiety, stress, and burnout.[46] Their life expectancy is reduced, and at least a third are depressed.[47,48,49] Encouraging caregivers to strengthen their social support system for the long term should be a basic component of OT intervention.[50] A basic occupational therapy plan for people with AD should include providing caregivers with information about progression of disease, referral to community resources, practical ideas for caregiving, and understanding of how the caregiving role is different from other family roles.[51]

The COTA/OTR team can formulate a maintenance program.[52] Contributing to a maintenance program may require COTAs to sensitize caregivers to the nature and progression of AD. An understanding of task breakdown and simplification, activity modification, behavioral interventions, supportive communications, and the need for flexibility is essential in maintenance programs.

TERMINAL STAGE ISSUES

Severe dementia, or terminal stage, is exhibited when the elder is oriented only to person and depends entirely on others for self-care. Defining the exact time of terminal, or end-stage, AD is difficult because of changes and variations in the disease process.[53] For example, Vernon appeared to have entered the terminal stage because he

had been refusing food for 2 weeks. When offered familiar "comfort" foods from his past and sweet foods, he suddenly started to eat again.

Many elders at the terminal stage of AD are kept in bed or positioned in wheelchairs or recliners. Unfortunately, those kept in bed often lie in the fetal position. These elders are dependent on others for basic life functions and display an almost total loss of communication skills or the ability to express pain.[54] To help make them more comfortable, COTAs may provide positioning suggestions and passive range-of-motion exercises. A caring touch, hand-over-hand movement, and various sensory activities may produce a response. Some people become ill with symptoms leading to pneumonia or other systemic problems shortly before death. This is an important time for supporting family members and staff caregivers.[50]

REIMBURSEMENT FOR SERVICES

A functional outcome must be meaningful, utilitarian, and sustainable over time. Currently, the maintenance of remaining abilities of elders with dementia, or any chronic illness, is not usually covered by third-party payers such as Medicare unless there is a need for "skilled" therapeutic coverage. Elders on Medicare Part A in Skilled Nursing Facilities under the Prospective Payment System (PPS) may qualify for therapy on the basis of their determined level of resources needed with the Resource Utilization Groups (see Chapter 6 for more details on the PPS system).[55] For elders on Medicare Part B, the COTA/OTR team may address cognitive and physical impairment related to functional performance. Medicare will reimburse for cognitive disabilities that require "complex and sophisticated knowledge to identify current and potential capabilities."[55] All levels of assistance from total to standby address both physical and cognitive components. Table 20-4 outlines the cognitive components only. Behavioral issues with cognitive impairment can be focused on if they require skilled OT services.[55]

The COTA/OTR team may suggest a short-range program on the basis of continuous functional support, especially if a change in functional status has occurred. Often, elders with AD who receive Medicare reimbursement for care have an initial evaluation from OT. A maintenance program is then developed by the therapists and carried out by facility staff. Medicare will reimburse if skilled OT is needed to evaluate a "complex" patient to increase function or safety, and then to train staff to carry out the program.[55] The OTR evaluates the elder and establishes the plan of care. The COTA may train caregivers to carry out the plan. OT practitioners may manage the elder for reevaluation when significant changes occur in functional status. As discussed in Chapter 6, memorandums from Medicare prevent automatic denials just because a person has the diagnosis of AD and mention benefits for therapeutic intervention with this diagnosis.[55]

TABLE 20-4

	Medicare Cognitive Levels of Assistance	
Assistance level	**Cognitive assistance**
Total assistance	Total assistance is the need for 100% assistance by one or more persons to perform all cognitive assistance to elicit a functional response to an external stimulation. A cognitively impaired patient requires total assistance when documentation shows external stimuli are required to elicit automatic actions such as swallowing or responding to auditory stimuli. Skills of an occupational therapist are needed to identify and apply strategies for eliciting appropriate, consistent automatic responses to external stimuli.
Maximal assistance	Maximum assistance is the need for 75% cognitive assistance to perform gross motor actions in response to direction. A cognitively impaired patient, at this level, may need proprioceptive stimulation and/or one-to-one demonstration by the occupational therapist because of the patient's lack of cognitive awareness of other people or objects.
Minimum assistance	Moderate assistance is the need for 50% assistance by one person or constant cognitive assistance to sustain/complete simple, repetitive activities safely. The records submitted should state how a cognitively impaired patient requires intermittent one-to-one demonstration or intermittent cueing (physical or verbal) throughout the activity. Moderate assistance is needed when the occupational therapist/caregiver needs to be in the immediate environment to progress the patient through a sequence to complete an activity. This level of assistance is required to halt continued repetition of a task and to prevent unsafe, erratic, or unpredictable actions that interfere with appropriate sequencing.
Standby assistance	Standby assistance is the need for supervision by one person for the patient to perform new procedures adapted by the therapist for safe and effective performance. A patient requires such assistance when errors are demonstrated or the need for safety precautions is not always anticipated by the patient.
Independent status	Independent status means that no physical or cognitive assistance is required to perform functional activities. Patients at this level are able to implement the selected courses of action, demonstrate lack of errors, and anticipate safety hazards in familiar and new situations.

The Physical Levels of Assistance are not included in this chart.
From Centers for Medicare and Medicaid Services (CMS). (2008). Medicare program integrity manual [WWW page]. Retrieved November 22, 2009, from www.cms.hhs.gov/manuals/downloads/pim83c06.pdf.

CONCLUSION

COTAs can make a unique contribution to elders with AD. COTAs can treat these elders from the initial stages of forgetfulness and poor judgment by offering strategies for continuing independence. COTAs may also provide advice about late-stage care by focusing on positioning, feeding, and responses to sensory activities. Understanding the changes that occur as dementia progresses challenges elders, caregivers, and families to pursue creative and supportive solutions for daily care. The holistic programs and care provided by COTAs support the abilities and well-being of elders. When offered occupation-focused care, elders with dementia can have meaningful lives.

CASE STUDY

Mildred is 78 years of age and has mid-stage AD. Mildred was formerly a teacher and experienced a happy family life with her husband of 58 years and their two sons. She has been widowed for the last 5 years. Mildred was originally brought to the special care unit where she currently resides when she was found wandering outside during the cold winter months.

At the special care unit the COTA helped assess Mildred's functional status. The COTA identified the following abilities:

Mildred follows one-step directions, responds to multisensory cueing, maintains strong socialization skills, and refers to her former profession by often mentioning her past role as a teacher. She also mentions her past interest in the activities of cooking and sewing.

Mildred functions at Allen's Cognitive Level 3. The COTA observed that she was forgetful, with limited instructional carryover. Mildred experiences problems with sequencing ADL functions. She often becomes anxious, which leads to combativeness during ADL functions, especially bathing. Other assessment findings included the inability to toilet independently and use multiple utensils with meals. Communication challenges included receptive and expressive understanding of words, especially nouns.

The COTA instructed all staff members who work with Mildred to consider her strengths, as well as her attention span deficits and feelings of depression, as she attempts to cope with her disease.

■ CASE STUDY QUESTIONS

1 Considering Mildred's case, how can visual triggers and written phrases be used to help Mildred be as independent as possible?
2 What anxiety-reducing approaches can be explored? What specific interventions can be used during bathing?

3 How can the COTA develop a system for sequencing Mildred's clothing?

4 What environmental issues might need to be addressed, especially in the bath/shower room?

5 What suggestions can be incorporated as mealtime interventions for promoting successful dining?

6 If Mildred can find the toilet, what strategies can enable her to remain continent?

7 How can the COTA use ADL functions as therapeutic modalities for reducing feelings of depression and helplessness?

8 How can the COTA make Mildred's care "person-centered" and "activity-focused"?

■ CHAPTER REVIEW QUESTIONS

1 In reference to the entire chapter, what are the basic symptoms of AD, and how do they affect elders with the disease and their caregivers?

2 Identify six ways to facilitate communication with elders who have dementia.

3 How can a functional assessment be used to develop intervention goals?

4 List three guidelines for the provision of ADL support to elders functioning at the mid-stage level of AD.

5 Outline six specific mealtime adaptations for elders with a short attention span.

6 List steps for getting dressed using task simplification.

7 What are possible antecedents and appropriate interventions for agitation?

8 Why do people with dementia wander, and how can the risk for elopement be decreased?

9 Give specific examples of ways that activity-focused care supports COTAs' interventions.

10 Describe strategies to adapt the activity of folding laundry to address the elder's cognitive, physical, psychosocial, and normalization needs.

REFERENCES

1. Alzheimer's Association, 2009. Alzheimer's disease facts and figures. Alzheimer's & Dementia 5 (3), 234-270.
2. Jolley, D., 2009. The epidemiology of dementia. Practice Nursing 20 (Suppl. 6), S4-S6.
3. Shackle, S., 2009. Alzheimer's: The facts. New Statesman 138 (4931), 29-37.
4. Alzheimer's Disease International, 2009. World Alzheimer's report 2009: Executive summary. Author, London, England.
5. Neugroschl, J., Sano, M., 2009. An update on treatment and prevention strategies for Alzheimer's disease. Current Neurology and Neuroscience Reports 9 (5), 368-376.
6. Leifer, B., 2009. Alzheimer's disease: Seeing the signs early. Journal of the American Academy of Nurse Practitioners 21 (11), 588-595.
7. Alzheimer's Association, 2009. What is Alzheimer's? Retrieved November 22, 2009, from http://www.alz.org/alzheimers_disease_what_is_alzheimers.asp.
8. Grossberg, G., Kamat, S., 2007. Alzheimer's: The Latest Assessment and Treatment Strategies. Jones & Bartlett, Sudbury, MA.
9. Caroli, A., Frisoni, G., 2009. Quantitative evaluation of Alzheimer's disease. Expert Review of Medical Devices 6 (5), 569-588.
10. Davatzikos, C., Xu, F., An, Y., Fan, Y., Resnick, S., 2009. Longitudinal progression of Alzheimer's-like patterns of atrophy in normal older adults: the SPARE-AD index. Brain: A Journal of Neurology 132 (8), 2026-2035.
11. Kurz, A., Perneczky, R., 2009. Neurobiology of cognitive disorders. Current Opinion in Psychiatry 22 (6), 546-551.
12. Chiappelli, F., Navarro, A., Moradi, D., Manfrini, E., Prolo, P., 2006. Evidence-based research in complementary and alternative medicine III: Treatment of patients with Alzheimer's disease. Evidence-Based Complementary and Alternative Medicine 3 (4), 411-424.
13. Smith, D., 2009. Treatment of Alzheimer's disease in the long-term-care setting. American Journal of Health-System Pharmacy 66 (10), 899-907.
14. American Occupational Therapy Association, 2008. Occupational therapy practice framework: Domain and process, 2nd ed. American Journal of Occupational Therapy 62, 625-683.
15. Edvardsson, D., Winblad, B., Sandman, P., 2008. Person-centered care of people with severe Alzheimer's disease: Current status and ways forward. Lancet Neurology 7 (4), 362-367.
16. Hellen, C.R., 1998. Alzheimer's Disease: Activity-Focused Care. Butterworth-Heinemann, St. Louis, MO.
17. Kitwood, T., 1998. Toward a theory of dementia care: Ethics and interaction. Journal of Clinical Ethics 9 (1), 23-34.
18. Fazio, L., 2007. Developing Occupation-Centered Programs for the Community, 2nd ed. Prentice Hall, New York.
19. Murray, L., Boyd, S., 2008. Protecting personhood and achieving quality of life for older adults with dementia in the U.S. health care system. Journal of Aging and Health 21 (2), 350-373.
20. Schmidt, K., Lingler, J., Schulz, R., 2009. Verbal communication among Alzheimer's disease patients, their caregivers, and primary care physicians during primary care office visits. Patient Education and Counseling 77 (2), 197-201.
21. Spector, A., Thorgrtimsen, L., Woods, B., Royan, L., Davies, S., Butterworth, M., et al., 2003. Efficacy of an evidence-based cognitive stimulation therapy program for people with dementia. British Journal of Psychiatry 183, 248-254.
22. Ballard, C., Corbett, A., Chitramohan, R., Aarsland, D., 2009. Management of agitation and aggression associated with Alzheimer's disease: Controversies and possible solutions. Current Opinion in Psychiatry 22 (6), 532-540.
23. Hopper, T., 2001. Indirect interventions to facilitate communication in Alzheimer's disease. Seminars in Speech and Language 22 (4), 305-315.
24. Small, J., Gutman, G., Makela, S., Hillhouse, B., 2003. Effectiveness of communication strategies used by caregivers of persons with Alzheimer's disease during activities of daily living. Journal of Speech, Language, and Hearing Research 46 (2), 353-367.
25. Bonder, B., Dal Bello-Hass, V., 2009. Functional Performance in Older Adults, 3rd ed. FA Davis, Philadelphia.
26. Farran, C., Gilley, D., McCann, J., Bienias, J., Lindeman, D., Evans, D., 2007. Efficacy of behavioral interventions for dementia caregivers. Western Journal of Nursing Research 29 (8), 944-960.
27. Gitlin, L., Corcoran, M., 2005. Occupational Therapy and Dementia Care: The Home Environmental Skills-Building Program for Individuals and Families. AOTA Press, Bethesda, MD.
28. Price, J., Hermans, D., Grimley-Evans, J., 2001. Subjective barriers to prevent wandering of cognitively impaired people. Cochrane Database of Systematic Reviews, Issue 1. Art. No.: CD001932.
29. Verkaik, J., vanWeert, J.C.M., Francke, A., 2005. The effects of psychosocial methods on depressed, aggressive, and apathetic

behaviors of people with dementia: A systematic review. International Journal of Geriatric Psychiatry 20, 301-314.

30. Barker, W., Luis, C., Harwood, D., Loewenstein, D., Bravo, M., Ownby, R., et al., 2005. The effect of a memory screening program on the early diagnosis of Alzheimer's disease. Alzheimer's Disease and Associated Disorders 19 (1), 1-7

31. de Jonghe, J., Wetzels, R., Mulders, A., Zuidema, S., Koopmans, R., 2009. Validity of the severe impairment battery short version. Journal of Neurology, Neurosurgery, and Psychiatry 80 (9), 954-959.

32. Dementia Care Specialists, 2006. Facilitating functional and quality-of-life potential: Strength-based assessment and treatment for all stages of dementia. Topics in Geriatric Rehabilitation 22 (3), 213-227.

33. Burns, T., Mortimer, J., 1993. The cognitive performance test: A new approach to functional assessment in AD. Journal of Geriatric and Psychiatric Neurology 7 (1), 46.

34. Austrom, M., Hartwell, C., Moore, P., Perkins, A., Damush, T., Unverzagt, F., et al., 2006. An integrated model of comprehensive care for people with Alzheimer's disease and their caregivers in a primary care setting. Dementia 5 (3), 339-352.

35. Evans, L., Cotter, V., 2008. Avoiding restraints in patients with dementia: Understanding, prevention, and management are the keys. American Journal of Nursing 108 (3), 40-49.

36. Brubacher, D., Zehnder, A.E., Monsch, A.U., et al., 2005. Assessment of everyday behavior in Alzheimer's disease patients: Its significance for diagnostics and prediction of disease progression. American Journal of Alzheimer's Disease and Other Dementias 20, 151-158.

37. Baum, C., Perlmutter, M., Edwards, D., 2000. Measuring function in Alzheimer's disease. Alzheimer's Care Quarterly 1 (3), 44-61.

38. Clare, L., Woods, B., 2003. Cognitive rehabilitation and cognitive training for early-stage Alzheimer's disease and vascular dementia. Cochrane Database of Systematic Reviews, Issue 4. Art.No.: CD003260. DOI: 10.1002/14651858.CD003260.

39. Dooley, N., Hinojosa, J., 2004. Improving quality of life for persons with Alzheimer's disease and their family caregivers: Brief occupational therapy intervention. American Journal of Occupational Therapy 58, 561-569.

40. Allen, C.K., 1985. Occupational Therapy for Psychiatric Diseases: Measurement and Management of Cognitive Disabilities. Little Brown, Boston.

41. Watson, R., Green, S., 2006. Feeding and dementia: A systematic literature review. Journal of Advanced Nursing 54, 86-93.

42. Whall, A.L., Black, M.E., Groh, C.J., et al., 1997. The effect of natural environments upon agitation and aggression in late stage dementia patients. American Journal of Alzheimer's Diseases 12, 216-220.

43. Sherratt, K., Thornton, A., Hatton, C., 2004. Music interventions for people with dementia: A review of the literature. Aging & Mental Health 8 (1), 3-12.

44. Alzheimer's Association, 2008. 2008 Alzheimer's disease facts and figures. Alzheimer's Association, Chicago.

45. Alzheimer's Association and National Alliance for Caregiving, 2004. Families care: Alzheimer's caregiving in the United States, 2004. Retrieved November 22, 2009, from http://www.alz.org.

46. Yaffe, K., Fox, P., Newcomer, R., Sands, L., Lindquist, K., Dane, K., et al., 2002. Patient and caregiver characteristics and nursing home placement in patients with dementia. JAMA 287, 2090-2097.

47. Adams, K., 2008. Specific effects of caring for a spouse with dementia: Differences in depressive symptoms between caregiver and non-caregiver spouses. International Psychogeriatrics 20, 508-520.

48. Arlt, S., Hornung, J., Eichenlaub, M., Jahn, H., Bullinger, M., Petersen, C., 2008. The patient with dementia, the caregiver, and the doctor: Cognition, depression, and quality of life from three perspectives. International Journal of Geriatric Psychiatry 23, 604-610.

49. Kim, Y., Schulz, R., 2008. Family caregivers' strains: Comparative analysis of cancer caregiving with dementia, diabetes, and frail elderly caregiving. Journal of Aging and Health 20, 483-503.

50. Mittelman, M.S., Roth, D.L., Clay, O.J., Haley, W.E., 2007. Preserving health of Alzheimer's caregivers: Impact of a spouse caregiver intervention. American Journal of Geriatric Psychiatry 15, 780-789.

51. Curry, L.C., Walker, C., Hogstel, M.O., 2006. Educational needs of employed family caregivers of older adults: Evaluation of a workplace project. Geriatric Nursing 27 (3), 166-173.

52. American Occupational Therapy Association, 1993. Occupational therapy roles. American Journal of Occupational Therapy 47 (12), 1087.

53. Goldberg, T., Botero, A., 2008. Causes of death in elderly nursing home residents. Journal of the American Medical Directors Association 9 (8), 565-567.

54. Mitchell, S., Teno, J., Kiely, D., et al., 2009. The clinical course of advanced dementia. New England Journal of Medicine 361 (16), 1529-1538.

55. Centers for Medicare and Medicaid Services, 2008. Skilled nursing facility prospective payment system refinements and consolidated billing guide. Retrieved November 22, 2009, from http://www.cms.hhs.gov/Manuals/.

chapter 21

Working with Elders Who Have Psychiatric Conditions

ANN BURKHARDT

KEY TERMS

mental well-being, mood disorders, anxiety disorders, panic disorder, posttraumatic stress disorder, acute stress disorder, schizophrenia, drug abuse, dual diagnosis, personality disorder, medication

CHAPTER OBJECTIVES

1. Understand the prevalence of mental illness among elders.
2. Discuss trends in approaches to support well-being, and circumvent the influences of diseases of meaning in daily life.
3. Become acquainted with psychiatric diagnoses common among institutionalized and community dwelling elders.
4. Describe the importance of considering both mental health and medical conditions when working with elders.
5. Identify assessments commonly used by occupational therapy (OT) practitioners with elders who have mental illness.
6. Describe intervention approaches commonly used with elders who have mental illness.

Current estimates about aging include expectations that the population of persons over age 65 will balloon to 71.5 million persons by 2030.[1] Public health and aging trends in the United States indicate that the major mental health disorders affecting people over age 65, many acquired as a part of the aging process, include anxiety disorders, depressive disorders, depression resulting in suicide, and dementia (such as Alzheimer's disease, Pick's disease, and Lewy body disease).

There are also many people who have had mental illness throughout their lives and who live into older age. Over 200 conditions are classified as mental illnesses, ranging from minor to severe, that are part of the lives of elders just as they are part of the lives of the general population. However, some of the most common mental illnesses of older adults include depression and schizophrenia.[2] As technology in health care has improved, people with chronic diseases and illnesses are living further into older age. Determining how this affects their lifestyle over time is an ongoing discovery.

Statisticians often group older adults into categories of the young aged/baby boomers (46-64), moderately older (65-79), and oldest old (80 and older).[3] With advances in health care and lifestyle, more and more people are surviving to over 100 years of age. The challenge that society now has is to manage health concerns for the masses that are aging. Health care financing falls short of adequate dollars to spend on older adults living into later life.

Historically, funding for intervention of mental illnesses has always fallen short in comparison to funding for other general medical and surgical conditions. When persons age and are classified as elders, and when they age with chronic illnesses such as a mental illness, the costs for their care can rise exponentially. Long-term use of antipsychotic medicines can affect a number of body functions. Neurological (such as tardive dyskinesia, parkinsonism, and others), hematological (such as pernicious anemia), and cognitive (such as dementia, delirium, and increase in clinical cognitive signs or symptoms, such as increased hallucinations) are some of the most devastating consequences that affect functional ability. When people who have mental illness enter old age, they often need additional personal and environmental facilitators to enable them to remain safely in their communities. Some may require homecare with or without group housing, some may require skilled care with supervision and assistance, whereas some may require institutionalization.

The current generation of people classified as elders also presents new social challenges. There are nearly 93 million unmarried Americans over age 18, representing roughly 42% of the adult population.[4] As of 2000, the most common household type in the United States is a person living alone.[5] People who are currently in their sixties and seventies are those who lived through the rock-and-roll revolution and the "summer of love" era of the late 1960s. They may be veterans of the Vietnam War, and some may have continued to serve in the military through the Desert Storm days of the 1990s. Posttraumatic stress disorder (PTSD) is common amongst veterans who saw active duty within war zones, although it also is present in people in the general population who lived through major terroristic events, such as for people living in New York City, Washington, DC, or in rural Pennsylvania during the September 11, 2001, attacks in the United States.[6] There are likely many different mental health issues this generation will face as they age related to their history of experimentation with drugs, other addictions (alcohol, prescription drugs, gambling, food, sex, and so on), changes in the meaning of family, cultural distancing, and changes in social mores. Many people in this age group may opt to live singly into older age.[7] This could create unique social management needs for them as they develop health concerns and require assistance to remain in place in the community. The oldest old still are the survivors of the Great Depression and World War II; the moderately older adults are those who lived through the Korean War. These generations had higher divorce rates than previous generations, and the divorce rates among older generation couples have been continually on the rise. People in this age group are twice as likely to break up their marriage than those of a decade back.[7] Many moved away from their immediate families, and this migration changed how they celebrated holidays and other life landmarks with their families, and how they coped with major life changes as they developed diseases and illnesses that required support from others to remain at home (person enablers). Social isolation is common. For some, "pseudo families," made up of non-blood related close friends, replaced the immediate family. Some experts believe this is leading to an exponential rise in the incidence of what the American Psychological Association's *Diagnostic and Statistical Manual* refers to as a "spiritual crisis."[8]

The challenge for OT practitioners is to meet clients where they are living and are currently engaged in occupation. It would be helpful for OT practitioners to have simple, straightforward assessments and potential interventions in mind to meet the needs of the growing numbers of seniors who will be living at home and in the community as well as in facilities in the future. Mental health practice in the social model is where OT has some of its strongest roots. Social systems within communities could become the most common venue for OT practice as more and more adults remain in community dwellings with support to remain in their homes.

It is estimated that nearly half of all Americans will be diagnosed with a mental health condition at some time in their lives.[9] So many older adults will need services in the future that it is anticipated there will not be enough OT practitioners to meet the demand. Further, the profession will be challenged to explore new models of intervention so that more people can benefit from services.

Consultancy models within community public health service delivery systems may be used with greater frequency in the future. There should be less reliance on third-party reimbursement as service delivery change occurs. OT must establish a continued presence in the work with people who are mentally ill so that services that honor the human need for occupation survive as change in the health care system takes place. Society, in general, and people served by OT, in particular, have historically valued the affect that participation in occupations has on quality of life and a sense of overall well-being. This recognition, however, has not been sufficiently explicit to guarantee its continuity.

ASSESSMENT

Occupational Therapy–Specific Assessments

Social interaction is core to a person's ability to engage in occupations and to participate in the life of a society. In addition, it is a significant predictor of quality of life.[10] The Evaluation of Social Interaction (ESI)[11] is an observational tool that assesses the quality of a person's performance of social interaction skills in natural contexts with typical social partners during involvement in any area of occupation. The skills measured by this assessment include items describing how a person empathizes, agrees, places self, expresses emotions, heeds, speaks fluently, replies, and clarifies, plus a number of other valued skills. The ESI is closely associated with the Assessment of Motor and Process Skills (AMPS).[12] Practical in its applied use, it appears to be a useful scale for application to home and community mental health models.

Kielhofner (2008)[13] suggested that perceived control is important for people's occupational performance. Eklund (2007)[14] found that perceived control was related to both activity level and satisfaction with daily occupations. A commonly used occupational performance measure tool in common usage that measures occupational performance and a client's satisfaction with their engagement and participation is the Canadian Occupational Performance Measure (COPM). Warren (2002)[15] studied the Canadian Model of Occupational Performance (CMOP) and the COPM in mental health practice and produced an OT assessment form that can be used in mental health practice.

The Activity Card Sort (ACS)[16] is a helpful tool for use with older adults in the community. When attempting to assess diversity of daily activity, loss of tasks over time, or lifestyle preferences, it is helpful to use a tool that prompts memory of familiar tasks and encourages sharing of current ability.[17] The ACS comes with an administration and scoring manual in paper and electronic form.

The Assessment of Motor and Process Skills (AMPS) is standardized for use with a variety of client populations, including individuals who have mental illness. The AMPS assesses a person's performance while doing a wide variety of instrumental activities of daily living (IADL). A person's performance is rated while they participate in several familiar tasks demonstrating a variety of motor and process (inclusive of cognitive) skills. Motor skills can be impaired in persons with mental illness. Sometimes, motor scores can change normally with age. However, if someone has lived a long time with schizophrenia, for example, he or she may have stiffness or other limitations in moving, bending, reaching, and flowing. Process skills include such things as attending, organizing, sequencing, questioning, accommodating, and benefiting, all of which can be impaired in people with chronic mental illness.[18]

Haertl and colleagues[19] studied the factors influencing satisfaction and efficacy of services at a free-standing psychiatric OT clinic. They found that a supportive therapeutic environment and an emphasis on the therapist–client relationship increased client and therapist satisfaction with OT mental health intervention. Highly valued services were associated with the therapeutic relationship, occupational engagement, skills training, and opportunities for socialization. It would appear that occupation-based measures are needed to demonstrate value to the consumer. While some commercially available multidisciplinary scales are readily available, intrinsic meaning and purpose to the client are well measured by OT-specific assessments only.

The Comprehensive Occupational Therapy Evaluation (COTE)[20] is used by OT practitioners to evaluate general, interpersonal, and task behaviors. This evaluation assesses client actions in structured and non-structured interactions and activities. It has inter-rater reliability and criterion validity.[21] The scale defines 25 behaviors that occur during occupations and that are based in OT practice. The scale can be used to evaluate or monitor patient progress, for interdisciplinary communication, and as a means of reporting progress in therapy to others. Ratings indicate improvement and readiness for discharge and are easily used in collaboration with other health professions within interdisciplinary teams.

The Kohlman Evaluation of Living Skills (KELS) is another OT-specific test that has been used successfully with older adults. The KELS has been found to have convergent validity with cognitive, affective, executive, and functional measures often used to determine older adults' ability to live safely and independently in the community. It is a practical screen for the capacity to live safely and independently among older adults.[22]

The Volitional Questionnaire (VQ) is an observational tool used by OT practitioners. It consists of 14 items and is used to assess motivation and the effect of the environment on volition. The VQ has criterion and construct validity and inter-rater reliability.[21]

Interdisciplinary Assessments

Measures of quality of life can give general insight into a person's sense of well-being. The Rand SF-36 Health Survey Questionnaire[23] consists of 36 questions that capture reliable and valid information regarding the participants' perceptions about their functional health status and well-being, including how well they are able to perform their daily activities. There is free public access to the assessment and the scoring form. This is a self-reported measure.

The Beck Anxiety Inventory (BAI) and the Beck Depression Inventory (BDI) are commonly used self-report questionnaires to determine the presence of anxiety or depression. The BAI is a 21-item questionnaire that distinguishes anxiety from depression. It has convergent and discriminate validity and internal consistency reliability.[21] The BDI is a questionnaire that has an overall depression score based upon content composed of cognitive, behavioral, and emotional symptoms. The BDI has internal consistency and test-retest reliability and concurrent and construct validity.[21] Both of the Beck indices are portable and easily used in community settings as well as in facilities.

The Mini Mental Status Examination (MMSE) is a short assessment used in a variety of practice settings and is commonly used with adults and older adults. The MMSE assesses cognitive status and basic mental functions,[21] such as short-term memory, object identification, ability to follow directions with several steps, ability to write from oral directions, and orientation. It has inter- and intra-rater reliability as well as concurrent, construct, predictive, and content validity.[24]

People who live through major medical events, such as a stroke or heart attack, in particular, also often have mental health diagnoses or conditions that become exacerbated. Gillen[25] studied coping during inpatient stroke rehabilitation and noted that the ability to cope with life circumstances is core to one's ability to have hope and to engage in occupation-based approaches. Gillen relied on the Brief COPE assessment[26] as an assessment that measures active versus avoidant coping strategies. Scales such as the Brief COPE may have implications for use by registered occupational therapists (OTRs) in screening coping ability as it applies to mental well-being.

These standardized assessments could all be used by both OTRs and certified occupational therapy assistants (COTAs). The interpretation of the tests and the influence on practice applications and anticipated outcomes require input from the OTR.

COMMON MENTAL HEALTH DISORDERS
Depression

Depression is the most common psychiatric disorder affecting people as they age.[27] The prevalence of clinically significant depressive symptoms ranges from 8% to 15% among community-dwelling elderly persons and is about 30% among the institutionalized elderly.[28] It is presumed that many more older adults are living with depression than what has been reported because they often do not seek help to treat depression if they have it. Older adults tend to underestimate the need to seek help for intervention of illnesses that they perceive to be the result of emotional states. In addition, caregivers often mistakenly believe that it is normal to experience depression in older age. Although many older people have periods of sadness and grief or temporary periods of feeling "blue" and lonely, these are usually transient experiences when they are not accompanied by depression. Living with depression usually results in changes in normal day-to-day function.

There are a variety of causes of depression. There are also many debates in the medical community about how some forms of depression may be monikers for other underlying diagnoses. For example, there is a "chicken and egg" phenomenological relationship between depression and cardiac disease.[29] People who are depressed have more frequent cardiac illness, and people who have cardiac illness have a greater incidence of depression. There is also a link between other chronic illnesses and the presence of depression. Neurological disorders of the brain can contribute to depression. An example of this is the link between Parkinson's disease and related disorders and the prevalence of depression.[30] Mental health, especially depression, is a major health indicator and focus of the Health People 2010 initiative.[31] Depression is essentially a major public health issue.

Depression is also referred to as a "disease of meaning" in recognition of issues beyond its physiological dimensions. People often become depressed by changes in life circumstances. This is sometimes referred to as *situational depression*. Some scholars theorize that diseases of meaning contribute to the development of physical illnesses themselves. Health practitioners who embrace this theory work to assist their clients in recognizing that some of their problems can actually make them stronger and lead toward health. OT practitioners can work toward helping clients manage the disease by shifting the focus from the symptoms toward what is causing stress or distress in the life circumstances of those elders who are experiencing the illness.[32]

Public health models, such as those proposed by the Harvard School of Public Health, have also researched the influence of pessimism or optimism on survival.[33] Their findings suggest that the avoidance of pessimism and actively trying to think optimistically can bolster one's outlook and prevent depression in the long term. There are several factors that can influence the incidence and severity of depression, including access to mental health resources, overcoming barriers to intervention (for example, cost of receiving care), mental health intervention utilization (for example, prescription drug therapy), and socioeconomic factors (for example, a person's level of education and his or her access to health insurance).[34]

Depression appears to have a negative effect on overall health. When people are depressed, their general health tends to suffer and they often develop comorbid conditions. Some comorbidity also tends to contribute to the development of depression. For example, the presence of chronic pain can lead to depression. Living with other acute or chronic illnesses and the impairments that accompany them can also contribute to the presence of depression.

Depression can be mild, moderate, or severe. It is estimated that over 21 million people in the United States are living with depression. It is the leading cause of disability.[35] In 2010, situational depression has increasingly been linked to major changes in the world economy that impact on people's quality of life. For example, after the recent economic crisis there has been an increase in the incidence of homicide and suicide.[36] The use of antidepressants by adults almost tripled between 1988 and 1994 and between 1999 and 2005. Ten percent of women age 18 and older and 4% of men now take antidepressants.[37]

Anxiety

Anxiety is another common mood disorder in older adults.[38] Use of supportive counseling and pharmaceutical therapy is common for people who have anxiety with accompanying mood disorders, such as depression. Anxiety disorders often accompany depressive episodes, particularly when the depression is situational as the result of major life events or changes in daily living. A commonly used scale in general hospitals to determine whether someone has anxiety and/or depression is the Hospital and Anxiety Depression Scale (HADS).[39] A systematic review of 747 research papers published in peer reviewed journals to determine the validity of the HADS determined that it consistently performed well in assessing the symptom severity of anxiety disorders and depression in somatic, psychiatric, and primary care patients and in the general population.[39] Most people today experience some form of anxiety day to day. However, when anxiety prevents or limits functioning, short-term intervention may be needed.

Suicide

Suicide is a possible result of depression, and older Americans are more likely to die by suicide than any other age group. There is also ethnic disparity concerning suicide. White older men are more likely to commit suicide than any other group: 49.8 suicide deaths per 100,000 persons.[37] Older men who are independent and have had a background of caregiving for another elder, usually a spouse, are at greatest risk for suicide in the United States.[40] This may be because they see what the person they care for is experiencing and they wish to avoid that possibility in their own futures. They often do not tell anyone that they are thinking about killing themselves, and they most often shoot themselves with a firearm.

Dementia

Dementia can arise from several underlying conditions. The most common form of dementia in the United States is Alzheimer's disease (AD). There are many variants of AD. One variant that is being diagnosed with greater frequency in the last few years is Lewy body disease (LBD).[41] LBD has elements of parkinsonism with the advance of dementia. In addition to the cognitive and neurobehavioral impairments, a person with LBD tends to have more visual hallucinations, tremor, aphasia, dysphagia, ballistic movements, and sleep disorder.

Dementia is characterized by the progressive loss of orientation to person, place, time, and circumstance. There is a loss of ability to calculate. Memory, especially short-term memory, eventually becomes severely impaired. People often develop other neurobehavioral impairments that increase in severity over time. Apraxia, aphasia, and disorientation (including topographical disorientation) all are prevalent features.[42] In later stages, people with AD tend to wander away from home. Home no longer looks familiar. Confusion can leave the person recalling home as being somewhere they have not lived since childhood. It is often helpful to ask them to tell you their address because they do not recognize errors in their ability to recall recent details of their lives. It is often possible to register individuals living in the community with Medic Alert and the local police department in the event that they wander and become lost.

AD can last for over a decade of a person's life. As the disease progresses, there is a growing need for caregivers' assistance with activity setup, cueing, and physical support. Lewy body disease tends to have a shorter life span prognosis and is accompanied by a degenerative movement disorder.[41] Over time people with dementia lack interest in food and eating and tend to develop swallowing impairments. Their life span may also be limited by advanced directives and advocacy by their designated proxy when impairments result in a failure to thrive without medical supports. Hospice services commonly follow people with dementia in the advanced stages.[43]

Alcoholism

Excessive alcohol use in the United States is the third leading cause of death related to lifestyle.[44] The extent of alcoholism among the elderly is debated, but the diagnosis and intervention of alcohol problems are likely to become increasingly important as the elderly population grows. Although alcoholism usually develops in early adulthood, the elderly are not exempt. In fact, physicians may overlook alcoholism when evaluating elderly patients, mistakenly attributing the signs of alcohol abuse to the normal effects of the aging process. Reports vary, but as many as 15% of men and 12% of women over age 60 may be hazardous drinkers, and 9% of men and 3% of women over age 60 may be alcohol-dependent.[45]

Alcoholism has both short-term and long-term health effects. There is probably a genetic risk for the propensity to become addicted to alcohol. Dependence tends to increase risk-taking behaviors. Immediate health risks and effects include impaired judgment and unintended injuries to self and to others. People have a tendency to drink and drive, which can lead to fatal traffic accidents and injury to self and others. There are higher incidences of domestic violence, child abuse, and sexual promiscuity amongst alcoholics, including elderly ones, than in the general population.[46,47] Long-term effects of alcoholism include neurological, cardiovascular, and psychiatric problems (depression, suicide ideation, and anxiety), increased cancer risk (mouth, throat, esophagus, liver, prostate, and breast), liver diseases (cirrhosis, alcoholic hepatitis, and alcohol use with hepatitis C), and gastrointestinal problems.[44] If alcohol is added to the equation of aging body systems and organs, people are at greater risk of injury (such as from falls). As the body ages and is less resilient as a result of aging, the damage caused to the body by alcohol as well requires more recovery effort from the body. Long-term problems can also include the development of secondary neurological and cognitive impairments.

Aging with Psychosis

Although people may develop psychosis at earlier ages, more people who have a diagnosis of psychosis are living into older age with continuing prevalence of the disease. People who have lived for decades of their lives with mental illnesses and psychosis may develop chronic problems in advanced age that are associated with long-term use of antipsychotic medicines.[48] Neurological disorders, such as tardive dyskinesia, can result. People have odd movements of their mouth and tongue (buccofacial mandibular) and neurological ticks (such as pill rolling). People with chronic psychosis may also develop dementia. As with other chronic, lifelong illnesses, people living with psychosis often require intermittent medical and psychological/psychiatric intervention at regular intervals throughout their lifetime. Access to care can circumvent the need for acute hospitalization and support a person through exacerbations over time.

Mood Disorders

Living with mood disorders can also persist across a lifetime. At times when the body undergoes major physiological shifts, the disorder may temporarily worsen (at menopause, for example). In old age, bipolar disorder is often mistaken for side effects of normal aging. Further, mood disorders often coexist with other common anxiety disorders, dysthymic disorder, alcoholism, and panic disorder.[49] Drugs used to treat mood disorders (for example, lithium) can influence the risk and development of blood related disorders, such as pernicious anemia. Some of these disorders can be life threatening. Intervention for pernicious anemia can be dramatic and includes procedures such as bone marrow transplantation.

Intervention planning considerations

Many clients in the United States have access to OT services for short intervals at a time. Elderly clients commonly receive services in inpatient settings. Acute care for mental illness in a hospital setting is very short term and often people with mental illness return to the same intervention setting over and over again, when they are in a crisis.[50] This is often referred to as a "revolving door" of care delivery. For example, people who are living with mood disorders, such as bipolar disorder, may require short-term, interval-dependent service access to care throughout their lifetime to successfully remain in their home and communities. Personnel in the settings that provide care to these consumers know them and recognize their immediate needs during hospitalization. OT practitioners in acute care settings, where clients are part of the revolving door, can often focus care on what clients need to be able to do safely, so that they can return home to the community. Sometimes, it is not possible to use standardized assessment to guide care.

Transitional services are also important. Opportunities for OT involvement in transitions may be underutilized. Often OT practitioners have the best insights into the lifestyle, habits, and rituals that people use as they live their daily lives. Meaning of habits and rituals may be very important and hold the key to successful transitions for persons living with mental illness in older age (Figure 21-1). OT practitioners can work with an older adult in a one-to-one, direct care relationship, provide education and problem solving in small group settings, work with caregivers of older persons with mental illness to develop strategies to help the family with transitioning, and serve the population and community by serving in advisory capacities to consumer-driven non-profit organizations, government, or media concerns. This is a developing area of practice and will require a concerted effort amongst clinicians, educators, and scientists in the field to establish efficacy in an evidence-based environment.

Care management models are another approach to keeping older persons at home with support. In such care models, OT practitioners may have a role in assisting with managing particular behaviors of elders. A major problem of many persons aging in the United States is the prevalence of clutter in homes.[51] Clutter may be a sign of a variety of diseases or disorders, including dementia or obsessive compulsive disorder. When the presence of clutter expands to hoarding, the disorder has increased in severity.[52] OT practitioners can work with the person and family to assist them with strategies for organizing the environment and day-to-day life, living space and lifestyle choices, habits and patterns to improve the physical environment, and to promote successful aging in place.

CASE STUDY

Louise is a 75-year-old woman diagnosed with depression. After being stabilized on an antidepressant at an acute care hospital, she was placed in a group home that specializes in the care of elders with mental illness. The residents are taken daily to a day intervention program, where a COTA provides the major part of the service. An OTR visits the center twice a week. Louise is a widow and has three married daughters and eight grandchildren. Sewing clothes for her daughters and grandchildren has always been important to Louise. She also has been a member of the same quilting club since the birth of her first child. A homemaker until age 45 years, she experienced the "empty-nest syndrome" after all of her daughters left for college or got married. She had been depressed then but not severely enough to require hospitalization. Her husband, a farmer, encouraged her to visit her sister, who lived in a large city. The change of scenery seemed to help her overcome the loss she felt. She returned from her visit to her sister's home and enrolled in a technical program for office workers. From ages 45 to 65 years she worked as a secretary at the local high school. At 65 years, she retired but continued to work as a substitute. Her husband lost their farm as a result of bank foreclosure and eventually accepted a position on a corporate farm. When Louise was 68 years old, her husband died of a sudden heart attack. She began to show symptoms of depression within a year. She reduced her activities, turning down jobs to fill in at the school, refusing to go out with her friends, declining to baby-sit her grandchildren, and quitting her quilting group. Her daughters did not become worried until they realized she was hoarding medication and planning suicide. They persuaded Louise to admit herself to the psychiatric unit of the regional hospital.

Although her medication was working at the time of her discharge from the acute care inpatient psychiatric unit, she

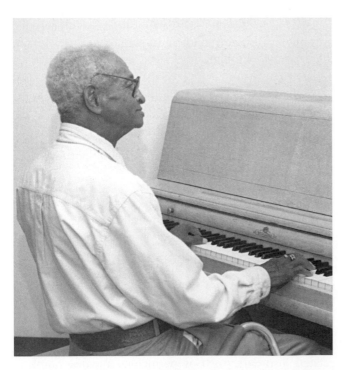

FIGURE 21-1   Music can help elders express their feelings.

had residual dysfunction in several self-care, socialization, and cognitive areas. Because all of her daughters lived more than 3 hours away, they agreed that Louise would stay in a group home until the family felt she could adequately take care of herself again. Fortunately, they were able to place her in a local group home with 24-hour supervision. The schedule of the group home included chair aerobics, weekend outings to the mall, a reminiscence group, and a crafts group that made stuffed toys for children with developmental disabilities. Louise also participated in a day intervention program 3 days a week. The family hoped that when Louise recovered sufficiently, she could resume her life in one of the assisted living units in a nearby housing development operated by her religious denomination.

Soon after Louise's arrival in the day intervention program, the COTA completed the COPM[53] with her. Louise identified priorities of some activities that she missed doing. Louise began crying as she discussed her grandchildren and her quilting group. She also discussed her difficulty with some activities of daily living (ADL) and especially with homemaking tasks. After consulting with the OTR, the COTA left a copy of an interest checklist[54] for Louise to fill out on her own. The COTA returned a day later and gave Louise the Allen Cognitive Level Test (see Chapter 7).[55] Louise scored at cognitive level 4.1 on the ACL, which meant that although she recognized an error, she could not correct it. Two days later, the COTA administered the Routine Task Inventory-2.[55] Louise also scored at cognitive level 4 on this test of ADL functions. This score meant she initiated grooming tasks and completed most of them; however, she neglected the back of her hair and neglected to clean up the bathroom after she bathed herself.[55]

Louise was able to find the mailbox in the group home when she wanted to mail letters to her daughters. However, she got lost easily when she attempted to walk unsupervised in the neighborhood. She was independent in toileting but got anxious when she had to use any restroom other than the one in her room or in the OT clinic. She usually remembered to ask the nurse for her medications. She was able to fix a sandwich in the kitchenette at the day intervention program, but she often burned the soup. The last time this happened she stated, "I can't do anything right anymore. I am just a burden to my daughters. They would be better off not having to worry about me." Although she could dress herself in the morning, she did not pay attention to whether her clothing matched or was appropriate for the weather.

After discussion with the OTR, the COTA explained her findings to Louise and to one of her daughters. The OTR, COTA, daughter, and Louise then planned for her participation in a daily ADL group session with the COTA to work on self-care and homemaking occupations. The plan included the use of self-cueing devices such as timers, environmental aids such as a neighborhood map, and a medication check-off sheet. These adaptations would be useful after discharge.

■ CASE STUDY QUESTIONS

1 Considering the case study described previously, which of Louise's behaviors might cause the COTA to think she was experiencing depression rather than dementia?
2 What other activities in the group home schedule might the COTA want to encourage Louise to attend?
3 What community resources could be used in guiding Louise's recovery?

■ CHAPTER REVIEW QUESTIONS

1 Why is it important to consider whether an elder has a mental illness in addition to other medical conditions for which they may have originally been referred to occupational therapy?
2 Explain three assessment tools that could be used to evaluate an elder's social and occupational functioning.
3 Explain two assessment tools that are commonly used to evaluate depression in elders.
4 What common symptoms of depression may go unrecognized in elders and why?
5 What kinds of intervention opportunities are there for occupational therapy practitioners working in transitional services for elders with mental illness?

REFERENCES

1. U.S. Department of Health & Human Services, 2010. Aging statistics: Administration on aging. Retrieved February 6, 2010, from http://www.aoa.gov/aoaroot/aging_statistics/index.aspx.
2. Mayo Clinic Staff, 2008. Mental illness. Retrieved February 7, 2010, from http://www.mayoclinic.com/print/mental-illness/DS01104/METHOD=print&DSECTION=all.
3. U.S. Census Bureau, 2008. Age data of the United States. Retrieved February 6, 2010, from http://www.census.gov/population/www/socdemo/age/agebyage.html.
4. U.S. Census Bureau, 2007. America's families and living arrangements: 2007. Retrieved February 7, 2010, from http://www.census.gov/prod/2009pubs/p20-561.pdf.
5. Hobbs, F., 2005. Examining American household composition: 1990 and 2000. U.S. Census Bureau. Retrieved February 7. 2010, from http://www.census.gov/prod/2005pubs/censr-24.pdf.
6. Ghafoori, B., Yuval, N., Gameroff, M.J., et al., 2009. Screening for generalized anxiety disorder symptoms in the wake of terrorist attacks: A study in primary care. Journal of Traumatic Stress 22, 218-226.
7. Ferguson, J., 2010. Shifting the Center: Understanding Contemporary Families, 4th ed. McGraw-Hill, New York.
8. Agrimson, L.B., Taft, L.B., 2009. Spiritual crisis: A concept analysis. Journal of Advanced Nursing 65, 454-461.
9. Kessler, R.C., Berglund, P., Dernier, O., et al., 2005. Lifetime prevalence and age of onset of distributions of DSM-IV disorders in the National Comorbidity Survey Replication. Archives of General Psychiatry 62, 593-602.
10. Rahman, A., Simmons, S., 2007. Measuring resident satisfaction more accurately: Two approaches. Nursing Homes: Long-Term Care Management 56 (5), 58-64.
11. Fisher, A., Griswold, L., 2008. The Evaluation of Social Interaction Manual, 2nd ed. AMPS Project International, Boulder, CO.
12. Fisher, A., Atler, K., Potts, A., 2007. Effectiveness of occupational therapy with frail community living older adults. Scandinavian Journal of Occupational Therapy 14 (4), 240-249.
13. Kielhofner, G. (Ed.). 2008. A Model of Human Occupation. Theory and Application, 4th ed. Lippincott Williams & Wilkins, Baltimore.
14. Eklund, M., 2007. Perceived control. How is it related to daily occupation in patients with mental illness living in the community? American Journal of Occupational Therapy 61 (5), 535-542.
15. Warren, A., 2002. An evaluation of the Canadian Model of Occupational Performance and the Canadian Occupational

Performance Measure in mental health practice. British Journal of Occupational Therapy 65 (11), 515-521.

16. Baum, C.M., Edwards, D., 2008. Activity Card Sort, 2nd ed. AOTA Press, Bethesda, MD.

17. Albert, S.M., Bear-Lehman, J., Burkhardt, A., 2009. Lifestyle-adjusted function: Variation beyond BADL and IADL competencies. Gerontologist 49, 767-777.

18. Fisher, A.G., Bernspång, B., 2007. Response to: A critique of the Assessment of Motor and Process Skills (AMPS) in mental health practice. Mental Health Occupational Therapy 12, 10-11. Retrieved April 19, 2010, from http://www.ampsintl.com/documents/MHOT%20March%202007.pdf.

19. Haertl, K., Behrens, K., Houtujec, J., Rue, A., Ten Hake, R., 2009. Factors influencing satisfaction and efficacy of services at a free-standing psychiatric occupational therapy clinic. American Journal of Occupational Therapy 63, 691-700.

20. Brayman, S.J., Kirby, T.F., Misenheimer, A.M., Short, M.J., 1976. Comprehensive occupational therapy evaluation scale. American Journal of Occupational Therapy 30, 94-100.

21. Law, M., McColl, M.A., 2010. Interventions, Effects, and Outcomes in Occupational Therapy: Adults and Older Adults. Slack, Thorofare, NJ.

22. Burnett, J., Dyer, C.B., Naik, A.D., 2009. Convergent validation of the Kohlman Evaluation of Living Skills as a screening tool of older adults' ability to live safely and independently in the community. Archives of Physical Medicine and Rehabilitation 11, 1948-1952.

23. The Rand Short Form 36 Survey, 2010. Retrieved April 19, 2010, from http://www.rand.org/health/surveys_tools/mos/mos_core_36item.html.

24. Molloy, D., Alemayehu, M.B., Roberts, R., 1991. Reliability of a standardized mini-mental state examination compared with the traditional mini-mental state examination. American Journal of Psychiatry 148, 102-105.

25. Gillen, G., 2006. Coping during inpatient stroke rehabilitation: An exploratory study. American Journal of Occupational Therapy 60, 136-145.

26. Carver, C.S., 1997. You want to measure coping but your protocol's too long: Consider the Brief COPE. International Journal of Behavioral Medicine 4 (1), 92-100.

27. Centers for Disease Control and Prevention, 2008. Depression in the United States' household population, 2005-2006. NCHS Data Brief 7, 1-8.

28. Beers, M., Jones, T., Berkwits, M., Kaplan, J., Porter, R., Bjelland, I., 2006. The Merck Manual of Geriatrics, updated edition. Merck & Co, West Point, PA.

29. Shah, S.U., White, A., White, S., Littler, W.A., 2004. Heart and mind: (1) Relationship between cardiovascular and psychiatric conditions. Postgraduate Medical Journal 80, 683-689.

30. Weintraub, D., Moberg, P.J., Duda, J.E., et al., 2004. Effect of psychiatric and other non-motor symptoms on disability in Parkinson's disease. Journal of the American Geriatrics Society 52, 784-788.

31. Snowden, M., Snowden, L., Frederick, J., 2008. Treating depression in older adults: Challenges to implementing the recommendations of an expert panel. Preventing Chronic Disease 5. Retrieved November 1, 2009, from http://www.cdc.gov/pcd/issues/2008/jan/07_0154.htm.

32. Jobst, K.A., Shostak, D. Whitehouse, P.J., 1999. Diseases of meaning, manifestations of health, and metaphor. Journal of Alternative and Complementary Medicine 5 (6), 495-502.

33. Center for Health Decision Science, 2010. Examples of models: Harvard School of Public Health. Available at http://chds.hsph.harvard.edu/About/Examples-of-Models.

34. Mental Health America, 2010. Ranking America's mental health: An analysis of depression across the states. Retrieved April 19, 2010, from http://www.nmha.org/go/state-ranking.

35. Laird, P., 2009. Feeling depressed and blaming the depression. Trinity Western University On-line Magazine. Retrieved April 19, 2010, from http://www.twu.ca/about/news/general/2009/money-and-mood.html.

36. Olfson, M., Marcus, S., 2009. National patterns in antidepressant medication treatment. Archives of General Psychiatry 66 (8), 848-856.

37. National Institute of Mental Health. 2008. The numbers count: Mental disorders in America. Retrieved April 19, 2010, from http://www.nimh.nih.gov/health/publications/the-numbers-count-mental-disorders-in-america/index.shtml.

38. Zigmond, A., Snaith, R., 1983. The Hospital Anxiety and Depression Scale. Acta Psychiatrica Scandinavica 67 (6), 361-370.

39. Bjelland, I., Dahl, A., Haug, T., et al., 2002. The validity of the Hospital Anxiety and Depression Scale: An updated literature review. Journal of Psychosomatic Research 52, 69-77.

40. Zanni, G., Wick, J., 2010. Understanding suicide in the elderly. Consultant Pharmacist 25 (2), 93-102.

41. NINDS, 2010. Dementia with Lewy bodies information page. Retrieved April 19, 2010, from http://www.ninds.nih.gov/disorders/dementiawithlewybodies/dementiawithlewybodies.htm.

42. Koedam, E., Lauffer, V., van der Vlies, A., van der Flier, W., Scheltens, P., Pijnenburg, Y., 2010. Early-versus late-onset Alzheimer's disease: More than age alone. Journal of Alzheimer's Disease 19 (4), 1401-1408.

43. Jones, B., 2009. Hospice disease types which indicate a greater need for bereavement counseling. American Journal of Hospice & Palliative Care 27 (3), 187-190.

44. Hoyer, W.J., Rudin, P.A., 2009. Adult Development in Aging, 16th ed. McGraw-Hill, Boston.

45. Merrick, E., Hodgkin, D., Garnick, D., Horgan, C., Panas, L., Ryan, M., et al., 2008. Unhealthy drinking patterns and receipt of preventive medical services by older adults. Journal of General Internal Medicine 23 (11), 1741-1748.

46. Cummings, S., Bride, B., Rawlins-Shaw, A., 2006. Alcohol abuse treatment for older adults: A review of recent empirical research. Journal of Evidence-Based Social Work 3 (1), 79-99.

47. Herrmann, N., 2007. Principles of geriatric psychopharmacology. In: Conn, D., Herrmann, N., Kaye, A., Rewilak, D., Schogt, B. (Eds.), Practical Psychiatry in the Long-Term Care Home, 3rd ed. Hogrefe & Huber, Ashland, OH.

48. Goldstein, B.I., Herrmann, N., Shulman, K.I., 2006. Comorbidity in bipolar disorder among the elderly: Results from an epidemiological community sample. American Journal of Psychiatry 163, 319-321.

49. Sirey, J., 2008. The impact of psychosocial factors on experience of illness and mental health service use. American Journal of Geriatric Psychiatry 16 (9), 703-705.

50. Gitlin, L.N., Schinfeld, S., Winter, L., Corcoran, M., Boyce A.A., Hauck W., 2002. Evaluating home environments of persons with dementia: Inter-rater reliability and validity of the Home Environmental Assessment Protocol (HEAP). Disability Rehabilitation 24, 59-71.

51. Ayers, C., Saxena, S., Golshan, S., et al., 2010. Age at onset and clinical features of late life compulsive hoarding. International Journal of Geriatric Psychiatry 25 (2), 142-149.

52. Law, M. (Ed.). 1998. Client-Centered Occupational Therapy. Slack, Thorofare, NJ.

53. Matsutsuyu, J.S., 1969. The interest checklist. American Journal of Occupational Therapy 24 (4), 32.

54. Allen, C., Earhart, C., Blue, T., 1992. Occupational Therapy Treatment Goals for the Physically and Cognitively Disabled. American Occupational Therapy Association, Rockville, MD.

55. Allen, C.K., 1985. Occupational Therapy for Psychiatric Diseases: Measurement and Management of Cognitive Disabilities. Little, Brown, Boston.

298

22

Working with Elders Who Have Orthopedic Conditions

BRENDA M. COPPARD, TYROME HIGGINS, KAROLINE D. HARVEY, AND RENÉ PADILLA

KEY TERMS

orthopedic, fracture, osteoarthritis, compound fracture, transverse fracture, spiral fracture, comminuted fracture, closed reduction, open reduction, internal fixation, external fixation, delayed union, nonunion, malunion, HemoVac, total hip replacement, arthroplasty, antiembolus hosiery, rheumatoid arthritis, wrist subluxation, ulnar drift, swan-neck deformity, boutonnière deformity, Nalebuff type I deformity, joint protection, work simplification, energy conservation

CHAPTER OBJECTIVES

1. Identify the causes of fractures in the elder population.
2. Identify terminology related to fractures and their management.
3. Describe the precautions required after a hip pinning and implications of such a procedure relative to occupational performance.
4. Describe the precautions required after a total hip replacement and the implications of such a procedure relative to occupational performance.
5. Identify adaptive equipment and modified methods of performance that benefit elders with hip fractures.
6. Identify the signs and symptoms of osteoarthritis, rheumatoid arthritis, and gout.
7. Describe the effects of osteoarthritis, rheumatoid arthritis, and gout on occupational performance.
8. Explain the principles of joint protection, work simplification, and energy conservation.

The two weeks I spent in rehab were tough, but I had to learn how to walk all over again, just like a baby! Not only did the physical therapist teach me how to walk, the occupational therapist taught me how to dress, and how to do things around the house. They presented me with all sorts of new gadgets that would help me in my daily living.

—Linda

Orthopedic problems are prevalent among elders. For example, an estimated 850,000 fractures occur annually in persons age 65 years or older.[1] One of every two women and one in eight men older than age 50 years will experience an osteoporosis-related fracture.[2] Orthopedic problems may result in elders being hospitalized for a surgical procedure, rehabilitation, and possibly being placed temporarily or permanently in a long-term care facility. Elders who sustain a hip fracture as a result of a fall have a 34% mortality rate within 1 year of the fracture.[3] The most common complications of elders who undergo orthopedic surgery include stroke, cardiac failure, and severe infection. There is a reported 10.1%

overall rate of mortality after orthopedic surgery for this population.[4]

The role of the certified occupational therapy assistant (COTA) and registered occupational therapist (OTR) team is to help maximize the occupational performance of elders who have orthopedic problems. Elders who would otherwise need to enter an extended care facility are often able to go home as a result of occupational therapy (OT) intervention. COTAs must be familiar with orthopedic conditions and their effects on occupational performance to ensure that appropriate evaluation and intervention are carried out. This chapter addresses orthopedic problems and conditions that contribute to these problems.

FRACTURES

Causes of Fractures

Causes of fractures include falls, trauma from automobile accidents, osteoarthritis, and metastatic carcinoma.[5] Other factors such as a current or previous smoking habit,[6] alcohol abuse,[7] diabetes,[8] and decreased level of physical activity also correlate with the incidence of fractures.[9]

The majority of fractures in elders result from falls.[10] Factors associated with falling include poor vision, orthostatic hypotension, poor balance, diminished mobility, side effects of medication, muscle weakness, neurological diseases, reduced alertness, urge incontinence, a cluttered home environment, and dementia.[11] (An in-depth examination of the causes of falls in elders is provided in Chapter 14.)

The number of elder drivers is increasing. For example, in 1995, about 9% of drivers in the United States were people age 70 years and older, and their number increased to 12% by 2010.[12] It is estimated that by 2020, 20% of all people who drive will be older than age 65 years.[13] Elders have greater rates of fatal crashes than younger drivers, and they do not deal well with complex traffic situations.[14] Trauma resulting from auto accidents accounts for a portion of the fractures seen in the elder population.

Elders are more likely to sustain fractures after a fall because of osteoporosis, osteomalacia, and the diminished ability to repair microfractures.[15] Stress fractures also can occur in elders who, for example, suddenly increase their levels of activity by jogging, walking farther than usual, or walking on a different terrain.[16]

Fractures may also be caused by cancer that has metastasized to bone. Although any cancer may metastasize to bone, metastases from carcinomas, particularly those that arise in the breast, lung, prostate, kidney, and thyroid, are most common. Metastatic lesions weaken the strength of bones and may lead to fractures.[17]

Types of Fractures

A fracture is a break in a bone. Although radiographs are used to diagnose the fracture, it does not reveal damage to soft tissues or cartilage. Fracture sites can disrupt the intraarticular, epiphyseal, metaphyseal, or diaphyseal portions of the bone. If a fracture occurs and dislocates a joint, it is a fracture-dislocation.[18]

Various terms are used to categorize fractures. A fracture is considered to be *compound* or *open* if the bone protrudes through the soft tissue and skin. If the soft tissue and skin are undamaged, the fracture is considered to be *closed* or *simple*. Different physical forces can result in certain types of fractures. A transverse fracture occurs as a result of a direct force, whereas a spiral fracture results from a circular or twisting force. A fracture that results in more than two bone fragments is a comminuted fracture. Figure 22-1 shows these various types of fractures.

Medical Intervention for Fractures

The goals of medical management of a fracture are to reduce pain and align the fracture for proper healing.[18] The fracture can be aligned with or without surgery. The process of manually realigning (sometimes using traction devices) and then casting a fracture is termed *closed reduc-*

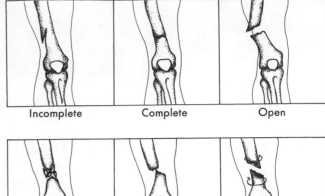
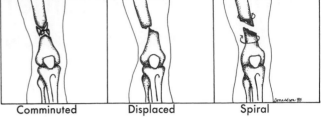

FIGURE 22-1   Types of fractures. *(Modified from Garland, J. J. (1979).* Fundamentals of Orthopaedics. *Philadelphia: WB Saunders.)*

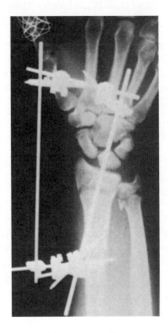

FIGURE 22-2   External fixator in place to maintain reduction. *(From Hunter, J., Mackin, E., & Callahan, A. (Eds.). (1995).* Rehabilitation of the Hand: Surgery and Therapy, *4th ed. St. Louis, MO: Mosby.)*

tion. The *open reduction* is a surgical procedure that is used to internally fixate the fracture site. Internal fixation is performed with the use of orthopedic nails, screws, pins, rods, or plates. When external fixation is used to align or reduce a fracture, the fixator device is attached with pins or wire, which is inserted through the soft tissues and into the bone (Figure 22-2). This device usually involves the use of screws and rods that are removed after the fracture has healed. The skin around placement sites

TABLE 22-1

General Recommended Pin Site Care

Frequency	1-2 times each day
Massage	Massage site area gently to prevent abnormal adhesions/scars
Crusts	Remove from site
Cleaning solution	Peroxide or saline
Dressing	Dry dressing, especially if oozing

Adapted from Sims, M., & Whiting, J. (2000). Pin-site care. *Nursing Times, 96*(48), 46.

of the rods or screws must be kept clean to prevent infection (Table 22-1).

COTAs also should be familiar with terminology relating to the healing of fractures. Three terms used to describe fractures that do not heal well are *delayed union, nonunion,* and *malunion*.[18] Delayed union describes a fracture that heals at an abnormally slow rate. Nonunion describes a fracture that has not healed within 4 to 6 months. Malunion describes a fracture in which the bone heals in a normal length of time but with an unsatisfactory alignment.

Complications After Fractures

Several complications can occur after a fracture.[18] Edema can lead to joint stiffness, and joint contractures often are caused by adhesions or prolonged immobilization. After a fracture, posttraumatic arthritis can occur in joints associated with or near the fracture site. Reflex sympathetic dystrophy is a syndrome that often occurs after minor injuries. The condition is believed to be related to the sympathetic nervous system and presents with severe pain, edema, stiffness, muscle atrophy, muscle spasms, contractions, and loss of bone mineralization. Myositis ossificans is the formation of heterotopic ossification near a traumatized area. The most common joints where heterotopic ossification forms are the arms, thighs, and hips.

Factors Influencing Rehabilitation

Several factors affect the outcome of rehabilitation efforts in elders who sustain fractures. Age is a predominant factor in rehabilitation.[19] Elders may need more time than younger persons to achieve their greatest levels of independence. For example, in elders, a comminuted fracture of the proximal humerus should be immobilized for the shortest period possible to reduce the chances of development of adhesive capsulitis or frozen shoulder. With a younger person, the threat of such a complication may not always be a concern.

The general condition of elders also affects the course of rehabilitation. For example, elders who are in shock or are unconscious require different intervention than those who are alert and oriented. In addition, past and current

medical conditions may affect the rehabilitation of elders who have fractures. Elders with congestive heart failure or chronic obstructive lung disease may be limited in their abilities to participate in endurance and strengthening activities. Furthermore, a large percentage of elders with fractures also have associated medical problems such as arthritis, hypertension, hearing impairments, heart disease, cataracts, orthopedic impairments, sinusitis, and diabetes.[20]

The presence of dementia often affects rehabilitation outcomes for elders with fractures. For example, teaching the integration of hip precautions or joint protection methods while engaging in self-care tasks to an elder with short-term memory deficits is difficult. (A detailed discussion of intervention considerations for elders who have dementia is presented in Chapter 20.)

Although hip fractures are the most common type of fracture sustained by elders, fractures of other bones also occur. COTAs should know the common fractures and general recommended intervention techniques (Table 22-2).

Hip fractures

Approximately 300,000 hip fractures occur annually in people older than age 65 years, and hip fractures are more common in women than in men.[21] Fractures of the hip are classified by the type and direction of the fracture line.

Hip fractures usually require an open reduction internal fixation, or pinning procedure. The open reduction internal fixation of the involved hip usually must be protected from excessive force through weight-bearing restrictions (Table 22-3). The open reduction internal fixation site is sutured shut, and a HemoVac may be used for about 2 days.[22] A HemoVac, which is connected to a suction machine, is a device that draws and collects drainage from the site. The HemoVac unit should not be disconnected for any activity and is usually removed by a registered nurse or a physician.

The amount of time required for a hip fracture to heal depends on the elder, the fracture site, the fracture type, and the severity of the injury. Most incisions for hip surgeries are 12 to 18 inches in length; however, some new surgical approaches that involve less cutting of muscle, tendons, and ligaments are being tested with the anticipation that the hospital length of stay will dramatically decrease.[23]

Many health care providers in hospitals follow a protocol or clinical pathway that outlines the timeframe for each professional's rehabilitation tasks.[24] Out-of-bed therapy activities for persons with hip pinnings are usually initiated 2 to 4 days after surgery.[19] Most function returns within 6 weeks to 6 months after the fracture occurs; most persons experience little improvement in function from 6 months to 1 year after sustaining a fracture.[25]

Weight-bearing restrictions for hip pinnings Depending on the type and severity of the fracture, the physician may restrict the amount of weight bearing allowed on the involved hip while the person is walking. Most

TABLE 22-2

General Recommended Intervention Techniques for Upper-Extremity Fractures

Fracture location	Precautions and/or contraindications	Acute injury treatment techniques	Treatment techniques after repair
Humeral	Keep elbow, wrist, and finger joints mobile or per physician's order; monitor for signs of edema; position upper extremity above heart if edema occurs and is not contraindicated for cardiac conditions; PROM is contraindicated; discontinue immobilizer or brace with physician's order.	Use shoulder immobilizer or plaster cast to immobilize; after 5 to 7 days, a humeral cuff brace can be used.	Begin AROM when acute pain is subsided to prevent stiffness; PROM is contraindicated; encourage isometric exercises during and after immobilization; Codman's exercises should be encouraged only in the absence of edema.
Elbow	Keep shoulder, wrist, and finger joints mobile or per physician's order; monitor for signs of edema; position upper extremity above level of heart if edema occurs and is not contraindicated for cardiac condition; PROM is contraindicated; discontinue immobilizer(s) with physician's order	A plaster cast or elbow conformer can be used to immobilize the elbow in 90 to 100 degrees of flexion; a sling also can be used.	Begin gentle, non-resistive AROM after removal of cast; perform AROM in a gravity-eliminated plane; PROM in the early stage is not advised; person may have difficulty regaining full elbow extension, but a functional arc should be regained for ADL.
Wrist (scaphoid)	Keep shoulder, elbow, and finger joints mobile or per physician's order; if an external fixator is in place, monitor sites for infection; clean pin sites with hydrogen peroxide; discontinue any splints with physician's order.	A plaster cast may be worn for 2 weeks to 2 months depending on the physician; a thumb spica splint can be used after the cast is removed to position the wrist in slight flexion and radial deviation.	When stabilized and cast is removed, AROM should begin to all wrist motions.
Colles' (distal radius)	Keep shoulder, elbow, and finger joints mobile or per physician's order; if an external fixator is in place, monitor sites for infection; clean pin sites with hydrogen peroxide; discontinue any splints with physician's order.	A volar wrist splint is used for positioning after plaster cast has or internal/external fixation is removed.	Begin ROM of wrist and forearm once a bony union has occurred and cast has been removed.

ADL, activities of daily living; AROM, active range of motion; PROM, passive range of motion; ROM, range of motion.
Physicians may vary these protocols.
Adapted from Daniel, M. S., & Strickland, L. R. (1992). *Occupational Therapy Protocol Management in Adult Physical Dysfunction.* Gaithersburg, MD: Aspen.

weight-bearing restrictions are observed for 6 to 8 weeks, during which time the person may use crutches or a walker to ambulate.[19] COTAs must be aware of any weight-bearing precautions before initiating therapy and should know the terminology related to weight-bearing restrictions (see Table 22-3).

JOINT REPLACEMENTS

Total Hip Replacements

Total hip replacements (THRs), or total hip arthroplasties (THAs), are often elective surgeries indicated for reducing pain and restoring motion for elders who have severe osteoarthritis, rheumatoid arthritis, or ankylosing spondylosis. Emergency THAs frequently follow traumatic injuries to the hip, such as after a motor vehicle accident

or fall. A hip replacement, or arthroplasty, may be full or partial. During a full hip arthroplasty, the hip's ball and socket are replaced with metal or metal and plastic prosthetic implants.[26] During a partial joint replacement, which is commonly used for fractures of the femoral neck and head, the femoral neck and head are replaced with a prosthesis. Hip prostheses last approximately 10 to 15 years or longer in 90% of elders.[27] When radiographs show evidence of loosening of the cement and the client is experiencing pain, a hip revision arthroplasty may be performed.[28]

The two basic surgical approaches for THRs are the anterolateral approach and the posterolateral approach.[29] When an anterolateral approach of surgery is used, elders must avoid adduction, external rotation, and extension of the operated hip. If a posterolateral surgical approach is

TABLE 22-3

Weight-Bearing Terminology

Term	Definition
No weight bearing (NWB)	No body weight is borne on the involved side.
Toe-touch weight bearing (TTWB)	No weight is borne on the heel; weight is borne on the toes only.
Partial weight bearing (PWB)	A partial amount of the body weight can be borne on the involved side; usually a percentage of body weight (for example, 50% PWB) or pounds (PWB with 50 lb) is stated.
Weight bearing at tolerance (WBAT)	Weight bearing is allowed to the extent that it does not cause the elder too much pain; the elder tolerates the weight bearing.
Full weight bearing (FWB)	Full body weight is borne on the involved side.

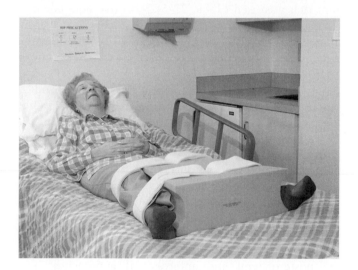

FIGURE 22-3 While the elder is supine, the elder's legs should be abducted with a wedge to prevent hip rotation and adduction.

used, elders should avoid flexion beyond 60 to 90 degrees, adduction, and internal rotation of the operated hip.[30] COTAs must be aware of which type of surgical approach was used to properly carry out OT intervention (Figure 22-3). COTAs also should note the position precautions for each surgical approach.

The movement precautions are usually observed for 6 to 12 weeks as indicated in a physician's order (Table 22-4).[30] Cemented THRs usually have no weight-bearing restrictions. When cement is not used, bony ingrowth is used to secure the prosthesis to the elder's bone. Often 6 to 12 weeks of weight-bearing restrictions are required when this type of prosthesis is used.[29]

TABLE 22-4

Motion Precautions for Clients Who Have Had a Total Hip Replacement

Approach	Position precautions
Anterolateral	1. Hip external rotation 2. Hip adduction 3. Hip extension
Posterolateral	1. Hip flexion beyond 90 degrees 2. Hip internal rotation 3. Hip adduction

After THA surgery, physicians often instruct clients to wear antiembolus hosiery. These thigh-high hose are worn 24 hours a day and removed during bathing only. Clients are instructed to wear this hosiery because it assists with blood circulation, prevents edema, and reduces the risk for deep vein thromboses. If an elder has not been instructed to wear these hose and complains of pain or swelling in the affected leg, the physician should be consulted immediately because it could be a sign of the presence of a thrombus. COTAs should be skilled in donning and doffing antiembolus hosiery because they may need to assist elders before bathing. If the hose are to be worn for a length of time, caregiver training should occur because it is often difficult for elders to perform this task independently.

Researchers show that there are several milestones during rehabilitation, including adherence to hip precautions; ambulating 100 feet with a mobility aid; independence with home exercise program; and requiring supervision only with toileting, transfers, and activities of daily living (ADL).[27]

Three areas reported in research studies that are important concerns for clients with THA are sexual activity, driving, and work return.[31] In a study of 86 clients with THA, 50% of preoperative clients reported experiencing difficulties with sexual activities because of hip problems, and 90% of these clients reported a desire for more information about sexual functioning after THA. The majority of clients (55%) resumed sexual activity within 2 months of the THA with physician approval and following positioning precautions. Most people report that the supine position during intercourse is the most comfortable.[31] (A detailed discussion of addressing sexuality with elders is presented in Chapter 12.)

After surgery, driving reactions normalize between 3 and 8 weeks if elders resume good leg control. Return to work activities is dependent on the amount of stress and torque on joints. Typically, elders must take off from work for 3 to 6 weeks after surgery.

A number of studies exist on appropriate leisure activities after a THA.[31] A survey of 28 orthopedic surgeons from Mayo Clinic recommended that activities such as cycling, golfing, and bowling are acceptable after a THA. Generally, many physicians counsel well elders to avoid participation in sports that impart high torque or stress on the hip joint, such as jogging. Often, active elders resume activities and athletics regardless of physician or therapist warnings.

Psychosocial issues after total hip replacement

A number of psychosocial issues may surface during an elder's rehabilitation after a hip replacement. Dealing with a chronic condition such as arthritis can be stressful and frustrating; many elders are required to deal with pain, swelling, and mobility limitations on a daily basis. Providing information on support groups may be beneficial to the elder.

After a THR, some elders find it difficult to abide by the position precautions. They may view these precautions as impediments to resuming the lifestyles they had before the procedure, especially when they had no predisposing medical conditions that limited activities. COTAs should be empathetic to the elder's concerns, but they must also help elders understand the rationale for

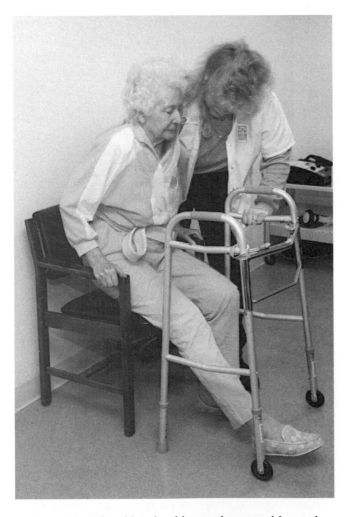

FIGURE 22-4 The elder should extend operated leg and bear weight on arms when coming into a standing position.

adhering to hip precautions (Figure 22-4). The COTA also should address the consequences of not following these precautions. COTAs may need to reassure elders that healing takes time and that involvement in activities may continue but usually with some modifications.

Many elders feel guilty or become anxious when they require assistance from family or friends.[32] Elders who are temporarily placed in an extended care facility while they heal may also find it difficult to accept assistance from nursing staff in the facility. Feelings of guilt are sometimes accompanied by financial worries about the cost of care. In addition, relocation to a new environment such as a hospital, extended care facility, or long-term care facility can be stressful.[33] COTAs should encourage elders to talk about their feelings. When possible, discussing the situation with elders before they are moved to a new facility is beneficial. In addition, the elder should be thoroughly oriented to the new facility.

Occupational therapy interventions

The specific intervention strategies and techniques used with an elder who has had a THA vary depending on whether the anterolateral or posterolateral surgical approach was used (Table 22-5). Adaptive equipment is typically supplied to patients regardless of approach. The most used piece of adaptive equipment tends to be the raised toilet seat, which often is used for at least 6 months after THA. Other pieces of equipment that participants reported to be helpful were the reacher, long-handled shoehorn, and sock aid; however, they did experience some difficulties in using them.

COTAs are involved in educating elders and their caregivers about proper and safe usage of adaptive equipment, observing hip precautions during functional activities, and making environmental adaptations. Laurel is a COTA who works in an acute care hospital and is involved in patient education. Before having a hip replacement, elders and their primary caregivers attend a class to prepare them to return home. Laurel reviews the precautions for both the posterolateral and anterolateral approaches. The elders bring clothing to practice using a dressing stick, reacher, sock aid, and long-handled shoehorn. Laurel has the elders practice transferring to and from a chair, couch, commode, and raised toilet seat. They also practice using reachers to retrieve items from the floor and cupboards. During one question-and-answer session, several elders expressed an interest in feeding their pets. Laurel asked a volunteer from her church to make pet feeders that could be easily lifted from the floor to the counter so that the elders could fill them with water and food without bending over (Figure 22-5). Laurel also reviews information in a notebook with elders and their caregivers that will be used as their home programs. After surgery, Laurel works with elders to review the dressing techniques and reinforces the information that they learned earlier in class. Laurel also makes recommendations for bathroom equipment that the elders may need to return home. Some elders have

TABLE 22-5

Occupational Therapy Interventions for Posterolateral and Anterolateral Approaches to Total Hip Replacement

Bed mobility	■ Abduct legs with wedge or pillows to prevent hip rotation and adduction.
Walking	■ Avoid pivoting on the leg that has been operated on.
	■ When approaching corners, take small steps in a circular fashion.
	■ If possible, take 10- to 15-minute walks four times per day 6 to 8 weeks after the operation.
	■ Walk at a slow, comfortable pace.
Chair transfers	■ Sit on chairs with firm seats, preferably with arm rests.
	■ Avoid low, soft chairs and rocking chairs.
	■ Extend leg that has been operated on, reach for arm rests, and bear some weight through arms when trying to sit down.
Commode chair transfers	■ Use a chair with a height that accommodates for hip flexion precaution.
For posterolateral approach	■ Wipe between legs while seated or wipe from behind while standing with caution to avoid internal rotation.
	■ Stand and face the toilet to flush.
For anterolateral approach	■ An over-the-toilet commode is usually used initially in the hospital and on discharge; elders usually have enough hip mobility to use a standard toilet seat.
	■ Avoid external rotation while wiping.
	■ Stand and face the toilet to flush.
Shower stall transfer	■ Use a nonskid mat to avoid slips and falls.
	■ Use a shower chair and grab bars.
Car transfer	■ Avoid bucket seats in small cars.
	■ Back up to passenger seat, hold onto a stable part of the car, extend the leg that has been operated on, and slowly sit in the car.
	■ Increase the seat height with pillows, if necessary.
	■ Avoid prolonged sitting in the car.
Lower extremity dressing	■ Sit on a chair or the bed's edge when dressing.
	■ Use assistive devices, if necessary, to observe precautions.
	■ Use a reacher or dressing stick in donning and doffing pants and shoes.
	■ Dress the leg that has been operated on first using a reacher or dressing stick to bring pants over the foot and up to the knee.
	■ Avoid crossing the operated lower extremity over the nonoperated lower extremity.
	■ Use a sock aid to don socks or knee-high nylons and a reacher or dressing stick to doff these items.
	■ Use a reacher, elastic shoe laces, and a long-handled shoehorn, if necessary.
	■ Use a long-handled sponge or back brush to reach the lower legs and feet safely, and use soap on a rope to prevent the soap from dropping (drill a hole into a bar of soap and thread a cord through the hole).
	■ Wrap a towel around a reacher to dry the legs.
	■ If a bath bench is used, place a damp towel on the seat to avoid sliding off of the bench.
	■ Consider a handheld shower extender.
Hair shampooing	■ Shampoo hair while seated until able to shower.
Leisure interests	■ Adapt and use long-handled tools when appropriate.
	■ Use stools when appropriate to avoid bending, squatting, and stooping.
Home management	■ Avoid heavy housework (e.g., vacuuming, lifting, and bed making).
	■ Practice kitchen activities; keep commonly used items at countertop level.
	■ Carry items in large pockets, a walker basket, a fanny pack, or a utility cart.
	■ Use reachers to grasp items in low cupboards, or pick up items off of the floor.
	■ Move frequently used items located low in cabinets and shelves to counter level.
	■ Keep a cordless phone with a belt clip close by at all times.
	■ Carry a water bottle with a belt holster.
	■ When initially recovering, place the television remote control, radio, telephone, medication, tissues, wastebasket, and water glass in the most convenient location.
	■ Before surgery, stock up on food that can be easily prepared or reheated.

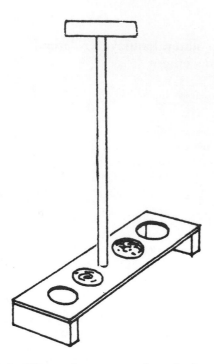

FIGURE 22-5 This easily constructed pet feeder allows elders to fill the water and food bowls without bending over. *(Courtesy Ron Connon).*

stated that it was helpful to be exposed to the information before surgery because it was harder for them to concentrate after surgery.

Knee Replacements

The knee joint has a large amount of synovium fluid, and thus one joint is often affected by rheumatoid and osteoarthritis.[20] Chronic knee pain may cause difficulty in ascending and descending stairs, squatting, walking, and jogging, thus affecting one's quality of life.

Nonsurgical intervention may include a variety of approaches, including medication, activity modification and exercise, braces, and weight reduction.[20] Nonsteroidal antiinflammatory drugs (NSAIDs) are often prescribed to reduce swelling and pain. Intraarticular injections are sometimes used when oral NSAIDs are ineffective.

Activity modification is targeted to minimize symptoms by avoiding high-impact activities. Maintaining a healthy body weight is difficult for people with knee pain because it often decreases their activities without changing their intake of calories. If possible, elders with knee pain should try to maintain a regular exercise program to maximize aerobic conditioning.

Physical therapists may provide braces to help active elders regain a sense of knee stability during activities. Such knee braces are helpful in the short term, but people tend not to use them on a day-to-day basis.[20] Surgical intervention includes a total knee joint arthroplasty or total knee replacement (TKR). Knee arthroplasties are best suited for sedentary persons older than age 65 years.[30]

Approximately 90% of TKRs are successful up to 10 years after surgery.

Rehabilitation after knee replacement

After a TKR, the knee is bandaged and changed 2 to 4 days after surgery. A HemoVac may be used and discontinued 2 to 3 days after surgery. To promote blood flow and decrease the chance of blood clot formation, the elder will likely wear thromboembolic disease (TED) hose. A knee immobilizer may be prescribed by some physicians. Others will prescribe the use of a continuous passive motion (CPM) machine,[30] which is designed to slowly and smoothly range the knee into flexion and extension. Physical therapists monitor the CPM unit and prescribe exercises to the elder.

Occupational and physical therapy services will work with elders to meet the following goals: transfer independently to and from bed, walk with crutches or a walker on a level surface, independently ascend and descend three stairs, independently carry out one's home exercise program, flex affected knee to 90 degrees, and extend knee to neutral. Other rehabilitation concerns of clients with TKRs include sexual activity, driving, and return to work. Many physicians do not discuss sexual activity related to the TKR. However, clients should be counseled to avoid sexual intercourse for 4 to 6 weeks after TKR. (See Chapter 12 for more specific information about resuming sexual activity after a TKR.) Resuming driving can occur as early as 3 weeks for some elders, whereas others are not ready to drive until 8 months after surgery. The ability to return to driving is dependent on exhibiting good leg control, limiting the use of narcotic pain relievers, and whether the overall recovery is unremarkable.[34] Returning to work is more difficult to predict and is dependent on the type of work. Typically patients return to work 3 to 6 weeks after their surgery.[34] Keep in mind these are generic timeframes; physicians may instruct their clients with different timeframes on the basis of the clients' conditions.

ARTHRITIS

Arthritis affects about 37 million of adults in the United States and is prevalent in nearly half of the elder population.[2] The self-reported prevalence of arthritis is greater among women than men, and for women age 45 years and older, arthritis is the leading cause of activity limitation.[35] Arthritis is also a leading predisposing condition for fractures.[36] Arthritis causes bone demineralization. The pain from arthritis limits people's activity, thus causing weight gain. These factors combined with environmental factors often result in falls or fractures.

More than 100 types of arthritis have been identified; the three most common types in the elderly population are osteoarthritis (OA), rheumatoid arthritis (RA), and gout.[35] Descriptions, causes, and symptoms of these three forms of arthritis are presented in Table 22-6.

Treatment for arthritis in elders can consist of any combination of therapy, medication, and surgery. Therapy

TABLE 22-6

Description of Osteoarthritis and Rheumatoid Arthritis

Condition	Definition	Cause	Symptoms
Osteoarthritis (degenerative joint disease)	A degenerative disease of cartilage with a secondary degeneration involving underlying bone	Possible biomechanical, inflammatory, and immunologic factors; secondary factors include congenital defects, trauma, inflammation, endocrine and metabolic disease, and occupational stress	Progressively developing pain, stiffness, and enlargement with limitation of motion; crepitus with PROM; commonly affects weight-bearing joints (hips, knees, cervical and lumbar spine, PIPs [enlargements or osteophytes in PIPs are often referred to as Bouchard's nodes], DIPs [enlargements or osteophytes in DIPs are often called Heberden's nodes], CMCs, and MTPs); joints appear red, tender, swollen; asymmetrical presentation; deformities of joints; pain often follows periods of overuse or extended inactivity
Rheumatoid arthritis	Chronic, systemic disease characterized by inflammation of the synovial tissue of joints; may involve the heart, lungs, blood vessels, or eyes	Unknown; seems to be of an unknown immune reaction in synovial tissue	Characterized by exacerbations and remissions; commonly affects weight-bearing joints (hips, knees, cervical and lumbar spine, PIPs, DIPs, CMCs, and MTPs); joints appear red, tender, swollen, and hot; usually a symmetrical presentation; deformities of joints (i.e., swan-neck, boutonnière); fusiform swelling in PIPs
Gout	Painful rheumatic disease affecting connective tissue, joint spaces, or both, caused by uric acid	Caused by deposits of needle-like crystals of uric acid in the connective tissue, joint spaces, or both	Characterized by swelling, redness, heat, pain, and joint stiffness; commonly affects the toes, ankles, elbows, wrists, and hands

CMC, carpometacarpal; DIP, distal interphalangeal; MTP, metatarsophalangeal; PIP, proximal interphalangeal; PROM, proximal range of motion.

may consist of the provision of physical therapy and OT. Medications commonly prescribed to elders who have arthritis are NSAIDs and cyclooxygenase-2 inhibitors (similar to NSAIDs but with fewer side effects). Performing surgery to replace joints is often a last resort.

COTAs must be aware of the physical restrictions and limitations that arthritis imposes on elders' activities. Interventions by the COTA/OTR team should focus on helping elders manage their symptoms more effectively in addition to modifying occupational tasks.

Common Problems Associated with Arthritis

Osteoarthritis of the knee affects approximately 60% of people older than age 65 years.[37] Limitations caused by knee OA include difficulty using stairs, squatting, and high-impact activities (i.e., running or jumping).[30] These activities can be quite painful and can reduce the quality of life for an active elder.

Upper extremity deformities caused by OA can be problematic. Osteophytes form in the fingers and base of the thumb. Although osteophytes are not painful, they are seen at the distal interphalangeal (DIP) (Heberden's nodes) and proximal interphalangeal (PIP) joints (Bouchard's nodes). Such nodes result in difficulty and pain

during pinching. In advanced stages, the thumb's carpal metacarpal (CMC) joint can subluxate and result in joint instability.

The hands are the most severely affected joints in RA. Often, the PIP joints present with fusiform swelling or spindle-like shape. Boutonnière and swan-neck deformities are also finger deformities that may result from RA. Nalebuff deformities are common to the thumb when affected by RA. Ulnar drift is often present in the metacarpophalangeal (MCP) joints of the hand, and the wrist may sublux volarly.

Gout commonly affects the toes, ankles, elbows, wrists, and hands. Swelling can cause the skin to become taut around the joint and make the area appear red or purple and be tender. These presentations, in turn, reduce joint mobility (NIA, n.d.).

Occupational Therapy Intervention

The primary goal of OT intervention is to improve the quality of life of elders with arthritis. Specific goals may include maintaining joint mobility or joint stability, preventing joint deformity, maintaining strength, maintaining or improving functional ability, maintaining a healthy balance of rest and activity, modifying performance of activities, and improving psychosocial acceptance and coping mechanisms.

Maintenance of joint mobility and stability

COTAs may develop an exercise program for the elder to keep arthritic joints moving. Such an exercise program should seek to minimize stress to all involved joints. Elders with arthritis often find that taking a warm bath or shower after waking up in the morning relieves joint stiffness, thereby making it easier to exercise and engage in other activities. Elders with arthritis may also find it helpful to use a paraffin bath before engaging in wrist and hand exercises. COTAs should demonstrate service competency when using physical agent modalities.

Joints requiring stability may warrant orthotic intervention. A carefully designed splint may provide stability to a joint and improve function. For example, discomfort in the CMC joint may be reduced by fabricating a hand-based thumb spica splint to support the CMC joint in a functional position.[38]

Prevention of joint deformity

COTAs must be aware of the common types of joint deformities that may develop as a result of arthritis. Deformities include wrist subluxation, ulnar drift of the MCP joints, swan-neck deformity, boutonnière deformity, and Nalebuff type I deformity of the thumb.

Volar subluxation of the wrist frequently occurs in elders who have arthritis. A wrist cock-up splint may aid the elder in maintaining better wrist alignment, which will promote function and reduce pain.[39] Ulnar drift, or ulnar deviation, of the MCP joints is another common deformity caused by arthritis. Ulnar drift is usually caused by the destruction and loosening of the radial collateral ligaments. Some experts suggest that the use of an ulnar drift splint may prevent further deformity.[38]

A swan-neck deformity of the finger results in PIP hyperextension with DIP flexion. A boutonnière deformity results in PIP flexion with DIP hyperextension. Both deformities can be splinted or surgically repaired with varying results. A Nalebuff type I deformity results in the metacarpal joint of the thumb flexed with hyperextension of the interphalangeal joint. A radial gutter thumb spica splint is often used for better positioning.[40]

To prevent further deformity, elders should be evaluated to determine whether they need splints that are appropriate for the deformity and activity level. In addition, elders should be taught joint protection techniques (Box 22-1).

Maintenance of strength

COTAs may be asked to develop graded strengthening programs for elders who have arthritis. These programs should include the principles of joint protection discussed previously. During periods of acute exacerbation of arthritis, elders should not engage in strengthening programs.

Improvement of functional ability

Functional ability can be improved through careful collaboration between the COTA, OTR, and the elder. This

---

BOX 22-1

Joint Protection Principles

- Respect pain. Monitor activities and stop to rest when discomfort or fatigue develops. For example, if kneeling or stooping to garden causes pain and stiffness, stop and rest. Next time, try sitting on a stool.
- Reduce stresses on joints. Use the largest joint possible for activities. For example, when using hands to push up from a seated position, push up with the palms, not the back of the fingers.
- Wear splints as prescribed to protect joints. For example, wear resting hand splints during exacerbation periods to reduce pain. Movements should be done in the opposite direction of deformity. For example, when wringing out a wash cloth, twist toward the radial side rather than the ulnar side.
- Avoid sustaining a strong, tight grasp. For example, use foam or a cloth wrapped around handles to relax the grip needed to manipulate an object.
- Avoid carrying and lifting heavy objects. For example, use a cart to move heavy objects. Distribute object weight evenly over many joints. For example, use both hands to handle a carton of milk.
- Limit the amount of time spent climbing, walking, and standing. For example, take an elevator or escalators; drive or use a walking aid; sit whenever possible.
- Avoid sustained flexion of the finger joints. For example, use a large sponge for cleaning; work with the fingers extended over the sponge rather than squeezing it.
- Avoid using heavy objects. For example, cook with lightweight pots and pans rather than heavy cast-iron pots and pans.

---

collaboration can help determine whether assistive equipment works well and is accomplishing the goal for which it was intended. For example, a rocker knife may allow the elder to continue to cut meat during meals. COTAs must observe how the elder handles the knife to ensure that the involved joints are protected as the knife is used and to ascertain that the knife actually cuts the meat.

Maintenance of life balance

Graded strengthening programs for elders who have arthritis are developed by OTRs and may be administered by COTAs. Assisting elders in achieving a balance between rest and activity is paramount. For example, elders are often tempted to schedule all activities during the morning hours with the hope of resting in the afternoon. However, a better balance is achieved when activities are scheduled throughout the day and an appropriate period of rest is incorporated after each activity. This type of schedule will help decrease the fatigue of elders and is less likely to lead

TABLE 22-7

Principles of Work Simplification and Energy Conservation

Pace	A moderate, slow pace is most productive; a slower pace is needed in a hot and humid atmosphere.
Rhythm	Working in a rhythmic manner saves energy and increases efficiency.
Eyes	Work in a well-lighted room, with local light for close work, and rest the eyes periodically.
Rest	Plan regular rest periods that are properly spaced during the day.
Body mechanics	Sit to work whenever possible; sit in a seat large enough to give full support; work with the elbows close to the body; if working at a table, the height of the table should be near the height of the elbows when they are bent at 90-degree angles.
Work areas	A place should be designated for all tools, utensils, and materials; materials should be located close to the area where they will be used.
Design of equipment	Handles of utensils and equipment should permit the maximum surface of the hand to come in contact with the handle; handles should be heat-resistant and built up as appropriate; handles that have impressions for the fingers should be used when possible; lightweight equipment should actually be light in weight.
Kitchen storage	Store supplies and utensils within easy reach; arrange the cupboards so that all articles are easy to see, easy to reach, and easy to grasp; store heavy equipment (e.g., stacks of plates and pans) on shelves that are easy to reach; use vertical dividers for dish storage, baking pans, trays, and lids; avoid clutter by eliminating or discarding unnecessary equipment.
Cooking	Use a cart for transporting food and dishes; slide heavy pots from the sink to the stove instead of lifting them; avoid holding containers or mixing bowls when preparing food; select equipment that can be used for more than one job.
Bed making	To avoid numerous trips around the bed, make one side completely and then the next side; if possible, keep the bed away from the wall; have the bed put on rollers if it must be moved.
Cleaning	When cleaning the bathtub, use long-handled brushes and sit on the edge of the bathtub; use a dust cloth on a long-handled stick for dusting baseboards and ceilings; have cleaning equipment available both upstairs and downstairs.

to an exacerbation of their conditions. In addition, elders will likely accomplish more during the day.

Modification of activity

Work simplification and energy conservation techniques often benefit elders who have arthritis (Table 22-7). These elders must attempt to distribute their energy output evenly over the number of tasks to be accomplished. Incorporating energy conservation and work simplification techniques into the elders' daily routines can assist them in maintaining a functional lifestyle.

Improvement of psychosocial well-being and coping mechanisms

The combination of acute and chronic pain, coupled with joint stiffness and immobility, can result in limitations of ADL such as dressing, and recreational and social outlets such as dancing. The population of elders who experience pain is challenged daily to use strategies that will enhance productive living. Elders who do not have coping and support systems will need assistance in developing such systems. COTAs may provide assistance by linking elders who have arthritis with community resources that can provide support and help elders develop coping mechanisms. Self-help courses sponsored by the Arthritis Foundation can provide social interaction. Alternative methods of pain control may include relaxation training, cognitive restructuring and modification, medication fading, and

social assertiveness training. The process of helping elders cope with arthritis must involve a multidisciplinary approach for chronic pain management to be successful.

CASE STUDY

Ford and Ida are meeting with a builder to design their retirement condominium. In planning the space, they have decided to consult with an agency that provides assistance for home design and modification for elders. They are awaiting a contact from the agency to schedule a meeting to begin plans for the new condominium.

One month previously, Ford fell during the nighttime in an attempt to go to the bathroom and sustained a hip fracture. Subsequently, he underwent an open reduction internal fixation and pinning of his right hip. Also, last year Ida had a TKA. Ida has considerable pain from RA. They hope to plan their ranch-style condominium to meet their current and future needs in relation to their health.

◼ CASE STUDY REVIEW QUESTIONS

1 List the precautions that Ford might need to follow after his hip pinning procedure.
2 List the ADL functions that will be directly affected by Ford's hip pinning procedure.
3 Describe the problems that Ida may be dealing with as a result of RA.
4 Name the wrist and hand deformities associated with RA that may be afflicting Ida.

5 Describe some possible causes for Ford's fall that should be investigated.

6 Describe the ways in which Ford's performance of ADL functions and his environment will need to be modified.

7 List appropriate recommendations for the living room, kitchen, bathroom, and bedroom for their new condominium.

▮ CHAPTER REVIEW QUESTIONS

1 Identify the most common causes of fractures in elders.

2 Why do elder women have a greater occurrence of orthopedic problems than elder men?

3 Why is it important for the COTA to have an understanding of the anterolateral and posterolateral approaches related to total hip replacements?

4 Identify two psychosocial issues that may have an effect on an elder after a total hip replacement.

5 Using joint protection techniques, explain how you would teach elders with arthritis in their hands to do the following:

  a Wash delicate clothing in the sink

  b Lift a child from a playpen

  c Use a computer

6 Explain how you would teach an elder energy conservation techniques during the following activities:

  a Removing groceries from the trunk of a car and taking them in the house

  b Vacuuming the floor

  c Cleaning the kitchen after a meal

REFERENCES

1. Centers for Disease Control, 1996. Incidence and costs to Medicare of fracture among Medicare beneficiaries age 65 years —United States, July 1991-June 1992. Morbidity and Mortality Weekly Report, 45 (41), 877-883.

2. National Institute of Arthritis and Musculoskeletal and Skin Diseases, 2010. Living with arthritis [WWW page]. http://www.niams.nih.gov/Health_Info/Arthritis/default.asp.

3. Min, L., Yoon, W., Mariano, J., Wenger, N., Elliott, M., Kamberg, C., et al., 2009. The vulnerable elders: 13 Survey predicts 5-year functional decline and mortality outcomes in older ambulatory care patients. Journal of the American Geriatrics Society 57 (11), 2070-2076.

4. White, A., Hashimoto, R., Norvell, D., Vaccaro, A., 2010. Morbidity and mortality related to odontoid fracture surgery in the elderly population. Spine 35, S146-S157.

5. Woolf, A., Akesson, K., 2009. Preventing fractures in elderly people. British Medical Journal 338 (7685), 89-96.

6. Söderqvist, A., Ekström, W., Ponzer, S., Pettersson, H., Cederholm, T., Dalén, N., et al., 2009. Prediction of mortality in elderly patients with hip fractures: A two-year prospective study of 1,944 patients. Gerontology 55 (5), 496-504.

7. Heuberger, R., 2009. Alcohol and the older adult: A comprehensive review. Journal of Nutrition for the Elderly 28 (3), 203-235.

8. Wolinsky, F., Bentler, S., Li, L., Obrizan, M., Cook, E., Wright, K., et al., 2009. Recent hospitalization and the risk of hip fracture among older Americans. Journals of Gerontology 64A (2), 249-255.

9. Moayyeri, A., Bingham, S., Luben, R., Wareham, N., Khaw, K., 2009. Respiratory function as a marker of bone health and fracture risk in an older population. Journal of Bone and Mineral Research 24 (5), 956-963.

10. McKay, C., Anderson, K., 2010. How to manage falls in community dwelling older adults: A review of the evidence. Postgraduate Medical Journal 86 (1015), 299-306.

11. Chen, J.S., Sambrook, P.N., Simpson, J.M., March, L., Cumming, R., Seibel, M., et al., 2010. A selection strategy was developed for fracture reduction programs in frail older people. Journal of Clinical Epidemiology 63 (6), 679-685.

12. Insurance Institute for Highway Safety, 2010. How many older drivers are there? Retrieved July 8, 2010, from http://www.iihs.org.

13. National Institute on Aging, 2010. Age page: Older drivers [WWW page]. URL http://www.nia.nih.gov/HealthInformation/Publications/drivers.htm.

14. Classen, S., Shechtman, O., Awadzi, K.D., Joo, Y., Lanford, D.N., 2010. Traffic violations versus driving errors of older adults: Informing clinical practice. American Journal of Occupational Therapy 64 (2), 233-241.

15. Kelsey, J., Samelson, E., 2009. Variation in risk factors for fractures at different sites. Current Osteoporosis Reports 4, 127-133.

16. Guadalupe-Grau, A., Fuentes, T., Guerra, B., Jose, A., 2009. Exercise and bone mass in adults. Sports Medicine 39 (6), 439-468.

17. Lipton, A., 2010. Bone continuum of cancer. American Journal of Clinical Oncology 33 (Suppl. 3), S1-S7.

18. Egol, K., Koval, K., Zuckerman, J., 2010. Handbook of Fractures, 4th ed. Lippincott Williams & Wilkins, Hagerstown, MD.

19. Sueki, D., Brechter, J., 2010. Orthopedic Rehabilitation Clinical Advisor. Mosby, Maryland Heights, MO.

20. Brotzman, B., Wilk, K., 2006. Handbook of Orthopedic Rehabilitation, 2nd ed. Mosby, St. Louis, MO.

21. Brauer, C., Coca-Perraillon, M., Cutler, S., Rosen, A., 2009. Incidence and mortality of hip fractures in the United States. Journal of the American Medical Association 302 (14), 1573-1579.

22. Kim, Y., 2006. Comparison of primary total hip arthroplasties performed with a minimally invasive technique or a standard technique: A prospective and randomized study. Journal of Arthroplasty 21 (8), 1092-1098.

23. Heinrich, S., Rapp, K., Rissmann, U., Becker, C., König, H., 2010. Cost of falls in old age: A systematic review. Osteoporosis International 21 (6), 891-902.

24. Parker, M., Handoll, H., 2006. Replacement arthroplasty versus internal fixation for extracapsular hip fractures in adults. Cochrane Database of Systemic Reviews 19 (2), CD000086.

25. Crotty, M., Unroe, K., Cameron, I., Miller, M., Ramirez, G., Couzner, L., 2010. Rehabilitation interventions for improving physical and psychosocial functioning after hip fracture in older people. Cochrane Database of Systematic Reviews, Issue 1, Art. No.: CD007624.

26. Hozak, W., Parvisi, J., Bender, B., 2009. Surgical Treatment of Hip Arthritis: Reconstruction, Replacement, and Revision. WB Saunders, Philadelphia.

27. Khan, F., Ng, L., Gonzalez, S., Hale, T., Turner-Stokes, L., 2008. Multidisciplinary rehabilitation programmes following joint replacement at the hip and knee in chronic arthropathy. Cochrane Database of Systematic Reviews, Issue 2, Art. No.: CD004957.

28. Parker, M., Gurusamy, K., Azegami, S., 2010. Arthroplasties (with and without bone cement) for proximal femoral fractures in adults. Cochrane Database of Systematic Reviews, Issue 6, Art. No.: CD001706.

29. McGann, W., 2006. Surgical approaches. In: Barrack, R., Booth, R., Lonner, J., McCarthy, J., Mont, M., Rubash, H. (Eds.), Orthopedic Knowledge Update: Knee and Hip Reconstruction. American College of Orthopedic Surgeons, Rosemont, IL, pp. 311-322.
30. Bhave, A., 2006. Rehabilitation after total hip and total knee replacement. In: Barrack, R., Booth, R., Lonner, J., McCarthy, J., Mont, M., Rubash, H. (Eds.), (2006). Orthopedic Knowledge Update: Knee and Hip Reconstruction. American College of Orthopedic Surgeons, Rosemont, IL.
31. Brander, V.A., Mullarkey, C.F., Stulberg, S.D., 2001. Rehabilitation after total joint replacement for osteoarthritis: An evidence-based approach. Physical Medicine and Rehabilitation 15 (1), 175-197.
32. Robnett, R., Chop, W., 2010. Gerontology for the Health Care Professional, 2nd ed. Jones & Bartlett, Sudbury, MA.
33. Alkema, G., Wilber, K., Enguidanos, S., 2007. Community- and facility-based care. In: Blackburn, J., Dulum, C. (Eds.), Handbook of Gerontology: Evidence-Based Approaches to Theory, Practice, and Policy. John Wiley & Sons, Hoboken, NJ.
34. Mullarkey, C.F., Brander, V., 2002. Rehabilitation after total knee replacement for osteoarthritis. Physical Medicine and Rehabilitation: State of the Art Reviews 16, 431-443.
35. Walker, J., Helewa, A., 2004. Physical Rehabilitation in Arthritis. WB Saunders, Philadelphia.
36. Gillespie, L.D., Gillespie, W.J., Robertson, M.C., Lamb, S.E., Cumming, R.G., Rowe, B.H., 2009. Interventions for preventing falls in elderly people. Cochrane Database of Systematic Reviews, Issue 2. Art. No.: CD000340. DOI: 10.1002/14651858CD000340.pub2.
37. Mikuls, T., 2010. Arthritis incidence: What goes down must go up? Arthritis and Rheumatism 62 (6), 1565-1567.
38. Riley, M.A., Lohman, H., Berger, S.M., Cavanaugh, M.T., Coppard, B.M., 2007. Splinting on elders. In: Coppard, B.M., Lohman, H. (Eds.), Introduction to Splinting, 2nd ed. Mosby, St. Louis, MO.
39. Lohman, H., 2007. Wrist immobilization splints. In: Coppard, B.M., Lohman, H. (Eds.), Introduction to Splinting. 2nd ed. Mosby, St. Louis, MO.
40. Lohman, H., 2007. Thumb immobilization splints. In: Coppard, B.M., Lohman, H. (Eds.), Introduction to Splinting. 2nd ed. Mosby, St. Louis, MO.

Working with Elders Who Have Cardiovascular Conditions

TONYA BARTHOLOMEW, JANA K. CRAGG, JEAN T. HAYS,
AMY MATTHEWS, CLAIRE PEEL, AND RENÉ PADILLA

KEY TERMS

cardiac rehabilitation, cardiovascular disease, heart rate, blood pressure, maximum
heart rate, metabolic equivalents, energy conservation, work simplification

CHAPTER OBJECTIVES

1. Identify the signs and symptoms of cardiac dysfunction.
2. Describe the phases of cardiac rehabilitation.
3. Recognize the role of occupational therapy in cardiac rehabilitation.
4. Describe assessments, intervention techniques, and precautions used with elders who have cardiac conditions.
5. Describe intervention approaches for elders with cardiac conditions in various treatment settings.

Joan is a certified occupational therapy assistant (COTA) who specializes in cardiac rehabilitation. She works closely with the cardiac team as she provides occupational therapy (OT) interventions. Mark is a COTA employed by a skilled nursing facility. He works with elders who have a variety of conditions. Many of the elders are admitted for specific reasons such as rehabilitation after a total hip replacement or stroke. Most have accompanying chronic illnesses, including cardiac conditions. Mark often informally consults with Joan when he has an intervention question about cardiac conditions because he does not have the same specialty experience that she has, and he values her expertise. This chapter focuses primarily on the role of COTAs in cardiac rehabilitation settings. However, intervention with elders who have cardiac conditions in other settings is also addressed.

Heart disease is the leading cause of death in the United States[1] and one of the most prevalent chronic conditions among older Americans.[2]

Cardiovascular disease refers to several types of heart conditions, which include (1) diseases that primarily affect the heart such as coronary artery disease and congestive heart failure, (2) circulatory problems involving peripheral vessels such as peripheral vascular disease, and (3) circulatory problems involving the cerebral circulation. This chapter focuses primarily on diseases in the first category: the heart.

BACKGROUND INFORMATION

During the aging process, the body experiences gradual changes. Although many of these changes are inevitable, studies show that some of the changes are less pronounced in elders who do not have cardiovascular diseases and associated risk factors.[2] This is especially true for elders who have lifestyles that include regular physical activity. However, most elders experience age-related changes in their cardiovascular systems, including changes in the heart muscle and vessels, peripheral vascular disease, and an increase in systolic pressure, which makes the heart work harder.[3] Most coronary diseases are related to lifestyle and family history, as well as age. Chronic cardiac conditions include hypertension, angina pectoris, congestive heart failure, and peripheral vascular disease. Heart disease often accompanies other illnesses or conditions such as diabetes or chronic obstructive pulmonary disease; therefore, the COTA should be aware of any additional precautions or contraindications associated with these diagnoses and cardiovascular disease.

Medical treatment varies according to the condition and other individual health factors. Thrombolytics are used to prevent muscle damage from heart attacks. Other common drugs are those used to treat hypertension, angina, heart failure, and dysrhythmias. The COTA should be aware of the medications that the patient is taking and the associated side effects. If conservative treatments involving medications are not effective, then surgical interventions may be necessary. Surgical treatments may include angioplasty or a bypass for damaged arteries. In rare cases, treatment may involve a heart transplant to replace heart muscle that is irreversibly damaged. Cardiac management may include electromechanical devices such as pacemakers to achieve a normal heart rate (HR) and rhythm.

Heart disease may begin with a loss of elasticity in the small vessels, causing the heart to work harder to maintain blood flow to organs. A change in the temperature in the extremities, cyanosis, or an increase in systolic blood pressure may indicate circulatory insufficiency.[4] Atherosclerosis is a condition in which lipid deposits accumulate on the walls of large and medium vessels.[5] This narrows the lumen of these vessels, which restricts blood flow. Atherosclerosis of coronary vessels can produce ischemia, which causes angina (chest pain), a myocardial infarction (MI), or both, which damages the heart muscle. Atherosclerosis of cerebral vessels can lead to a cerebrovascular accident, or stroke. A change in the structure of the heart valves, either from viral illness or aging, may result in heart failure, a condition in which the heart cannot deliver enough oxygen to peripheral tissues.

Valvular disease may be heard as a murmur during a routine examination. When the left side of the heart fails, fluid accumulates in the lungs, causing exertional dyspnea, orthopnea, paroxysmal nocturnal dyspnea, dyspnea at rest, pulmonary edema, weakness, and fatigue.[4] When the right side of the heart fails, blood backs up in the periphery, causing systemic venous congestion, dependent edema, upper right quadrant pain, anorexia, nausea, bloating, and fatigue.[6] Many elders with cardiovascular disease lose the ability to perform physical activities and lose independence in their daily skills.[2]

PSYCHOSOCIAL ASPECTS OF CARDIAC DYSFUNCTIONS

Cardiac dysfunction can have profound psychosocial implications on elders and their significant others. All elders react differently to a cardiac event, experiencing a wide range of emotions, including anxiety, depression, denial, and helplessness,[7] but most progress through many stages of adjustment. Initially, the anxiety produced by fear of death, discomfort, dependence, and disability can have a profound effect and produce overwhelming feelings. Some elders demonstrate this anxiety in behavioral changes and may act out or become agitated. This level of anxiety places a physiological demand on the cardiac system at a time when rest is important. Elders experiencing a rapid change in their care status may also have difficulty with anxiety; as a result, anti-anxiety medications are often used to assist them. However, anti-anxiety medications can have unwanted side effects and lead to additional stress. Elders should be encouraged to voice their feelings and work with the health care team to alleviate their fears about the course of events. Good communication and supportive staff members are the key elements in reducing elders' anxiety levels.[8] Fear of another cardiac event can impair functional levels, especially in the early rehabilitation phase. Education and therapeutic intervention can help alleviate these fears. Once stable, elders should be encouraged to begin ambulation and self-care activities following the guidelines established by the registered occupational therapist (OTR). This helps to eliminate the helplessness elders may feel after a cardiac event. The longer that these two elements are delayed, the more helpless elders may feel, which can reinforce the disability.[7,8] (Chapter 12 includes a discussion of ways to address the sexual concerns of elders with heart disease.)

As elders begin to regain some strength and control over their activity, the denial of risk related to the disease may become evident. Denial gives some elders the mechanism necessary to cope with the cardiac event. This particular phase may be more prevalent in elders with coronary disease because the symptoms and characteristics associated with this disease are vague. COTAs must not try to break through the denial phase too soon. Facing the realities of the situation may be overwhelming and may create stress-related physical and emotional complications. COTAs can help elders by instructing them to monitor their performance carefully, thus reducing the risk for another cardiac event.

Some elders become depressed after a cardiac event. Inactivity and anxiety may trigger depression. Depression and anxiety combined can have a long-term effect on the elder's physical and emotional well-being. Patients with depression are less likely to resume normal activity and are at an increased risk for death.[7]

COTAs can play a strong role in addressing the psychosocial aspects of cardiac disease by educating elders about the expected outcomes after a cardiac event. Relaxation training and lifestyle education are key elements in achieving emotional well-being. Informing the family of risks and precautions can assist elders in the transition to the home environment and ensure that elders have the best chance to regain their status in the home and community.[9]

EVALUATION OF ELDERS WITH CARDIAC CONDITIONS

COTAs working with elders who have had cardiac events or who have chronic cardiac conditions should be able to monitor vital signs. It is important that COTAs accurately determine HR and take blood pressure (BP) during activities. Guidelines for HR and BP responses are typically written as treatment precautions. To determine the HR, COTAs should palpate the elder's pulse at the wrist, count the number of beats felt for 15 seconds, and then multiply this number by 4. This will provide a baseline HR in beats per minute (bpm) before the elder engages in activity.

Although HRs vary, a normal baseline HR ranges between 60 and 100 bpm.[9] Maximum HR corresponds with performing maximal levels of exertion that involve large muscle groups in rhythmic activities, such as walking and cycling. One method of predicting maximum HR is by subtracting the elder's age from 220. This figure is multiplied by 0.6 to predict the appropriate HR response for normal activity.[10] For example, a 78-year-old woman's predicted maximum HR would be 142 bpm (220 − 78 = 142). Her HR appropriate for activity would be 85 (0.6 × 142 = 85 bpm). Signs and symptoms, such as dyspnea, must be considered when using formulas to predict activity HR values. Elders should perform activities in a symptom-free range. Some medications (beta-blockers, verapamil, and diltiazem) blunt the usual HR in response to exercise, especially in elders; therefore, watching symptoms is especially important.[11] In the first phase of cardiac rehabilitation, patients are often on continuous pulse oximetry. The COTA should be careful to ensure that the patient is maintaining pulse and oxygen saturation levels within the range set by the physician.

Likewise, the BP should be taken if a physician has so ordered or if the elder has symptoms of distress such as shortness of breath, dizziness, weakness, or cyanosis. Elders with hypertension should be monitored for excessive increases in the BP or orthostatic hypotension, which may occur as a side effect of medications. BP values greater than 140/90 mm Hg indicate mild hypertension, and those greater than 160/100 mm Hg indicate moderate hypertension.[12] BP is considered hypotensive if the systolic BP is less than 90 mm Hg. Hypotension can be associated with dizziness and light-headedness or, in severe cases, circulatory inadequacy of the extremities.[9] In the presence of a shunt for renal dialysis, the BP should be read on the opposite limb. Renal shunts are fragile and cannot withstand the pressure produced by the BP cuff (sphygmomanometer) during BP monitoring. For training, COTAs should practice monitoring HR and BP with an instructor before performing care.

The COTA/OTR team should be able to perform a basic bedside activities of daily living (ADL) evaluation as part of the initial evaluation. This might include having the elder perform oral care, grooming tasks, washing of the upper body, and dressing. COTAs working with elders who have decreased endurance and low activity tolerance caused by cardiac disease may use metabolic equivalents (METs) as a basis for estimating the energy expended when performing an activity. The MET table provided along with HR and BP responses can help COTAs determine the cardiovascular stress and amount of work performed for specific tasks (Table 23-1).[13,14,15] Further areas to be assessed are grip strength, muscle strength, and bed mobility. The OT should also assess the patient's cognitive abilities to ensure that the patient will be able to comprehend the education and interventions that the COTA is teaching.

INTERVENTIONS, GOALS, AND STRATEGIES

For interventions to be effective, COTAs must understand the functional levels that are used to classify elders with cardiac disease. There are four functional categories for cardiac disease (Table 23-2). Knowing the categories allows COTAs to make adjustments in elders' rehabilitation programs. The four phases of cardiac rehabilitation describe where the elder is in the recovery process (Table 23-3).

COTAs need to be aware of activities that can be stressful to the heart. Such activities include isometric and upper extremity activities, especially if performed at a level above the heart. The stress on the heart is reflected by the elder's HR and BP responses, as well as other signs and symptoms. Consequently, any activity that produces excessive increases in HR and BP may overstress the heart (Box 23-1).

The primary goal of any cardiac rehabilitation program is to return elders to their maximum functional capacities. The COTA/OTR team must design an individualized rehabilitation program for each elder. Although the phases of rehabilitation follow certain key steps, each elder's progress will be different. Psychosocial aspects, family support, age, and medical status, as well as the desire to participate in the rehabilitation program, affect progression. A rehabilitation intervention plan for OT with MET allowances for specific activities is useful (see Table 23-1).

BOX 23-1

When to Stop Activity and Seek Medical Help

If any of the following symptoms lasts more than a few minutes before, during, or after the activity program, the elder should stop activity and seek medical help:

- Nausea
- Extremely heavy breathing
- Uncomfortable pressure, squeezing, fullness, or pain in the center of the chest that lasts more than a few minutes
- Severe fatigue
- Extreme sweating, breaking out in cold sweat
- Discomfort in the upper body (arms, neck, jaw, or stomach) during activity
- Light-headedness
- Unexplained low heart rate or dramatically higher rate than the target heart rate
- Drop in systolic blood pressure or failure of systolic blood pressure to rise
- Excessively high blood pressure (over 240/100 mm Hg)

Adapted from Streuber, S., Amsterdam, E., & Stebbins, C. (2006). Heart rate recovery in heart failure patients after a 12-week cardiac rehabilitation program. *American Journal of Cardiology, 97*(5), 694-698.

TABLE 23-1

	Santa Clara Valley Medical Center's Metabolic Equivalents After Myocardial Infarction and After Open Heart Surgery	
Stage	**Occupational therapy**	
In ICU or on ward	General mobility (bed mobility, transfers to the commode, and position changes) with energy conservation techniques (environmental setups, equipment, and pacing)[13]	
1-2 METs	Sedentary leisure tasks with arms supported (reading, writing, playing cards)[13] Standing tasks (seconds to 2 minutes)[13] Simple hygiene, semi-recline sitting position[13] Standing tasks (3 to 5 minutes)[13] Bedside bathing (assist with feet and back)[13] Bathroom privileges[13] Light leisure tasks such as keyboarding at a computer[13] Writing[14] Billiards[14] Needlework[15]	
2-3 METs	Standing tasks (5-30 minutes)[13] Sustained upper extremity (UE) activity (2-30 minutes)[13] Total body bathing at sink[13] Total hygiene, bathing, dressing at sink[13] Total body mobility: bending for small objects, retrieval training[13] Moderate leisure tasks[13] Walking at a slow or moderate pace[14] Driving[14] Playing the piano or other musical instrument[15] Using a sewing machine[15]	
3-4 METs	Shower transfers[13] Total showering task (hair washing, total body washing, drying, and dressing)[13] Simple homemaking tasks such as meal preparation[13] Energy conservation techniques with activity such as cleaning windows[13] Walking at a pace of 3 miles per hour[14] Doing laundry[15] Ironing[15] Vacuuming[15]	
4-5 METs	Pushing a light power mower[13] Dance[13] Raking leaves[13] Climbing stairs[14] Slow swimming[14] Washing windows[15]	
5-6 METs	Digging in a garden[13] Sex[13] Fishing[13] Hiking[14] Jogging[14] Shoveling snow[15] Most sports involving running (e.g., basketball, softball)[15]	

ICU, intensive care unit; MET, metabolic equivalent.

Phase I

Phase I consists of the period of inpatient hospitalization. Most referred elders are in the acute phase after undergoing surgery or experiencing MI. Other elders are referred for atypical chest pain. Beginning in phase I, elders are evaluated by an OTR. During the evaluation, the COTA/OTR team reviews the medical chart to obtain information on medical history and current cardiac status, and they interview the elder to determine lifestyle and personal goals for rehabilitation. During phase I, OT practitioners and elders work toward developing a discharge plan on the basis of the elder's individual needs and lifestyles. Goals for meeting each of the stages in phase I are discussed (see Table 23-1). Activities and educational

TABLE 23-2

The Four Functional Categories of Cardiac Disease

Class I	Elders with cardiac disease but without resulting limitations of physical activity. Ordinary physical activity does not cause undue fatigue, palpitation, dyspnea, or anginal pain.
Class II	Elders with cardiac disease resulting in slight limitation of physical activity; they are comfortable at rest. Ordinary physical activity results in fatigue, dyspnea, palpitation, or anginal pain.
Class III	Elders with cardiac disease resulting in marked limitation of physical activity; they are comfortable at rest. Less than ordinary physical activity causes fatigue, dyspnea, palpitation, or anginal pain.
Class IV	Elders with cardiac disease resulting in inability to perform any physical activity without discomfort. Symptoms of cardiac insufficiency or of anginal syndrome may be present even at rest. If any physical activity is undertaken, discomfort increases.

From New York Heart Association. (1979). *Nomenclature and Criteria for Diagnoses of Diseases of the Heart and Great Vessels*, 8th ed. Boston: Little, Brown.

TABLE 23-3

The Three Phases of Cardiac Rehabilitation

Phase I	This phase occurs in the acute phase of hospitalization for the cardiac event. Elders qualifying for cardiac rehabilitation must be stable after event as determined by physician(s).
Phase II	Elder enters a program designed to regain former functional and performance level. Focus is on increasing duration and intensity of physical activity to achieve health benefits and to increase cardiorespiratory fitness.
Phase III	Elder enters a maintenance phase of cardiac rehabilitation. This phase is indefinite in length and involves periodic evaluations.

information are introduced as the rehabilitation process begins. Activities and exercises are initially low level. Early in phase I, COTAs educate elders regarding the need for balancing their lifestyles, which includes stress reduction techniques. Elders are also educated to accommodate for changes in their health status. Using the occupational behavioral model of work, rest, and play, COTAs can introduce the concepts of energy conservation and work simplification while providing bedside intervention.[16] This gives elders the ability to regain some of their self-care and dignity while learning to work with their limitations after a cardiac event. COTAs can build rapport and support continued rehabilitation by carefully monitoring physiological responses, signs, and symptoms and structuring activities to prevent elders from feeling fatigue.

METs help establish parameters for functional activities. One MET, the oxygen consumed by the body at rest, is equal to approximately 3.5 ml O_2/kg body mass per minute. To translate this concept into an activity level, it takes 1.5 METs to write a letter in bed with the arms supported.[9] Most self-care activities range from 1.5 to 3.5 METs, and, although this may seem to be light work, it can be physically demanding for some elders. In some rehabilitation settings, OT does not intervene in cardiac rehabilitation until the elder is able to perform light work (1.5 to 2 METs) without symptoms of dyspnea, palpitation, or angina during or after activity. Once elders are at this level, they can attempt activities required to return home and can independently perform most self-care activities. During phase I, elders are reevaluated to determine whether additional equipment or education is necessary so that they are able to return home and conduct functional activities with safe and appropriate HR, electrocardiogram (ECG), and BP responses.

Phase II

Phase II, often referred to as the recovery, or healing, phase, is the period immediately after hospitalization.[16] Elders receive rehabilitation through home health or outpatient clinic services. An elder's functional performance during self-care activities is evaluated by monitoring the resting pulse and peak pulse during a task and then measuring the recovery time to a resting pulse once the activity is terminated. The elder's status is monitored during the activities by measuring HR, BP, ECG, and respiratory responses before, during, and after task completion. The course of treatment and the elder's progress are determined by the physiological responses during activities and the estimated MET level for activities. During this phase of rehabilitation, education and training continue for modifications of risk factors and monitoring of the elder's general health.[17]

Phase III

Once elders are able to tolerate increased MET activities at greater than 3.5 METs with safe and appropriate HR, BP, and ECG responses, they are ready to move into phase III of rehabilitation. At this level of function, elders ideally have been under the care of a cardiac rehabilitation team for 2 to 3 months. Goals of phase III programs include increasing activity duration and intensity to a level sufficient to elicit cardiorespiratory training adaptations while assisting elders in making necessary lifestyle changes.[17] Phase III of cardiac rehabilitation requires elders to be more responsible for self-monitoring and to react appropriately if signs or symptoms of a recurring cardiac event become evident. Elders in phase III programs typically

TABLE 23-4

Assistive Devices and Rationale for Use	
Item(s)	**Rationale**
Long-handle reacher Long-handle shoehorn Sock aid Elastic shoelaces Long-handle bath sponge	These items prevent the need to bend more than 90 degrees forward flexion in trunk. This may be a precaution for bypass surgery to reduce strain over incision. Limiting trunk flexion to 90 degrees facilitates breathing by allowing full excursion of the diaphragm.
Bath bench	Allows patient to sit during bathing.
High stool	Allows patient to sit during household tasks, such as food preparation and ironing.

attend outpatient programs two or three times per week. These sessions provide opportunities for therapists to evaluate function and performance and to facilitate progression of activity programs. Providing elders with the education and techniques necessary to maintain their new lifestyles allows them to be more successful at self-monitoring. Elders are often counseled to make dietary changes, to stop smoking, and to increase physical activity levels. COTAs are in a position to reinforce lifestyle changes. Continued training in energy conservation and the use of assistive devices is provided to elders at functional levels III and IV. In outpatient clinics, elders can also receive training in a simulated work environment to provide guidelines for returning to a job or for avocational interests.

ENERGY CONSERVATION, WORK SIMPLIFICATION, AND OTHER EDUCATION

During OT, elders receive education on energy conservation, work simplification, and cardiac status monitoring.[16] Energy conservation is not only important for the elder's well-being, but also it is a safety monitor for routine tasks. In the acute portion of cardiac rehabilitation, this component allows elders to set the pace of their self-care routines. Energy conservation begins with basic task analysis, which includes identifying the main steps in the task, analyzing the way the task is performed, and determining the tools or skills needed to perform the task. Once analyzed, the next component of work simplification is added. Having elders perform basic grooming at the bedside is an example of ADL energy conservation. Using the bedside table, with arms propped for energy conservation, the elder can perform grooming with all of the supplies and a basin of water on the table (Figure 23-1). Elders may need to be educated to take rest breaks during the task if they experience dyspnea or an increase in HR beyond the established parameters. The task can be simplified with a complete setup of supplies, including the removal of all caps from grooming supplies and the provision of a lightweight electric razor, if appropriate. With the elder in the semi-reclined position in bed, this task

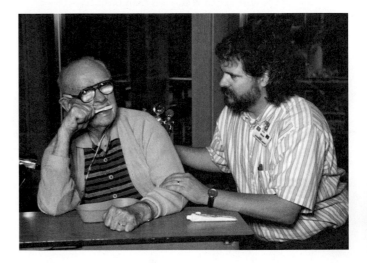

FIGURE 23-1 Elders should perform oral care with arms propped on a table.

can be accomplished with no more than 1.5 METs. Other ADL functions are analyzed in the same manner, with the therapist identifying ways to reduce the energy expenditure (energy conservation) and minimize steps to perform the task (work simplification). The addition of assistive devices may be an added benefit (Table 23-4). (See Chapter 12 to learn about addressing sexuality aspects of ADL with heart disease.)

Elders should be educated to pace themselves during activities to reduce fatigue. The work–rest–work principle is important for elders to maintain in the acute phase, especially when denial is an issue. Elders in denial about their cardiac disease may want to prove they are well by overworking or pushing themselves, placing unnecessary stress on their damaged hearts.

INTERVENTION WITH ELDERS WITH CARDIAC CONDITIONS IN OTHER SETTINGS

The chapter has focused primarily on cardiac rehabilitation when cardiac disease is the primary diagnosis. However, COTAs may encounter elders who have cardiac problems, perhaps as one of many chronic conditions, in settings such as nursing homes, outpatient clinics, or at home. Elders with acute cardiac conditions eventually may be transferred from the cardiac rehabilitation setting to another setting for further rehabilitation. In these settings, COTAs who are not formally trained in cardiac rehabilitation need to be aware of treatment approaches and precautions. Elders with cardiac conditions in any setting need to be educated on work simplification and energy conservation. The optimal approach is to demonstrate work simplification and energy conservation during the performance of meaningful tasks.

The primary recommendation for all elders with cardiac conditions is to monitor responses to activity by measuring HR, BP, and respiratory rate at rest, during activity, and during recovery. Activities that elicit excessive increases in HR or BP or that elicit abnormal signs and symptoms should not be performed or should be modified to ensure appropriate responses. Elders who have had coronary artery bypass graft surgery are often given lifting restrictions. Recommendations vary by physician and often include not lifting more than 10 lb for at least 1 month after surgery. Lifting precautions may also be recommended for elders who have had a procedure involving catheterization of the femoral artery, such as angioplasty and stent placement. Lifting guidelines for these procedures, determined by the elder's physician, are based on the elder's lifestyle and physical status and the specific procedures performed.[9]

Recognition of distress signals is vital in any setting when working with elders with cardiac dysfunction. Primary signs and symptoms are chest pain, shortness of breath, cyanosis, sweating, fatigue, weakness, and confusion. Elders with cardiac dysfunction often complain of burning or pressure in the chest or of upper extremity, jaw, or cervical pain. These symptoms may occur with elders who have congestive heart failure, dysrhythmias, or a history of MI or angina.[4] If elders demonstrate or report any of these symptoms, the COTA should monitor their BP, HR, and ECG readings for changes in medical status. Any abnormal sign or symptom should be documented and discussed with the OTR and other health care professionals.

Another key area is the type of medication that elders with cardiac or BP problems are taking. Anticoagulants are commonly used for elders who have hypertension or who have had a cerebrovascular accident or hip or knee replacement surgery. Nitroglycerin is a common medication for elders with angina pectoris. Table 23-5 lists commonly prescribed medications. Knowledge of which medications elders are taking and their side effects is important to any therapist, but especially to those who perform therapy services through a home health agency or in a community setting.

TABLE 23-5

Examples of Common Medications and Potential Side Effects

Condition	Medication category (examples)	Side effects
Angina pectoris	Nitrates (nitroglycerin, isosorbide dinitrate) Beta-blockers (atenolol, propranolol) Calcium channel blockers (verapamil, diltiazem)	Headache, orthostatic hypotension, dizziness Bradycardia, depression, fatigue Peripheral edema
Heart failure	Cardiac glycosides (digitalis, digoxin) Diuretics (furosemide) Ace inhibitors (enalapril, captopril)	Cardiac dysrhythmias, GI distress, CNS disturbances Electrolyte disturbances, volume depletion Skin rash
Hypertension	Beta-blockers (atenolol, metoprolol) Diuretics (hydrochlorothiazide) Calcium channel blockers (verapamil, diltiazem) Ace inhibitors (enalapril) Alpha-blocker (prazosin) Centrally acting SNS antagonists (clonidine) Vasodilators (hydralazine)	Bradycardia, depression, fatigue Volume depletion, electrolyte imbalance Peripheral edema Skin rash Reflux, tachycardia, orthostatic hypotension Dry mouth, dizziness, drowsiness Reflux, tachycardia, dizziness, orthostatic hypotension, weakness, headache
Dysrhythmias	Sodium channel blockers (quinidine, lidocaine) Beta-blockers Drugs that prolong repolarization (amiodarone) Calcium channel blockers (verapamil)	Cardiac rhythm disturbances Bradycardia Pulmonary toxicity, liver damage Bradycardia, dizziness, headache
Acute MI	Narcotic analgesic (morphine) Platelet-aggregation inhibitors (aspirin) Thrombolytics (streptokinase, tissue plasminogen activator)	Sedation, respiratory depression, GI distress GI distress Excessive bleeding

ACE, angiotensin-converting enzyme; CNS, central nervous system; GI, gastrointestinal; MI, myocardial infarction; SNS, sympathetic nervous system.

CASE STUDY

Adelle, who is 79 years old, is receiving OT in an acute care hospital setting after a coronary bypass graft. Her medical history includes type II diabetes mellitus, hypertension, peripheral vascular disease, and iron deficiency anemia. Her occupational history includes interests in growing tomatoes and volunteering at her church, where she answers the telephone and sends welcome letters to new members. She lives alone in a home with three stairs. Some adaptations have been made in the home environment such as a tub/shower combination on the main level next to her bedroom. Adelle would like to remain independent with doing self-care and light homemaking tasks, managing her health, and gardening. Her son and daughter live nearby and drive her to appointments, shopping, and social activities. Her friends from her church visit weekly and they tend to her garden together. Adelle's niece helps her with vacuuming and cleaning the bathroom.

Trina, the COTA, has been educating Adelle on energy conservation and work simplification techniques. They have practiced pacing self-care activities in bed and have discussed techniques for gardening and cooking simple meals when she returns home. Trina has also provided Adelle with handouts and a home program. Adelle will be receiving home health OT, and Trina will be communicating with the home health OTR to update her on Adelle's progress and goals in the acute care hospital program.

■ CASE STUDY REVIEW QUESTIONS

Describe how the HR for activity should be determined in Adelle's case.

1 How would Adelle's endurance for dressing be calculated? Discuss when it can be increased.
2 What tools or equipment could be provided to simplify her self-care and home-making tasks?
3 What are three activities that Adelle should avoid? Why are these activities contraindicated?
4 What would be important for Trina to report to the home health OTR?
5 What recommendations should the COTA make for home health?
6 How does Adelle's support affect her overall health?
7 What health management techniques would be important for Adelle to engage in?

■ CHAPTER REVIEW QUESTIONS

1 Describe the impact that anxiety may have on an elder's ability to perform occupations.
2 Explain the role that COTAs play in addressing the psychosocial aspects of cardiac disease.
3 Describe how maximum HRs and activity HRs are determined.
4 Describe what is involved in the evaluation of elders with cardiac conditions.
5 Describe why evaluating cognition is important.
6 Describe the four functional categories of cardiac disease.
7 Describe the four phases of cardiac rehabilitation.
8 What is a MET, and how can the MET system be used in cardiac rehabilitation?

9 Describe how energy conservation and work simplification are used in elders with cardiac conditions.
10 What should COTAs do for elders who report symptoms of angina pectoris while washing their hair?
11 Identify a method of energy conservation for elders while dressing their lower extremities.

REFERENCES

1. Centers for Disease Control and Prevention, 2010. Heart disease [WWW page]. http://www.cdc.gov/HeartDisease/index.htm.
2. Federal Interagency Forum on Aging-Related Statistics, 2008. Older Americans 2010: Key indicators of well-being. U.S. Government Printing Office, Washington, DC.
3. Hardaway, B., Tang, W., 2008. Heart failure with systolic dysfunction. In: Griffin, B., Topol, E. (Eds.), Manual of Cardiovascular Medicine. 3rd ed. Lippincott Williams & Wilkins, Philadelphia.
4. Silverstein, A., Silverstein, V., Nunn, L., 2006. Heart Disease. Twenty-First Century, Minneapolis, MN.
5. George, S., Lyon, C., 2005. Pathogenesis of atherosclerosis. In: George, S., Johnson, J. (Eds.), Atherosclerosis: Molecular and Cellular Mechanisms. Wiley-VCH, Weinheim, Germany.
6. Lipsky, M., Mendelson, M., Havas, S., Miller, M., 2008. American Medical Association Guide to Preventing and Treating Heart Disease. John Wiley & Sons, Hoboken, NJ.
7. Jonker, A., Comijs, H., Knipscheer, K., Deeg, D., 2009. The role of coping resources on change and well-being during persistent health decline. Journal of Aging & Health 21 (8), 1063-1070.
8. Taylor, R., Dalal, H., Jolly, K., Moxham, T., Zawada, A., 2010. Home-based versus centre-based cardiac rehabilitation. Cochrane Database of Systematic Reviews Issue 1, Art. No.: CD007130.
9. Huntley, N., 2006. Cardiac and pulmonary diseases. In: Radomski, M., Trombly, C. (Eds.), Occupational Therapy for Physical Dysfunction. 6th ed. Lippincott Williams & Wilkins, Baltimore.
10. American Association of Cardiovascular and Pulmonary Rehabilitation. 2006. Cardiac Rehabilitation Resource Manual. Human Kinetics, Champaign, IL.
11. Wenger, N., 2008. Current status of cardiac rehabilitation. Journal of the American College of Cardiology 51, 1619-1631.
12. Muntner, P., Krousel-Wood, M., Hyre, A., Stanley, E., Cushman, W., Cutler, J., et al., 2009. Antihypertensive prescriptions for newly treated patients before and after the Main Antihypertensive and Lipid-Lowering Treatment to Prevent Heart Attack Trial Results and Seventh Report of the Joint National Committee on Prevention, Detection, Evaluation, and Treatment of High Blood Pressure Guidelines. Hypertension 53, 617-623.
13. Reed, K., 2003. Quick Reference to Occupational Therapy, 2nd ed. Pro-Ed, Austin, TX.
14. Mazzini, M., Stevens, G., Whalen, D., Ozonoff, A., Balady, G., 2008. Effect of an American Heart Association "Get with the Guidelines" program-based clinical pathway on referral and enrollment into cardiac rehabilitation after acute myocardial infarction. American Journal of Cardiology 101, 1084-1087.
15. Adams, A., Hubbard, M., McCullough-Shock, T., Simms, K., Cheng, D., Hartman, J., et al., 2010. Myocardial work during endurance training and resistance training: A daily comparison, from workout session 1 through completion of cardiac rehabilitation. Baylor University Medical Center Proceedings 23 (2), 126-129.

16. LaPier, T., Wintz, G., Holmes, W., Cartmell, E., Hartl, S., Kostoff, N., et al., 2008. Analysis of activities of daily living performance in patients recovering from coronary artery bypass surgery. Physical & Occupational Therapy in Geriatrics 27 (1), 16-35.

17. Wu, S., Lin, Y., Chen, C., et al., 2006. Cardiac rehabilitation vs. home exercise after coronary artery bypass graft surgery: A comparison of heart rate recovery. American Journal of Physical Medicine & Rehabilitation 85 (9), 711-717.

chapter 24

Working with Elders Who Have Pulmonary Conditions

ANGELA M. PERALTA, SHERRELL POWELL, AND DAVID PLUTSCHACK

KEY TERMS

chronic obstructive pulmonary disease, chronic pulmonary emphysema, chronic bronchitis, bronchiectasis, energy conservation, work simplification

CHAPTER OBJECTIVES

1. Define chronic obstructive pulmonary disease.
2. Identify common symptoms of chronic obstructive pulmonary disease.
3. Identify the psychosocial effect of chronic obstructive pulmonary disease on elders.
4. List conditions that affect the sexual functioning of elders with chronic obstructive pulmonary disease.
5. Describe assessment and intervention for elders with chronic obstructive pulmonary disease.

Jennifer is a certified occupational therapy assistant (COTA) who works in a large rehabilitation hospital in the South Bronx section of New York City. Her clients are from lower socioeconomic backgrounds. Many of them are factory workers and manual laborers. Jennifer has noticed a marked increase in the number of referrals to occupational therapy (OT) of elders who have chronic obstructive pulmonary disease (COPD) as a secondary diagnosis. These elders are finding it difficult to carry out their activities of daily living (ADL) because of the debilitating effects of COPD. On reviewing their social histories, Jennifer found that many of these elders worked with a variety of chemicals and that many of them were heavy smokers. Some of the major problems these elders deal with include difficulty engaging in self-care activities, a decreased level of endurance, chronic fatigue, and an inability to engage in leisure activities. Like many elders with COPD, some of them report a fear of not being able to breathe because of frequent episodes of shortness of breath.

COPD, along with other respiratory conditions, can be seen in elder residents of nursing homes, usually as a secondary diagnosis. Regardless of the setting, COTAs working with elders who have COPD and other respiratory diagnoses must be aware of the causes, symptoms, and OT interventions. When addressing elders with pulmonary conditions or issues related to respiratory system function COTAs should consider the Occupational Therapy Practice Framework for all aspects of the person's life (2nd ed.) (AOTA, 2008).

CHRONIC OBSTRUCTIVE PULMONARY DISEASE

COPD is a general disease that can include chronic pulmonary emphysema and chronic bronchitis. A debate arises whether to include chronic severe asthma within the COPD definition. Current research shows pathological differences between COPD and asthma. However, individuals with chronic severe asthma show similar debilitating symptoms as individuals with COPD, and therefore this diagnosis will also be included within the chapter.[1] Chronic bronchitis and emphysema affect the upper and lower respiratory tracts and are characterized by cough, expectoration, wheezing, sputum production, and dyspnea.[1] These symptoms occur first with exercise and later when the elder is at rest. Asthma, which is characterized by an increased responsiveness of the bronchi to various stimuli, results in bronchoconstriction, inflammation of the mucosa, and an increased amount of secretions.[2,3] COPD is associated with airflow obstruction, which may be accompanied by airway hyperreactivity and may be partially reversible.[4-6] Clinical symptoms of COPD vary, depending on the severity and duration of the diseases.

Chronic Bronchitis

Chronic bronchitis is defined as the presence of a chronic productive cough and sputum production for at least 3 months out of a year for a 2-year period.[4] One symptom of chronic bronchitis is hypersecretion of mucus in the respiratory tract in individuals for whom other causes, such as infection, have been ruled out.[1,7] The sputum of a person with chronic bronchitis is usually thick yellow to gray. A deep, productive cough is the main symptom of this disease. Other symptoms include shortness of breath, wheezing, a slightly elevated temperature, and pain in the upper chest that is aggravated by cough.

A person may have a mild form of chronic bronchitis for many years. Individuals with mild chronic bronchitis may have only a slight cough in the morning after being inactive at night. This cough can become aggravated after the person has an acute upper respiratory tract infection. As the condition progresses, obstructive and asthmatic symptoms appear, together with dyspnea. Chest expansion becomes diminished, and scattered rales and wheezing are frequently heard.[8]

Bronchiectasis, a permanent dilation of the bronchi, is the most common complication of bronchitis. Bronchiectasis is often associated with bronchiolectasis, a dilation of the bronchiole. Such dilation occurs as a result of persistent inflammation inside the airways. The dilated bronchi and bronchiole are filled with mucopurulent material that stagnates and cannot be cleared by coughing. Infection then spreads into the adjacent alveoli, and recurrent episodes of pneumonia are common. Clubbing of the fingers often develops in elders with this condition.[9]

Chronic Pulmonary Emphysema

Emphysema is a chronic condition characterized by the permanent enlargement of the air spaces distal to the terminal bronchioles. Emphysema is accompanied by the destruction of the alveolar walls and causes the lungs to lose elasticity, resulting in decreased airflow.[10,11] This decreased airflow results in dyspnea. Elders with emphysema have no bronchial obstruction or irritation that would cause them to expectorate.[8] The inability to exhale the carbon monoxide that is trapped in the lungs causes the chest to overexpand, a condition referred to as *barrel chest*.[12] The elder must hunch forward while holding onto a stable object to engage the auxiliary respiratory muscles during breathing. These elders manage to oxygenate their blood by hyperventilating, which prevents cyanosis and anoxia.[10]

Asthma

Asthma is defined as a reversible airway disease characterized by an increased responsiveness of the trachea and the bronchi to various stimuli. Asthma is displayed by a widespread narrowing of the airways that changes in severity either spontaneously or as a result of therapy. During an acute attack, pronounced wheezing occurs because of difficulty in inhaling and exhaling air. Dyspnea, tachypnea, and chest tightness may also occur. In severe cases, the elder experiencing an asthmatic attack may also perspire profusely.[5,13]

PSYCHOSOCIAL EFFECT OF CHRONIC OBSTRUCTIVE PULMONARY DISEASE

Rehabilitation of elders with COPD should include both medical management and assistance in coping with the debilitating effects of this chronic condition. As with any chronic condition, elders adapt in different ways. Some elders accept and adapt to the changes in energy level and other accompanying symptoms of COPD. For other elders, coping with symptoms of COPD may be a frustrating and depressing experience. Furthermore, elders with COPD often have additional stressors in their lives, such as the loss of a spouse and close friends, changes in their living situation, a decrease in financial status, the loss of productivity, a lack of family support, the inability to perform ADL functions, and the loss of general body function.[14,10]

Weakness and fatigue associated with COPD may require changes in living situations, including a move to a higher level of assistive living. As with any move, emotional adaptations are required. Often elders with COPD seek to live in a different environment where they believe the air is cleaner or they can breathe better; however, they may find that such a move is not the solution to their problem because it cuts them off from a social support network. A sense of isolation may cause an increase in anxiety and may lead to depression.

Additional problems related to decreases in finances may arise for elders. The primary source of income for some elders is Social Security payments. Funds obtained from this source may not be sufficient to pay for medications or home health services, if needed. However, the prescription medication benefit available from Medicare (Part D) with improvements made with health reform may provide some assistance with medication purchases. The situation can be particularly frustrating for elders with COPD who are insured by Medicare because they will not be reimbursed for rehabilitation care unless they have a change in functional status.

In addition, elders with COPD may have a sense of loss of productivity if they are unable to engage in activities that provided enjoyment in previous years. Social isolation because of concerns about a decreased energy level, shortness of breath, oxygen usage, coughing, and sputum production may contribute to depression. Elders may become afraid that engaging in any type of physical activity may cause an increase in shortness of breath. This can lead to a cycle of fear and ultimately a need for more oxygen. Some elders with COPD also experience frustration because of a decline in their abilities to perform ADL functions as a result of a decreased level of endurance. Finally, some elders with COPD may have other chronic problems such as decreased vision, or perhaps a general decline in other body systems. All of these stressors could contribute to anxiety and depression.

Over time some elders with COPD begin to realize that a change in emotional status, whether positive or negative, has a direct effect on the respiratory system.

Fear of expressing any type of emotion becomes a reality. This situation can further perpetuate a state of isolation. These elders may rationalize, "If I cannot express my emotions, then I will stay by myself." This position may be misinterpreted by others as hostility or aloofness, thereby creating more isolation.

SEXUAL FUNCTIONING

Elders with COPD may experience some loss of sexual functioning.[15] Factors that may affect sexual functioning are shortness of breath, a decreased level of endurance, and a lack of desire. Changes in self-concept can also affect sexuality. Some men may have difficulty maintaining or obtaining an erection, perhaps because of fears of sexual failure. However, impotence can be the result of many causes, including side effects of medication. Therefore, elders who are impotent should contact their physicians. Fear of sexual failure because of shortness of breath is one of the most common causes of sexual inactivity among elders with COPD. Engaging in sexual activity involves an increase in the breathing rate. For many elders the fear of suffocation or not being able to increase the depth of breathing is a major concern that inhibits their ability to engage freely in sexual activity.[16,17] COTAs can address some of the sexual functioning concerns of these elders by being open to discussing these concerns during intervention. Providing energy conservation suggestions may be beneficial, such as encouraging elders to have sexual relations when they are most rested. (A more in-depth discussion of ways to address sexual concerns with elders is provided in Chapter 12.)

OCCUPATIONAL THERAPY ASSESSMENT AND INTERVENTION PLANNING

COTAs contribute to the evaluation process of elders with COPD and collaborate with registered occupational therapists (OTRs) in intervention planning. ADL functions and productive and leisure activities are often the primary areas of concern because of the disabling effects of COPD.[15] A study of 100 individuals with COPD found that the most common reported symptoms from COPD were dyspnea (shortness of breath), fatigue, xerostomia (dry mouth), coughing, and anxiety.[18] Elders may experience the most disabling symptoms of COPD, such as dyspnea and fatigue, when engaging in ADL and leisure activities. These symptoms, together with anxiety and depression related to the chronic illness, perpetuate the vicious cycle of inactivity. The deconditioning and muscle weakness that occur from inactivity make it increasingly difficult for elders to perform necessary ADL functions to be independent in the home and community.[14,19]

The OTR and COTA consider client factors when assessing the effects of COPD on function.[15] Client factors such as sensory function and pain are assessed to determine tactile impairment. Perceptual skills are assessed to determine an elder's response during episodes of dyspnea, particularly if they become dizzy. Neuromuscular and movement-related functions are assessed to determine physical tolerance and endurance, shortness of breath on exertion, muscle strength, range of motion, and posture. Higher level cognition is assessed to determine the elder's knowledge of the disease and accompanying problems. The elder's judgment, problem-solving skills, ability to generalize learning, and awareness of safety hazards are evaluated. Global mental functions such as energy and drive, temperament, and personality are considered. Psychosocial ability is assessed to determine the elder's psychological, social, and self-management skills. Elders with COPD may experience feelings of hopelessness, anxiety, depression, withdrawal from social activities, and dependency on a spouse or caregiver.[20,21] Impairment in any of these areas directly affects the elder's ability to engage in self-care, work, and leisure activities.

COTAs must be aware of certain precautions during intervention (Box 24-1). Knowing the various symptoms associated with COPD is important, such as shortness of breath and asthma, as well as the environmental irritants that can affect the elder's ability to breathe. These irritants can include cigarette smoking, dust from woodworking activities, and fumes that arise from activities such as copper tooling. Other irritants include talcum powder, certain perfumes, and poor air quality in the clinic.

OT intervention is geared toward increasing independence in functional activities by improving strength and endurance through resistive activities (Box 24-2). Reconditioning programs such as the metabolic equivalents (METs) that are used with individuals who have cardiac conditions are often also used with patients with

BOX 24-1

Safety Considerations

- Individuals with COPD are often unconditioned and present with muscle weakness, which puts them at risk for injuries and falls. Be very observant during intervention and *think safety*.
- Strenuous activity and overexertion can be life threatening to elders with COPD or asthma. Stop activities that cause nausea, dizziness, fatigue, dyspnea, or chest pain.
- Engaging in exercise and activity may activate debilitating effects of COPD and asthma, such as dyspnea, fatigue, and wheezing. COTAs must be aware of these symptoms and monitor the patient accordingly. Asthmatic attacks are life-threatening occurrences, and precautions must be taken when dealing with these patients.
- Recognize the effect that the environment may have on the elder. Smoke, pollution, dust, and other environmental irritants can trigger COPD symptoms and asthmatic attacks.

BOX 24-2

Intervention Gems

- Collaborate with the elder and the OTR to formulate an intervention plan that will be beneficial for the individual. Intervention should focus on increasing the elder's independence in everyday activities. Consider client functions[15] as you make your intervention plan.
- Retrain ADL tasks using energy conservation and work simplification techniques to complete them. Have the elder demonstrate these techniques. The elder will need to take breaks during and between ADL tasks. Environmental modifications and adaptive equipment can also be used by the elder to successfully complete ADL tasks.
- Reconditioning through strengthening and exercise is a necessity with elders who have COPD. The METs program is a valuable reconditioning program. Low-impact exercise can be used with patients with COPD as a precursor to meaningful occupations.
- Demonstrate and educate the elder on the effectiveness of the two breathing techniques described in the chapter, *pursed-lip* breathing and *diaphragmatic* breathing. Recognize and address psychosocial issues that the elder may have in relation to the COPD.

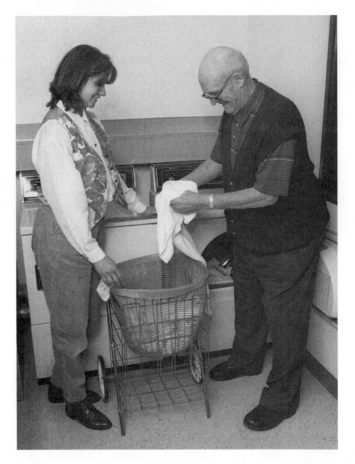

FIGURE 24-1 A COTA observes an elder practice energy conservation and work simplification techniques as he does laundry.

COPD.[14,19,22] (A more in-depth discussion of the use of METs to guide activity prescriptions is provided in Chapter 23.) Low-impact exercise places minimum stress on joints and is easier to perform than high-impact activities. Exercise programs should include functional activities that target the upper body, and they should be designed to increase the strength of respiratory muscles. Activities should be stopped if nausea, dizziness, fatigue, increased shortness of breath, or chest pain develops.

Energy conservation and *work simplification* techniques are used with elders who are predisposed to fatigue (Figure 24-1). COTAs should actually try these techniques with elders rather than simply provide them with education sheets. Energy conservation and work simplification techniques should include scheduling rest periods in between activities, sitting whenever possible, reducing or eliminating steps, pushing rather than pulling, and analyzing an activity before starting it. Having all of the supplies for ADL functions within easy reach to avoid unnecessary trips is also beneficial. Time management is a technique that teaches elders to plan daily activities so that rest periods are "built in" to avoid some of the complications of COPD. Good time management skills may make the difference between a full, active life and a sedentary one.

Elders must develop the problem-solving skills needed to identify that they are no longer able to perform a task in the customary way and when to change the process.

Adaptive equipment such as a reacher, a cart to carry heavy items, and a motor scooter for outdoor activities can assist with function. In addition, COTAs can encourage elders to become involved in social activities. Teaching stress reduction techniques can help encourage elders to have a sense of independence.

The COTA/OTR team may also reinforce breathing techniques taught in the respiratory therapy program, such as pursed-lip breathing and diaphragmatic breathing (Figure 24-2). According to Spencer,[23] "Pursed-lip breathing creates a resistance to the flow of air out of the lungs and slows down the breathing rate. This technique is used with stressful activities to avoid shortness of breath. Diaphragmatic breathing decreases the cost of breathing and enables the elder to engage in purposeful activities." COTAs working with elders who have COPD must become efficient at administering oxygen and must be prepared to assist with controlled coughing, breathing, and other procedures.

CONCLUSION

COPD is a common disease in the United States, especially among elders. COTA/OTR teams are becoming

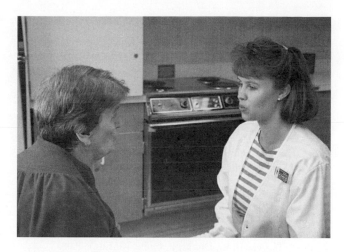

FIGURE 24-2 COTAs often must reinforce techniques such as pursed-lip breathing during activity.

increasingly proactive in the intervention of this debilitating disease. They provide intervention to elders with COPD in a variety of settings. OT intervention is geared toward the restoration of self-care skills, instruction in the pacing of daily activities, and the restoration of physical capabilities. COTAs are instrumental in teaching compensatory techniques to be used in the performance of ADL functions and in the selection and use of assistive devices and adaptive equipment. COTAs may also become involved in teaching energy conservation and work simplification techniques. Addressing stress management may be a part of therapy; this may also help reinforce respiratory therapy breathing techniques. Ultimately, the goal of OT with elders who have COPD is to maximize their level of independence as they adjust to living with a chronic condition.

CASE STUDY

Rose is a 70-year-old woman who was recently discharged from the hospital after being treated for pneumonia. She has a 20-year history of COPD. Rose's most current hospitalization greatly compromised her health. Rose has been a widow for 25 years. She has one son who lives in the area but is not very involved in her life. "He is afraid that I may need him to fix something. I wish that I would see him more often as I do enjoy his company," Rose stated.

Rose enjoys needlework, and her concern for the environment is evident in the extensive recycling she does in her home. She previously went out into the community three or four times a month for doctor appointments, shopping, and socializing with friends. She does not drive and relies on others for transportation.

Rose was independent in ADL and in instrumental activities of daily living (IADL) before her hospitalization. Her primary care physician ordered home health at discharge, and the OTR completed the initial evaluation. Maritza is a COTA who has been working in home health for 5 years and will manage Rose twice a week for 3 weeks. Initially, Rose is concerned about how she will be able to complete her daily routine

now that she is on oxygen 24 hours a day and her endurance is severely limited.

Maritza and Rose discuss the occupational tasks that Rose wants to complete independently. They identify that it would be best to start with basic self-care activities incorporating energy conservation. Maritza reviews handouts on energy conservation for Rose to refer to later. She then has her practice the techniques while engaged in activities. For example, she places a chair in the bathroom for her to sit in while undressing, dressing, and for resting. Maritza instructs Rose in using pursed-lip breathing techniques during self-care tasks. Maritza saw photos of Rose posted in her home and observed that she took pride in her appearance. Low endurance and a fixed income have prevented Rose from visiting the beauty salon, so Maritza suggests that she purchase a wig. Rose embraces the idea.

Maritza provides a commode that Rose can use over the toilet and next to her bed at night. Other bathroom equipment includes a handheld shower and a tub transfer bench. The shower doors are removed and replaced with a shower curtain to help Rose transfer safely to the tub.

Rose becomes independent in ADL using energy conservation techniques. She figures out ways to get around safely in her home while managing the oxygen hose. She reports difficulty with food preparation and the desire to address that area in intervention. Subsequently, Maritza completes a kitchen evaluation and finds that cooking is difficult and unsafe. Rose tires easily, forgets about food in the oven, and leaves food out to spoil. She has lost interest in eating nutritious meals. Maritza suggests that Rose receive Meals on Wheels.

Rose expresses an interest in continuing her recycling activities. The recycling bins are located on the porch floor, and she has difficulty reaching them. Maritza moves a small picnic table close to the door, places the recycling bins on top of it, and labels the bins for easy identification. The picnic table allows Rose to work at a proper work height. A neighbor boy who visits frequently volunteers to take the bins to the curb on a weekly basis. At discharge Rose is able to function safely in her environment and plans to pursue public transportation so she can move about the community because she is interested in taking a needlepoint class at a local craft store.

■ CASE STUDY QUESTIONS

1 Why did Maritza instruct Rose in pursed-lip breathing techniques while transferring?
2 What are the physical and psychological benefits of Rose wearing a wig?
3 Why is it important to practice energy conservation techniques during activities?
4 Describe how Rose could use energy conservation during two other activities.

LEARNING EXERCISE: UNDERSTANDING THE EFFECTS OF COPD

Complete the following activity as an individual or in groups, and answer the questions at the end of the activity.

Activity

1. Complete an ADL or a simple exercise, such as jumping jacks or walking up or down stairs.

2. Next, breathe through a standard straw for 30 seconds without breathing through your nose while attempting to complete the same ADL or simple exercise. (The straw simulates having a breathing problem.)

Answer the following questions based on the simulation of a breathing problem, using a straw while doing an activity:

1. How would having a breathing problem affect your daily routine?
2. What areas of occupation would be affected?
3. What psychosocial factors would be present?
4. What interventions would you consider using with an individual with COPD after completing this activity?

This activity was adapted from Clark, C. (2004). Catching your breath: How does it feel to have lung disease? Retrieved, from http://www.raft.net/ideas/Catching%20 Your%20Breath.pdf.

■ CHAPTER REVIEW QUESTIONS

1 Describe some physiological factors that may affect elders with COPD.

2 Describe precautions to be aware of when working with elders with COPD.

3 Describe community resources that would be useful for elders with pulmonary conditions.

REFERENCES

1. Global Initiative for Chronic Obstructive Lung Disease, 2009. Global strategy for the diagnosis, management, and prevention of chronic obstructive pulmonary disease (Updated 2009). Medical Communications Resources. Retrieved from http://www.goldcopd.org/Guidelineitem.asp?l1=2&l2=1&intId=2003.

2. Buc, M., Dzurilla, M., Vrlik, M., Bucova, M., 2009. Immunopathogenesis of bronchial asthma. Archivum Immunologiae Et Therapiae Experimentalis 57 (5), 331-344. doi:10.1007/s00005-009-0039-4.

3. Pauwels, R.A., 2000. National and international guidelines for COPD: The need for evidence. Chest 117 (Suppl. 2), 20S-22S.

4. Anthonisen, N., Manfreda, J., 2004. Epidemiology of chronic obstructive pulmonary disease. In: Crapo, J.D., Glassroth, J., Karlinsky, J.B., King, T.E. Jr. (Eds.). Baum's Textbook of Pulmonary Diseases, 7th ed. Lippincott Williams & Wilkins, Philadelphia, pp. 203-222.

5. Baum, G., 1997. Textbook of Pulmonary Diseases. JB Lippincott, Philadelphia.

6. Donohue, J., San Pedro, G., 2005. Chronic obstructive pulmonary disease. In: George, R.B., Light, R.W., Matthay, M.A., Matthay, R.A. (Eds.). Chest Medicine: Essentials of Pulmonary and Critical Care Medicine. Lippincott Williams & Wilkins, Philadelphia, pp. 163-182.

7. Keith, J., Novak, P. (Eds.), 2001. Mosby's Medical, Nursing, and Allied Health Dictionary, 6th ed. Mosby, St. Louis, MO.

8. Petty, T.L. 2001. Early diagnosis of COPD: National Lung Health Program in the United States. Program and abstracts of 67th Annual Scientific Assembly of the American College of Chest Physicians.

9. Damjanov, I., 2006. Pathology for the Health Professions, 3rd ed. Elsevier Saunders, Philadelphia.

10. Pauwels, R.A., Buist, A.S., Calverley, P.M., Jenkins, C.R., Hurd, S.S., 2001. Global strategy for the diagnosis, management, and prevention of chronic obstructive pulmonary disease. NHLBI/WHO Global Initiative for Chronic Obstructive Lung Disease (GOLD) Workshop summary. American Journal of Respiratory and Critical Care Medicine 163, 1256-1276.

11. Simon, H., Zieve, D., 2009, April. Chronic Obstructive Pulmonary Disease (Rep. No. 70). Nidus Information Services, New York.

12. Piper, T., Lukens, R., Dirckx, J., Cadle, K. (Eds.), 2008. Stedman's Medical Dictionary for the Health Professions and Nursing, 6th ed. Lippincott Williams & Wilkins, Philadelphia.

13. U.S. Department of Health and Human Services (DHHS), 2007, August 28. Expert panel report 3: Guidelines for the diagnosis and management of asthma (Rep. No. 3). Retrieved from http://www.nhlbi.nih.gov/guidelines/asthma/asthgdln.pdf.

14. Bonder, R., Wagner, B., 2001. Functional Performance in Older Adults. FA Davis, Philadelphia.

15. American Occupational Therapy Association, 2008. Occupational therapy practice framework: Domain and process, 2nd ed. American Journal of Occupational Therapy 62, 625-683.

16. Habraken, J., Pols, J., Bindels, P., Willems, D., 2008, December. The silence of patients with end-stage COPD: A qualitative study. British Journal of General Practice 58 (557), 844-849.

17. Hodgkin, J.E., Bartolome, R., Gerilynn, L., 2000. Pulmonary rehabilitation: Guidelines to success. Lippincott Williams & Wilkins, Boston.

18. Blinderman, C., Homel, P., Billings, A., Tennstedt, S., Portenoy, R., 2009, July. Symptom distress and quality of life in patients with advanced chronic obstructive pulmonary disease. Journal of Pain and Symptom Management 38 (1), 115-123.

19. Dean, E., De Andrade, A.D., 2009. Cardiovascular and pulmonary function. In: Bonder, B.R., Bello-Haas, V.D. (Eds.). Functional Performance in Older Adults. FA Davis, Philadelphia, pp. 85-100.

20. American Psychiatric Association, 2000. Diagnostic and Statistical Manual of Mental Disorders, 4th ed. Association, Washington, DC.

21. Nazir, S., Erbland, M., 2009. Chronic obstructive pulmonary disease: An update on diagnosis and management issues in older adults. Drugs & Aging 26 (10), 813-831.

22. Matthews, M., 2006. Cardiac and pulmonary disease. In: McHugh Pendleton, H., Schultz-Krohn, W. (Eds.). Pedretti's Occupational Therapy: Practice Skills for Physical Dysfunction, 6th ed. Mosby Elsevier, Philadelphia, pp. 1139-1156.

23. Spencer, E.A., 1993. Functional restoration: Implementation of occupational therapy with adults. In: Hopkins, H.L., Smith, H.D. (Eds.). Willard and Spackman's Occupational Therapy. JB Lippincott, Philadelphia.

Working with Elders Who Have Oncological Conditions

LESLIE BRUNSTETER-WILLIAMS

KEY TERMS

cancer, metastasis, pathological fracture, myelosuppression, cachexia, fatigue

CHAPTER OBJECTIVES

1. Identify four common oncological diagnoses associated with aging.
2. Discuss cancer treatment provided to elders with cancer and the associated side effects.
3. Describe the role of occupational therapy (OT) with the elder cancer patient, and list three different approaches that might be used with them.

4. Identify three common complications that elders receiving cancer treatment often face, and discuss the impact of these on the OT intervention process.
5. Describe modified approaches to daily occupations that might be used by the certified occupational therapy assistant (COTA) when working with an elder who has cancer.

Hannah is a COTA who works for an agency that provides relief coverage for two OT departments in acute-care hospitals in a large city. After arriving at work and receiving an orientation to the department, she reviews the charts of the patients with whom she will be working. She notices that five of the eight patients are elders on the oncology or cancer unit of the hospital, and three of them appear to be currently undergoing chemotherapy for the disease. She learns that those who are receiving chemotherapy have limited tolerance to activity and greater susceptibility to infections. She plans to allow time before her intervention to review the special precautions with this group of patients and collaborate with the other team members to provide the best intervention possible while insuring the patients' safety.

People with cancer are living longer.[1] As the population of those over age 65 grows, the number of people living with cancer will also increase within this group. Health care providers need to recognize the problems encountered by those living with this disease.

OVERVIEW OF CANCER WITH THE ELDER POPULATION

Nearly 13% of the total U.S. population was age 65 years or older in 2009.[2] At the current rate of our population growth, this group has been predicted to increase to 36% by 2020, approaching a total of 55 million people.[2] With this expanding population of elders, it is important to look at diseases directly associated with the process of

aging. Cancer occurs most frequently in this group and ranks second only to heart disease as the leading cause of death in the United States.[3] It is important that health care providers become adept at recognizing and dealing with health problems and treatment issues faced by elders with cancer. COTAs have a valuable role in contributing to improved quality of life of the elder with cancer. Specific strategies and interventions will follow in this chapter.

Age is the single highest risk factor for the development of cancer. From ages 60 to 69, one in six men and one in ten women have the probability of developing cancer, but the risk increases after age 70 to one in three for men and one in four for women.[3] According to a report by the American Cancer Society,[3] there were 970,000 total new cases of cancer reported from 2000 to 2004. Although this reflects a large number of people who are dealing with cancer, it is important to note that the current national trend in cancer incidence and death rates appears to be declining.[4] While the decrease in incidence appears to be the result of changes in screening, diagnostic techniques, and the reduction in exposure to environmental risk factors, such as smoking cessation, the decrease in death rates is reflective of those issues in addition to more effective disease treatment options.

COMMON CONDITIONS

In the chapter, we will be considering four types of cancer that are associated with aging: breast, colorectal, lung, and

TABLE 25-1

5-Year Relative Survival Rates of Common Cancer Diagnoses

Diagnosis/site	5-Year relative survival rates (1999-2005)	Median age at diagnosis
All sites	66.1%	66
Lung/bronchus	15.6%	71
Colorectal	65.2%	71
Breast	89.1%	61
Prostate	99.7%	68

Adapted from National Cancer Institute SEER. Cancer statistics review 1999-2005 tables and graphs. Retrieved from the National Cancer Institute (SEER), http://seer.gov/statistics/.

prostate. In Table 25-1, these four types of cancer are listed in relation to their 5-year survival rates and the median age at diagnosis.

Lung Cancer

Since the early 1950s, lung cancer has been the most common cause of death among men and women, and, in 2002, the incidence of lung cancer in women surpassed that in men.[5] According to the Surveillance Epidemiology and End Results survey, between 2002 and 2006 the median age at diagnosis for cancer of the lung and bronchus was 71 years.[6] As one ages, the risk of developing lung cancer increases, rising to a high of 31.4% between ages 65 and 74.[6] There are two major types of lung cancer: small cell lung cancer (SCLC) and non-small cell lung cancer (NSCLC). It is also possible for lung cancer to occur with characteristics of both, in which case it is known as mixed small cell/large cell carcinoma. The more common of the two types is non-small cell cancer, which accounts for 87% of total lung cancers.[5] This type of cancer tends to spread, or metastasize, to other parts of the body more slowly than small cell carcinoma, which spreads more quickly and is more likely to be found in other organs of the body. The major cause of lung cancer is smoking, which has been linked to both types of lung cancer in men and women, although, interestingly, women appear to have a higher rate than men of those lung cancers that are not associated with smoking. Lung cancer has also been shown to be caused by other occupational exposures, such as radon, asbestos, and uranium.[5]

Upon the initial diagnosis of lung cancer, the oncologist determines the prognosis and the best course of treatment available according to a process called *staging* in which it is determined whether the cancer has spread to other parts of the body. Generally, three levels are described: localized (within lungs), regional (spread to lymph nodes), and distant (spread to other organs).[5] Unfortunately, only 16% of lung cancer cases are diagnosed at an early or localized stage, which would increase the probability of an improved 5-year survival (see Table 25-1). The difficulty in an early diagnosis is that the symptoms associated with lung cancer, such as coughing with mucous production, do not occur until the advanced stages of the disease.[5] However, there are newer tests being developed such as low-dose spiral computed tomography (CT) and molecular markers in sputum that show promise for earlier detection, thus improving treatment responses.[5]

The treatment of lung cancer may include chemotherapy, surgery, or local radiation therapy. Due to the limits in the early diagnosis of this disease, combination chemotherapy with or without radiation therapy is more commonly used than surgical resection of the primary tumor because, as noted previously, the cancer has often already spread at the time of the initial diagnosis.

Breast Cancer

Breast cancer is currently the most common type of cancer in women and is second to lung cancer as the cause of cancer-related deaths in American women.[7] There has been a recent increase in an early-stage breast cancer diagnosis, likely resulting from increased public awareness, improved screening, and technology.[7] Between 2002 and 2006 the median age of breast cancer diagnosis was 61 years old.[6] As women age, the risk for developing this disease increases, and we now know that between ages 50 and 70, about 5.57% of all women in the United States will develop breast cancer.[6] As the number of people over age 65 in our country continues to climb, it is expected that by the year 2030 nearly 60% of them will be women.[8] Therefore, a large proportion of the oncologist's practice will include older women with breast cancer.[9] It is important that this population be given an opportunity to participate in clinical trials for cancer treatment and thus be offered the best options for treatment.

At the time of diagnosis of breast cancer, the specific type of breast cancer involved will be determined with a biopsy done either through a fine-needle aspiration of the mass or lumpectomy (removal of the mass). At that point, the pathology and the stage of disease can be determined, and decisions can be made regarding recommended treatment. Surgery, radiation therapy, cytotoxic chemotherapy, and hormonal therapy are all treatment choices with potential side effects that may compound already present comorbidities. Hormonal therapy is a treatment option often used with the older population with breast cancer. This has been shown to be of particular benefit with tumors that are estrogen-receptor positive (ER-positive), meaning that the tumor is likely to be stimulated to grow by the presence of estrogen. A common endocrine or anti-estrogen drug used with breast cancer patients is tamoxifen, which has been studied extensively in older women with breast cancer. Some studies have reported a complete or a partial response in 75% of those women treated with this drug alone.[9]

Prostate Cancer

Prostate cancer is currently the most common cancer diagnosed in men age 70 years and older, but, because tumors confined to the prostate are often diagnosed early, the 5-year survival rate is high in this group (see Table 25-1).[3] Between 2002 and 2006 the median age at the time of diagnosis of prostate cancer was 68 years old.[6] It is estimated that there are over 2 million men living in the United States with prostate cancer.[6] The high 5-year survival rate in this group appears to be a result of the use of the prostate specific antigen (PSA) blood test as well as of other improved treatments of the disease itself.[10] Nonmodifiable risk factors for prostate cancer include age, African American race, and a positive family history of prostate cancer.[10] There are also risk factors that men can control or modify, thus reducing the risk, such as diet, smoking habits, exercise, and large body size.[10]

The treatment of prostate cancer may include radiation, surgery, hormonal (or androgen deprivation therapy), and cytotoxic chemotherapy. All types of treatment carry with them a potential for adverse side effects, and when determining the best option for each patient, the oncologist considers each individual's quality of life and anticipated longevity in the decision-making process.

Colorectal Cancer

Colorectal cancer is currently the third most common cancer in both men and women in our country.[3] Between 2002 and 2006, the median age at the time of diagnosis was 71 years old.[6] The overall rate for colorectal cancer survival is improving because of enhanced screening, which yields earlier diagnoses with localized disease staging. The screening procedure for this disease can include detection and removal of colorectal polyps before they become cancerous, thus helping reduce the mortality and advanced-stage diagnosis. The greatest predictor of survival and treatability of this cancer is finding the cancer at an early stage. Surgery, which can be curative but sometimes results in a colostomy, is commonly part of the treatment regimen. However, the presence of comorbidities in the elder population may preclude this option. There is increasing evidence that although older patients maintain high function, they often are not treated with the same surgery as younger groups, and they receive less aggressive treatment based on their age alone.[11]

Adjuvant chemotherapy, either alone or in combination with radiation, may be used before or after surgery in cases where the cancer has spread locally to the bowel wall or metastasized to the lymph nodes.[3] As in other types of cancer associated with aging, there is a need to expand clinical studies for colorectal cancer to include people over age 65 to make the best treatment available to them and to those people for whom it will most likely prove successful.[12]

The risk factors for colorectal cancer include increased age, family history, the presence of inflammatory bowel disease, or a personal history of colorectal neoplasms.[3] Screening for this disease in persons with an average risk may include flexible sigmoidoscopy, in which the left side of the colon is visualized. The fecal occult blood test (FOBT), in which a specimen is taken from three consecutive stools to detect the presence of blood, can indicate early presence of the disease. Finally, a colonoscopy, which allows a view of the entire colon, is the most effective screening tool. The American Cancer Society currently recommends that a colonoscopy be done once every 10 years beginning at age 50 for people with an average risk of the disease.[3]

CANCER METASTASIS

Metastasis occurs when malignant or cancerous cells spread from the primary site (or site of origin) to other organs or systems in the body. This spread may be local, occurring in tissues or organs adjacent to the primary tumor site, or distant, traveling to another site in the body. This movement takes place through blood vessels and the lymphatic system at a microscopic level. Common sites of metastasis include breast cancer to bone, lungs, or brain; lung cancer to brain, liver, or bone; prostate cancer to bone; and colorectal cancer to the liver or lungs.

Lung metastasis may be seen secondary to breast cancer and is sometimes found in progressed colorectal cancer. When the lungs are involved in either primary cancer or metastasis, pulmonary functions may change, altering the patient's functional capacity and respiratory potential during daily activities and functional mobility. Rehabilitation efforts can be of benefit in these situations, working to maximize the patient's functional abilities with adaptive approaches, pacing, and the utilization of correct body mechanics.

Skeletal, or bone, metastasis may occur secondary to breast, prostate, or colorectal cancers. If weight-bearing bones are affected, the structures become weakened, thus resulting in the potential for breaking. This is referred to as *pathological fractures*. A pathological fracture may occur with very little actual weight or pressure being applied to the bone, but, because of its weakened support system, a break occurs. For example, if the elder's humerus has a metastatic lesion, performing a daily task such as emptying the trash or picking up a grocery bag could precipitate a fracture at that site. If the upper extremity is affected by a fracture, immobilization, surgical reduction, or radiation therapy may be used to improve bone healing and function. During this time, the elder may have only one upper extremity available for use and will require training in one-handed activities of daily living (ADL). If the hip or femur is involved, surgical repair or total hip replacement may be necessary to restore joint integrity and enable the person to resume weight bearing on the hip joint (Chapter 22 further describes orthopedic interventions). Depending upon which surgical approach is used in the hip surgery, there may be post-surgical precautions in movement, such as hip flexion, adduction, or abduction, and limited weight bearing, which must be followed for proper healing to occur. Therefore, the COTA's intervention should include instruction in ADL with needed adaptive equipment to achieve modified independence in lower extremity activities such as dressing and bathing while adhering to the necessary hip precautions. If metastasis involves the spinal column, pain can limit reaching and bending during ADL. Medical treatment may include epidural nerve blocks, radiation treatments, or surgical stabilization of the spine. In these cases, OT efforts should include teaching correct body mechanics in ADL and instrumental activities of daily living (IADL) to protect the spine and to prevent further damage.

Brain metastasis is a common complication of late-stage breast cancer and is also sometimes seen in lung cancer.[13] The symptoms may include headache, nausea, vomiting, mental status changes, seizures, or motor paresis similar to that seen in stroke victims. Medical approaches used to manage this problem include radiation therapy, surgery, and chemotherapy. Impaired balance or ataxia, upper or lower extremity weakness, and impaired cognition may become apparent in these elders, and OT should include one-handed, self-care tasks and safety in ADL through fall prevention strategies and strengthening exercises.

CANCER TREATMENT AND SIDE EFFECTS

Advances in treatment protocols are constantly being made based upon clinical trials. However, data from these trials do not always represent the elderly population.[14] If chronological age is used as the criteria for subjects in these trials, the older patients with cancer are often excluded by virtue of their age alone. This seems ironic in that the most common diagnoses of cancer are age-related. However, there are assessments that oncologists and nurse practitioners use in cancer settings that more clearly identify those cancer patients who are appropriate for certain types of cancer treatment and determine the best course of action available for older patients. For example, the Comprehensive Geriatric Assessment (CGA) considers areas such as function, physical performance, comorbidity, nutrition, social support, cognition, and depression.[14] Another example is the Barthel Index, which is an observational tool frequently used with stroke patients but may also be used with cancer patients.[15] The Karnofsky Performance Status Scale measures functional ability of patients with cancer, requiring the oncologist's assessment of the patient's abilities.[15] A disadvantage of using assessments such as these is that they are time-consuming to complete. Further, not all assessments have been validated for use with the older population with cancer.[15] Hopefully inclusion of the aging population into more clinical trials will increase as these screenings are further used and results extrapolated.

Currently, standardized treatment protocols established from clinical trials are devised for the younger population, who inherently have less comorbidity and are less susceptible to the complications from cancer treatment than elders. Comorbidities that may be present with the older patient, such as hypertension, arthritis, gait imbalance, or chronic lung disease, and visual, cognitive, or hearing impairments make aggressive treatment of older cancer patients a challenge.[16] There are also changes that take place in the body during the normal aging process, such as declines in peripheral nerve functioning, muscle strength, and muscle mass. Because of these issues, the patient's tolerance to established protocols can be impaired, further supporting the need for inclusion of these considerations when protocols are created.

Surgery, radiation therapy, and cytotoxic chemotherapy are frequently applied cancer treatments. The side effects of each vary, depending on which part of the body is involved and the dosage administered. Body image changes or loss of bodily functions may result from surgery, requiring that attention be focused on the patient's ability to adapt or modify activities that are impacted. Radiation therapy (RT) is applied to nearly one half of all patients with cancer at some time in the course of their illness.[17] RT can be used alone or in conjunction with surgery or chemotherapy. If used preoperatively, RT can lessen the extent of surgery required, a helpful option with the older population. It may also be used as a curative treatment in the early stages of a disease or as a palliative treatment, improving comfort and control of adverse symptoms in more advanced stages of cancer. Recent studies show that RT is beneficial and generally well tolerated by most elderly patients, and chronological age should not be a reason to avoid its use.[17] Systemic chemotherapy may be used for any of the previously mentioned cancer diagnoses. When making decisions about which chemotherapeutic agents to use with this population, the oncologist considers factors such as quality of life, costs to the patient, management of potential toxicities, and associated physiological changes that take place with age in their patients.[12] The side effects of chemotherapy will depend upon the drug used and dosage given. They may include peripheral neuropathy, alopecia (loss of hair), body image changes, fatigue, and myelosuppression (impairment of the body to produce normal white blood cells, red blood cells, or platelets). Table 25-2 describes cancer treatment side effects and the implications for OT intervention.

PSYCHOSOCIAL ASPECTS OF ONCOLOGICAL CONDITIONS/IMPLICATIONS FOR OCCUPATIONAL THERAPY

Psychosocial issues arise as the elder cancer patient begins the process of dealing with the diagnosis of cancer and enters the initial phase of treatment. These issues should be acknowledged by all health professionals involved in the patient's care. Fear of the unknown, depression, and worry about the impact of the disease on the ability to

TABLE 25-2

Complications Related to Cancer and Its Treatment

Complication	Clinical symptoms	OT intervention implications
Granulocytopenia (decreased white blood cells)	Increased susceptibility to infection	Adhere to universal precautions; good hand washing technique, frequent cleaning of equipment, wearing of mask if in reverse isolation; treatment in client's room
Thrombocytopenia (decreased platelets)	Easily bruised, potential for bleeding, CNS bleeding	Avoidance of sharp objects, resistive exercises, participation in less strenuous activities
Anemia (decreased red blood cells)	Easy fatigue, shortness of breath	Frequent rest periods, client monitored for fatigue, treatment modified according to client's tolerance
Fatigue	Mild to moderate shortness of breath; decreased tolerance with task completion; poor interest in initiating activities	Pacing techniques in all activity; gradation of physical activities or strengthening exercises as tolerated
Hypercalcemia (excessive calcium in blood; normal level: 8-10.5 mg/dL Ca)	Confusion, giddiness, mental status changes, drowsiness, polyuria, polydipsia	Consultation with physician before beginning activity, reality orientation
Hyperkalemia (abnormally high level of potassium)	Weakness, paralysis, ECG changes, renal disease if severe	Decrease in physical demands of treatment
Airway obstruction (emergent situation caused by tumor impingement on trachea)	Coughing, SOB, acute difficulty breathing	Immediate notification of medical staff
Increased intracranial pressure (caused by primary tumor or metastatic lesion in the brain)	Headaches, blurred vision, nausea or vomiting, seizure	Avoidance of physically active tasks requiring fine vision, quiet environment for treatment
Spinal cord compression (caused by tumor impingement on spinal cord)	Back pain, leg pain or weakness, sensory loss, bowel or bladder retention	Consultation with physician before treatment, avoidance of resistive exercise, extreme care in client transfers, immediate notification of any changes in sensation or strength
Skin desquamation (breakdown of outer layer of skin)	Open ulcers on skin, fragile epidermis	Protection of skin surfaces during treatment, avoidance of abrasive contact
Cardiac toxicity (decreased cardiac output or function)	Limited cardiovascular tolerance, SOB, dizziness	Selection of activities that do not exceed client's tolerance, monitoring of client's pulse and blood pressure during treatment
Peripheral neuropathy (impaired sensory pathways in upper or lower extremities)	Impaired sensation; loss of coordination; unsteady gait, foot-drop	Adaptive equipment, splints, compensation techniques

CNS, central nervous system; ECG, electrocardiogram; OT, occupational therapy; SOB, shortness of breath.

maintain one's previous level of activity and function often come with the diagnosis of cancer. Anger over having to experience this at all may also arise. It is not uncommon for elder cancer patients to be fearful of the pain associated with cancer, which in some cases of advanced disease may have precipitated the diagnosis. Uncontrolled pain can limit activity tolerance and accelerate feelings of loss of control. A sense of control is a basic human need which, if lost, can negatively impact an elder's quality of life.[18] COTAs are in a unique position to use active listening, develop a trusting relationship with the patient, and give supportive responses while encouraging the elder to express concerns, anxieties, and fears.

As a trusting relationship develops, it is important that the COTA provide information to the patient and family, as appropriate, about the treatment and potential side effects because it can alleviate anxieties and fears. If elders sense that they have greater knowledge about the illness and treatment, they may also feel empowered during this potentially very difficult life experience.

Although financial implications may not be the first concern that comes to mind when one receives the diagnosis of cancer, it soon becomes an important one for many elders.[3] Some elders who have modest incomes are able to get Medicaid and may have the majority of their costs covered, but many people remain who must face cancer without adequate health insurance coverage. This can result in delays or limited access to treatment and a significant financial burden. Sadly, if elders had consistent coverage for adequate screenings, or better access to health care throughout their lives in the first place, the need for cancer treatment could have been prevented altogether or diagnosed at an earlier stage, reducing financial burden and struggle.

Adverse side effects may bring about changes in the patient's body image and self-confidence. If alopecia occurs because of chemotherapy or total brain irradiation, the patient may tend to avoid social situations because of a decreased comfort level around other people. Avoidance of previous social opportunities that had given the person a sense of fulfillment may create a void in life and remove opportunities for receiving emotional support during this difficult time. Women may have difficulty adjusting to the loss of a breast after a mastectomy and experience changes in their feelings about femininity and sexuality. The COTA may want to refer these elders to community or hospital-based support groups for breast cancer survivors.

If myelosuppression occurs because of cytotoxic chemotherapy, the bone marrow is limited in production of necessary white and red blood cells and platelets. This, in turn, results in increased susceptibility to opportunistic infection, anemia (which can cause increased fatigue), or easy bruising and bleeding. In the case of decreased white blood cells (granulocytopenia), elders may need to limit their contacts with other people to prevent infection. In doing this, feelings of isolation may increase. COTAs should adhere to universal precautions during intervention, include frequent hand washing, and include the use of antibacterial wipes on equipment during intervention. COTAs can work with patients to explore interests and encourage solitary activities such as putting photos in albums, which promotes reminiscence, communicating with friends and family through e-mail or letter-writing, or developing a new meaningful hobby that can be done at home. With the growth of Internet-based communities, online support groups may be a practical option for socialization.[19] Impaired platelet production (thrombocytopenia) makes a person prone to bleeding, and activities with sharp tools or resistive strengthening exercises should be limited to protect skin and maintain muscle integrity. If there is a decrease in red blood cells (anemia), activities will need to be paced well because the elder's physical tolerance to activity will be limited. Because of these blood count-related issues, it is important that the COTA check their clients' daily blood counts in the medical record for changes that may preclude intervention or require modifications to the plan.

The National Comprehensive Cancer Network has defined cancer-related fatigue as a "distressing persistent, subjective sense of tiredness or exhaustion related to cancer or cancer treatment that is not proportional to recent activity and interferes with usual functioning."[20] While fatigue is the most common chronic complication of chemotherapy,[20] it has also been associated with surgery and radiation therapies. When it occurs, it can result in significant limitations in an elder's ability to engage in the occupations of value in their life, limiting mobility, working ability, and social interactions, thus eroding their physical, social, and spiritual well-being.[18] These areas directly impact one's quality of life. Providing social support and referring to community resources that may offer assistance in daily activities may be of benefit during this period.

As the cancer treatment continues, the chronic nature of the disease and the impact it has on the entire family system become evident. Daily routines and schedules may require changing to include required medical appointments for treatment and blood work. Periodic radiographic scans and tests are necessary to assess one's response to treatment. Elders often face problems with transportation to and from clinics for regular treatment, which compounds the already present stress and anxiety about the potential recurrence of the disease.

If the cancer recurs, feelings of denial, anger, and loss of control resurface. Uncertainty about the future may become a concern, and fear of dying can reappear. If the disease recurrence results in the loss of functional ability, family roles may require change. Cancer impacts the entire family, and its effect on the family and caregiver is clearly evident throughout all stages of the illness.[21] It is important to recognize the caregiver's needs and provide support and assistance as changes are made in family roles. An example of how this can occur is the case of an elder female with breast cancer and metastasis to the lumbar spine with subsequent pain while lifting or bending. Up to this time maintaining laundry duties and shopping have been her responsibilities at home, while her husband performed the meal preparations and clean up. She may now need her husband to assume parts of the laundry and shopping duties that require lifting and carrying loads, while she may in exchange have to perform some meal preparation and clean up (see Chapter 11 for a discussion of caregiver and family issues).

In most communities there are cancer support and self-help groups that can be of benefit to elders with cancer and their families. One of the most effective means of support given to a person dealing with the chronic nature of cancer comes from others who are dealing with the same issues. The health care team should refer to these community groups and support options whenever the need is identified. Examples of these include Reach to Recovery (for people who have undergone breast surgery), the American Cancer Society, the local YMCA or YWCA (for supervised indoor exercise or swim programs), and hospital-based support groups. There are many online support websites, including those that offer connections with other survivors. Examples of these include www.CancerHopeNetwork.org, www.csn.cancer.org, and www.cancer.org.

Quality of life is a concept that has increasingly been studied by professionals from diverse perspectives, often in search of definitive parameters to better assess the cancer patient's appropriateness for treatment, tolerance to treatment, and outcome success. Four areas often included in definitions of quality of life are related to physical, psychosocial, social, and spiritual well-being.[18] Elders' perceptions of their functional status can influence their feelings of self-worth and emotional adjustment and, therefore, impact their ability or desire to seek out needed social support. It is because of this dynamic that achieving the highest functional level possible becomes a primary goal in OT intervention.

Family support and education are critical when elders reach the end stage of the cancer process. The team must identify needed home care services, including therapies, a home attendant if indicated, and possible respite care for the primary caregiver. It is important that the COTA include the caregiver in the assessment of the patient's needs and in planning of care, relating to this person(s) as a contributing team-member. At the end-stage of the disease, referral to hospice/palliative care should be made to help alleviate suffering while maintaining the elder's dignity. All services provided should be coordinated to be ever-mindful of maintaining the emotional adjustment and support of the entire family.

OCCUPATIONAL THERAPY INTERVENTION

Evaluation and Intervention Planning

As Hannah, a COTA, prepares for her interventions of the day, she reviews the OT evaluation and history information for each patient, which was gathered at the time of the initial visit. This helps her familiarize herself with any obstacles or safety concerns that may inhibit the patient's functional independence and will need to be addressed by her intervention. Hannah will need to pay particular attention to the prior level of function of each patient, keeping it in mind as she instructs the patient in self-care tasks with the use of adaptive equipment, if needed, to work toward achieving the prior level of function.

When beginning the evaluation process with the elder cancer patient, a holistic approach is ideal. As stated earlier, health and well-being are directly impacted by the physical, functional, emotional, and social domains. OT intervention should be personally tailored to the stage of the disease—early diagnosis, treatment phase, recurrence—and in the end stage for the palliation of symptoms. The first step is a thorough review of the patient's medical/surgical records. This should include past medical history to identify comorbidities, current medical progress notes, treatments being provided, lab results (checking blood values to monitor possible myelosuppression), and radio-

graphic reports (checking for potential skeletal or other organ metastasis).

After reviewing the medical record, the registered occupational therapist (OTR), the COTA, and the elder collaborate to perform the evaluation. The focus of the assessment is the patient's functional status, but incorporated into this must be his or her emotional level of adjustment, perceptions of that functional status, and areas of concern/distress that may impact functional status. Family or caregiver concerns should also be assessed as early as possible. This process provides an understanding of the elder's occupational history and experiences, patterns of daily living, interests, values, and needs.[22] With this information, the OTR, COTA, and the client and caregivers, as appropriate, collaborate to identify priorities of intervention. Participation in daily occupations suitable for the elder is included, and through observation, the activity demands can be noted, problems that hinder success are recognized, and targeted outcomes are identified—for example, observing the elder ambulating to the bathroom with a walker, performing a toilet transfer, toileting skills, clothing management, hygiene and returning to a chair incorporates safety, fine-motor performance in daily activities, balance, cognitive sequencing, and functional tolerance. As deficits are noted in the elder's performance of the activity, they are included in the intervention plan. Throughout the evaluation process, it is important to communicate with the elder's family and/or caregivers. This provides assurance that the details of the home environment and prior occupational history are accurate and enables the OTR and COTA to have a clear understanding of all durable medical equipment (DME) or adaptive equipment that may be present in the home, including information about its use before the referral to OT. Standardized, objective assessments, such as sensorimotor assessments, may be helpful in the evaluation process and should be used whenever possible. Shortened length of stay and increasing time constraints in the acute-care settings require a general "functional" assessment of the strength, range of motion, or cognitive abilities needed for the performance of daily occupations.

As noted earlier, the OTR, COTA, elder, and caregivers collaborate to develop the intervention plan. The plan includes objective and measurable goals, a timeframe for planned achievement, and specific OT interventions that will be implemented to achieve these goals. Communication with other team members is important to provide the most comprehensive plan possible. As intervention progresses, the COTA and the OTR have ongoing communication to discuss complications and the elder's tolerance to intervention, thus making modifications or changes as needed. It is important with this patient population that each day before OT intervention, the COTA reviews the medical record, checking lab, radiology tests, physicians' orders and progress notes, to ensure that the patient's blood counts continue to allow for active involvement in intervention, and that there are no new developments in disease spread that may compromise the patient's abilities/safety in OT intervention. During the course of therapy, involvement and education of the family members and caregivers are important to provide them with an increased understanding of their elder's capabilities and the level of assistance that will be needed after discharge. Whenever possible, instruction and inclusion of family members within the intervention session are helpful. This provides the family with education about proper body mechanics, giving them increased comfort in their assistance of the patient and safe use of needed adaptive equipment or DME to be used at home. If it becomes apparent during this process that changes in family roles may be necessary, the COTA can provide support to all as this unfolds.

From the beginning of the evaluation process throughout intervention provision, the COTA must be mindful of the discharge plan, anticipated home care needs, equipment needs, and assistance required in the elder's care. To ensure multidisciplinary communication, it is important to identify what the best "next step" is from the OT perspective in the elder's discharge destination. A written recommendation in the daily progress note should be made, noting, for example, "Home with home health" or "Skilled nursing stay is needed for ..." or "Inpatient rehabilitation stay is recommended." It is understood that this recommendation is from the perspective of OT, incorporating safety issues and the current functional performance capacity of the client as observed in the OT intervention sessions. The format for this will vary, depending upon the setting and documentation guidelines used there.

Goals and Interventions

Hannah is treating a 75-year-old man with prostate cancer that has metastasized to his spine and pelvis, resulting in pain with forward flexion and prolonged standing. By instructing him in the use of a shower bench and long-handled sponge, he is now able to bathe seated, reaching his lower body without bending, thus limiting stress on his skeletal system. Because this intervention occurred in the hospital, Hannah knows it is important to coordinate home health efforts with the multidisciplinary team, recommending grab bars in his shower at home, and referring to home health OT follow-up with training after the needed equipment is in place. Hannah and the OTR confer about local equipment source options to help decrease out-of-pocket expenses incurred by the patient, and this information is relayed to the patient and caregiver.

The purpose of OT intervention is to "assist the client in reaching a state of physical, mental, and social well-being; to identify and realize aspirations; to satisfy needs; and to change or cope with the environment."[22] As we consider these concepts with elder cancer patients, we are reminded about the importance of achieving maximal functional independence in meaningful daily occupations as allowed within the limits of the disease. It is through this process that we establish our goal of improving the elder's quality of life. To meet this goal, COTAs aim at improving the elder's abilities in areas of meaningful occupations through training in ADL, such as bathing, bowel and bladder management, dressing, feeding, functional mobility, personal hygiene and grooming, personal device care (such as hearing aids, orthotics, adaptive equipment), or toileting, and IADL, such as care or supervision of others at home, care of pets, communication management (such as the use of a computer), meal preparation and cleanup, shopping for groceries, or community mobility. If adaptive equipment or an orthotic device is needed as a part of the intervention, education of the family and the client is important to ensure appropriate fit and compliance with the device. If muscle weakness prevents progress in intervention, COTAs may include strengthening exercises to increase functional capacity.

As noted, fatigue is a common problem among elders with cancer, being found almost universally in elders receiving chemotherapy.[20] With the identification of fatigue as a major impairment, the use of energy conservation techniques becomes an important component of OT intervention. COTAs may issue a written handout for energy conservation and work simplification in daily activities to the client, provide instruction, and observe demonstration by the client of these principles. It is through performance in daily activities while using the modified pacing techniques that the elder can learn how to better tolerate those activities required during their day. Adaptation of body mechanics in performing daily activities is important in the case of an elder with bone disease, which increases his susceptibility to pathological fractures (see Box 25-1). Educating the client and family in modified positions for daily activities can increase tolerance for the activities, decrease pain during the activities, and lower the risk of sustaining a fracture during the task.

It is well known that as one ages, the risk of falls increases.[23] Because of their age, elders with cancer are at increased risk for falls. Falls are associated with intrinsic factors, such as arthritis, depression, muscle weakness, or cognitive impairment, and extrinsic factors, such as uneven walking surfaces, inadequate lighting, throw rugs, improper footwear, or clothing.[23] COTAs have an opportunity to intervene in both areas to help prevent falls. Maximizing the client's tolerance to daily activities through energy conservation techniques and modified body mechanics with adaptive equipment use can help modify intrinsic fall risk, and working to adapt the home environment by improving lighting, removing throw rugs, and repositioning furniture to make a clear path, can aide in modifying extrinsic fall risk (Table 25-3). Providing the client with strengthening exercises, thus improving proprioception, can also aide in decreasing fall risk. Chapter 14 contains a discussion of fall prevention with elders.

Sometimes OT intervention may necessitate the use of orthotic devices designed to protect and support joints,

BOX 25-1

Body Mechanics to Decrease Stress on Bones and the Skeletal System

- Pain may arise from sitting in one position for prolonged periods, therefore change positions frequently.
- While working at a desk or table, make sure the work surface is the correct height so your shoulders are not raised or lowered, and your neck is not bent forward.
- While sitting for activities, place a small pillow or rolled towel at your lower back for added support. Also, keep your knees higher than your hips by using a low stool to slightly raise your feet.
- Stooping and bending are not advised, but if you must perform a task in a bent position, interrupt the position at regular intervals before the pain starts. This may be done by standing upright or sitting down briefly.
- Avoid bending your neck backward; you may need to rearrange your kitchen to prevent reaching and looking up for items on high shelves.
- While driving, move the seat forward enough to keep your knees bent and back straight. Using a small pillow or supportive roll behind your lower back may be helpful while sitting in the car.
- When moving from lying to a sitting position, use a log-rolling technique: roll on your side, bring your legs up toward your chest, then as you swing your legs off the bed, push up with your arms.

- Usually a good firm bed with support is desirable. If your bed is sagging, slats or plywood supports between the mattress and base will help add firmness.
- Slide objects rather than lifting or carrying, and push instead of pull objects when able.
- When performing daily tasks with equipment or tools, use lightweight tools. Stand near the work, rather than reaching for the activity.
- Avoid sitting or lying on low surfaces. Use foam or pillows to raise the seat with chairs or beds.
- Sit rather than stand while working whenever possible. Any activity longer than 10 minutes should be done sitting.
- Whenever lifting, follow these rules:
  Stand close to the object.
  Concentrate on using the small curve, or lordosis, in your lower back.
  Bend at your knees and keep your back straight.
  Get a secure grip and hold the load as close to you as possible.
  Lean back slightly to stay in balance, and lift the load by straightening your knees.
  Take a steady lift, and do not jerk.
  When upright, shift your feet to turn and avoid twisting the lower back.

maintain functional position, alleviate pain, support fractures, promote healing, and improve functioning. Examples of devices frequently seen are lumbosacral supports, arm elevators, slings, arm immobilizers, splints, and braces. COTAs may need to fabricate an upper or lower extremity splint, which positions the extremity in a functional position while providing needed joint support. After making the splint and fitting it, the COTA should instruct the client regarding the purpose of the device, proper fit, techniques for donning and doffing, wearing schedule, skin inspection techniques, and care of the device or support. If caregivers will be needed to assist the elder in donning the splint or device, it is important to include them in the teaching, allowing their participation to proper fit and wearing after discharge. There are many pre-fabricated splints and orthoses available on the market, and it is important that the COTA have knowledge of cost-saving options or sources when recommending these devices to provide the best care at the lowest possible cost to the client.

If and when the disease progresses, changes can occur that limit the client's physical capacity to perform previously accomplished daily activities, and, at this time, alterations in family roles may be needed. For example, if an elder female with breast cancer has a new onset of metastasis found in her femur, she may need to learn the proper techniques for ambulating with a cane or walker and

incorporate the use of this assistive device in her daily activities. It may be important to get assistance in grocery shopping and housework from family members, while she is able to maintain her role as menu planner, grocery list compiler, and checkbook manager for the family. Throughout this process of role adaptation, it is very important that the client and family all are involved in discussing potential changes, and everyone is aware of the client's abilities and limitations. With the use of empathetic listening, respect for the family's dilemma, and a trusting relationship during this period, potentially difficult situations can be resolved.

An integral part of the COTA perspective includes recognition of the client's emotional needs, while meeting his or her physical challenges. COTAs draw from their psychological and supportive perspectives as well as problem-solving skills when helping their clients manage change.[24] It is in recognizing the emotional needs of clients and caregivers that we can truly serve elders with cancer and their families. Psychological issues, including feelings of fear, lack of self-confidence, loss of control, and stress, have been reported as having a major impact upon elders with cancer.[21] With the use of relaxation exercises, such as visual imagery or deep breathing, clients can achieve increased feelings of control and manage their fear and anxiety in a positive manner. The therapeutic use of touch reaffirms acceptance and counters potential

TABLE 25-3

Checklist for Fall Prevention for Elders at Home

Area	Considerations	Possible interventions
Floors	Do you have a clear path to walk around furniture?	Ask someone to move the furniture so your path is clear.
	Are there any throw rugs on the floor?	Remove rugs, or use non-slip backing so the rugs won't slip. If you use a walker, remove rugs from the home because they can catch on the walker and cause a fall.
	Are there objects (e.g., books, shoes, boxes, papers) on the floor?	Pick up things that are on the floor. Always keep objects off of the floor.
	Are there wires or lamp cords on the floor that you must walk over?	Tape electrical cords and wires to the wall to prevent tripping on them. An electrician may need to install another outlet.
Stairs and steps	Are there papers, shoes, or other objects on the stairs?	Remove all objects from the stairs.
	Is there a light over the stairway?	Have an electrician install an overhead light at the top and bottom of the stairs.
		Make sure you have a light switch at the top and bottom of the stairs, and preferably a switch that glows for nighttime.
	Are the handrails loose or broken? Are they on both sides of the stairs?	Make sure handrails are on both sides of the stairs and as long as the stairs.
Kitchen	Are the most frequently used items on high shelves?	Move frequently used items to lower shelves. (Keep these at waist level.)
	Is your step-stool unsteady?	It is best not to use a step-stool, but if you must, get one with a bar to hold onto.
		Never use a chair as a step-stool.
Bathroom	Is the tub or shower floor slippery?	Place a non-slip rubber mat on the floor of the tub or shower.
	Is there a grab bar in place near the tub or shower for stability when entering?	Have a carpenter install a grab bar inside the tub or next to the shower.
	Is it difficult to get up from the toilet?	Consider a toilet riser or having a grab bar installed near the toilet to help in rising from the toilet.
Bedroom	Is there a light near the bed within easy reach?	Place a lamp close to the bed where it is easy to reach.
	Is the path dark from your bed to the toilet?	Use a night-light to see where you are walking during the night.

Adapted from Centers for Disease Control and Prevention. (2009). Check for safety: A home fall prevention checklist for older adults. www.cdc.gov/Home and Recreational Safety/Falls/Checklist for Safety.

feelings of rejection that may be triggered by alopecia or loss of hair following chemotherapy or total brain irradiation. Before instituting this intervention, the OTR/COTA team must verify the cultural appropriateness of touch for the elder. The COTA may provide or suggest a scarf, cap, or turban and help supply the client with local source options for these products. The use of such items can minimize decreased self-esteem, enabling the client to continue much needed social connections, thus receiving support from friends and family.

Hannah has a patient with breast cancer on her intervention list who had a recent right humeral pathological fracture diagnosed on x-ray. The orthopedist's recommendation was to immobilize the patient's upper extremity with an orthotic immobilizer for 8 weeks, during which time the patient will also receive radiation therapy to the area. The patient is right-handed, very frightened and anxious about the potential for further damage if she moved her arm "in the wrong way." Hannah instructs the patient in adaptive dressing and bathing techniques, teaching one-handed techniques, using her non-dominant hand to perform these tasks. Hannah realizes that reassurance and psychological support are important throughout this process to alleviate the patient's anxiety, increase her attention on the task, and enable her to retain the information she is learning. Hannah allows the patient time to express her fears, listening and responding with gentle support and encouragement. Hannah includes the patient's husband in her intervention, instructing both of them in the method of donning and doffing the immobilizer for bathing, the care of the immobilizer, proper fit, and skin inspection techniques.

Special Considerations in Intervention Planning and Implementation

One of Hannah's patients is a 64-year-old man with a recent diagnosis of lung cancer, who is recovering from a surgical thoracotomy for the removal of the tumor. As Hannah enters his room, she finds him sitting on the edge of the bed, on 8 liters of oxygen per nasal cannula. He is very short of breath and appears quite anxious. He states he is "tired of not being able to do anything," and that he has been unable to walk 20 feet to the bathroom for toileting and bathing tasks because of his poor endurance and breathing difficulty. He states he has lost control of his life and is so nervous he "wishes he would just die now." Hannah maintains good eye contact with him, listening to his fears, and acknowledging how frightening his situation must be. She discusses with him the option of using pursed-lip breathing techniques and muscle relaxation techniques to decrease feelings of anxiety and gain control over his breathing. They then perform the relaxation exercise, with the patient seated in a chair at bedside. She provides him with energy conservation techniques in writing to use in his daily routine, incorporating frequent rests, using modified body mechanics, and the use of adaptive devices, such as a bath bench, to maximize his tolerance during bathing. Through the demonstration of the relaxation exercise and performance of the proper transfer technique with the bath stool the patient learns that he is able to accomplish these tasks and feels an increased sense of control in his life. After completing this intervention, Hannah communicates to the nurse and the social worker what the patient has stated about his death so that all of the team members can maintain an awareness of this patient's emotional needs.

There are unique considerations that one should be mindful of while working with elder cancer patients. Cachexia is sometimes seen with this population during the course of the disease and intervention. This condition presents itself with malnutrition, muscle atrophy, weakness, and loss in body mass, and occurs because of biochemical abnormalities and loss of appetite. With decreased nutritional intake there is less energy, inactivity, and a downward spiral begins. In this situation, it is difficult to increase the elder's activity level, and the COTA should be aware of the current nutritional status of the client during the intervention course. Strategies used to help cope with fatigue, such as lifestyle management, planning, and energy conservation techniques are useful approaches in these situations.

The presence of depression with fatigue is common in elders with cancer, and sometimes depression can prevent participation in the intervention process or contribution to establishing one's goals of intervention. It is important that the COTA recognize when additional psychological support/counseling is needed and help facilitate formal psychological interventions, if indicated.

Inactivity may occur because of the cancer process itself or to the treatment of the disease. In the normal aging process there is a decrease in muscle mass and strength as well as reduced peripheral nerve functioning.[16] Certain chemotherapeutic agents are known to bring with them the potential for neurotoxicity and myotoxicity, which results in impairments of muscles and the sensory nerves. Issues such as peripheral neuropathy and muscle weakness can have devastating consequences for elders, who may no longer be able to perform their daily living activities without assistance. Recent evidence suggests that increasing physical activity of elders with cancer can decrease cancer fatigue, improve physical functioning, and enhance the quality of life.[18] The COTA can institute a supervised exercise program to carefully progress the client's activity as tolerated, incorporating seated ADL and pacing techniques with the activities.

Lymphedema sometimes develops following lymph node resections in breast cancer patients but can also occur with lymph node removal in the inguinal area in other types of cancer. This swelling takes place because of an abnormal collection of protein-rich fluid and may be present in the upper or lower extremities (Figure 25-1). The retrieval of lymph nodes following the diagnosis of breast cancer is important to accurately identify the stage of the cancer, thus affording the client the best options for treatment. However, the interruption of the normal

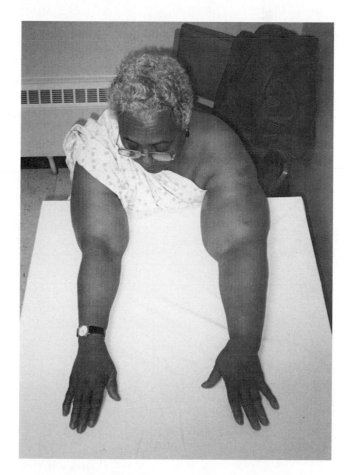

FIGURE 25-1 Lymphedema is swelling that results from the abnormal accumulation of protein-rich fluid. This condition is sometimes seen after lymph node removal or radiation treatment for breast cancer.

lymph system and fluid drainage increases the risk of lymphedema. When present, this problem may also bring pain, chronic inflammation, or fibrosis. At any degree of severity, lymphedema can impair the elder's ability to wear certain types of clothing, and it often reduces self-esteem, body-image, and thus quality of life. OT interventions may include applying pressure to the extremity with compression garments or bandages, exercise, massage therapy (known as manual lymph drainage), and sequential pumps. Treatment can improve skin texture and sensation, overall appearance, decrease limb girth, and increase functionality. In conjunction with the physical interventions, OT intervention should include education of the client about lymphedema prevention strategies, skin protection techniques, and early identification of potential infection. It is hoped that with the recent use of sentinel node dissection (a surgical technique that results in fewer lymph nodes being removed) and new surgical and radiation techniques, we will see a reduction in the presence of this problem (Table 25-4).

It is important for the COTA to collaborate with the OTR during the intervention process and modify or advance goals as the client progresses. However, if disease progression causes loss of function, the intervention goals may need to be modified to accommodate changing needs with additional adaptations. It can be empowering to the client to have the opportunity to make decisions about daily routines or activity adaptations, thus restoring a sense of control during a difficult time. Encouragement, reassurance, and effective communication with both the client and family members are essential in this process to ensure a therapeutic transition.

Following an intervention session with a 70-year-old patient with prostate cancer, Hannah realizes that his tolerance was limited and prevented the completion of the planned upper extremity Thera-Band exercises that had previously been used as an intervention. The patient's medical record shows that he has completed his second course of chemotherapy and the prognosis is hopeful, but his level of physical tolerance has diminished in the last

TABLE 25-4

OT Intervention Gems	
Problem	**OT intervention option**
Inability to reach lower extremities for dressing due to spinal metastasis or joint replacement surgery	■ Instruct in use of a reacher, long-handled shoehorn, sock aid for dressing ■ Have patient demonstrate modified techniques in dressing
Limited use of one upper extremity for bathing, dressing, cooking tasks	■ Instruct in adapted long-handled sponge for bathing ■ Teach one-handed techniques for dressing ■ Use adapted cutting board, rocker knife, or Dycem matting for cooking tasks
Anxiety or fear inhibiting patient's attention/participation in therapy	■ Deep breathing techniques ■ Visual imagery or relaxation exercises ■ Therapeutic use of touch ■ Active listening techniques
Increased susceptibility to infection; decreased immune response	■ Universal precautions and frequent hand washing ■ Develop interest in solitary activities (photo album development, needlework, computer games)
Upper extremity weakness	■ Thera-Band exercise program ■ Progressive resistive exercise as tolerated
Decreased endurance in ADL and IADL	■ Participation in functional tasks while standing, such as meal preparation, grooming tasks at the vanity ■ Progress time as tolerated
Fall history; risk of falls/fractures	■ Issue/instruct in Fall Risk Reduction handout ■ Performance in bathing, dressing, or kitchen task while using techniques ■ Modify extrinsic fall risk factors at home by including family/caregiver in education ■ Strengthening exercises
Shortness of breath, weakness in ADL	■ Pursed-lip breathing techniques ■ Energy conservation techniques
Upper extremity lymphedema	■ Compression bandaging ■ Manual lymphatic drainage ■ Lymphedema prevention strategies in ADL ■ Skin protection techniques ■ Sequential pumps

several days. Hannah discusses this with the OTR and together they modify the plan of care to include progressively more strenuous activities, working toward increasing his tolerance. They put together a written program beginning with sitting activities and eventually toward standing and then activities that include walking and carrying household items. They instruct the patient to follow the program at home and discuss how and when he can progress the activities on his own after discharge. Hannah also communicates the recommendation to the social worker for OT follow-up at home, which provides ongoing monitoring of the patient's progress and strengthening after discharge.

Discharge Planning

Because of the current short length of stays in hospitals and the push for early discharge, the process of discharge planning begins at the time of evaluation and continues with each subsequent OT intervention session. There should be an ongoing discussion with the elders, their families, and the multidisciplinary team members about the client's abilities, need for assistance, and recommendations for post-acute rehabilitation, discharge, or home health care follow-up. It is helpful to have a multidisciplinary team meeting to discuss the client's progress and for the care team to effectively communicate to one another concerns or issues that may need to be addressed before discharge. The COTA should anticipate home equipment needs of the elder and with the elder, family, and durable medical equipment (DME) provider to ensure that important equipment is in place for the client's safety at home. Provision of any needed equipment should include thorough instructions by the COTA to both the client and caregiver on the setup, use, and care of the equipment. If a caregiver will be needed to assist the elder with any daily activities, practice of the caregiver in the task, such as bathing or transfers, is helpful during a therapy session before discharge. Referral to home health OT services may be made to ensure a seamless transition to home, providing the family and client with supervised instruction within their own home. Strengthening programs may be used, and adaptations of the home environment should be recommended as needed to improve safety of the elder.

CASE STUDY

At the end of the day, Hannah has one more patient to work with. Carol is a 68-year-old woman who was diagnosed with small cell carcinoma of the lung one month ago. At that time, she underwent left lower lung lobectomy for removal of the primary tumor and has been recovering well from that surgery, although she continues to have shortness of breath with exertion in activities. She has now been re-admitted to the hospital with left sided weakness and behavior changes as reported by her husband, including poor attention span and occasional impaired judgment. An MRI scan of the brain reveals a right hemispheric lesion, and a stereotactic brain biopsy shows it to be a metastatic lesion secondary to the primary

lung cancer. Carol has begun radiation therapy treatments to the brain, and her oncologist has ordered "OT to evaluate and treat as indicated."

During the OT assessment, the OTR and Hannah learned that Carol and her husband live in a two-story home. The master bedroom and bath are on the second floor, although there is a guest bedroom and bath on the main level. Before her illness, Carol had been the primary cook and housekeeper. She had also maintained the family finances while her husband managed the yard, was the primary driver, and worked part-time as a consultant for a non-profit agency. During the brief time she was home after her initial lung surgery, Carol fell once while getting out of the shower. Fortunately, she was not injured. She had continued to perform her own self-care tasks, but with increasing difficulty because of recent one-sided weakness on her dominant left side. Her husband had begun to assist her with her daily activities intermittently. She had been walking without an assistive device.

A functional sensorimotor assessment of Carol's upper extremities shows that her right upper extremity function is within functional limits with both strength and active range of motion (AROM). Her left upper extremity appears to have 3+/5 muscle strength throughout with AROM within functional limits. Sensation appears intact, but mild left neglect is present during functional activities. During toileting and shower transfers, Carol moves impulsively and has two episodes of loss of balance during which she catches herself, preventing a fall. During a discussion of this, Carol denies any imbalance, stating she really "does just fine." She also denies any previous falls at home. During the evaluation of her ADL performance, Carol exhibits increased shortness of breath, requiring frequent rest periods. However, she is able to maintain her blood oxygen saturation level above 90% without additional oxygen throughout the tasks. She requires minimal assistance for dressing and bathing because of decreased left upper extremity strength and increased fatigue. She is very anxious to return home with her husband and is cooperative but minimizes the need for therapy.

◼▮ CASE STUDY QUESTIONS

1 In the previous case study, identify daily occupations that Hannah should include in the OT intervention to help with improving Carol's independence and endurance.
2 What adaptations could be incorporated in the bathroom to improve Carol's safety at home while bathing, toileting, and performing grooming tasks?
3 What techniques could be used to maximize Carol's independence and tolerance to her daily occupations and leisure activities at home?
4 What instructions and/or suggestions need to be provided to Carol and her husband to help prevent falls in the future? Are there any suggestions related to the home architecture to consider?
5 How can Hannah assist Carol and her husband in modification of their roles at home to allow Carol to maintain a contributory family role now and in the future?
6 What needs of Carol's should Hannah communicate to the other team members during discharge planning to ease the transition from hospital to home?
7 What other special considerations in intervention apply to Carol?

■ CHAPTER REVIEW QUESTIONS

1 What types of precautions should a COTA use when working with an elder who has prostate cancer with bone metastasis to his spine?
2 What should a COTA suggest to help an elder female who has recently lost her hair from chemotherapy?
3 If cancer-related fatigue is preventing an elder from performing his own bathing without assistance, what approaches could be used to improve his independence?
4 What information should a COTA gather before treating the elder with cancer?
5 Why is the elder's participation in daily activities important in achieving the OT intervention goals?
6 What is the ultimate goal of OT intervention with an elder who has cancer?
7 What approaches can the COTA use to help the elder who is experiencing anxiety, depression, or fear of the unknown?
8 At what point in the intervention process should the COTA be contributing to the discharge process with the other team members?

REFERENCES

1. Horner, M., Ries, L., Krapcho, M., Neyman, N., Aminou, R., Howlader, N., et al. (Eds.), 2009. Seer cancer statistics review, 1975-2006, National Cancer Institute. Bethesda, MD. http://seer.cancer.gov/csr/1975-2006/, based on November 2008 SEER data submission, posted to the SEER website.
2. U.S. Department of Health and Human Services., 2005. Administration on aging: A profile of older Americans. URL http://www.aoa.dhhs.gov.
3. American Cancer Society., 2008. Cancer facts and figures. Society, Atlanta, GA.
4. Jemal, A., Thun, M., Ries, L., Howe, H., Weir, H., Center, M., et al., 2008. Annual report to the nation on the status of cancer, 1975-2005, featuring trends in lung. Journal of the National Cancer Institute 100 (23), 1672-1694.
5. American Lung Association., 2008. Lung cancer. American Lung Association Lung Disease Data:, 2008. [URL page]. www.lungusa.org.
6. National Cancer Institute, 2009. What you need to know about lung cancer. Washington, D.C.: U.S. Department of Health and Human Services / National Institutes of Health.
7. McArthur, H., Hudis, C., 2007. Adjuvant chemotherapy for early-stage breast cancer. Hematology/Oncology Clinics of North America 21 (2), 207-222.
8. U.S. Census Bureau., 2008. Table 3. Percent distribution of the projected population by selected age groups and sex for the United States: 2010 to 2050 (NP2008-T3). http://www.census.gov/population/index.html. Source: Population Division, U.S. Census Bureau.
9. Dittus, K., Muss, H., 2007. Management of the frail elderly with breast cancer. Oncology (Williston Park) 21 (14), 1727-1734.
10. Chan, J., Feraco, A., Shuman, M., Hernandez-Diaz, S., 2006. The epidemiology of prostate cancer—with a focus on nonsteroidal anti-inflammatory drugs. Hematology/Oncology Clinics of North America 20 (4), 797-809.
11. Amemiya, T., Oda, K., Ando, M., Kawamura, T., Kitagawa, Y., Okawa, Y., et al., 2007. Activities of daily living and quality of life of elderly patients after elective surgery for gastric and colorectal cancers. Annals of Surgery 246 (2), 222-228.
12. Berger, N.A., Savvides, P., Koroukian, S.M., Kahana, E.F., Deimling, G.T., Rose, J.H., et al., 2006. Cancer in the elderly. Transactions of the American Climatological Association 117, 147-156.
13. Nguyen, T., Abrey, L., 2007. Brain metastases: Old problem, new strategies. Hematology/Oncology Clinics of North America 21 (2), 369-388.
14. Rodin, M.B., Mohile, S.G., 2007. A practical approach to geriatric assessment in oncology. Journal of Clinical Oncology 10; 25 (14), 1936-1944.
15. Gosney, M.A., 2005. Clinical assessment of elderly people with cancer. Lancet Oncology 6 (10), 790-797.
16. Visovsky, C., 2006. The effects of neuromuscular alterations in elders with cancer. Seminars in Oncology Nursing 22 (1), 36-42.
17. Mell, L., Mundt, A., 2005. Radiation therapy in the elderly. Cancer Journal 11 (6), 495-505.
18. Luctkar-Flude, M., Groll, D., Tranmer, J., et al., 2007. Fatigue and physical activity in older adults with cancer. Cancer Nursing 30 (5), E35-E45.
19. Meier, A., Lyons, E., Frydman, G., Forlenza, M., Rimer, Barbara, K., 2007. How cancer survivors provide support on cancer-related Internet mailing lists. Journal of Medical Internet Research 9 (2), e12.
20. Luciani, A., Jacobsen, P., Extermann, M., et al., 2008. Fatigue and functional dependence in older cancer patients. American Journal of Clinical Oncology 31 (5), 424-430.
21. Kealey, P., McIntyre, I., 2005. An evaluation of the domiciliary occupational therapy service in palliative cancer care in a community trust: A patient and carers perspective. European Journal of Cancer Care (Engl) 14 (3), 232-243.
22. American Occupational Therapy Association, 2008. Occupational therapy practice framework: Domain and process, 2nd ed. American Journal of Occupational Therapy 62 (6), 625-683.
23. Rao, S.S., 2005. Prevention of falls in older patients. Am Fam Physician 72 (1):81-88.
24. Vockins, H., 2004. Occupational therapy intervention with patients with breast cancer: A survey. European Journal of Cancer Care (Engl) 13 (1), 45-52.

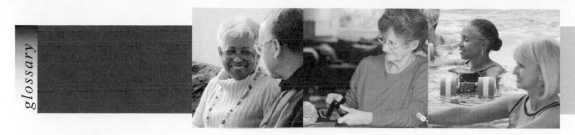

Glossary

A

acalculia Form of aphasia characterized by the inability to solve simple mathematic calculations.

acetylcholine A neurotransmitter substance widely distributed in body tissues with the primary function of mediating synaptic activity of the nervous system and skeletal muscles.

acute Beginning abruptly with marked intensity or sharpness, then subsiding after a relatively short period.

ageism Prejudice or discrimination against a particular age group, particularly the elderly.

aging in place Living where the elders have lived for years, typically not in a health care environment, using products, services, and conveniences that allow them to remain home as circumstances change. Elders continue to live in the home of their choice safely and independently as they get older. Livability can be extended through the incorporation of universal design principles, telecare, and other assistive technologies.

amyloid Combining form: starch of polysaccharide nature or origin.

angina Spasmodic choking or suffocative pain; currently used almost exclusively to denote angina pectoris.

angioplasty The reconstruction of blood vessels damaged by disease or injury.

ankylosing spondylitis A chronic inflammatory disease of unknown origin that first affects the spine and adjacent structures and commonly progresses to cause eventual fusion of the involved joints.

anosognosia An abnormal condition characterized by a real or feigned inability to perceive a defect, especially paralysis, on one side of the body; possibly attributable to a lesion in the right parietal lobe of the brain.

anoxia An abnormal condition characterized by a lack of oxygen.

antecedent Something that comes before something else; a precursor.

anticholinergic Agents pertaining to the blockade of acetylcholine receptors that result in the inhibition of the transmission of parasympathetic nerve impulses.

antihistamines Any substance capable of reducing the physiologic and pharmacologic effects of histamine, including a wide variety of drugs that block histamine receptors. Many such drugs are readily available as nonprescription medications for the management of allergies.

antioxidant A chemical or other agent that inhibits or retards oxidation of a substance to which it is added.

arrhythmias Variations from the normal rhythm, especially of the heartbeat.

atrophy A wasting or diminution of size or physiologic activity in a part of the body because of disease or other influences.

axis I Psychiatric disorder usually diagnosed in infancy, childhood, or adolescence, excluding mental retardation.

axis II Psychiatric personality disorder and mental retardation.

B

Baby Boomers Persons who were born between 1946 and 1964. The Baby Boomer generation makes up nearly 20% of the North American population.

benzodiazepines A group of psychotropic agents, including tranquilizers, prescribed in the treatment of insomnia and to alleviate anxiety.

bradycardia A circulatory condition in which the myocardium contracts steadily but at a rate of less than 60 contractions a minute.

bronchiole A small airway of the respiratory system extending from the bronchi into the lobes of the lung.

C

calcification The accumulation of calcium salts in tissues.

cataract A progressive condition of the lens of the eye characterized by loss of transparency.

catastrophic sudden downturn A pattern of medical and nursing care that involves intensive, highly technical life support care of an acutely ill or severely traumatized patient.

chronic Developing slowly and persisting for a long time, often for the remainder of the individual's lifetime.

cochlea A conic, bony structure of the inner ear, perforated by numerous apertures for passage of the cochlear division of the acoustic nerve.

cohort A collection or sampling of individuals who share common characteristics, such as individuals of the same age or sex.

collagen A protein consisting of bundles of tiny reticular fibrils that combine to form the white, glistening, inelastic fibers of the tendons, the ligaments, and the fascia.

contralateral Affecting or originating in the opposite side of a point of reference, such as a point on the body.

contrast sensitivity The ability to distinguish the borders of objects as they degrade in contrast from their backgrounds.

cyanosis Bluish discoloration of the skin and mucous membranes caused by an excess of deoxygenated hemoglobin in the blood or a structural defect in the hemoglobin molecule.

cytology The study of cells, including their formation, origin, structure, function, biochemical activities, and pathology.

cytotoxic chemotherapy Any pharmacologic compound that inhibits the proliferation of cells within the body.

D

decubitus ulcer stage III Stage characterized by broken skin, loss of skin, loss of full thickness of skin, possible damage to subcutaneous tissues, and possible serous or bloody drainage.

decubitus ulcer stage IV Stage characterized by formation of a deep, crater-like ulcer, loss of the full thickness of skin, and destruction of subcutaneous tissues; exposure of fascia, connective tissue, bone, or muscle underlying the ulcer, causing possible damage; an inflammation, sore, or ulcer over a bony prominence.

deleterious Harmful or dangerous.

detrusor urinae muscle A complex of longitudinal fibers that form the external layer of the muscular coat of the bladder.

developmental stages A perspective that sees continuity between phases of adult development, although during each phase there may be qualitative differences in behavior. There are a number of different views about the way in which psychological and physical development proceed throughout the lifespan.

diabetic retinopathy A disorder of retinal blood vessels characterized by microaneurysms, hemorrhage, exudates, and the formation of new vessels and connective tissue.

diaphragmatic breathing A type of breathing exercise that patients are taught to promote more effective aeration of the lungs; movement of the diaphragm downward during inhalation and upward with exhalation.

diplopia Double vision.

DNA (deoxyribonucleic acid) A large nucleic acid molecule found principally in the chromosomes of the nucleus of a cell that carries genetic information.

dopamine A naturally occurring sympathetic nervous system neurotransmitter that is the precursor of norepinephrine.

DRG (diagnosis-related group) A group of patients classified for measuring delivery of care in a medical facility; used to determine Medicare payments for inpatient care.

durable power of attorney for health A document that designates an agent or proxy to make health care decisions for a patient who is unable to do so.

dyspnea Shortness of breath or a difficulty in breathing that may be caused by certain heart conditions, strenuous exercise, or anxiety.

E

eccentric viewing A technique in which a person views objects by directing his or her gaze to an area just adjacent to the target object to compensate for a scotoma involving the fovea or macula. This position allows the desired target to be focused on a healthy area of retina.

edema The abnormal accumulation of fluid in interstitial spaces of tissues, such as in the pericardial sac, intrapleural space, peritoneal cavity, and joint capsules.

elastin A protein that forms the principal substance of yellow elastic fibers of tissue.

embolus A foreign object, a quantity of air or gas, a bit of tissue or tumor, or a piece of thrombus that circulates in the bloodstream until it becomes lodged in a vessel.

endocarditis An abnormal condition that affects the endocardium and the heart valves and is characterized by lesions caused by a variety of diseases.

erosion The wearing away or gradual destruction of a mucosal or epidermal surface as a result of inflammation, injury, or other effects; usually marked by the appearance of an ulcer.

esthesia Sensitivity or feeling.

exertional dyspnea Shortness of breath during exertion or exercise.

expectoration The ejection of mucus, sputum, or fluids from the trachea and lungs by coughing or spitting.

G

gastrostomy Surgical creation of an artificial opening into the stomach through the abdominal wall; performed to feed a patient who has cancer of the esophagus or a tracheoesophageal fistula, or one who is expected to be unconscious for a long period.

Generation X The generation following the post–World War II baby boom, especially people born in the United States and Canada from the early 1960s to the late 1970s.

Generation Y The generation following Generation X, especially people born in the United States and Canada from the early 1980s to the late 1990s.

generational cohort The group of individuals born within a similar time period who experience the same events within the same time or historical interval.

geriatrics The care of elderly people based on the integration of knowledge of gerontology and chronic disease.

gerontology The comprehensive study of aging and how it affects individuals—physically, socially, psychologically, and economically.

glaucoma An abnormal condition of increased pressure inside the eyeball, often leading to damage to tissues of the eye and vision loss if untreated.

glomerular filtration The renal process whereby fluid in the blood is filtered across the capillaries of the glomerulus and into the urinary space of Bowman's capsule.

glycogen A polysaccharide that is the major carbohydrate stored in animal cells.

gracilis The most superficial of the five medial femoral muscles.

H

health The condition of being sound in body, mind, or spirit; also a general condition of well-being or flourishing.

health care proxy A person designated to make health care decisions for a patient who has become incapacitated.

hemi-inattention (also referred to as **hemi-neglect, neglect syndrome, unilateral neglect syndrome**) A disregard or lack of attention for one side of a person's visual space. Inattention to the left visual space is much more common than inattention to the right.

hemiparesis (hemiplegia) Paralysis of one side of the body.

hemorrhage An escape of blood from the blood vessels.

heterotopic ossification A nonmalignant overgrowth of bone, frequently occurring after a fracture, that is sometimes confused with certain bone tumors when visualized on x-ray film.

hypercalcemia Greater than normal amounts of calcium in the blood, most often resulting from excessive bone resorption and release of calcium, as occurs in hyperparathyroidism, metastatic tumors of bone, Paget's disease, and osteoporosis.

hyperesthesia An extreme sensitivity of one of the body's sense organs, such as pain or touch receptors of the skin.

hyperglycemia A greater than normal amount of glucose in blood.

hypertonicity Excessive tone, tension, or activity.

hypotonicity Lower or lessened tone or tension in any body structure, as in paralysis.

I

IADL Instrumental activities of daily living, including health management, community living skills, safety management, and home management.

illness An unhealthy condition of body or mind.

intergenerational Being or occurring between generations.

intermediary A Blue Cross plan, private insurance company, or public or private agency selected by health care providers to pay claims under Medicare.

intrinsic Originating from or situated within an organ or tissue.

ipsilateral Pertaining to the same side of the body.

irradiation Exposure to any form of radiant energy such as heat, light, and x-ray.

J

jejunostomy A surgical procedure to create an artificial opening to the jejunum through the abdominal wall.

L

Lewy bodies Concentric spheres found inside vacuoles in midbrain and brainstem neurons in patients with idiopathic parkinsonism, Alzheimer's disease, and other neurodegenerative conditions.

lumen A cavity or channel within any organ or structure of the body.

M

macular degeneration A progressive deterioration of the macula of the retina and choroid of the eye.

malabsorption syndrome A complex of syndromes resulting from disorders in the intestinal absorption of nutrients, characterized by anorexia, weight loss, abdominal bloating, muscle cramps, bone pain, and steatorrhea.

motor planning The ability to plan and execute coordinated movement.

mucopurulent Characteristic of a combination of mucus and pus.

mucosa Mucous membrane.

myelosuppression The inhibition of the process of production of blood cells and platelets in the bone marrow.

N

nasogastric tube Any tube passed into the stomach through the nose.

neurons Functional cells of the nervous system.

O

oculomotor control The ability to move the eyes together in a coordinated fashion.

ombudsman A person who investigates and mediates patients' problems and complaints regarding hospital services.

opacification Making something opaque.

orthopnea An abnormal condition in which a person must sit or stand to breathe deeply or comfortably; usually accompanies cardiac and respiratory conditions.

orthostatic hypertension Abnormally low blood pressure occurring when an individual assumes a standing posture; also called postural hypotension.

ossification The development of bone.

osteoarthritis A form of arthritis in which one or many joints undergo degenerative changes, including subchondral bony sclerosis, loss of articular cartilage, and proliferation of bone and cartilage in the joint, forming osteophytes.

osteomalacia An abnormal condition of the lamellar bone characterized by a loss of calcification of the matrix, resulting in softening of the bone, accompanied by weakness, fracture, pain, anorexia, and weight loss.

P

palliative Therapy designed to relieve or reduce intensity of uncomfortable symptoms, but not to produce a cure.

parenteral nutrition The administration of nutrients by a route other than through the alimentary canal, such as subcutaneously, intravenously, intramuscularly, and intradermally.

Parkinson's disease A slowly progressive, degenerative, neurological disorder.

paroxysmal nocturnal dyspnea A sudden onset of shortness of breath while sleeping.

pharynx A tubular structure in the throat about 13 cm in length that extends from the base of the skull to the esophagus and is situated just in front of the cervical vertebrae.

Pick's disease A form of presenile dementia occurring in middle age that produces neurotic behavior and the slow disintegration of intellect, personality, and emotions.

polyuria The excretion of an abnormally large quantity of urine.

presbycusis A loss of hearing sensitivity and speech intelligibility associated with aging.

psychodynamics The study of the forces that motivate behavior.

R

RNA (ribonucleic acid) A nucleic acid found in both the nucleus and the cytoplasm of cells that transmits genetic instructions from the nucleus to the cytoplasm.

S

scotoma An area of the retina where vision is depressed or absent.

sedative hypnotics A class of drugs that reversibly depresses the activity of the central nervous system, used chiefly to induce sleep and to allay anxiety.

semi-Fowler's position Placement of the patient in an inclined position, with the upper half of the body raised by elevating the head of the bed approximately 30 degrees.

senile Pertaining to or characteristic of old age or the process of aging, especially the physical or mental deterioration accompanying aging.

sinusitis An inflammation of one or more paranasal sinuses.

stent A compound used in making dental impressions and medical molds.

strabismus A condition in which an eye is deviated from its normal position and is not aligned with the other eye.

subacute Somewhat acute; between acute and chronic.

subluxation A partial abnormal separation of the articular surfaces of a joint.

supraglottic swallow Coordinated muscular contractions of swallowing in the region of the mouth and pharynx.

syncope A brief lapse in consciousness caused by transient cerebral hypoxia.

synovium Synovial membrane; the inner layer of an articular capsule surrounding a freely movable joint.

T

thrombophlebitis Inflammation of a vein, often accompanied by formation of a clot.

thrombotic stroke Obstruction by a thrombus of the blood supply to the brain, causing a cerebrovascular accident.

thrombus An aggregation of platelets, fibrin, clotting factors, and the cellular elements of the blood attached to the interior wall of a vein or artery.

trachea A nearly cylindrical tube in the neck composed of cartilage and membrane that extends from the larynx at the level of the sixth cervical vertebra to the fifth thoracic vertebra, where it divides into two bronchi.

tracheobronchial tree An anatomical complex including the trachea, bronchi, and bronchial tubes that conveys air to and from the lungs and is a primary structure in respiration.

Traditionalists The generational cohort that adheres to or advocates adherence to tradition or traditionalism (and orientation of a society toward old established values and institutions).

U

urodynamic The study of the hydrology and mechanics of urinary bladder filling and emptying.

utilitarianism A doctrine stating that the purpose of all action should be to bring about the greatest happiness for the greatest number of people and that value is determined by utility; often applied in the distribution of health care resources, such as in decisions regarding the expenditure of public funds for health services.

V

Valsalva maneuver Any forced expiratory effort against a closed airway, such as when an individual holds the breath and tightens the muscles in a concerted, strenuous effort to move a heavy object or change position in bed.

valvular heart disease An acquired or congenital disorder of a cardiac valve characterized by stenosis and obstructed by valvular degeneration and regurgitation of blood.

visual acuity The clearness or sharpness of vision, typically measured in Snellen equivalents, such as 20/20.

visual field The visual surround that can be seen when one looks straight ahead.

vital capacity A measurement of the amount of air that can be expelled at the normal rate of exhalation after a maximum inspiration; represents the greatest possible breathing capacity.

BIBLIOGRAPHY

American Psychiatric Association, 2000. Diagnostic and Statistical Manual of Mental Disorders, fourth ed. Text Revision. The Association, Washington, DC.

Anderson, K.N., Anderson, L.E., Glanze, W.D., 2008. Mosby's Medical, Nursing, and Health Dictionary, eighth ed. St. Louis, Mosby.

McDonough, J.T., 1994. Stedman's concise medical dictionary, second ed. Williams & Wilkins, Baltimore.

Miller, B.F., Keane, C., 1987. Saunders's Encyclopedia and Dictionary of Medicine, Nursing, and Allied Health, fourth ed. WB Saunders, Philadelphia.

Miller, B.F., Keane, C., 2005. Encyclopedia and Dictionary of Medicine, Nursing, and Allied Health, seventh ed. WB Saunders, Philadelphia.

Taber's Cyclopedic Medical Dictionary, 2009. twenty-first ed. FA Davis, Philadelphia.

Index

A

AARP. *See* American Association of Retired Persons
Abandonment, 150-151
Abstinence, 156. *See also* Sexual activity
Accommodation, 206. *See also* Vision
Accreditation Standards for Educational Program for the Occupational Therapy Assistant, 121-122
ACL. *See* Allen Cognitive Levels
ACS. *See* Activity Card Sort
Activities of daily living (ADL), 4
  AD and, 283-284, 284t-285t
  assistance with, 8
  dementia and, 283-284
  health promotion program and, 58
  oncological conditions and, 336
  sexual function and, 155
Activity. *See also* Exercise
  arthritis and modifying, 309, 309t
  levels, 47, 47f
  medications and, 175-177, 176t
  theory, 23, 24f
    OT and, 24-25
  well-being promoting, AD and, 285-286
Activity Card Sort (ACS), 292
Acuity, decreased, 221-222, 222f-223f
AD. *See* Alzheimer's disease
ADA. *See* Americans with Disabilities Act
ADL. *See* Activities of daily living
Adult care options, 9
Adult day care, 9, 118-119
Adult foster care, 9, 111-112
Aesthetic appearance, aging and, 33-34
Age
  cancer and, 329
  chronological, 43-44
  middle, 26
  myths, 14-17, 43-48
  old, 6
  status awarded people due to, 129
Aged population. *See* Elder population
Ageism, 14-17, 129
  health care system and, 16
  language encouraging, 16
  reflection questions about, 16, 16b
Age-related macular degeneration (ARMD), 215-216
Aging, 31-33
  aesthetic appearance and, 33-34
  biological theories of, 21-22
    genetic, 21-22
    nongenetic, 22
  brain, 263
  changes, 32-33, 32f
  driving and, 202, 206
  emotions associated with, 48
  facts about, 43-48
  genetic theories of
    free radical theory, 22
    neuroendocrine theory, 22
    somatic mutation theory, 22
  health and, 4-5
  hearing conditions associated with, 230-232, 231t
  learning and, 44-45

Aging (*Continued*)
  losses associated with, 48
  mobility and, 202
  myths about, 43-48
  nongenetic, 21
  physical illness and, 4-5
  in place, 9-10
  population, 7-8
    COTA services, 32
    cultural diversity in, 121-133
  primary, 32-33
  process, 31-41
    cardiopulmonary system and, 35-36
    case study of, 39
    cognition and, 36-37
    immune system and, 36
    integumentary system and, 33-34, 34f
    kinesthetic changes and, 38
    medications and physiology of, 170
    neuromusculoskeletal system and, 34
    physiology and, 170
    sensory system, 37-38
    skeletal system and, 34-35
    somatosensory changes and, 38
  programmed, 21-22
  psychological aspects of, 43-52
    case study and, 50-51
  with psychosis, 295
  secondary, 32-33
  social theories of, 22-28
    activity, 23, 24f
    continuity theory, 23-25
    disengagement theory, 23
    Erikson's theory of human development, 25-26, 25t
    exchange theory, 27-28
    holistic life span theory, 28
    life span/life course theory, 25, 25b
    Peck's stages of psychosocial development, 26-27, 26t, 27f
  stages of, 5-7
    mid old, 6, 6f
    old old, 6-7
    young old, 6
  stressors associated with, 48, 48b
  successful, 56-57, 56b
  swallowing changes and, 254t
  symptoms associated with, 61
  trends, 3-19
    COTAs and, 11
    OT practice and, 11-12, 11f
  visible changes and, 32-33, 32f, 34f
  vision and effects of, 214-215, 214f, 215t
  well, 53-67
    case study of, 53, 54f
  well-being and, 4-5
Alcoholism, 295
Allen Cognitive Levels (ACL), 92-95, 93t-94t
Alzheimer's disease (AD)
  behavior analysis, 279, 280t-281t
  behavior observation form, 279, 281f
  behavior profile, 279, 279b
  behavioral aspects of, 278-282

Alzheimer's disease (*Continued*)
  difficult, 279
  typical, 278-279
  case study, 287-288
  causes, 276-277
  communication and, 277-278, 278b
  connectedness and, 278b
  incidence, 275
  intervention, 282-286
    adapted environments and, 284-285
    ADLs and, 283-284, 284t-285t
    caregivers and, 286
    COTAs and, 282-286
    implementing, 282-283
    observations, screening and assessment for, 282
    planning of, 282
    well-being promoting activities and, 285-286
  pacing and wandering, 280t-281t
  psychosocial aspects of, 278-282
  reimbursement for services, 286, 287t
  stages, 275-276, 276t
  terminal stage issues, 286
  treatments, 276-277
  working with elders who have, 275-289
    occupation-focused care for, 277-282
    person-centered care for, 277-282
Ambulation, CVAs and, 269
American Association of Retired Persons (AARP), 26-27, 156
American Occupational Therapy Association (AOTA), 9-10, 142-143
Americans with Disabilities Act (ADA), 204-205
AMPS. *See* Assessment of Motor and Process Skills
Antiembolus hosiery, 303
Anxiety, 294
  BAI, 293
  HADS, 294
  reduction, sources of, 128
AOTA. *See* American Occupational Therapy Association
Aphasia, 271-272
Apraxia, 271
ARMD. *See* Age-related macular degeneration
Arthritis, 306-309, 307t
  common problems associated with, 307
  OT interventions, 307-309
    activity modification and, 309, 309t
    coping mechanisms and, 309
    functional ability improvement and, 308
    joint deformity prevention and, 308, 308b
    joint mobility/stability maintenance and, 308
    life balance maintenance and, 308-309
    psychosocial well-being and, 309
    strength maintenance, 308
  sexuality and, 164
Aspiration, 259
Assessment of Communication and Interaction Skills, 100-101
Assessment of Motor and Process Skills (AMPS), 100-101, 292-293
Assessment of Occupational Functioning, 100-101

Assisted living facilities, 9
  costs, 10
  COTAs working in, 113-115, 114t
Assistive hearing devices, providing, 236-237, 237f
Asthma, 324
Attitude self-analysis, 131, 131b
Awareness, 136-143

B

Baby Boomers, 6, 14
BAI. *See* Beck Anxiety Inventory
Balanced Budget Act (BBA), 70
BBA. *See* Balanced Budget Act
BDI. *See* Beck Depression Index
Beck Anxiety Inventory (BAI), 293
Beck Depression Index (BDI), 293
Behavior
  AD, 278-282
    difficult, 279
    typical, 278-279
  analysis, 279, 280t-281t
  observation form, 279, 281f
  profile, 279, 279b
  questionnaire, prevention, 63, 64b
Beliefs, 131, 132b
  medications and, 173
Benign paroxysmal positional vertigo (BPPV), 196
Best practice, opportunities for, 103-120
Biofeedback, incontinence, 246
Biological changes
  falls and, 196-197
  learning and, 44-45
Biological theories of aging, 21-22
  genetic, 21-22
  nongenetic, 22
Bladder training, incontinence, 246
Blood pressure (BP), 314-315
Board and care homes, 9
Bodily functions, medications and, 173
Body alignment, CVAs and, 267-268, 268b
Body scheme disorder, 271
BP. *See* Blood pressure
BPPV. *See* Benign paroxysmal positional vertigo
Brain, aging, 263
Breast cancer, 330, 338. *See also* Oncological conditions
  lymphedema and, 339-340, 339f
Brief COPE assessment, 293
Bronchiectasis, 324
Bronchitis, chronic, 323-324

C

Cachexia, 339
Canadian Model of Occupational Performance (CMOP), 292
Canadian Occupational Performance Measure (COPM), 292
Cancer. *See also* Oncological conditions
  age and, 329
  breast, 330, 338
    lymphedema and, 339-340, 339f
  colorectal, 331
  depression and, 339
  education, 335
  in elder population, 329
  emotional needs and, 337-338
  fall risk and, 336, 338t
  fatigue related to, 334
  inactivity and, 339
  lung, 330
  lymphedema and, 339-340, 339f
  metastasis, 331-332

Cancer (*Continued*)
  prostate, 331, 340-341
  recurrence, 334
  role adaptation/changes and, 337
  support/self-help groups for, 334-335
  treatment/side effects, 332, 333t
CAPS. *See* Certified Aging in Place Specialists
Cardiopulmonary system, 35-36
Cardiovascular conditions, 315, 317t
  background information, 313-314
  case study, 320
  education, 318
  energy conservation, 318, 318f, 318t
  evaluation of elders with, 314-315, 316t
  falls and, 197
  goals, 315-318
  medical treatment, 313-314, 315b
  medication, 319, 319t
  OT interventions, 315-318
    settings, 318-319
  phase I, 316-317
  phase II, 317
  phase III, 317-318
  psychosocial aspects of, 314
  rehabilitation, 315, 317t
  strategies, 315-318
  work simplification, 318
  working with elders who have, 313-321
Cardiovascular system function, medication and, 175
Caregivers
  AD interventions and, 286
  COTA's roles for facilitating, 147-148
  dementia interventions and, 286
  dysphagia, eating/nutrition concerns and, 259
  family, 146
  informal, 146
  medication administration and, 179, 180b
  stresses, 148-149, 149b, 149f
    reducing, 150b
  working with, 145-154
    case study of, 151-153
Cataracts, 215
Centenarians, 8-9
Centers for Medicare and Medicaid Services (CMS), 73-74, 80-81. *See also* Medicaid; Medicare
Cerebrovascular accidents (CVAs)
  case study, 272
  cognitive dysfunction and, 272
  CT evaluation, 264-266
    motor assessment and, 265-266
    psychosocial skills and, 266
    sensory assessment and, 266
    swallowing assessment and, 266
  hypertonicity and, 267, 269f
  incidence, 263
  language and, 271-272
  neurological deficits after, 264, 264t
  OT intervention, 266
    ambulation and, 269
    body alignment and, 267-268, 268b
    case study of, 266
    emotional adjustment and, 272
    hemiplegic upper extremity and, 269-270, 271f
    motor deficits and, 266-272, 267f
    shoulder-hand syndrome and, 270, 270f
    visual-perceptual-cognitive deficits, 271-272
  outcome, 264, 265t
  risk factors, 264
  sexuality and, 162-163
  shoulder-hand syndrome and, 270, 270f
  working with elders who have had, 263-274
Certified Aging in Place Specialists (CAPS), 9
Certified nursing assistants (CNAs), 186

Certified occupational therapy assistant (COTA), 3
  abuse/neglect and, reporting, 151
  action and ethical problems, 141-143
  AD interventions and, 282-286, 284t-285t
  aging population and services provided by, 32
  aging trends and, 11
  caregivers and, roles for facilitating, 147-148
  Cognitive Disabilities Model and, 95
  communication, 147, 147b
  cultural/diversity sensitivity and, 125-126
  deciding what should happen, 139-141
  dementia interventions and, 282-286
  discussing ethical problems, 140-141
  dysphagia and role of, 251-252
  eating concerns and role of, 251-252
  elder medication use and implications for, 170-172, 170t-171t
  elder population, image of, 4
  ethical concerns, 136
  ethical reflection, 140
    free writing and, 140, 140b
  families and, roles for facilitating, 147-148
  generational characteristics and, 14, 14b, 15f
  gustatory system impairment and, 37-38
  health promotion and role of, 63-65
  intergenerational concepts, 12
  issues related to, 108-109
  medications and, 170-172, 170t-171t, 179, 181b
  nutritional concerns and role of, 251-252
  olfactory system impairment and, 37-38
  oncological condition evaluation/intervention planning and, 335-336
  OTRs and, 104, 107-108
  public policy and, 80, 80b
  reporting mistakes, 142
  restraint reduction and role of, 186
    assessment and, 186
    consultation and, 186, 187t-188t
  sexual education and role of, 161
  THA OT interventions and, 304-306, 306f
  wellness and role of, 63-65
  working with elders in various settings, 109-119
    adult day care and, 118-119
    adult foster homes and, 111-112
    assisted living facility, 113-115, 114t
    free standing hospice and, 116-118, 117f
    geropsychiatric unit and, 109-110
    home health agency and, 115-116, 115f
    IRFs and, 110-111, 110f
    SNFs and, 112-113, 113f
Chemotherapy, cytotoxic, 334. *See also* Oncological conditions
Chronic bronchitis, 323-324
Chronic illness, 4-5, 49. *See also* Physical illness
Chronic obstructive pulmonary disease (COPD), 323-324
  asthma, 324
  chronic bronchitis, 323-324
  chronic pulmonary emphysema, 324
  effects of, understanding, 327-328
  productivity and, 324
  psychosocial effect of, 324-325
Chronic pulmonary emphysema, 324
CLASS. *See* Community Living and Assistance Services and Support Program
Client autonomy, 136
Client-centered therapy, 5
CMOP. *See* Canadian Model of Occupational Performance
CMS. *See* Centers for Medicare and Medicaid Services
CNAs. *See* Certified nursing assistants
Cochlear implants, 230-231, 231f. *See also* Hearing impairments

Code of Ethics, 121-122, 138
Cognition, 36-37
  disorders, medications, 172
  dysfunction, CVAs and, 272
  falls and, 197
  Medicare cognitive levels of assistance, 287t
Cognitive Disabilities Model, 86, 92-96
  ACL, 92-95, 93t-94t
  in use, 96
Cognitive level, 95. *See also* Allen Cognitive Levels
Cognitive style, 126-127
Cohort(s), 4
  elder, 4, 7-8
  generational, 12-14, 13t
Colorectal cancer, 331. *See also* Oncological
  conditions
Communication
  AD and, 277-278, 278b
  effective, 147, 147b
  elder, improving, 234-236, 235t, 236b
  style, 129-130
  understanding and being understood, 277-278
Community
  cancer support groups, 334-335
  elders in, 8-10, 8f
  mobility, 202-209
    alternative transportation and, 204-205, 205f
    options for, 202-203, 203b
    pedestrian safety and, 203-204, 203b
    safe driving and, 206-208
  retirement, 54
Community Living and Assistance Services and
  Support Program (CLASS), 79
Comprehensive Occupational Therapy Evaluation
  (COTE), 293
Computer technology, elder usage of, 11-12, 11f
Connectedness, AD and, 278b
Conservatism, 46-47, 47f. *See also* Politics
Continence. *See also* Incontinence
  anatomy, 242
  case study, 248-249
  clothing adaptations/management and, 248
  environmental adaptations and, 247-248, 247b, 247t
  etiology, 242
  physiology, 242
  strategies for maintaining, 241-249
Continuity theory, 24-25
Continuous passive motion (CPM) machine, 306
Contrast sensitivity, reduced, 224, 224b
COPD. *See* Chronic obstructive pulmonary disease
Coping mechanisms, arthritis, 309
COPM. *See* Canadian Occupational Performance
  Measure
COTA. *See* Certified occupational therapy assistant
COTE. *See* Comprehensive Occupational Therapy
  Evaluation
Counseling, sexual activity, 160-162
CPM machine. *See* Continuous passive motion
  machine
Cultural diversity
  in aging population, 121-133
  in elder population, 124-125, 124f
  issue of, 123-130
  overview, 121
  valuing, 124
Culture, 121-123
  ethnicity and, 123
  learning, 122-123
  levels of, 123
  OT and, 121-122
  OT interventions and sensitivity to, 125-126
  shared, 122
CVAs. *See* Cerebrovascular accidents
Cytotoxic chemotherapy, 334

D

Dark adaptation, 206-207. *See also* Vision
Death, leading cause of, 56, 56t
Decision making
  capacity, 136
  ethical, 136, 143, 143b
  locus of, 127-128, 128f
Deep venous thrombosis (DVT), 264
Dementia, 295. *See also* Alzheimer's disease
  case study, 287-288
  characteristics, 295
  course, 275-276
  intervention, 282-286
    adapted environments and, 284-285
    ADLs and, 283-284
    caregivers and, 286
    implementing, 282-283
    observations, screening and assessment for, 282
    planning of, 282
    well-being promoting activities and, 285-286
  progression, 295
  reimbursement for services, 286, 287t
  terminal stage issues, 286
  working with elders who have, 275-289
Demography
  aged population growth, 7-12, 7f
  economic, 10-11
Depression, 293-294
  BDI, 293
  cancer and, 339
  causes, 294
  HADS, 294
  physical health and, 294
  preventing, 294
  situational, 294
Diabetic retinopathy, 218
Diaphragmatic breathing, 326
Dietary concerns, 257-258. *See also* Nutrition
  dysphagia and dietary modifications, 258
  physiological changes and, 258
  structural changes and, 258
Disabled persons
  ADA, 204-205
  disabled parking placard for, 204
  transportation for, 205, 205f
Disease prevention, 53-67. *See also* Physical illness
Disengagement theory, 23
Disuse syndrome, 61
Diversity
  case study, 130-131
  cognitive style and, 126-127
  communication style and, 129-130
  among elder population, 4
  OT interventions and sensitivity to, 125-126
Dizziness, 196
Driving, 202, 202f
  aging and, 202, 206
  disabled parking placard for, 204
  education, 207, 207f
  hearing loss and, 207
  physical changes and, 207
  safe, 206-208
    case study of, 208-209
    equipment for, 208, 208t
    evaluation of, 207-208
  sense dimension of, 206
  vision and, 206
DVT. *See* Deep venous thrombosis
Dysphagia, 251-262
  assistive devices for, 256
  case study, 260-261
  COTA's role in, 251-252
  diet modifications, 258
  environmental concerns and, 253-254, 254f

Dysphagia (*Continued*)
  etiology, 252-253
  intervention strategies, 253-260, 255b
    direct, 256-257
  nursing/caregiver instruction for, 259
  positioning techniques, 254-256, 255f-256f
  precautions, 258-259

E

Eating concerns, 251-262
  assistive devices for, 256
  case study, 260-261
  COTA's role in, 251-252
  environmental concerns and, 253-254, 254f
  feeding program, managing, 259-260
  intervention strategies, 253-260, 255b
    direct, 256-257
  normal swallow and, 252, 252f
  nursing/caregiver instruction for, 259
  positioning techniques, 254-256, 255f-256f
  precautions, 258-259
EC. *See* Ethics Commission
Economic demographics
  elder population, 10-11
  public policy and, 10
  Social Security and, 10
Education
  cancer and, 335
  cardiovascular conditions and, 318, 318f
  driving, 207, 207f
  health, 65
  level, elder, 8
  restraint reduction, 185
  sexual, 160-162
Ego, preoccupation/transcendence, 27
Elder(s)
  activity levels, 47, 47f
  AD and, working with, 275-289
  advocacy for, 79-80
  cardiovascular conditions and, working with,
    313-321
  chronic illness adaptation and, 4-5
  chronological age and, 43-44
  communication, improving, 234-236, 235t, 236b
  in community, 8-10, 8f
  computer technology usage and, 11-12, 11f
  conservatism, 46-47, 47f
  continence in, strategies for maintaining, 241-249
  COTAs working with, in various settings, 109-119
  dementia and, working with, 275-289
  dysphagia, 251-262
  eating concerns, 251-262
  education level, 8
  ethical aspects in work with, 135-144
  ethics and care of, 135-136
  exercise, 43-44, 44f
  federal funds for, 10
  grandchildren raised by, 11
  hearing impaired, working with, 229-239
  intelligence, 44-45
  medications and
    factors affecting risk of, 169-170
    use of, 169-181
  nutritional concerns, 251-262
  oncological conditions and, working with, 329-342
  orthopedic conditions and, working with, 299-311
  overweight, 59-61
  prevention and health promotion, 61-63, 61t
  productivity, 45-46, 46f
  psychiatric conditions in, working with, 291-298
  public policy for, regulation of, 69-82
  pulmonary conditions and, working with, 323-328
  senile, 47-48

Elder(s) (*Continued*)
  sexual activity, 155-167
  sexual functioning, myths about, 156-158
  underweight, 59-61
  vision impaired, working with, 213-227
    case study of, 213-214
  in workforce, 11, 45-46, 46f
Elder abuse
  emotional or psychological, 150-151
  physical, 150-151
  reporting, 142
  self-abuse, 150-151
  sexual, 150-151
  signs and symptoms of, 151, 152t
    recognizing, 150-151
Elder Locator, 142-143
Elder neglect, 150-151
Elder population
  aging of, 7-8
  cancer in, 329
  centenarians, 8-9
  COTA's image of, 4
  diversity in, 4
    cultural, 124-125, 124f
  economic demographics, 10-11
  ethnic groups in, 124, 124f
  female, 7
  groups of, 291
  growth of, demographical data and, 7-12, 7f
  living arrangements, 9-10
  myths about, 14-17
  poverty rate, 10-11
  STDs among, 159
  stereotypes about, 14-17
Emotions
  aging-associated, 48
  cancer and, 337-338
  CVAs and, 272
Emphysema, chronic pulmonary, 324
Endurance, improving, 35
Energy conservation, 336
  cardiovascular conditions and, 318, 318f, 318t
  pulmonary conditions and, 326, 326f
Environment
  fall causes in, 195-196, 196f
  hazards, 195-196, 196f
Environmental adaptations
  AD and, 284-285
  continence and, 247-248, 247b, 247t
  dementia and, 284-285
  dysphagia, eating/nutritional concerns, 253-254, 254f
  fall prevention and, 199-200
  restraint reduction and, 186-189, 189f
Equality/inequality, issues of, 128-129
Erectile dysfunction, 156-158. *See also* Sexual function
Erikson, Erik, 25-26
Erikson's theory of human development, 25-26, 25t
ESI. *See* Evaluation of Social Interaction
Ethic(s), 135-144
  Code of, 121-122, 138
  cost-driven strategies, 135-136
  COTAs and, 136
  decision making, 136
    tips for, 143, 143b
  elder care and, 135-136
  health care and, 136
  laws and, 137-138
  OT and, 138-139
Ethical consideration, 136, 136b
Ethical problems, 137
  COTA and discussing, 140-141
  COTAs and action for, 141-143
  examples, 137b
  individual involved in, 137

Ethics Commission (EC), 142-143
Ethnic groups/ethnicity
  in aged population, 124, 124f
  culture and, 123
  poverty rates and, 10
Ethnocentricity, 123
Evaluation of Social Interaction (ESI), 292
Exchange theory, 27-28
Exercise
  elders and, 43-44, 44f
  fall OT interventions and, 199
  seated, 58-59, 59f
Expanded Routine Task Inventory (RTI), 95
Expressive aphasia, 271-272

F
Facilitating Growth and Development Model, 86, 90-92, 91t
  in use, 91-92
Faiths, 125f
Fall(s)
  causes, 195-197, 195b
    biological, 196-197
    cardiovascular, 197
    cognitive, 197
    environmental, 195-196, 196f
    functional, 197
    musculoskeletal, 196-197, 197f
    neurological, 196-197, 197f
    psychosocial, 197
    sensory, 196
  evaluation, 197-198
  fear of, 58-59
  fractures from, 300
  injuries related to, 195
  OT interventions
    exercise-based, 199
    institutional, 200
    multifactorial, 200-201, 201b
  prevention, 194-202
    case study, 202
    environmental assessment/modifications and, 199-200
    evidence for, 198
    interventions for, 198-201
    outcomes of, 201-202
  risk
    assessment of, 198-199
    cancer and, 336, 338t
    factors, 195-197, 195b
    reduction of, 198-199
  spatial relationships and, difficulty with, 196
  vestibular disorders and, 196
  vision impairments and, 196
Families
  cancer support in, 335
  care, 9
  caregivers, 146
    stresses and, 148-149, 149b-150b, 149f
  COTA's roles for facilitating, 147-148
  long-term care provided by, 146
  resources, 149-150, 151f
  role changes in, 148-150
    family resources and, 149-150, 151f
  working with, 145-154
    case study of, 151-153
Fear of falling, 58-59
Fecal incontinence. *See* Incontinence
Fecal occult blood test (FOBT), 331
Federal funds
  for elders, 10
  institutionalization and, 10
Feeding programs, managing, 259-260
Figure ground perceptions, poor, 271

FIM. *See* Functional Independence Measure
Finances
  exploitation, 150-151
  income sources, 324
  oncological conditions and, 333-334
FIs. *See* Medicare Fiscal Intermediaries and Carriers
FOBT. *See* Fecal occult blood test
Food pyramid, 59, 59t. *See also* Nutrition
Forgetfulness, 45
Fractures, 299-302
  causes, 299-300
    fall as, 300
  closed, 300, 300f
  closed reduction, 300-301
  complications after, 301
  compound, 300, 300f
  delayed union, 301
  fixation, 300-301, 300f
  hip
    rehabilitation and, 301-302, 303t
    weight-bearing restrictions and pinnings for, 301-302, 303t
  malunion, 301
  medical intervention, 300-301, 300f
  nonunion, 301
  open, 300, 300f
  open reduction, 300-301
  pathological, 331-332
  rehabilitation-influencing, 301-302
  simple, 300, 300f
  types, 300, 300f
  upper-extremity, 301, 302t
Free radical theory, 22
Free standing hospice, 116-118, 117f
Functional ability improvement, arthritis and, 308
Functional Independence Measure (FIM), 78

G
Generational characteristics, 14, 14b, 15f
Generational cohorts, 12-14, 13t
Generational sexual attitudes/values inventory, 157
Genetic theories, 21-22
  programmed aging, 21-22
Geriatric population. *See* Elder population
Geriatrics, 4
Gerontology, 4
Geropsychiatric unit, 109-110
Glare, 206-207. *See also* Vision
Glaucoma, 216-218, 217f, 218b
Grandchildren, elders raising, 11
Grief process, 49
Gustatory system, 37-38

H
HADS. *See* Hospital and Anxiety Depression Scale
HCFA. *See* Health Care Financing Administration
Health, 4-5
  education, 65
  OT and enhancing, 57
  risk factors, 55, 55t
  risks, occupational engagement/participation and effects of, 57-59
  sensory system impairment and, 37
  societal views, 56
Health care
  ageism and, 16
  ethical decision making, 136
  policies, trends in federal, 79
  practice, errors in, 142
  public regulated sources, 71-72
  reform, 79
  U.S. trends in, 70-72
    policies and, 79

Health Care Education Reconciliation Act of 2010, 79
Health Care Financing Administration (HCFA), 190
Health promotion, 53-67
  COTA's role in, 63-65
  occupation and, 58
  OT practice and, 55-61
  prevention and, 61-63, 61t
    primary, 62
    secondary, 62-63
    tertiary, 62-63
  programs, 57-58
Healthy People 2010, 32, 56
Healthy People 2020, 32
Healthy population, 56-57
Hearing impairments
  aging-associated, 230-232, 231t
  assistive hearing devices, providing, 236-237, 237f
  case study, 238
  driving and, 207
  psychosocial aspects of, 232
  rehabilitation and, 232-233, 233f, 234b
  working with elders who have, 229-239
Heart disease, 163-164, 314. See also Cardiovascular conditions
Heart rate (HR), 314-315
Hematological system function, 175
Hemianopsia, 271
Hemiplegic upper extremity
  CVAs and, 269-270, 271f
    movement and, 270
  one-handed dressing techniques, 270-271
  voluntary control of, 270, 271f
HemoVac, 301
Hip replacement. See Total hip replacements
Holistic life span theory, 28
Home health
  agency, COTAs working in, 115-116, 115f
  Medicare coverage for, 75-78
Homebound, 75-78
Homosexuality, 158. See also Sexuality
Hospital and Anxiety Depression Scale (HADS), 294
HR. See Heart rate
Hypertonicity, CVAs and, 267, 269f

I

IADL. See Instrumental activities of daily living
ICF, 16
Immune system, 36
Immunological system function, medication and, 175
Immunosenescence, 36
Inactivity, cancer and, 339
Income sources, 324
Incontinence
  biofeedback for, 246
  bladder training for, 246
  fecal, 241-243
    bowel profile for, 245, 246f
    cost of, 242
    prevalence of, 241-242
  functional, 243, 248
  habit training for, 245
  interdisciplinary team strategies, 243-247
  MDS, 243, 244f
  nocturnal, 242
  OBRA and, 243
  OT interventions for, 245
  overflow, 243
  pelvic floor exercises for, 246-247
  prompted voiding for, 245
  related research, 243
  skin erosion and, prevention of, 248
  timed voiding for, 245
  urinary, 241-242

Incontinence (Continued)
  bladder profile for, 245, 246f
  cost of, 242
  prevalence of, 241-242
  stress, 242-243
  types of, 242-243
  urge or urgency, 242
Information processing, cognitive style and, 126-127
Informed consent, 136
Injury risk factors, 7-8
Inpatient rehabilitation facilities (IRFs)
  COTAs working in, 110-111, 110f
  Medicare in, 78
Inpatient Rehabilitation Facility Patient Assessment Instrument (IRF-PAI), 78
Institute of Medicine (IOM), 32
Institution(s). See also Skilled nursing facilities
  fall prevention and, 200
  rules, 137-138
Institutionalization, 8, 10
Instrumental activities of daily living (IADL), 58, 292-293
Integumentary system, 33-34, 34f
Intelligence
  elder, 44-45
  stereotypes, 45
Intergenerational commonalities and differences, 3-4
Intergenerational concepts, 12-14
IOM. See Institute of Medicine
IRF-PAI. See Inpatient Rehabilitation Facility Patient Assessment Instrument
IRFs. See Inpatient rehabilitation facilities
Ischemic strokes, 263-264. See also Cerebrovascular accidents

J

Joint
  deformity, arthritis and preventing, 308, 308b
  mobility/stability, arthritis and, 308
Joint replacement, 302-306
  knee replacements, 306
  sexuality and, 164
  THRs, 302-306

K

Kegel exercises. See Pelvic floor exercises
KELS. See Kohlman Evaluation of Living Skills
Kinesiological Model, 86
Kinesthetic changes, 38
Knee replacements, 306
  nonsurgical interventions, 306
  rehabilitation after, 306
Kohlman Evaluation of Living Skills (KELS), 293
Kubler-Ross, Elisabeth, 49

L

Language, CVAs and, 271-272. See also Communication
Laws, ethics and, 137-138
LBD. See Lewy body disease
LCDs. See Local coverage determinations
Learned helplessness, 49-50
Learning. See also Education
  age-related changes in, 44-45
  biological changes affecting, 44-45
Leisure time, 46. See also Retirement
Lewy body disease (LBD), 295
Licensure laws, 143
Life balance, arthritis and maintaining, 308-309
Life expectancy, 31
Life Span Perspective, 33, 38
Life span/life course theory, 25, 25b

Lifestyle factors, 56-57, 56b
Living arrangements, 9-10
  adult care options, 9
  adult day care, 9, 118-119
  adult foster care, 9, 111-112
  assisted living facilities, 9-10, 113-115, 114t
  board and care homes, 9
  family care, 9
  personal care, 9
  retirement communities, 9, 54
Llorens's Facilitating Growth and Development Model, 86, 90-92, 91t
Local coverage determinations (LCDs), 73-74
Longevity, 56
Long-term care, family-provided, 146
Losses, aging-associated, 48
Low vision, 225. See also Visual dysfunction/impairment
Lung cancer, 330. See also Oncological conditions
Lymphedema, 339-340, 339f

M

MACs. See Medicare administrative contractures
Macular degeneration, 215-216, 216b
Malnutrition, 251
Managed care, SNF, 79
Material exploitation, 150-151
Maturity, characteristics of, 90, 92t
MDS. See Minimum data set
Medicaid, 11, 70-71, 78-79
Medicare, 11, 70-72
  cognitive levels of assistance, 287t
  COPD and, 324
  coverage, 75, 75t
  home health services, 75-78
  in IRFs, 78
  OT coverage, 73
  OT practice and, 71-72
  Part A, 71-72, 72t
    SNFs and, 75
  Part B, 72
    therapy cap for, 72
  Part C, 79
  regulations, related, 74
  skilled/unskilled therapy and, 73, 74t
  wheelchair guidelines, 191
Medicare administrative contractures (MACs), 73-74
Medicare Fiscal Intermediaries (FIs) and Carriers, 73-74
Medicare Reimbursement, 71-72, 286, 287t
Medication(s)
  activity demands and, 175, 176t
  aging process, physiology and, 170
  cardiovascular condition, 319, 319t
  caregivers and administration of, 179, 180b
  case study, 179-181
  client factors, 173-175
    bodily functions and, 173
    mental functions and, 173-174
    neuromusculoskeletal and movement-related functions, 174-175
    sensory functions and pain, 174, 174f
    skin and related structure functions and, 175
    speech function and, 175
    values, beliefs, and spirituality, 173
    voice function and, 175
  cognitive disorders, 172
  common, used by elders, 170, 171t
  COTA and, 170-172, 170t-171t, 179, 181b
  elder use of, 169-181
  erectile dysfunction, 158
  OT process and, 175-177, 176t
  pain, 171-172
  polypharmacy, 170

Medication(s) (*Continued*)
  problems, strategies for minimizing, 172-173
  psychiatric disorders, 172
  psychosocial disorders, 172
  risks, in elders, 169-170
  side effects, 171t
  sleep disturbances, 172
  swallowing of, 259
  terminology, 170, 170t
Mental function, medications and, 173-174
Mental health disorders, common, 293-296. *See also*
    Psychiatric disorders
  aging with psychosis, 295
  alcoholism, 295
  anxiety, 294
  dementia, 295
  depression, 293-294
  intervention planning considerations and, 296,
    296f
  mood disorders, 295-296, 296f
  suicide, 294
Metabolic equivalents (METs), 325-326
Metastasis, cancer, 331-332
METs. *See* Metabolic equivalents
MI. *See* Myocardial infarction
Mid old, 6, 6f
Middle age, Peck's stages of, 26
Mini Mental Status Examination (MMSE), 293
Minimum data set (MDS), 75, 76f-77f, 243, 244f
Mixed urinary incontinence (MUI), 243. *See also*
    Incontinence
MMSE. *See* Mini Mental Status Examination
Mobility
  age-related changes and, 202
  community, 202-209
    alternative transportation and, 204-205, 205f
    options for, 202-203, 203b
    pedestrian safety and, 203-204, 203b
    safe driving and, 206-208
  considerations, 183-212
  fall prevention and, 194-202
  functional, falls and, 197
  restraint reduction and, 183
  wheelchair seating/positioning, 191-194
Model of Human Occupation, 96-101
  external environment layers, 96, 97f
  internal organization and, 97-98, 97f
    habituation in, 98
    mind-brain-body performance in, 98, 99t-100t
    volition in, 98
  in use, 101
Mood disorders, 295-296, 296f
  intervention planning considerations and, 296, 296f
Motor deficits, 266-272, 267f. *See also* Assessment of
    Motor and Process Skills
Movement-related functions, medication and,
    174-175
MUI. *See* Mixed urinary incontinence
Multifactorial interventions, fall prevention, 200-201,
    201b
Muscle strength, improving, 35
Musculoskeletal conditions, falls and, 196-197, 197f
Myelosuppression, 334
Myocardial infarction (MI), 163

N

NAHB. *See* National Association of Home Builders
    Remodelers Council
Nalebuff type I deformity, 308
National Association of Home Builders Remodelers
    Council (NAHB), 9
National Board for Certification in Occupational
    Therapy (NBCOT), 143

National Center on Elder Abuse (NCEA), 150-151.
    See also Elder abuse
Naturally Occurring Retirement Communities
    (NORC), 9
NBCOT. *See* National Board for Certification in
    Occupational Therapy
NCEA. *See* National Center on Elder Abuse
Neuroendocrine theory, 22
Neurogenic detrusor overactivity, 242
Neurological deficits
  falls and, 196-197, 197f
  after stroke, 264, 264t
Neurological insult, visual dysfunction after,
    218-219, 219b
Neuromusculoskeletal functions, medication and,
    174-175
Neuromusculoskeletal system, 34
Nocturnal incontinence, 242
Nongenetic aging, 21
Nongenetic theory, 22
NORC. *See* Naturally Occurring Retirement
    Communities
Nutrition
  food pyramid, 59, 59t
  integumentary system and, 34
  obesity and, 60
  overweight elders, 59-61
  personal factors associated with, 59-60, 60t
  poor, 59-60, 60t
  underweight elders, 59-61
  weight and, 59-61
Nutritional concerns, 251-262
  assistive devices for, 256
  case study, 260-261
  COTA's role in, 251-252
  dietary concerns and, 257-258
  dysphagia, 259
  environmental concerns and, 253-254, 254f
  feeding program, managing, 259-260
  OT intervention strategies, 253-260, 255b
    direct, 256-257
  positioning techniques for, 254-256, 255f-256f
  precautions, 258-259

O

OA. *See* Osteoarthritis
OAA. *See* Older Americans Act
Obesity, 60. *See also* Weight
OBRA. *See* Omnibus Budget Reconciliation Act
Occupation
  areas of, 87-89, 88t
  engagement/participation in, 56
    health risks and effects on, 57-59, 58f
    enjoyment of participation in, 58
  health promotion and, 58
  performance, factors influencing, 146
  sense of purposefulness and, 58, 58f
Occupational Case Analysis Interview and Rating
    Scale, 100-101
Occupational Performance History Interview,
    100-101
Occupational therapy (OT), 3
  activity demands and, 106
  activity theories and, 24-25
  areas of occupation and, 105-106
  client factors and, 106
  context, environment and, 106
  continuity theories and, 24-25
  culture and, 121-122
  CVA, evaluation, 264-266
  domain of, 87, 87f, 104-106, 105t
  ethical options, 138-139
  evaluation, 106-108

Occupational therapy (*Continued*)
  health enhancement and, 57
  Medicare coverage, 73
  oncological conditions and, 332-335
  outcome, 106-108
  payment, 72-73
  performance patterns and, 106
  performance skills and, 106
  practice, 32
    aging trends and, 11-12, 11f
    framework for, 104
    health promotion and, 55-61
    implications for, 12
    Medicare and, 71-72
    wellness and, 55-61
  practice models, 85-102
    overview of, 86-101
  practitioners, 104
  process, 89, 106-107, 107t
    medications and, 175-177, 176t
  psychiatric conditions assessment and, 292-293
  pulmonary conditions assessment and, 325-326
  retirement community transition and, 54
  self-medication and, 173
Occupational Therapy Ethics Standards, 138. *See also*
    Ethics
Occupational Therapy Practice Framework, 86-90
  activity demands and, 89
  areas of occupation, 87-89, 88t
  client factors, 87-89
  Cognitive Disabilities Model, 86, 92-96
  Domain and Process, 16, 121-122
  environments and, 89
  Facilitating Growth and Development Model, 86,
    90-92, 91t
  Model of Human Occupation, 96-101
  OT process, 89
  performance skills, 87-89, 88t
  in use, 90
Occupation-focused care, 277-282
Ocular pathologies, specific, 215-218
  ARMD, 215-216
  cataracts, 215
  diabetic retinopathy, 218
  glaucoma, 216-218, 217f, 218b
  macular degeneration, 215-216, 216b
Oculomotor dysfunction, 223-224
Old age, 6
  Peck's stages of, 26-27
Old old, 6-7
Older Americans Act (OAA), 70, 79
Older population. *See* Elder population
Olfactory system, 37-38
Omnibus Budget Reconciliation Act (OBRA), 70, 74,
    138
  incontinence and, 243
  restraint use and, 183-184
Oncological conditions
  cancer metastasis, 331-332
  cancer treatment/side effects, 332, 333t
  case study, 341
  common, 329-331, 330t
  financial implications and, 333-334
  OT, 332-335
  OT interventions, 335-341
    discharge planning, 341
    evaluation/intervention planning and, 335-341
    gems for, 339-340, 340t
    goals/interventions, 336-338, 337b
    special considerations in planning/
      implementation of, 338-341
  psychosocial aspects of, 332-335
  working with elders who have, 329-342
One-handed dressing techniques, 270-271

Orientation, reality, 277
Orthopedic conditions
    arthritis, 306-309
    case study, 309-310
    fractures, 299-302
    joint replacements, 302-306
    prevalence, 299
    surgery for, complications of, 299
    working with elders who have, 299-311
Orthotic devices, 336-337
Osteoarthritis (OA), 306, 307t. See also Arthritis
    common problems associated with, 307
Osteoporosis, 35
OT. See Occupational therapy
OT interventions, 72-73, 73t, 106-108
    AD, 282-286
    arthritis, 307-309
    cardiovascular condition, 315-319
    culture sensitivity and, 125-126
    CVA, 266
    dementia, 282-286
    diversity sensitivity and, 125-126
    dysphagia, 253-260, 255b
    eating concerns, 253-260, 255b
    fall prevention, 198-201
    goals, 89
    incontinence, 245
    mental health disorders, planning considerations
        for, 296, 296f
    mood disorders, planning considerations for, 296,
        296f
    nutrition concerns, 253-260, 255b
    oncological conditions, 335-341
    pulmonary condition planning of, 325-326,
        325b-326b
    restraint reduction, 189-190
    strategies, 89
    THA, 304-306, 305t, 306f
    vision impairments and, 220-221, 222b
OTRs. See Registered occupational therapists
Overflow incontinence, 243
Overweight elders, 59-61. See also Weight

P

PACE. See Program for All-Inclusive Care of the
        Elderly
Pacing, AD and, 280t-281t
Pain, medications, 171-172, 174
Pathological fractures, 331-332
Patient Protection and Affordable Care Act, 79
Peck, Robert, 26-27, 26t, 27f
Pedestrian safety, 203-204, 203b, 204f
Pelvic floor exercises (Kegel exercises), 246
Permission, Limited Information, Specific
        Suggestions, and Intensive Therapy Model
        (PLISSIT), 160-161, 161b
Personal care, 9
Peson-centered care, 277-282
Physical health
    alcoholism and, 295
    depression and, 294
    elder sexuality and effects of, 162-165
Physical illness, 4-5, 49
    chronic, 4-5
    stressors associated with, 49, 49b
Physical restraints. See Restraints(s)
Physiological changes
    dietary concerns and, 258
    driving and, 207
    normal age-related, 158-159, 159b
Physiological functioning, wheelchair seating/
        positioning and, 192-193
Physiology, aging process and, 170

Plaques, 276-277
PLISSIT. See Permission, Limited Information,
        Specific Suggestions, and Intensive Therapy
        Model
Politics, elders and, 46-47, 47f
Polypharmacy, 170
Poverty
    elder, 10-11
    ethnic groups and, 10
    rate, 125
PPS. See Prospective payment system
Preferences, 131, 132b
Preferred retinal locus (PRI), 223
Presbyopia, 215
Pressure sores, wheelchair, 192
PRI. See Preferred retinal locus
Primary prevention, 62
Productivity, COPD and, 324
Program for All-Inclusive Care of the Elderly
        (PACE), 7
Programmed aging, 21-22
Prospective payment system (PPS), 70, 75, 78b,
        286
Prostate cancer, 331, 340-341. See also Oncological
        conditions
Psychiatric disorders. See also specific disorders
    assessment, 292-293
        interdisciplinary, 293
        OT-specific, 292-293
    case study, 296-297
    classification, 291
    common, 293-296
    intervention, funding for, 291
    medications, 172
    working with elders who have, 291-298
Psychosis, aging with, 295
Psychosocial development
    Erikson and, 26
    Peck's stages of, 26-27, 26t, 27f
Psychosocial disorders, medications, 172
Psychosocial issues
    AD and, 278-282
    of cardiac dysfunctions, 314
    cardiovascular conditions and, 314
    of COPD, 324-325
    falls and, 197
    hearing impairments and, 232
    of oncological conditions, 332-335
    restraint reduction, 189
    THR and, 304, 304f
    vision impairments, 214
Psychosocial skills, CVAs and evaluation of, 266
Psychosocial well-being, 309
Public policy
    advocacy for elders and, 79-80
    changes, keeping up with, 80-81
    COTAs and, 80, 80b
    economic demographics and, 10
    for elders, regulation of, 69-82
    health care trends, U.S., 70-72
    introductory concepts, 70
    OT payment and intervention, 72-73, 73t
    payment systems, 74
    skilled/unskilled therapy, 73, 74t
    SNFs and, 74
Pulmonary conditions
    case study, 327
    COPD, 323-324
    diaphragmatic breathing, 326
    energy conservation, 326, 326f
    OT assessment and interventional planning,
        325-326, 325b-326b
    pursed-lip breathing, 326, 327f
    sexual functioning and, 325

Pulmonary conditions (Continued)
    work simplification, 326, 326f
    working with elders who have, 323-328
Purposefulness, occupation and sense of, 58, 58f
Pursed-lip breathing, 326, 327f

R

RA. See Rheumatoid arthritis
Rand SF-36 Health Survey Questionnaire, 293
Receptive aphasia, 271-272
Registered occupational therapists (OTRs), 5. See
        also Occupational therapy
    COTAs and, 104, 107-108
    wheelchair seating/positioning assessment, 191
Respiratory system function, medication and, 175
Restraints(s)
    guidelines regarding, 184
    negative effects, 183-184, 184b
    OBRA and, 183-184
    reduction, 183
        activity alternatives, 189
        assessment, 186
        case study of, 190
        consultation, 186, 187t-188t
        COTAs' role in, 186
        education and, 185
        environmental adaptations, 186-189, 189f
        OT intervention, 189-190
        philosophy behind, 184-185
        policy for, 185
        program for, establishing, 184-186
        psychosocial approaches to, 189
        successful, steps for, 185-186, 185b
Retirement, 46. See also Naturally Occurring
        Retirement Communities
    communities, 9
    transition to, 54
Rheumatoid arthritis (RA), 34-35, 306, 307t
    common problems associated with, 307
Role adaptation/changes
    cancer and, 337
    family, 148-150
        caregiver stresses and, 148-149, 149b-150b, 149f
        family resources and, 149-150, 151f
RTI. See Expanded Routine Task Inventory

S

Sarcopenia, 35
Scooters
    pedestrian safety and, 203, 204f
    transport of, 204
Seated exercise, 58-59, 59f
Secondary prevention, 62-63
Self-abuse, 150-151
Self-medication. See also Medication(s)
    assistive aids for, 177-179
        calendars as, 177
        commercial, 177-178
        homemade, 178-179
        insulin holders as, 178
        medication diary as, 178-179, 178t
        pill crushers as, 178
        pill splitters as, 178
        pill storage boxes/storage boxes as, 177-178,
            177f
        storage cups as, 179, 179f
        talking/shaking alarms, watches, prescription
            bottles as, 178
    OT process and, 173
    program, 179
Self-neglect, 150-151
Senescence, 5-6

Senility, 47-48
Sensory assessment, CVA, 266
Sensory functions
    driving and, 206
    falls and, 196
    medications and, 174, 174f
Sensory Integration Model, 86
Sensory system, aging, 37-38
    gustatory, 37-38
    olfactory, 37-38
Sexual activity
    counseling, 160-162
    intervention gems and, 162b
    role play exercises, 164-165
    safety considerations, 161-162
Sexual attitudes/values inventory, 157
Sexual education, 160-162
    COTAs' role in, 161
    intervention in, role of, 159-160
    PLISSIT and, 160-161, 161b
    role of intervention in, 159-160
Sexual function, 155
    myths about elders and, 156
        discussion of, 156-158
    pulmonary conditions and, 325
Sexual response, physiological changes and, 158-159,
    159b
Sexuality, 155, 156f
    arthritis and, 164
    CVAs and, 162-163
    generational sexual attitudes/values inventory, 157
    health conditions and effects on, 162-165
    heart disease and, 163-164
    joint replacement and, 164
    myths about geriatric, 158
    in nursing facilities, addressing, 160, 160f
    personal values assessment, 157
    physiological changes and, normal age-related,
        158-159, 159b
    values about, 156
Sexually transmitted diseases (STDs), 159
Shearing, wheelchairs and, 192
Shoulder-hand syndrome, 270, 270f
Situational depression, 294
Skeletal system, 34
Skilled nursing facilities (SNFs)
    COTAs working in, 112-113, 113f
    Medicare A in, 75
    payment system, prospective, 75-79
        managed care, 79
        Medicaid, 78-79
        Medicare in IRFs, 78
        OAA and, 79
        PPS, 75, 78b
        public policy and, 74
    sexuality in, addressing, 160, 160f
Skin and related structure functions, medications
    and, 175
Skin breakdown, wheelchair seating/positioning and,
    192
Skin erosion, incontinence and prevention of, 248
Sleep disturbances, medications and, 172
SNFs. See Skilled nursing facilities
Social interaction, psychiatric condition assessment
    and, 292
Social Security, 5-6, 70-71
    economic demographics and, 10
    payments, 324
Social support, need for, 48-49
Somatic mutation theory, 22
Somatosensory changes, 38
Spatial relationships, difficulty with, 196, 271
Speech function, medications and, 175
Spirituality, medications and, 173

State Regulatory Board, 143
STDs. See Sexually transmitted diseases
Stereotypes
    aged, 14-17
    intelligence, 45
Strength maintenance, arthritis and, 308
Stress urinary incontinence (SUI), 242-243. See also
        Incontinence
Stresses, caregiver, 148-149, 149b, 149f
    reducing, 150b
Stressors
    aging-associated, 48, 48b
    physical illness, 49, 49b
Strokes. See Cerebrovascular accidents
SUI. See Stress urinary incontinence
Suicide, 294. See also Depression
Swallowing
    aging and, 254t
    CVAs and evaluation of, 266
    esophageal phase, 252
    medications, 259
    normal, 252, 252f
    oral phase, 252
        interventions during, 257
    oral preparatory phase, 252
    pharyngeal phase, 252
        interventions during, 257
    phases of, 252, 253f
    straws and, 259
    structures, changes in, 252, 254t

T
Tangles, 276-277
TED. See Thromboembolic disease
Temperature regulation, 34
Tertiary prevention, 62-63
Thera-Band exercises, 340-341
Therapeutic fibs, 277-278
Third-party payers, 286. See also Medicare
Thrombocytopenia, 5
Thromboembolic disease (TED), 306
THRs. See Total hip replacements
Time, use of, 129
Tinnitus, 231
Total hip replacements (THRs), 302-306
    antiembolus hosiery, 303
    movement precautions, 303, 303t
    OT interventions, 304-306, 305t, 306f
    psychosocial issues, 304, 304f
    surgical approaches, 302-303, 303f
Traditionalists, 10, 12-14
Transportation. See also Driving
    community mobility and alternative, 204-205, 205f
    disabled persons, 205, 205f
Truth, what is accepted as, 127

U
Undernourishment, 251
Underweight elders, 59-61. See also Weight
Urinary incontinence. See Incontinence

V
Value system, 127-129, 131, 132b
    anxiety reduction and, sources of, 128
    equality/inequality and, issues of, 128-129
    locus of decision making and, 127-128, 128f
    medications and, 173
    use of time, 129
Valvular disease, 314
Vertigo, 196
Vestibular disorders, falls and, 196

Viagra, 158
Vision
    driving and, 206
    field of, 206, 223
Visual attention/scanning, impaired, 224
Visual dysfunction/impairment
    addressing, settings for, 225
    aging and, 214-215, 214f, 215t
    case study, 226
    contrast sensitivity and, reduced, 224, 224b
    decreased acuity and, 221-222, 222f-223f
    environmental adaptation basics, 225, 226b
    falls and, 196
    after neurological insult, 218-219, 219b
    ocular pathologies and, specific, 215-218
    oculomotor dysfunction, 223-224
    principles of intervention, 220-221, 222b
    psychosocial effects, 214
    visual attention/scanning, impaired, 224
    visual-perceptual deficits and, higher level, 224
    Warren's hierarchy for addressing, 219-220, 220b,
        220f, 221t
    working with elders who have, 213-227
Visual-perceptual deficits, higher level, 224
Visual-perceptual-cognitive deficits, 271-272
Voice function, medications and, 175
Volitional Questionnaire (VQ), 293
VQ. See Volitional Questionnaire

W
Walkers, pedestrian safety and, 203
Wandering, AD and, 280t-281t
Warren's hierarchy, 219-220, 220b, 220f, 221t
Wear and tear theory, 22
Weight
    nutrition and, 59-61
    personal factors associated with, 59-60
Weight-bearing, hip fractures and, 301-302, 303t
Well-being, 4-5
    AD interventions and, 285-286
    dementia interventions and, 285-286
    psychosocial, arthritis OT interventions and, 309
Wellness
    COTA's role in, 63-65
    OT practice and, 55-61
    program, 63, 65b
Wheelchair(s)
    assessment, 191
    measurement, 192, 193f
    Medicare guidelines and, 191
    outcome satisfaction, 191
    pedestrian safety and, 203
    seat depth, 192
    seating/positioning, 191-194
        assessment of, 191, 194, 194b
        physiological functioning and, 192-193
        poor, negative impacts of, 193, 193t
        pressure sores and, 192
        shearing and, 192
        skin breakdown and, 192
    selection, 191-192
    sling-upholstered, 193-194
    transport of, 204
Whistle-blowing, 142
Work simplification. See also Occupation
    cardiovascular conditions and, 318, 318f
    pulmonary conditions and, 326, 326f
Workforce, elders in, 11, 45-46, 46f

Y
Young old, 6
Youth, American society and, 17